Dementia

PUBLISHING FOR THE WORLD
125 Years
THE JOHNS HOPKINS UNIVERSITY PRESS

Dementia

Presentations, Differential Diagnosis, and Nosology

Second Edition

Edited by

V. Olga B. Emery, Ph.D.
Department of Psychiatry, Dartmouth Medical School, Lebanon, New Hampshire
Faculty of Medicine, Harvard Medical School, Boston, Massachusetts

and

Thomas E. Oxman, M.D.
Departments of Psychiatry and of Community and Family Medicine, Dartmouth Medical School
Lebanon, New Hampshire

The Johns Hopkins University Press
Baltimore and London

Printed in the United States of America on acid-free paper
9 8 7 6 5 4 3 2 1

The Johns Hopkins University Press
2715 North Charles Street
Baltimore, Maryland 21218-4363
www.press.jhu.edu

Library of Congress Cataloging-in-Publication Data

Dementia : presentations, differential diagnosis, and nosology / edited by V. Olga B. Emery and Thomas E. Oxman.—2nd ed.
p. ; cm.
Includes bibliographical references and index.
ISBN 0-8018-7156-5 (hardcover : alk. paper)
1. Dementia.
[DNLM: 1. Dementia—diagnosis. 2. Dementia—classification.
WM 220 D376383 2003] I. Emery, V. Olga B. II. Oxman, Thomas E.
RC521 .D4557 2003
616.'3—dc21 2002009445

A catalog record for this book is available from the British Library.

To our parents, who taught us respect for mind,
and
to our spouses and children, whose cooperation made this work possible

Contents

List of Contributors *xi*
Acknowledgments *xv*
List of Abbreviations *xvii*
Introduction *xix*

PART ONE: Background, Concepts, and Diagnostics

1 Boundaries between Normal Aging and Dementia: Perspectives from Neuropsychological and Neuroimaging Investigations 3
Laura A. Flashman, Heather A. Wishart, Thomas E. Oxman, and Andrew J. Saykin

2 The Spectrum of Dementias: Construct and Nosologic Validity 31
Thomas E. Oxman

3 Diagnostic Procedures for Dementia 61
Christopher J. Patterson and A. Marc Clarfield

PART TWO: Alzheimer Dementias

4 The Neuropathology of Alzheimer Dementia 89
Jerzy Wegiel, Thomas Wisniewski, Barry Reisberg, and Wayne Silverman

5 Neural Inflammatory Mechanisms in Alzheimer Syndrome 121
Edith G. McGeer and Patrick L. McGeer

6 Clinical Subgroups of Alzheimer Disease 139
Magnus Sjögren, Anders Wallin, and Kaj Blennow

7 Progressive Aphasia, Frontotemporal Dementia, and Other "Focal Dementias" 156
Howard S. Kirshner

8 "Retrophylogenesis" of Memory in Dementia of the Alzheimer Type: A New Evolutionary Memory Framework 177
V. Olga B. Emery

PART THREE: Vascular Dementias and Subcortical Dementias

9 Cortical and Frontosubcortical Dementias: Differential Diagnosis 239
Frédéric Assal and Jeffrey L. Cummings

10 Noninfarct Vascular Dementia: The Spectrum of Vascular Dementia and Alzheimer Syndrome 263
V. Olga B. Emery, Edward X. Gillie, and Joseph A. Smith

11 The Relationship of Hypertension to Vascular Dementia 291
Shotai Kobayashi

12 Vascular Dementias and Alzheimer Disease: Differential Diagnosis 306
Tuula Pirttilä, Timo Erkinjuntti, and Vladimir Hachinski

13 Acquired Immunodeficiency Syndrome Dementia Complex 336
Richard W. Price

PART FOUR: Depressive Dementias

14 Depressive Dementia: A "Prepermanent Intermediate-stage Dementia" in a Long-term Disease Course of Permanent Dementia? 361
V. Olga B. Emery and Thomas E. Oxman

15 Depressive Dementia: Cognitive and Biological Correlates and Course of Illness 398
George S. Alexopoulos

16 The Nondepressive Pseudodementias 417
Perminder Sachdev and Sharon Reutens

17 Neurobiology of Major Depression in Alzheimer Disease 444
George S. Zubenko

PART FIVE: Conclusions and Future Directions

18 Approaches to the Treatment of Dementing Illness 463
Thomas E. Oxman and Robert B. Santulli

19 The Spectra of the Dementias 490
V. Olga B. Emery and Thomas E. Oxman

Index 523

Contributors

George S. Alexopoulos, M.D., Professor, Department of Psychiatry, Weill Medical College of Cornell University, White Plains, New York

Frédéric Assal, M.D., International Scholar, Department of Neurology, UCLA School of Medicine, Los Angeles, California

Kaj Blennow, M.D., Ph.D., Professor, Department of Clinical Neuroscience, Sahlgren's University Hospital, Mölndal, Sweden

A. Marc Clarfield, M.D., FCPC, FRCP, Professor, Faculty of Medicine, Ben Gurion University of the Negev, Israel; Adjunct Professor, Division of Geriatric Medicine, McGill University, Montreal, Quebec, Canada

Jeffrey L. Cummings, M.D., Augustus Rose Professor of Neurology and Professor of Psychiatry and Biobehavioral Sciences, UCLA School of Medicine, Los Angeles, California

Timo Erkinjuntti, M.D., Ph.D., Professor, Department of Neurology, University of Helsinki, Finland

Laura A. Flashman, Ph.D., Associate Professor, Department of Psychiatry, Dartmouth Medical School, Lebanon, New Hampshire

Edward X. Gillie, M.D., Retired; formerly Chair, Department of Geriatric Medicine, Manchester Veterans Affairs Medical Center, Manchester, New Hampshire; Faculty of Medicine, Harvard Medical School, Boston, Massachusetts

Vladimir Hachinski, M.D., FRCP(C), MSC, DSC, DMHC, Professor, Department of Clinical Neurological Sciences, University of Western Ontario, London, Ontario, Canada

Howard S. Kirshner, M.D., Professor and Vice Chair, Department of Neurology, Vanderbilt University School of Medicine, Nashville, Tennessee

Shotai Kobayashi, M.D., Ph.D., FAJSIM, FACP, FRCP, Professor and Chair, Department of Internal Medicine III, Shimane Medical University, Shimane, Japan

Edith G. McGeer, Ph.D., OC, Emerita Professor, Kinsmen Laboratory of Neurological Research, Department of Psychiatry, University of British Columbia, Vancouver, British Columbia, Canada

Patrick L. McGeer, M.D., Ph.D., FRCP(C), OC, Emeritus Professor, Kinsmen Laboratory of Neurological Research, Department of Psychiatry, University of British Columbia, Vancouver, British Columbia, Canada

Christopher J. Patterson, M.D., FRCP(C), Professor, Division of Geriatric Medicine, Department of Medicine, Faculty of Health Sciences, McMaster University, Hamilton, Ontario, Canada

Tuula Pirttilä, M.D., Ph.D., Professor, Department of Neurology, University of Kuopio, Kuopio, Finland

Richard W. Price, M.D., Professor of Neurology, University of California, San Francisco; Chief, Neurology Service, San Francisco General Hospital, San Francisco, California

Barry Reisberg, M.D., Ph.D., Professor, Department of Psychiatry, New York University School of Medicine, New York, New York

Sharon Reutens, M.B.B.S., FRANZCP, Consultant Psychiatrist, Royal Prince Alfred Hospital; Neuropsychiatry Fellow, Neuropsychiatric Institute, Prince of Wales Hospital, Sydney, Australia

Perminder Sachdev, M.D., Ph.D., FRANZCP, Professor of Neuropsychiatry, University of New South Wales; Director, Neuropsychiatric Institute, Prince of Wales Hospital, Randwick, New South Wales, Australia

Robert B. Santulli, M.D., Assistant Professor, Department of Psychiatry, Dartmouth Medical School, Lebanon, New Hampshire

Andrew J. Saykin, Psy.D., Professor, Departments of Psychiatry and Radiology, Dartmouth Medical School, Lebanon, New Hampshire

Wayne Silverman, Ph.D., Chair, Department of Psychology, New York State Institute for Basic Research in Developmental Disabilities, Staten Island, New York

Magnus Sjögren, M.D., Ph.D., Associate Professor, Institute of Clinical Neuroscience, Goteborg University, Sahlgrenska University Hospital, Mölndal, Sweden

Joseph A. Smith, M.D., Chair, Department of Radiology and Diagnostic Imaging, Manchester Veterans Affairs Medical Center, Manchester, New Hampshire

Anders Wallin, M.D., Ph.D., Professor, Institute of Clinical Neuroscience, Sahlgrenska University Hospital, Mölndal, Sweden

Jerzy Wegiel, V.D.M., Ph.D., Acting Chair, Department of Pathological Neurobiology, New York State Institute for Basic Research in Developmental Disabilities, Staten Island, New York

Heather A. Wishart, Ph.D., Assistant Professor, Department of Psychiatry, Dartmouth Medical School, Lebanon, New Hampshire

Thomas Wisniewski, M.D., Ph.D., Associate Professor of Neurology, Pathology, and Psychiatry, Aging and Dementia Center, New York University Medical Center, New York, New York

George S. Zubenko, M.D., Ph.D., Professor, Department of Psychiatry, University of Pittsburgh School of Medicine, Pittsburgh, Pennsylvania

Acknowledgments

It has been our privilege to work with this volume's pioneering and eminent authors as they pulled together what is known about the dementias. They have explored the frontiers of the dementias with great knowledge, thoroughness, and originality. It has been our privilege to prepare and edit this volume on presentations, differential diagnosis, and nosology of the dementias with our readers in mind, hoping to make this work as interesting and useful for the readers as it has been for the editors.

We wish to acknowledge Henryk M. Wisniewski, M.D., Ph.D., Nelson M. Butters, Ph.D., and Leslie G. Kiloh, M.D., authors of our first edition whose groundbreaking, seminal work continues its widespread influence on dementia research and theory. We also wish to acknowledge Wendy A. Harris, JHUP Medical Editor, for her knowledgeable suggestions and work on the manuscript. Further, we wish to acknowledge our debt to Cynthia A. Hewitt, Department of Psychiatry, Dartmouth Medical School, for her dedication and tireless assistance in the research, reference, and executive aspects of this project. Finally, we wish to acknowledge the library staff of the Matthews-Fuller Health Sciences Library of Dartmouth Biomedical Libraries for their invaluable cooperation and assistance.

Abbreviations

AACD	age-associated cognitive decline
AAMI	age-associated memory impairment
AD	Alzheimer disease
ADC	AIDS dementia complex
Apo	apolipoprotein
APP	amyloid precursor protein
AS	Alzheimer syndrome
BD	Binswanger disease
CBGD	corticobasal ganglionic degeneration
CDR	Clinical Dementia Rating (scale)
CJD	Creutzfeldt-Jakob disease
CNS	central nervous system
CT	computerized tomography
DAT	dementia of the Alzheimer type
DLB	dementia with Lewy bodies
DS	Down syndrome
FAST	Functional Assessment Staging
fMRI	functional magnetic resonance imaging
FSCD	frontosubcortical dementias
FTD	frontotemporal dementia
HD	Huntington disease
IBGC	idiopathic basal ganglia calcification
LS	lacunar state
MCI	mild cognitive impairment
MID	multiinfarct dementia
MMSE	Mini-Mental State Examination
MRI	magnetic resonance imaging
MS	multiple sclerosis
MSA	multiple system atrophy
NSAID	nonsteroidal anti-inflammatory drug
PD	Parkinson disease
PET	positron emission tomography
PS	presenilin
PSP	progressive supranuclear palsy
SCD	subcortical dementia
SD	standard deviation

SPECT	single-photon emission computed tomography
TNF	tumor necrosis factor
VaD	vascular dementia
WD	Wilson disease

Introduction

This volume is an empirical, clinical, theoretical, and nosological discussion of the causes, presentations, differential diagnosis, and treatment of the dementias. It advances a spectrum approach: each dementing disorder involves a spectrum, an array of varied but related presentations that form a continuous series. The Alzheimer-type dementias, vascular dementias, depressive dementias, frontotemporal dementias, Creutzfeldt-Jakob dementia, schizophrenic dementia, AIDS/HIV dementia complex, as well as other cortical and frontosubcortical dementias (including progressive supranuclear palsy, primary progressive aphasia, Parkinson disease, Pick complex, corticobasal degeneration complex, motor neuron disease, Fahr disease, and others) are discussed in the context of a spectrum. Also, the boundaries between normal aging and the dementias, subcortical and cortical dementias, focal diseases and diffuse or generalized diseases, dementias and "pseudodementias" are examined from the vantage point of a continuity paradigm.

In addition to using a spectrum approach as an integrating organizational principle, this book is singular in its emphasis on and development of nosology as a critical tool in furthering explanation and treatment of the dementias. Recommendations are made pertaining to systematic classification, or nosology, of the dementias. Weaknesses of present nosology are described and levels of organization for future nosology are outlined. The hierarchic relationship between dementia subtypes is delineated as it pertains to nosology.

This volume emphasizes the need to add a diachronic component to both research and clinical work on the dementias. Approaches to the investigation and treatment of the dementias are apt to fail without a long-term perspective. By definition, dementias are disorders that evolve over time, and they cannot be understood or realistically treated using a static or synchronic view.

More people are living longer nowadays. Furthermore, the proportion of people who survive beyond the age of 75 years (the "old-old") has increased in developed nations (National Academy on an Aging Society 2000). Dementia is correlated with age, and, accordingly, the incidence and prevalence of dementia are increasing (see chaps. 2, 3, 10, 14, and 15). The question has been raised whether dementia is an inevitable part of the extension of life, but despite increased interest by health professionals in the relationships between the dementias, pseudodementias, and normal aging, our understanding of the spectra of the dementias is inadequate. No other book-length consideration of the topic exists, particularly one that includes the pseudodementias as part of the varied but intersecting continua of the dementias. This volume addresses the need for information on the presentations of and differential diagnosis between the dementias, as well as between the dementias and pseudodementias, and their interrelationships.

Historically, *dementia* (derived from the Latin root *de mens*) is a descriptive term denoting an observable decline in mental abilities. During the nineteenth century, the term was increasingly used to emphasize an etiologic dimension, becoming restricted to denote deteriorating mental capacity due to organic causes. Esquirol and others considered dementia to be a severe, acquired, irreversible form of intellectual deterioration secondary to organic brain disease. States of dementia in elderly individuals were described by Esquirol, and by the end of the nineteenth century, brains of elderly persons with dementia had been examined by histologic methods and lesions had been demonstrated. Alzheimer and Pick found histologic lesions in patients with early-onset disorder that resembled those of the "senile" elderly patients described by Esquirol (Alexander and Selesnick 1966).

Today's definition of dementia is consistent with this historical conceptualization but more specified. Current nosology describes dementia as a syndrome due to organic causes, the essential feature of which is the development of multiple cognitive deficits that include memory impairment and at least one of the following cognitive disturbances: aphasia, apraxia, agnosia, or disturbance in executive function (World Health Organization 1992, 1993; American Psychiatric Association 1994, 2000). Diagnostic criteria require that cognitive deficits be severe enough to cause impairment in occupational or social function and demonstrate a decline from a previously higher level of function (World Health Organization 1992, 1993; American Psychiatric Association 1994, 2000).

It has been almost a decade since the first edition of this book was published. Although that edition remains au courant and even cutting-edge, there have been many important advances in knowledge about the nature and treatment of the dementias. This second edition contains three new chapters, which present groundbreaking material relating to the role of inflammation in the pathogenesis of dementias of the Alzheimer type (DAT) (chap. 5), a phylogenetically based model of the intrinsic memory deficit of DAT (chap. 8), and the nature and treatment of AIDS/HIV dementia (chap. 13). Even though many chapters are organized around clinical material, in this second edition each chapter contains a new section entitled "Clinical Conclusions." The material of each chapter is refocused and presented through the vantage point or lens of clinical applications in this section.

More than half the chapters, while still having the same lead author, have changes in coauthorship, with resulting material that is on the frontier of knowledge with new perspectives. All chapters introduce and synthesize new material, some of which includes: (1) comparisons between Alzheimer-type dementias and Down syndrome, with discussion of shared pathogenesis; (2) new data and a paradigm shift pertaining to genetic factors crosscutting several dementias; (3) introduction of the concept of "prepermanent dementia" in the long-term disease course and conversion to "permanent dementia"; (4) conceptualization of a "depression-executive dysfunction syndrome"; (5) exploration of the roles of inflammation and cystatin C at the interface of vascular dementia and DAT; (6) introduction of a new nosologic category of schizophrenic dementia; (7) material on how to treat Binswanger dementia to prevent progression; (8) functional magnetic resonance imaging (fMRI) data relating to the continuum of normal aging and dementia; and (9) review of new medications and treatments for the dementias. Following is a brief description of core concepts and new material chapter by chapter.

Background, Concepts, and Diagnostics

The first section of this volume consists of three chapters that provide background concepts and a comprehensive review of clinical diagnostic procedures. Chapter 1 revolves around the boundaries between normal aging and early dementia. Hence, dementia is defined initially in terms of a normative aging baseline. This chapter reviews the most recent neuropsychological and neuroimaging findings that characterize the continuum from normal aging to dementia. Concepts defined as part of the continuum include *successful aging*, *age-associated memory impairment*, *age-associated cognitive decline*, *mild cognitive impairment*, and *dementia*. Criteria for these differing levels of cognitive impairment are discussed in the context of structural imaging data relating to neuroanatomic and neuropsychological changes in aging and dementia.

Chapter 2 deals with major issues pertaining to the validity and reliability of dementia constructs. Criteria and measures for dementia are outlined. The chapter presents a set of interrelated criteria for identifying dementia as a syndrome. Cognitive impairment, functional impairment, and neuropathology constitute a central or first-order triad in criteria for dementia. Second-order modifiers are described that center around severity and disease course. The concept of dementia as a threshold phenomenon is explored. Current prevalence figures and other recent data are used to explicate controversies related to validity of dementia constructs. The impact of validity issues on sociology of medical knowledge and conclusions is discussed. Key research questions and directions are outlined.

Chapter 3 presents new material from the most recent Canadian Consensus Conference on Diagnostic Procedures for Dementia and constitutes a practical conclusion for the background section of this volume. Table 3.3 is very important in that it provides a comprehensive list of the commonly used drugs and medications that can result in cognitive impairment. Iatrogenic factors in the pathogenesis of dementia have been largely unexplored. The material of chapter 3 serves to bring this neglected dimension of medicine into focus. Finally, although several subsequent chapters are oriented toward specialists, the majority of patients with dementing disorders are seen first, and sometimes only, by primary care physicians. Accordingly, we felt it important to include this chapter on diagnostic procedures viewed from the perspective of the primary care physician.

Alzheimer Dementias

The second section of this book consists of five chapters providing an empirical, theoretical, and clinical update on causes, presentations, differential diagnosis, and treatment of the most studied and most prevalent class of dementias: the dementias of Alzheimer type (DAT) (Lobo et al. 2000; Lyketsos et al. 2000; Gauthier and Ferris 2001). Dementias of the Alzheimer type are characterized using neuropathology, neuropsychology, clinical symptomatology, and personal and family history.

Chapter 4 presents an update on the neuropathology of dementia of the Alzheimer type. A broad spectrum of brain changes is discussed, including accumulation of fibrillar amyloid-β protein in plaques and vessels, neurofibrillary degeneration, and synaptic and neuronal loss. Neuropathologic diagnostic criteria for DAT are outlined and evaluated. New data and explanations are presented relating to the pathogenesis and pathomechanisms of DAT. For example, a detailed description of the processing of the amyloid-β protein precursor gene on chromosome 21 is integrated into the pathogenetic explanation, as are intracellular accumulation of amyloid-β peptides and extracellular fibrillar amyloid deposition. Further, the chapter discusses clinicopathological correlations in DAT, which are important for understanding memory deficit. Finally, the chapter presents new material on DAT in people with Down syndrome, discussing the pathogenesis and pathomechanisms underlying both syndromes.

Chapter 5 is a new chapter and presents material suggesting neural inflammation mechanisms play a major role in the conversion of dementia of the Alzheimer type from a relatively benign pathology to a malignant inflammatory disorder. Postmortem data reveal a state of chronic inflammation in affected regions of the brain of persons with DAT. Immunohistochemical studies indicate many inflammatory markers newly appear or are upregulated in affected regions of the brain of persons with DAT. The chapter describes the function of a chronically activated complement system in the membrane attack complex, which inserts only into viable cells, making holes in them and causing death. A distinction is introduced between autoimmune disorders and "autotoxicity" disorders. *Autotoxicity* is a pathomechanism of the phylogenetically more primitive innate immune system, whereas *autoimmunity* is a pathomechanism of the adaptive immune system. Chapter 5 proposes that autotoxicity is a critical variable in the pathogenesis of DAT. It suggests that anti-inflammatory agents might slow the process of DAT. This chapter points out that more than twenty epidemiological studies show that persons taking nonsteroidal anti-inflammatory drugs have a greatly reduced incidence of DAT.

Chapter 6 introduces evidence for clinical subgroups of dementia of the Alzheimer type. It emphasizes that diagnostic criteria sometimes incorrectly give the impression that DAT is a relatively homogeneous disorder. The chapter revolves around introducing genetic, neuropathological, neuropsychological, and clinical evidence that Alzheimer disorder is not a singular, homogeneous disorder, but rather has great heterogeneity and is better characterized as a syndrome with subgroups. The heterogeneity of DAT is particularly apparent when two specific spectra are considered: (1) the early-onset versus late-onset spectrum, and (2) the spectrum between persons with prominent temporoparietal symptoms versus those with minimal or absent temporoparietal symptoms. Within the parameters of these spectra, two subgroups are identified by the authors. Type I is characterized by early age at onset, severe memory disturbances, predominant parietal symptoms, low frequency of vascular factors, normal blood-brain barrier, and low frequency of white matter changes on computed tomography. Type II is characterized by late age at onset, global decline in cognitive functions, no or mild parietal symptoms, high frequency of episodes of confusion, mildly impaired blood-brain barrier function, and high frequency of white matter changes on computed tomography. Parameters for additional subgroups are discussed, with special focus on recent genetic parameters for subgroups identified in familial DAT.

Chapter 7 describes unusual patterns of neurodegenerative diseases that mimic focal brain disorders. Because of symptomatic focality, these disease patterns are differentiated from classical "diffuse" dementing illnesses, such as DAT. Neurodegenerative disease patterns in which language deterioration is the predominant presenting feature are defined. Primary progressive aphasia is shown to be a syndrome produced by several different pathological substrates. The relationships between primary progressive aphasia and Pick disease, corticobasal degeneration, and Creutzfeldt-Jakob disease are explicated. Further, Pick complex is described as an overarching syndrome encompassing a number of diseases with shared features of focal onset, frontotemporal neuronal loss, gliosis, and relative absence of senile plaques and neurofibrillary tangles. Pick complex is contrasted with DAT. Clinical and diagnostic criteria are outlined and discussed in the context of neuropathologic findings. Atypical subgroups of Alzheimer syndrome are examined, including those with myoclonus or extrapyramidal symptoms. The theoretical and clinical significance of atypical dementia presentations is discussed. The spectrum of focal and diffuse lesions is in the foreground of this chapter. The critical function of edema, disrupted cortical connections, and diaschisis is discussed in the context of the spectrum of focal-diffuse lesions.

Chapter 8 is new to this edition and introduces a new memory framework to account for the memory deficits of dementia of the Alzheimer type. Memory is redefined in a phylogenetic context as a critical adaptational tool enabling an organism to retain information so every minute of existence won't require a de novo response to same or similar challenges. Accordingly, it is posited that memory is a phylogenetically evolved structural and functional set of systems enabling organisms to interact more efficiently and flexibly in physical and social environments. An evolutionary memory framework is introduced consisting of the three phylogenetically based tiers of *motor (movement) memory*, *emotional memory*, and *higher cortical (neocortical) memory*. The three tiers of memory are evaluated in DAT with the finding that there exists an inverse correlation between phylogenetic memory development and memory preservation in DAT: the earlier and more primitive the memory system, the better preserved it remains in DAT. Hence, motor memory is better preserved than emotional memory in DAT, and both motor memory and emotional memory are better preserved than higher cortical (neocortical) memory. Put another way, memory systems located in brain regions that evolve earlier appear to remain best preserved in DAT. Thus, motor memory (subcortical) is better preserved in DAT than neocortical memory. Further, chapter 8 develops a new conceptualization of the neocortical tier of memory with six stages defined: stage 1 (sensory); stage 2 (selection, recode, encode); stage 3 (new learning); stage 4 (delayed new learning); stage 5 (old learning or knowledge); and stage 6 (overlearned knowledge). This chapter presents evidence that in addition to the inverse correlation between phylogenesis and memory preservation in DAT (i.e., the earlier in evolution, the better preserved), there is an inverse correlation between the ontogenetic development of the six neocortical stages of memory and preservation in DAT (i.e., the earlier to develop in the life span, the better preserved). The memory framework developed in this chapter enables new theoretical and clinical understandings of the fundamental nature of memory as applied to DAT disease progression across time. The reader will come to understand that the disease process of DAT involves a fundamental evolutionary and developmental retrogression (Emery 1985, 1988, 1999, 2000) or, in terms coined in chapter 8, *retrophylogenesis* and *retro-ontogenesis* disease course in the context of phylogenetic and ontogenetic development, respectively. In consequence, the clinician or family member of a person with DAT can anticipate specific memory decrements before they occur and plan accordingly.

Vascular Dementias and Subcortical Dementias

The third section of this book describes and defines presentations of dementias other than dementias of the Alzheimer type, with special focus on the vascular dementias (VaD) and subcortical dementias. These are compared and contrasted with DAT. The spectra of VaD and subcortical dementias are important not only in their own right, but also because of the difficulties that currently exist regarding construct validity, nosology, and, more pragmatically, differential diagnosis and co-occurrence with and at the interface of Alzheimer syndrome. These chapters systematically present diagnostic criteria that will help the reader distinguish among the different kinds of dementia. The authors of this section introduce new perspectives, paradigms, and much-needed clarification relating to cognitive deterioration in vascular disorders. Vascular dementia is reconceptualized in this section. Additionally, a chapter on AIDS/HIV dementia has been added to this edition. Usually, chapters on AIDS/HIV dementia do not find their way into volumes focused on geriatric organic brain syndromes. Precisely for this reason, we sought out a foremost pioneer and expert in the field of AIDS/HIV to contribute to this volume because the greatest learning occurs with shifting of paradigms and breaking of circumscribed mental sets. The chapter on AIDS/HIV dementia is included in this section because of dominant subcortical components in the AIDS dementia complex.

Chapter 9 reviews the cognitive and behavioral characteristics of frontosubcortical dementias (FSCD) and compares them to features of the cortical dementias, particularly dementias of the Alzheimer type. The main etiologies of FSCD and associated neurologic features are summarized with special emphasis for clinicians. Also, recent data on the pathophysiology of FSCD are discussed, focusing on the basal ganglia and frontal lobes. Attention and concentration, language and speech, visuospatial functions, memory, executive functions, and bradyphrenia are looked at in the context of pathophysiologic substrates, as are neuropsychiatric features such as mood changes, personality changes, and psychosis. The centrality of these dimensions for the clinician in the differential diagnosis of dementias is brought into focus. Diseases leading to the common pathway of FSCD are described. The importance of differential diagnosis is emphasized in relation to rationally based treatments and medications for FSCD. For example, even though the present medical culture fosters use of acetylcholinesterase inhibitors, the authors point out this class of medications has not been proven to benefit FSCD and has negative side effects. More basic research and clinicopathologic correlations are needed to improve diagnostic criteria and quality of care.

Chapter 10 redefines and broadens the nosologic construct of vascular dementia to include what is termed *noninfarct vascular dementia:* vascular dementia caused by underlying vascular factors other than cerebral infarction. Data from investigations in a broad spectrum of vascular disorders are summarized and analyzed. The data indicate that cerebral infarction is not the only path to the final common pathway of VaD. Vascular disease without cerebral infarction results in a continuum of cognitive impairment, with one end of this continuum represented by the concept of noninfarct VaD. Data are presented that implicate arteriosclerosis and hypertension/hypotension in the distal causality of VaD. It is argued that infarcts don't come out of nowhere, and a *preinfarct state* is conceptualized. Persons with vascular disease in a preinfarct state are often nosologically forced into the Alzheimer category, where they don't belong. Vascular dementia has the characteristics of a syndrome and appears to be caused by a number of underlying mechanisms; to equate VaD with any single subtype is invalid. Further, chapter 10 develops the thesis that VaD and Alzheimer syndrome constitute a spectrum. New data on vascular factors underlying pathogenetic mechanisms of both VaD and Alzheimer syndrome are discussed, including the role of activated complement cascade and activated microglia as part of inflammation of brain tissue common to both syndromes. Also, the common pathogenetic mechanisms of deposition of amyloid-β protein by microvessels and damaged cerebral capillary ultrastructure are discussed. Vascular disorders leading to VaD are found to span the cortical-subcortical spectrum. The authors conclude that a spectrum perspective results in a concomitant wider treatment spectrum.

Chapter 11 contains important information for the clinician on how to diagnose and treat Binswanger disease. New clinical and empirical data are described which relate to a ten-year treatment period for persons with Binswanger disease during which cognitive function was successfully maintained without further deterioration. Also in the chapter, relationships between hypertension, white matter findings on brain imaging, and VaD are discussed. Relationships between blood pressure and neuroradiologic findings are presented. The ambiguity of leukoaraiosis and its relation to normal aging and Alzheimer-VaD spectrum is discussed. The Alzheimer-vascular dementia spectrum is further defined by introducing the intriguing relationships of different types of amyloid. Amyloid deposition in cerebral vascular walls of persons with DAT is described. The possible relation between amyloid angiopathy with cystatin C deposition and recurrent cerebral hemorrhage is evaluated. Thus, cystatin C appears to be an underlying factor at the interface of VaD and DAT.

Along with chapters 10 and 11, chapter 12 breaks new ground in probing the function of noninfarct factors in the causal chain of vascular events leading to vascular dementia. The material of these chapters represents a research frontier at the interface between VaD and DAT. Noninfarct factors leading to VaD that are explored as part of the chapter include hypoperfusion, vessel wall changes leading to blood-brain barrier or carrier dysfunction, and possible dysfunction of the oligodendrocytes leading to defective myelination. Also, incomplete infarcts and functional inactivity of nerve cells because of ischemia are discussed in their pathogenetic relation to VaD. Vascular dementia is defined as an overarching syndrome composed of at least two subtypes: cortical and subcortical vascular syndromes. A number of specific vascular mechanisms that underlie VaD are described. Chapter 12 pioneers at the interface between VaD and DAT with new data and theoretical explanation bridging the two syndromes. The spectrum of cognitive impairment is evaluated in the context of the VaD-Alzheimer spectrum. Finally, *leukoaraiosis, a term* coined by one of the chapter authors in previous work, is explored in terms of the function, structure, and correlates of leukoaraiosis.

Chapter 13, on acquired immune deficiency syndrome/human immunodeficiency virus dementia, is new in this edition. This chapter informs the reader incrementally and provides the reader with a broader perspective on the spectra of the dementias. What is brought into high relief with this chapter is the nagging question usually not sufficiently in the foreground, as to whether some infectious agent plays a role in the multifactorial causality of any number of other dementias. The chapter provides a highly informed description of the nature, presentations, differential diagnosis, disease course, and medical management of the cognitive impairments of AIDS/HIV dementia. Neurologic complications of HIV-1 infection and AIDS are detailed, as is the medical management of these neurologic complications. Chapter 13 includes a discussion of early neurologic complications of acute HIV-1 infection; neurologic complications during the "asymptomatic" phase of systemic HIV-1 infection; and asymptomatic HIV-1 infection of the central nervous system. A variety of central nervous system disorders in the period after initial HIV-1 infection are described and reported frequencies given. During the phases of acute infection with seroconversion and middle "asymptomatic" period of "clinical latency," principal pathogenetic mechanisms appear to involve immunopathology, either through triggering autoimmune reactions or resulting from host responses to ongoing HIV-1 infection. Late nervous system involvement by HIV-1 is also detailed. In late stages of HIV-1 infection, when immune defenses have been severely compromised and systemic complications begin to accumulate, the nervous system becomes highly susceptible to a wide array of disorders. These may involve all levels of the neuraxis, including meninges, brain, spinal cord, peripheral nerve, and muscle. Major clinical manifestations of the AIDS dementia complex are described. The AIDS dementia complex has strong subcortical components affecting cognition, motor performance, and behavior.

Depressive Dementias

Many psychiatric disorders can result in a dementialike presentation. Historically, disorders that appear degenerative but with treatment or passage of time appear to reverse have been called "pseudodementias." This historical category can be conceptualized as an overarching category with many subtypes (Emery 1988; Emery and Oxman 1992, 1997). Regardless of etiology, most discussions of this syndrome tend to dichotomize dementia and pseudodementia with parameters of irreversibility-reversibility and structural, organic versus functional, nonorganic etiology. The contributors to this volume hold that a dichotomous approach to the dementias and pseudodementias is not productive and that a continuity framework is more useful for understanding and treating the presentations that are described. This section of the volume includes a reconceptualization of the pseudodementias. The usual dichotomies between the pseudodementias and degenerative dementias are rejected.

Chapter 14 is a theoretical, empirical, clinical, and nosological discussion of the depression-dementia spectrum, which involves an array of varied but related presentations. Depressive disorders form a prototypic and substantial core of the historical category of pseudodementia. The terms *depressive dementia, depressive pseudodementia, dementia syndrome of depression*, and *major depression with depressive dementia* are synonymous. The chapter posits that depressive dementia is not a "pseudo"dementia, but real. Depressive dementia is reconceptualized, with new terms coined, as a *prepermanent dementia* and *intermediate-stage dementia* in the multiphasic, morphogenetic, long-term disease course between major depression without dementia and, what is to date, "permanent dementia." Recent empirical and clinical evidence is presented that reveals depressive dementia is only "initially reversible" and that in a significant number of cases, depressive dementia later converts into an irreversible, permanent dementia. Accordingly, depressive dementia represents a transitional stage in the conversion of an initially-reversible or prepermanent dementia into a permanent, end-stage dementia, such as DAT. Recent neurophysiological and neuropsychological research is reviewed which points to the organic pathogenetic substrates underlying depressive dementia. Further, chapter 14 defines five prototypical groups that comprise the depression-dementia spectrum. The interrelationship between depression and dementia is explored within the context of the continuum of these five prototypic groups and found to be "curvilinearlike" as a function of a threshold for central cholinergic function below which expression of clinical depression is not possible. The critical question is raised as to why some and not other cases of depressive dementia devolve into permanent, irreversible dementia. The possible role of anticholinergic antidepressants is brought into focus as one possible factor, in this case iatrogenic, in a multifactorial process.

Chapter 15 includes an update of cognitive and biological correlates and course of illness of depressive dementia. The "initial reversibility" of depressive dementia is discussed in the context of differential diagnostic correlates. Recent data are presented which evidence major depression as a risk factor for dementia. On the foreground of research, the chapter contains a conceptualization of a *depression-executive dysfunction syndrome*, which appears to be descriptive of at least a subset of persons with late-life depressive dementia. The syndrome is characterized by impaired activities of daily living, reduced interest in activities, psychomotor retardation, and suspiciousness, and has a slow, unstable response to classical antidepressants. Data from physiological and neuropsychological studies provide evidence for right hemisphere dysfunction in depression. The construct of executive function includes such parameters as planning, organization, foresight, judgment, control, and management of time. It is suggested that the pathogenesis of late-life "depression-executive dysfunction" might stem from frontostriatal dysfunction.

Even though there have been very few investigations of depressive dementia per se, it becomes clear from what limited data exist that depressive dementia is a heterogeneous syndrome. There appear to be at least two modal patterns in which depressive dementia could constitute one phase in a long-term multiphasic disease course. One such possible multiphasic disease course involves a progression from major depression without dementia to depressive dementia, which after some years develops into a degenerative dementia of the Alzheimer phenotype. This modal pattern crosscuts subcortical and cortical parameters. It is this modal pattern which forms the central content of chapter 14. In contrast, chapter 15 conceptualizes a second modal disease pattern, which appears to be predominantly "subcortical," beginning with depression without dementia and devolving into a depressive dementia which years later becomes an "irreversible" dementia of a VaD phenotype (see chap. 9).

Chapter 16 discusses the nondepressive pseudodementias. The utility and validity of the construct of pseudodementia are discussed. Pseudodementia as a simulation of dementia is described, with the question raised as to whether competent simulation of dementia is possible. Recent data are provided casting light on malingering, factitious disorder, and dissociative (hysteric) pseudodementia. Hysterical puerilism, or hysterical infantilism, is discussed. Ganser syndrome is defined in its relation to pseudodementia. Further, pseudodementia is described when it is part of other primary psychiatric disorders, such as manic pseudodementia. Schizophrenic pseudodementia is reconceptualized as schizophrenic dementia in analogue to the model of depressive dementia. Recent evidence for organic brain abnormalities in schizophrenia is presented. Recent data consistent with the construct of schizophrenic dementia include evidence of decreased gray matter in the hippocampus, amygdala, parahippocampus, superior temporal gyrus, and thalamus. Further, data are presented revealing changes in the frontotemporal cortex to include decreased neural cell size. A comprehensive review of fMRI studies of schizophrenia is provided in the context of the concept of schizophrenic dementia. The lack of empiric data on many of the "pseudodementias" is shown to be problematic; the need for future research on these disorders is clear.

Chapter 17 presents the most recent material on the neurobiology of major depression in dementia of the Alzheimer type (DAT). Postmortem data on neuropathologic and neurochemical correlates of major depression in DAT are analyzed. The methodologies and results of four major neuropathologic investigations of major depression in DAT are compared; primary variables considered include the locus ceruleus (noradrenergic), substantia nigra (dopaminergic), dorsal raphe (serotonergic), basal nucleus of Meynert (cholinergic), senile plaques, neurofibrillary tangles, norepinephrine, dopamine, serotonin, and choline acetyltransferase. Further, clinical features of age at onset and duration of dementia are considered in comparisons of results of the four major investigations. In the context of DAT, the studies compared suggest that major depression describes a clinically and pathologically distinct subgroup of persons who have degenerative changes in brainstem aminergic nuclei, especially the locus ceruleus, which are disproportionate to those that occur in the cerebral cortex. This subgroup of persons with DAT and major depression also evidences a relative preservation of the basal nucleus of Meynert. Chapter 17 also introduces a phenotypic characterization of six susceptibility alleles in fifty autopsied DAT cases with a comparison of clinical, histopathologic, and neurochemical features associated with each allele. The pioneering work of this chapter's author on the concept of minimum neurotransmitter thresholds for the occurrence of depression is developed.

Throughout this section on the depressive dementias, the authors probe, empirically, theoretically, and clinically, the questions of if and how depressive illness itself causes depressive dementia, and in turn, why so many cases of depressive dementia appear to convert into degenerative dementia. Historically, the affective disorders have not been conceptualized as having a connection with "organic" brain syndromes. The association between major depression without dementia, depressive dementia, and neurodegenerative "permanent dementia" represents a new research and clinical focus. Whether depression without dementia, and its possible devolution into depressive dementia, represents a risk factor for permanent dementia; or whether the cognitive deficits of depression represent an early preclinical phase of permanent dementia are questions that bring into focus two sides of a fundamental continuity or spectrum relationship. Two sides of the same coin, one being the obverse of the other; these issues point to a fundamental connection between depression and dementia, which was historically not known. This breakthrough perspective will contribute to a better understanding of both.

Conclusions and Future Directions

The concluding section consists of a chapter that updates medication and treatment approaches to the dementias, as well as a chapter that distills and integrates the preceding material.

Chapter 18 involves an extensive description of the most current medications in use for the differing dementing illnesses; the efficacy of different medications is evaluated. The chapter also comprehensively discusses nonmedication treatment approaches or adjuncts. Treatment issues are delineated in the context of the dementia presentations discussed in prior material and their often ambiguous transitions. The chapter emphasizes that any dementia syndrome is treatable, even if its underlying cause is, at least to date, nonreversible or permanent. In such cases, the focus of treatment is excess disability (Reifler and Sherrill 1990). In addition to evaluating medications for cognitive impairments, the chapter discusses various treatment approaches to noncognitive symptoms, such as loss of impulse control and disrupted sleep.

Chapter 19 concludes the volume using the material of preceding chapters to examine the relationships and ambiguous transitions in the spectra of the dementias. This chapter emphasizes the volume authors' perspective that both Alzheimer dementia and VaD represent overarching superordinate nosologic categories comprised of subtypes. Alzheimer disorder is a heterogeneous syndrome with clinical subgroups, and needs to be better represented in nosology. Alzheimer dementia cannot be understood or rationally treated if conceptualized as a homogeneous, singular disease entity. In this volume, dementia(s) of the Alzheimer type (DAT), Alzheimer disease(s) (AD), and Alzheimer syndrome are synonyms. Further, the validity of VaD as a construct has been compromised for the past thirty years by the equation of the totality of VaD with what should have been conceptualized as only one subtype, multiinfarct dementia. This chapter points to the need for nosologic revision such that VaD is represented as an overarching superordinate category comprised of subtypes, including the newly conceptualized category of *noninfarct vascular dementia.* In the same vein, chapter 19 discusses the plurality of presentations for other dementia syndromes or complexes and also examines the interrelatedness between depressive dementia as a *prepermanent, intermediate-stage dementia* and permanent, nonreversible dementias. The newly conceptualized synonymous categories of *prepermanent dementias, intermediate-stage dementias,* and *transitional dementias* are discussed and evaluated. In view of the theoretical, clinical, and empirical contributions of our distinguished authors in preceding chapters, we highlight some of the challenges to current concepts about the dementias and suggest the use of a spectrum approach to understand the relationships of interest. The construct utility and nosologic validity of different dementia terms are evaluated, and recommendations are made for future nosologic classification.

To the best of our knowledge, there is currently no other comprehensive approach to the spectra of the dementias and their presentations, interrelationships, differential diagnosis, and nosology. In view of the increasing number of health care professionals involved in the evaluation and treatment of cognitive disorders, we hope that this book will increase understanding, be of some practical use, and serve as a heuristic stimulus for meaningful research.

REFERENCES

Alexander, F., and S. Selesnick. 1966. *The History of Psychiatry.* New York: Harper and Row.

American Psychiatric Association. 1994. *Diagnostic and Statistical Manual of Mental Disorders.* 4th ed. Washington, D.C.: American Psychiatric Association.

American Psychiatric Association. 2000. *Diagnostic and Statistical Manual of Mental Disorders.* 4th ed., text revision. Washington, D.C.: American Psychiatric Association.

Emery, V.O.B. 1985. Language and aging. *Experimental Aging Research Monograph Series* 11 (1).

Emery, V.O.B. 1988. *Pseudodementia: A Theoretical and Empirical Discussion.* Cleveland: Case Western Reserve University School of Medicine.

Emery, V.O.B. 1999. On the relationship between memory and language in the dementia spectrum of depression, Alzheimer syndrome, and normal aging. In *Language and Communication in Old Age: Multidisciplinary Perspectives,* edited by H. Hamilton. New York: Garland Publishing, pp. 25–62.

Emery, V.O.B. 2000. Language impairment in dementia of the Alzheimer type: A hierarchical decline? *International Journal of Psychiatry in Medicine* 30:145–64.

Emery, V.O.B., and T.E. Oxman. 1992. Update on the dementia spectrum of depression. *American Journal of Psychiatry* 149:305–17.

Emery, V.O.B., and T.E. Oxman. 1997. Depressive dementia: A transitional dementia? *Clinical Neuroscience* 4:23–30.

Gauthier, S., and S. Ferris. 2001. Outcome measures for probable vascular dementia and Alzheimer's disease with cerebrovascular disease. *International Journal of Clinical Practice* 120:29–39.

Lobo, A., L. Launer, L. Fratiglioni, et al. 2000. Prevalence of dementia and major subtypes in Europe: A collaborative study of population-based cohorts. *Neurology* 54:S4–9.

Lyketsos, C., M. Steinberg, J. Tschanz, et al. 2000. Mental and behavioral disturbances in dementia: Findings from the Cache Country Study on Memory in Aging. *American Journal of Psychiatry* 157:708–14.

National Academy on an Aging Society. 2000. *Challenges for the Twenty-first Century: Chronic and Disabling Conditions.* Washington, D.C.: Gerontological Society of America, pp. 2–5.

Reifler, B., and K. Sherrill. 1990. Dementias: Reversible and irreversible. In *Review of Psychiatry,* vol. 9, edited by A. Tasman, S. Goldfinger, and C. Kaufman. Washington, D.C.: American Psychiatric Press, pp. 220–32.

World Health Organization. 1992. *The ICD-10 Classification of Mental and Behavioral Disorders: Clinical Descriptions and Diagnostic Guidelines.* Geneva, Switzerland: World Health Organization.

World Health Organization. 1993. *The ICD-10 Classification of Mental and Behavioral Disorders: Diagnostic Criteria for Research.* Geneva, Switzerland: World Health Organization.

Part I / Background, Concepts, and Diagnostics

CHAPTER ONE

Boundaries between Normal Aging and Dementia

Perspectives from Neuropsychological and Neuroimaging Investigations

Laura A. Flashman, Ph.D.,
Heather A. Wishart, Ph.D.,
Thomas E. Oxman, M.D.,
and Andrew J. Saykin, Psy.D.

Recent research has advanced our understanding of the boundary between normal aging and dementia. In addition to illuminating changes associated with both normal and abnormal aging, researchers have identified a group of individuals whose cognitive deficits place them in an intermediate position on the continuum between normal aging and dementia. The study of the continuum is complicated by remarkable variability across individuals and domains of functioning. Aging is characterized by both decremental and incremental changes (Albert 1988). As a result, the range and standard deviation for almost any variable of interest increase with age (Rowe and Wang 1988). Emerging evidence from studies of neurogenesis indicates regenerative potential in the adult human brain (Kempermann and Gage 1999; Horner and Gage 2000; Shihabuddin et al. 2000) and possible neural recruitment (Reuter-Lorenz, Stanczak, and Miller 1999) that may be associated with successful cognitive aging or recovery from brain insults.

Concepts and Criteria

A common terminology is necessary for characterizing the cognitive profiles associated with normal aging and various types of abnormal aging.

Normal and Successful Aging

Normal aging has been conceptualized as the typical changes in behavior that occur with age (Schroots and Birren 1993). The common conception has been that subtle declines in cognition occur as part of the normal aging process. However, studies have included individuals with other age-associated conditions, such as cardiovascular disease or diabetes, which can affect cognition. More recently, some researchers examined normal elderly individuals without age-associated medical conditions, and evidence is emerging that their cognition can remain relatively stable, at least until about 85 years of age (e.g., Emery 1985; Schaie and Willis 1991; Hickman et al. 2000; Snowdon 2001). The critical question is whether systematic or regular changes occur with age in the absence of and independent of disease. Addressing this question, a classical investigation by Birren and colleagues, which has been reliably replicated, found that even optimally healthy individuals between ages 65 and 91 showed significantly slower psychomotor speed than did young adults; this age-related psychomotor slowing in the absence of any disease was found to have a negative impact on cognitive measures that required fast response (Birren, Woods, and Williams 1980; Salthouse 1985; Spirduso and MacRae 1990; Schaie and Willis 1991). Concomitantly, these optimally healthy disease-free elderly individuals evidenced slowing of electrical activity of the brain, or EEG changes, as a function of normal aging (Birren 1965; Birren, Woods, and Williams 1980; Schaie and Willis 1991). Shedding additional light on this issue, recent studies provide new insights on the aging brain, with evidence that neural regeneration and functional brain reorganization may help to preserve cognition during the aging process (Kempermann and Gage 1999; Reuter-Lorenz, Stanczak, and Miller 1999; Shihabuddin et al. 2000). Psychosocial factors that may contribute to successful cognitive aging include diet, exercise, no substance abuse (e.g., alcohol, illegal drugs, prescription drugs), social involvement, and very importantly, mental activity and new learning (see chaps. 3 and 19) (e.g., Baltes and Baltes 1990; Baltes 1993; Nicolas et al. 2001).

Age-associated Memory Impairment

Initially used to refer to the "benign forgetfulness" (Kral 1958, 1962) frequently reported as healthy individuals grow older, the term *age-associated mem-*

ory impairment (AAMI) was introduced in 1986 by a National Institute of Mental Health work group (Crook et al. 1986). While the original concept of benign forgetfulness was defined without formal psychometric testing and criteria, it assumed that some gradual cognitive change with aging is normal. The formal criteria developed by the 1986 work group included: (1) age 50 or older; (2) subjective decline or loss in memory function; (3) performance at least one standard deviation (SD) below the mean of young adults on memory tests; (4) preserved intellectual ability; (5) failure to meet the criteria for depression; and (6) failure to meet the criteria for dementia. Using these criteria, however, at least one study (Smith et al. 1991) showed that a very large percentage of the older population would be classified as having AAMI.

Age-associated Cognitive Decline

The term *age-associated cognitive decline* (AACD) has been used to describe a group of older individuals in which multiple domains of cognition may be mildly compromised relative to younger individuals (Levy 1994). As is the case for AAMI, the use of young adults as the reference group for AACD means that many older adults will be classified as having AACD, yielding little discriminative or predictive value to the classification (Shah, Tangalos, and Petersen 2000).

Mild Cognitive Impairment

The term *mild cognitive impairment* (MCI) has been used to describe the group of older individuals who have greater than expected memory impairment for their age, but do not meet the criteria for dementia (Petersen 2000). Unlike AAMI and AACD, the reference group for a diagnosis of MCI is composed of age-matched peers. Mild cognitive impairment generally presents with subjective memory difficulties of insidious onset. In fact, subjective cognitive complaints can be a harbinger of dementia even before the development of demonstrable cognitive deficits, particularly in highly educated individuals (Jonker, Geerlings, and Schmand 2000). When these complaints are corroborated by an informant, they are more likely to be borne out on further clinical evaluation. As time progresses, the forgetfulness becomes more frequent and significant. In spite of these developing memory problems, social and occupational functioning are relatively preserved. Nonmemory cognitive domains are relatively spared in MCI, as originally defined, but in practice may fall slightly below age- and education-based normative data. For example, speed of processing and cognitive flexibility may be subtly impaired (Petersen 2000).

The formal criteria for mild cognitive impairment include: (1) significant memory complaints, such as a chronic forgetting of important information, preferably corroborated by an informant; (2) memory impairment on standardized tests relative to age- and education-matched healthy controls (at least 1.5 SD below the mean); (3) otherwise normal cognitive function; (4) normal activities of daily living; and (5) failure to meet the criteria for dementia (Flicker, Ferris, and Reisberg 1991; Petersen et al. 1999).

Unlike the concept of age-associated memory impairment, the underlying assumption of the construct of mild cognitive impairment is that the memory impairment is not normal and that there is an increased likelihood of progression to dementia, particularly dementia of the Alzheimer type (DAT). Current estimates indicate conversion rates from MCI to DAT of between 6% and 25% per year (Petersen et al. 2001), with most studies falling in the range of 10–15% per year (Flicker, Ferris, and Reisberg 1991; Tierney et al. 1996; Bowen et al. 1997; Devanand et al. 1997; Petersen et al. 1999, 2001). This contrasts with the 1–2% per year rate at which DAT develops in the normal elderly population. Petersen and colleagues (1999) reported that up to 40% of individuals diagnosed with MCI convert to DAT within four years, and Morris et al. reported a conversion rate of more than 80% in individuals followed for 9.5 years.

Given the high likelihood of progression to dementia of the Alzheimer type in individuals with mild cognitive impairment, early identification and diagnosis may be important (Almkvist and Winblad 1999). While it is not yet clear who will or will not convert to DAT, several potential risk factors have been identified. Prominent among them is the presence of the apolipoprotein E (ApoE)-4 allele. ApoE is a marker initially studied as a risk factor for cardiovascular disease. It is involved in the normal regulation of phospholipid metabolism and cholesterol and may play a role in neural repair. Identified cognitive predictors include subtle decreases on verbal memory tested over time in longitudinal studies (Collie et al. 2001) and failure to benefit from cueing at recall (Petersen et al. 1994). Neuroimaging predictors include mesial temporal lobe changes, such as decreased volume of the hippocampus (Jack et al. 1999) and entorhinal cortex (Fox et al. 1996; Juottonen et al. 1998, 1999; Jack et al. 1999; Killiany et al. 2000). Magnetic resonance imaging or other techniques such as functional neuroimaging may be useful to distinguish those persons with MCI who will develop DAT from those who will not (Celsis 2000). The trajectory of decline in memory and medial temporal lobe volume is likely to be predictive of conversion to DAT (e.g., Chen et al. 2001).

As more researchers have become involved in studying mild cognitive impairment, it has become clear that it is not a homogeneous disorder (Ritchie, Artero, and Touchon 2001). For example, Petersen et al. (1999) distinguished between two types of MCI. They used the term *amnestic MCI* to describe the variant that progresses to DAT, and differentiated this from nonamnestic MCI. We will limit our discussion to the more widely recognized amnestic variant of MCI, which has been most addressed in the available literature. Future research on nonamnestic MCI will be important; this entity may progress to Pick, Lewy body, frontotemporal, or other types of dementia.

Dementia

Various criteria are used to diagnose dementia and to characterize its severity (see chap. 2 for more detail). For example, the fourth edition of the *Diagnostic and Statistical Manual of Mental Disorders* (DSM-IV), published by the American Psychiatric Association (1994), specifies three main criteria for dementing disorders: (1) memory impairment and impairment of at least one other cognitive domain (e.g., aphasia, apraxia, agnosia, executive dysfunction); (2) sufficient severity to lead to impairment in social or occupational functioning; and (3) decline from a previously higher level of functioning. Table 1.1 compares the criteria for MCI and dementia.

A widely adopted scale that covers these multiple dimensions of the diagnostic criteria is the Clinical Dementia Rating (CDR; Berg 1988; Morris 1993). The CDR quantifies the severity of dementia in six domains: memory, orientation, judgment and problem solving, community affairs, home and hobbies, and personal care. Ratings are based on the report of individuals, a spouse or other caregiver, and all available information (tab. 1.2). Clinical Dementia Rating scores range from 0 (healthy adult) to 3 (severe dementia).

Dementia can result from a number of etiologies, including dementia of the Alzheimer type, Lewy body disease, vascular insults, human immunodeficiency virus, Parkinson disease, Huntington disease, and Pick disease. It can also result from a number of general medical conditions, some of which are at least partially reversible (e.g., depression, hypothyroidism, and vitamin B_{12} deficiency; see chap. 3). See also chapters 6, 7, and 9–18 for discussions of the many types of dementia and their diagnosis and treatment. For the remainder of this chapter, the discussion is confined to DAT.

Table 1.1. Comparison of criteria for mild cognitive impairment and dementia

Domain	Mild Cognitive Impairment (Amnestic Type)	Dementia
Type of cognitive decline	Subjective and objective* memory impairment; preservation of other cognitive domains	Memory and at least one other cognitive domain
Social and occupational functioning	Preserved	Impaired
Comparison to individual's baseline	Decline in memory	Decline in cognition and activities of daily living (ADLs)

*At least 1.5 SD below age- and education-based normative data.

Table 1.2. Clinical Dementia Rating (CDR) scores

Score	Diagnostic Category	Cognition/Memory Impairment
0.0	Healthy elderly person	Normal for age
0.5	"Questionable dementia" MCI (Petersen et al. 2001) or "very mild" AD (Morris et al. 2001)	Memory mildly impaired; no other cognitive impairment, or slight impairment in other cognitive domains, instrumental activities of daily living (ADLs), and ADL care
1.0	Mild dementia (meets criteria for dementia)	Memory moderately impaired; mild to moderate disorientation to time or location; moderate impairment of judgment and problem solving, some assistance required with community affairs, functioning at home, and self-care
2.0	Moderate dementia	Severe memory loss with only highly learned material retained; rapid forgetting of new information; severe disorientation to time or place, severe impairment of judgment/problem solving; no independent functioning outside home; severely impaired function in independent ADLs and ADLs
3.0	Severe dementia	Profound memory loss; oriented to person only; unable to engage in independent problem solving; no independent functioning in or outside home; full assistance required for basic ADLs

Cognition and Cognitive Testing

As noted above, the diagnoses of mild cognitive impairment and dementia of the Alzheimer type both require the presence of memory impairment. To distinguish between MCI and DAT, it is important to determine the degree and course of memory impairment, the presence or absence of additional domains of cognitive dysfunction, and the impact of cognitive problems on the individual's daily functioning (for review, see chap. 2; Petersen et al. 1997, 1999; Collie and Maruff 2000; Petersen 2000).

The report of the Quality Standards Subcommittee of the American Academy of Neurology (Knopman et al. 2001) describes methods of assessing cognition for the evaluation of dementia. The subcommittee recommended the use of both screening instruments and neuropsychological evaluations in the diagnostic process. In general, brief screening tests, such as the Mini-Mental State Examination (MMSE; Folstein, Folstein, and McHugh 1975) or the Dementia Rating Scale (Mattis 1988), which assess multiple cognitive domains, have reasonable sensitivity and specificity for the early stages of DAT (Butters, Salmon, and Butters 1994). Some screening tests have a relatively wide range of item difficulty levels and can therefore also be used to track cognitive changes over the years (Butters, Salmon, and Butters 1994). However, very brief measures such as the MMSE have limited sensitivity and range, especially for individuals with a high baseline level of functioning.

Neuropsychological evaluations are highly accurate at discriminating dementia of the Alzheimer type from normal aging (Becker et al. 1994). A comprehensive neuropsychological evaluation of a person with dementia or suspected dementia includes a clinical interview and history of the presenting cognitive problem and related background medical and demographic information. Interview of a reliable informant is an important part of the comprehensive evaluation. A number of cognitive domains are assessed as a standard part of a neuropsychological assessment; those most frequently found to be impaired in persons with DAT are described briefly below. As noted above, in both DAT and MCI, the core deficit is memory impairment out of proportion to that seen in healthy older adults. To distinguish between MCI and mild DAT, examination of other cognitive domains and functional status is crucial.

Memory Impairment

The initial presenting symptom of dementia of the Alzheimer type is usually insidiously progressive memory impairment (Morris 1996; Troster 1998). The memory impairment exhibited in DAT has been the focus of substantial research, as it is the most distinguishing feature of the disease. Specific components of memory (see definitions below) are differentially affected as a function of the stage of DAT. Episodic and semantic memory were originally distinguished by Tulving and Donaldson (1972), and both are impaired early in DAT, with episodic memory perhaps showing the earliest changes. In contrast, other components such as procedural memory may remain relatively unaffected until later in the disease (e.g., Kaszniak 1986; Poon et al. 1986; Shimamura 1989, 1990; Birren and Schaie 1990; Carlesimo and Oscar-Berman 1992).

Episodic Memory

Episodic memory refers to the ability to learn and remember new contextual information. In MCI and DAT, episodic memory is often affected, and can be characterized by failure of consolidation and rapid forgetting. This can be assessed using measures of new verbal and nonverbal learning, for example, learning a list of words (California Verbal Learning Test; Delis et al. 1987) or recalling short stories or geometric designs (Wechsler Memory Scale; Wechsler 1987). Measures of delayed recall and forgetting are highly discriminative for persons with DAT and normal controls, but less discriminative for mild DAT and moderate DAT (Welsh et al. 1991, 1992; Becker, Lopez, and Butters 1996; Gray and Della Sala 1996; Gabrieli 1998).

Semantic Memory and Language

Semantic memory is defined as long-term memory for culturally shared general knowledge about words, concepts and symbols, their associations, and rules for their manipulation (Butters et al. 1987; Farah et al. 1997). It is increasingly apparent that persons with DAT also show deficits in semantic memory. Semantic memory is affected early in the disease course in the majority of cases (Hodges and Patterson 1995). This feature was listed by Alois Alzheimer in 1907 as part of the core cluster of symptoms of DAT. Relevant contemporary studies indicate naming deficits or semantic errors such as word substitutions on picture naming tasks in persons with DAT (Hodges, Salmon, and Butters 1991). Measures of word generation can also be used to assess semantic memory. Persons with DAT perform more poorly when asked to generate words belonging to a particular category than when asked to generate words beginning with a particular letter (Butters et al. 1987; Salmon, Heindel, and Lange 1999); while this is not a pure language measure (e.g., it also assesses the ability to initiate and to retrieve words, which can be considered executive functions), the distinction between poorer ability to generate categorical knowledge versus general word knowledge also supports the notion of a breakdown of, or inability to access, the network of semantic knowledge and meaningful associations (Chertkow and Bubb 1990). Johnson and Hermann (1995) and Saykin et al. (1999) reported deficits in persons with early DAT on category exemplar decision-making tasks such as recognizing that "vehicle-bus" match while "vehicle-carrot" do not.

Attention and Working Memory

Basic attentional capacity is generally spared in dementia of the Alzheimer type until later stages. More complex forms of attention, such as the ability to sustain or direct attention, are impaired earlier in DAT. Recently, impairment of working memory has also been identified as an early problem in DAT (Lange et al. 1995; Belleville, Peretz, and Malenfant 1996; Collette et al. 1997). *Working memory* refers to the ability to hold information in mind, or "on-line," while retrieving or processing other relevant information (Baddeley 1986; Baddeley and Hitch 1994). Impairment in this domain may also contribute to the deficits found in a variety of other cognitive functions, such as speed of information processing and semantic and episodic memory, since attention and working memory are important for encoding, consolidation, and retrieval (Craik and Kester 2000).

Executive Ability

Executive ability refers broadly to a set of behaviors that enable people to engage in goal-directed activities. They include organization and sequencing, planning, mental flexibility, judgment, and abstract reasoning. Many neuropsychological tests of executive abilities tap more than one of these skills. Some of these measures, such as the Wisconsin Card Sorting Test (Heaton et al. 1993), are more complex and are appropriate for assessing subtle changes in MCI or mild DAT. Others assess more basic executive functions and are suitable for the middle stage of the disease. For example, basic measures of judgment such as that included in the Neurobehavioral Cognitive Status Examination (Schwamm et al. 1987) examine the ability to solve everyday problems.

Visuospatial/Constructional and Visuoperceptual Abilities

Visuoperceptual and spatial abilities affect important practical functions, such as recognizing faces or finding one's way around a store or neighborhood. Constructional deficits are evident in drawing, copying, and reproduction of simple figures or designs. Neuropsychological tests of these abilities are frequently timed. Because of the documented slowing of speed of processing with age (Spirduso and MacRae 1990), older participants often perform more poorly than younger subjects on such measures. In individuals with DAT, there are changes in the actual understanding of spatial relations and three-dimensional perception. As the disease progresses, even simple two-dimensional copying or figure matching can become impaired (Moss and Albert 1988).

Praxis

Praxis refers to the ability to carry out skilled intentional movements and can affect everyday functions such as dressing. Apraxia can be tested through observation of single and sequential movements of the mouth, hand, and body. Apraxia typically manifests in middle to later stages of DAT, when the memory and other higher-level cognitive deficits are already apparent.

Other

Tests of instrumental activities of daily living skills are often helpful in differential diagnosis, and deficits have been related to brain structure and function (Souder, Saykin, and Alavi 1995). Further, measures of depression (e.g., Geriatric Depression Scale or Beck Depression Inventory) and vascular involvement (Hachinski 1990) are likely to help with differential diagnosis.

In summary, as noted above, many screening instruments are available for the initial assessment of cognitive impairment associated with mild cognitive impairment and early dementia of the Alzheimer type that clinicians can use in their office. Among the most commonly used are the Mental Status Questionnaire (Kahn et al. 1960), the Memory-Information-Concentration Test (Blessed, Tomlinson, and Roth 1968), the Short Portable Mental Status Questionnaire

(Fillenbaum, Landerman, and Simonsick 1998; Pfeiffer 1975), and the MMSE (Folstein, Folstein, and McHugh 1975). Even when individuals perform normally on these tests, comprehensive neuropsychological evaluation may be indicated to rule out more subtle cognitive changes, especially in those persons with subjective and informant-endorsed complaints, and in those individuals with presumed very high premorbid (or baseline) intelligence.

Neuroanatomy

The mean brain weight of normal young adult males varies from approximately 1300 to 1380 grams (Duckett 1991). With normal aging, the average brain weighs 7–8% less than the average brain of a middle-aged adult (Tomlinson 1977; Lauter 1985); however, there is considerable variability among individuals that may be due to the fact that "normal" study populations are not always rigorously screened for medical conditions that might also impact on the brain. Normal aging is associated with subtle changes in brain structure, including generally mild cortical atrophy and ventricular enlargement. Region-specific studies show greater neuronal decreases in some areas, including the superior frontal and temporal gyrus, precentral gyrus, visual cortex, locus ceruleus, substantia nigra, basal nucleus of Meynert, and cerebellar Purkinje cells (Lauter 1985).

In primary degenerative dementia, the decrease in brain weight is as much as 10% more than that seen in normal aging (Terry and Davies 1983). As in normal aging, atrophy and eventual cell loss is region-specific in DAT. Brains from persons with DAT demonstrate greater neuronal loss in frontal and temporal regions (Mountjoy et al. 1983). Subcortical nuclei including the locus ceruleus and basal nucleus of Meynert also show greater cell loss in DAT, but this may be more typical in those with a younger age of onset (Iversen 1987). The dominant theory of DAT has been related to loss of cholinergic cells, but recent findings of upregulation of choline acetyltransferase activity in MCI and mild DAT may extend this model to include compensatory changes (DeKosky et al. 2002). The pathology of DAT includes neurofibrillary tangles, senile plaques, and synaptic loss, as well as more pronounced cortical atrophy appearing as sulcal and ventricular enlargement disproportionate to age. Structural brain changes have been reported not only early in the disease, but also in persons with MCI. Medial temporal structures, including the hippocampus and entorhinal cortex, are particularly vulnerable in the earliest stages of DAT.

Structural Imaging

An important advance in the evaluation of people with suspected dementia of the Alzheimer type is the use of structural imaging to assess in vivo neuroanatomical changes. This technique can also be used in conjunction with neuropsychological test data to better understand the relationship between the structural brain changes and the cognitive deficits that characterize the disease.

Hippocampus

Integrity of the hippocampus has been strongly implicated in episodic memory (Squire 1992). Magnetic resonance imaging studies indicate substantial hippocampal atrophy in DAT, even in the very early stages of the disease (Jack et al. 1992; Scheltens et al. 1992; Killiany et al. 1993; Laakso et al. 1995; Johnson et al. 1998). In contrast, the hippocampus is spared significant aging effects through the seventh decade of life in healthy normals (Bigler et al. 1997). Studies of hippocampal atrophy in patients and healthy controls have reported age-related volume changes (i.e., greater volume loss with increased age) only in healthy controls. In contrast, in persons with MCI and DAT, volume reductions were not related to age (de Leon et al. 1997; de Toledo-Morrell et al. 1997). Although minimal longitudinal data are available, Jack, Petersen, and Xu (1998, 2000) reported significant annual decline in hippocampal volume in healthy older adults; persons with MCI showed somewhat greater rates of decline, while persons with DAT showed the greatest decline. Furthermore, within the control and MCI groups, clinical decline was related to greater rates of hippocampal atrophy.

Several studies have examined the relationship between hippocampal volume and cognitive functioning. For example, de Leon et al. (1997) found that after controlling for age, education, and immediate memory, a significant correlation was found between delayed memory and hippocampal atrophy in normal controls, but not in individuals with MCI (subjects with DAT were too impaired to be studied). In contrast, Convit et al. (1997) reported a relationship between delayed memory function and hippocampal volume in both healthy controls and persons with MCI. This may reflect the degree of impairment in the population with MCI in the de Leon study, since these relations become harder to detect as cognitive impairment becomes more severe. General cognitive measures such as the MMSE did not distinguish between normal controls and participants with MCI, and had no relationship to hippocampal volume. This lack of association has also been reported in persons with DAT (de Toledo-Morrell et al. 1997). Wilson et al. (1996) reported that hippocampal formation volume was associated with a delayed recall measure, but not with immediate recall, and with an object-naming test in persons with DAT. Medial temporal region volumes have been found to be correlated with delayed memory performance in persons with DAT (Kohler et al. 1998) and in elderly individuals without dementia (Golomb et al. 1994; Convit et al. 1997).

Entorhinal Cortex

Recent evidence strongly suggests that one of the earliest changes in dementia of the Alzheimer type is neurofibrillary tangles in the entorhinal cortex (Braak, Braak, and Bohl 1993). Measurement of the entorhinal cortex may provide a useful marker for early diagnosis (Bobinski et al. 1999). MRI studies show significant reductions of entorhinal cortex volume in DAT (Pearlson et al. 1992; Desmond et al. 1994; Juottonen et al. 1998; Krasuski et al. 1998). Entorhinal cortex volume is reduced even in persons with MCI compared to controls on MRI (Xu et al. 2000) and postmortem evaluation (Kordower et al. 2001). Baseline volumes of the entorhinal cortex predict conversion from MCI to DAT (Fox et al. 1996; Jack et al. 1999; Killiany et al. 2000). Juottonen et al. (1998) reported a significant correlation between left entorhinal cortex volume (corrected for whole brain size) and MMSE scores in persons with DAT.

Other Structural Changes

Other investigators have demonstrated the importance of measuring whole brain volume (Fox and Rossor 1999; Fox, Warrington, and Rossor 1999) to differentiate dementia of the Alzheimer type from healthy controls. White matter lesions (Barber et al. 1999; Wolf et al. 2000; DeCarli et al. 2001; Farkas and Luiten 2001) and metabolite changes (for review, Valenzuela and Sachdev 2001) may also be helpful for distinguishing between healthy controls and individuals with MCI and DAT. These measures may prove to be useful early indicators of conversion from MCI to DAT.

In summary, quantitative structural neuroimaging has revealed prominent and progressive cortical atrophy in dementia of the Alzheimer type starting in the earliest stages of the disease, with particular involvement of mesial temporal structures including entorhinal cortex and hippocampus observed even in mild cognitive impairment. In clinical practice, detailed evaluation of MRI findings in very mild cases may be of particular interest for early diagnosis (Soininen et al. 1994; Parnetti et al. 1996; Convit et al. 1997, 2000; de Toledo-Morrell et al. 1997; Jack et al. 1997). A promising new direction in structural neuroimaging of MCI and DAT is voxel-based morphometry (Ashburner and Friston 2000; Chung et al. 2001), a technique involving analysis of white matter, and cerebrospinal fluid tissue compartments on a voxel-by-voxel basis. Voxel-based morphometry may increase the clinical applicability of volumetric assessment in the early detection of at-risk individuals and those with early stages of dementia. Other promising techniques include functional neuroimaging methods.

Functional Imaging

Functional imaging methods used in research on aging, mild cognitive impairment, and dementia of the Alzheimer type include single-photon emission computed tomography (SPECT), positron emission tomography (PET), and functional magnetic resonance imaging (fMRI). Positron emission tomography and single-photon emission computed tomography use radioisotope tracers to detect brain metabolism or blood flow. Functional magnetic resonance imaging is a method that indicates regions of activation by detecting changes in blood oxygenation in capillaries. Normally, brain metabolism, blood flow, and neuronal activity are tightly coupled. The extent to which this relationship is altered in normal aging and DAT requires further investigation (D'Esposito et al. 1997; Ross et al. 1997; Johnson et al. 2001).

Functional imaging research involves several types of study design. Resting state studies examine metabolism or activity in various regions of the brain without engaging the participants in a particular activity or cognitive task. Other studies correlate resting state activation with neuropsychological status on tests completed outside of the scanner. Finally, activation studies examine patterns of brain activity associated with cognitive activities in which the participant engages during scanning.

Resting State Single-photon Emission Computed Tomography and Postitron Emission Tomography Studies

Numerous resting state positron emission tomography studies of regional cerebral metabolic rates for glucose and oxygen indicate hypometabolism in all association cortices in dementia of the Alzheimer type, with temporoparietal regions generally most affected early in the disease (Herholz 1995; Pietrini et al. 2000; Coleman 2001). Bilateral hippocampal hypometabolism has also been reported in some (Perani et al. 1993) but not all (Ishii et al. 1998) studies. By contrast, primary sensory and motor areas and subcortical gray matter show relative metabolic preservation (Herholz 1995; Pietrini et al. 2000). Even in persons with early stages of DAT or with MCI, a similar pattern of hypometabolic regions has been demonstrated (Haxby et al. 1990; see Almkvist and Winblad 1999 for review). Using PET, DeSanti and colleagues (2001) showed metabolic reductions in both MCI and DAT relative to healthy age-matched controls. Metabolic reductions in the hippocampus and anterior parahippocampal gyrus discriminated persons with MCI from controls, whereas more widespread reductions in temporal regions of interest discriminated persons with DAT from those with MCI.

The general pattern of affected brain regions on positron emission tomography remains relatively stable over time. The degree of hypometabolism is modestly correlated with disease severity (Parks, Haxby, and Grady 1993). Herholz and colleagues (1999) showed a relation between the degree of glucose hypometabolism at baseline and subsequent progression in DAT. In persons with mild cognitive deficits at study entry, the presence of severely impaired metabolism predicted a 4.7 times greater rate of progression relative to individuals whose metabolism was intact or only mildly impaired.

Significant relations have been demonstrated between the metabolic reductions in association cortex and neuropsychological impairment (Parks, Haxby, and Grady 1993). Using SPECT, Grossman et al. (1997) showed a relation between semantic memory and reduced perfusion in the left inferior parietal and superior temporal regions. PET studies have demonstrated patterns of cerebral glucose metabolism consistent with expected brain-behavior relations in DAT; for example, individuals with predominantly left hemispheric hypometabolism of association cortices showed greater verbal than visuospatial impairment (Grady et al. 1990). A recent advance is the use of special PET radioligand binding techniques to detect the level of cholinesterase activity in dementia of the Alzheimer type (Kuhl et al. 1999).

Functional Activation Studies

Functional activation studies examine patterns of brain activation that occur during task performance. There are very few functional activation studies of memory in DAT or MCI, and they are mainly limited to the milder end of the disease spectrum. One hypothesis that has been addressed in some PET activation studies posits a shift in activation from expected foci to a more widespread cortical distribution during cognitive task performance in persons with DAT compared to healthy controls (e.g., Becker et al. 1996; Woodard et al. 1998). This may reflect compensatory recruitment of remaining neural resources; however, studies to date have not ruled out loss of inhibitory neural processing leading to abnormally widespread activation (Saykin et al. 1999).

Several studies have shown abnormalities of mesial temporal activation on functional magnetic resonance imaging in persons with dementia of the Alzheimer type performing episodic memory encoding tasks (e.g., Rombouts et al. 2000). Small et al. (1999) reported diminished mesial temporal lobe activation in persons with DAT relative to controls. They also examined a group of older adults with isolated memory impairment; these individuals showed activation patterns that were either similar to those of persons with DAT, or that involved isolated hypoactivation of the subiculum. Kato, Knopman, and Liu (2001) compared fMRI activation patterns for patients with mild DAT and young and old controls; all participants activated visual cortex, but DAT patients failed to activate entorhinal, other temporal, and frontal regions.

Saykin et al. (1999) employed functional magnetic resonance imaging to study semantic and episodic memory processing in a sample of patients with mild dementia of the Alzheimer type. During semantic memory tasks, both patients and controls activated inferior frontal regions, particularly of the left hemisphere. The spatial extent of activation was increased in the group with DAT. Additional right frontal activation was observed in the patients with mild DAT. During an episodic memory (recognition) task, there was an absence of prefrontal activation in persons with DAT compared to controls, with greater activation in the medial temporal region than in controls. Together, these findings suggest that brain activation is not simply diminished as a function of DAT, but may also increase, and that spatial shifts in activation can occur. In fact, increased activation in inferior frontal brain regions subserving semantic memory that were directly related to the extent of local atrophy in persons with DAT have been reported (Johnson et al. 2000). Therefore, alterations in activation may be adaptive as a compensatory mechanism, a possibility that deserves further investigation using functional neuroimaging methods. In another study, Saykin et al. (2000) correlated structure and function, and found that degree of hippocampal atrophy predicted frontal lobe activation during episodic memory.

Analyses of functional connectivity provide a new means of analyzing functional magnetic resonance imaging or positron emission tomography data to examine disruption in normal patterns of coactivation of brain regions within a functional circuitry (Friston et al. 1993). Antuono, Li, and Jones (2000) reported preliminary evidence of disrupted functional connectivity within the hippocampus of individuals with DAT. The degree of disruption of functional connectivity was greater than that in healthy controls, while persons with MCI had an intermediate level.

Event-related functional magnetic resonance imaging, a relatively new technique, permits comparison of brain activation patterns for each individual during successful performance of a task compared to unsuccessful performance (Brewer et al. 1998; Wagner et al. 1998). Using an event-related analysis of successful and unsuccessful performance, we found that healthy controls showed greater right medial temporal activation when listening to items they would later correctly recognize compared to items they did not remember (Saykin, et al. 1999). By contrast, persons with DAT failed to show the same degree of differential activity in this area.

A small number of studies have shown functional magnetic resonance imaging alterations in individuals at risk for dementia of the Alzheimer type. For example, Smith et al. (1999) showed diminished temporal fMRI activation during language tasks in individuals at risk for DAT. Similarly, Bookheimer et al. (2000) reported changes on fMRI in individuals at genetic risk for DAT.

In summary, resting state studies reveal lowered metabolism in association cortices, particularly in the temporoparietal region. Studies employing cognitive challenges during scanning have provided a complex pattern of findings, involving not only reduced activation, but also enlarged and shifted areas of activation in patients relative to controls. Whether the more widespread activation is due to a compensatory mechanism, a loss of inhibitory neural processing, or some other as yet unidentified process remains unanswered. Both structural and functional neuroimaging have provided rich insights into the neuroanatomic and neurophysiological changes in the brain in MCI and DAT. Future research integrating analyses of brain structure, brain activation patterns, and cognitive performance is likely to further illuminate brain-behavior relations (see chap. 2) and mechanisms of impairment and compensation in MCI and DAT.

Clinical Conclusions

Using an evidence-based review of the literature, the Quality Standards Subcommittee of the American Academy of Neurology made three levels of recommendation for clinical practice related to the diagnosis and evaluation of individuals with mild cognitive impairment and dementia (Knopman et al. 2001; Petersen et al. 2001): *standards* were based on patient management strategies reflecting the highest degree of clinical and empirical certainty; *guidelines* reflected moderate certainty; and *options* were noted when evidence of clinical utility was minimal or inconclusive.

Even as recently as 1994, when the American Academy of Neurology published the prior practice guidelines, issues of early detection were not addressed. In the current review (Petersen et al. 2001), discussions of early detection and the boundary between normal aging and dementia were prominent. The legitimacy of MCI and related diagnostic entities as a point in the transition from normal aging to dementia is supported by the members of the committee. The committee (Petersen et al. 2001) recommended as guidelines that clinicians evaluate and monitor individuals with mild cognitive impairment for early identification and intervention, by using both screening instruments and neuropsychological evaluation as appropriate.

The report from the Quality Standards Subcommittee (Knopman et al. 2001), reviewing procedures for the evaluation of dementia, supported both the DSM and National Institute of Neurologic and Communicative Disorders and Stroke—Alzheimer's Disease and Related Disorders Association criteria as reliable and valid for the diagnosis of Alzheimer dementia (guideline). Consensus panels differ with regard to the utility of neuroimaging as standard practice in the evaluation of dementia (e.g., in the primary care setting—Patterson et al. 2001, see chap. 3—versus the specialty setting—Knopman et al. 2001).

Cognitive and neuroanatomic changes occur as part of the aging process. These changes can clearly be distinguished from those associated with moderate to severe dementia. What is less clear is the boundary between the detectable changes of normal aging and the corresponding changes in MCI and early dementia. Recent recognition of MCI as a diagnostic entity has helped to clarify an early stage in the transition from normal aging to dementia. Given recent and emerging treatments for memory disorders, early detection of MCI and DAT will be increasingly important. A comprehensive clinical evaluation that includes standardized cognitive assessment and structural neuroimaging techniques, when indicated, is currently recommended as standard practice. There is an emerging consensus that cholinesterase inhibitors and, possibly, vitamin E should be considered for the treatment of DAT and may help individuals with MCI, particularly those who show evidence of decline on serial assessment. The results of ongoing clinical trials should clarify prospects for early intervention in the near future.

ACKNOWLEDGMENTS

The authors would like to thank the following people for their contributions: Kathleen Baynes, Denette Babcock, Leslie Baxter, Cheryl Brown, Matt Beyea, Sterling Johnson, and Jennifer Stone Ramirez. We thank the Alzheimer's Association (IIRG-99-1653), the National Institutes of Aging (AG 19771-01), and the Ira DeCamp Foundation for support of our research in this area.

REFERENCES

Albert, M.S. 1988. General issues in geriatric neuropsychology. In *Geriatric Neuropsychology*, edited by M.S. Albert and M.B. Moss. New York: Guilford Press.

Almkvist, O., and B. Winblad. 1999. Early diagnosis of Alzheimer dementia based on clinical and biological factors. *European Archives of Psychiatry and Clinical Neuroscience* 249 (Suppl. 3):S3–9.

American Psychiatric Association. 1994. *Diagnostic and Statistical Manual of Mental Disorders*. 4th ed. Washington, D.C.: American Psychiatric Association.

Antuono, P., S.-J. Li, and J. Jones. 2000. A functional MRI index as a biological marker for Alzheimer's disease. Paper read at American Academy of Neurology.

Ashburner, J., and K.F. Friston. 2000. Voxel-based morphometry: The methods. *NeuroImage* 11:805–21.

Baddeley, A.D. 1986. *Working Memory*. Oxford: Clarendon Press.

Baddeley, A.D., and G.J. Hitch. 1994. Developments in the concept of working memory. *Neuropsychology* 8:485–93.

Baltes, P.B. 1993. The aging mind: Potential and limits. *Gerontologist* 33:580–94.

Baltes, P.B., and M.M. Baltes. 1990. Psychological perspectives on successful aging: The model of selective optimization with compensation. In *Successful Aging: Perspectives from the Behavioral Sciences*, edited by P.B. Baltes and M.M. Baltes. Cambridge: Cambridge University Press.

Barber, R., P. Scheltens, A. Gholkar, et al. 1999. White matter lesions on magnetic resonance imaging in dementia with Lewy bodies, Alzheimer's disease, vascular dementia, and normal aging. *Journal of Neurology, Neurosurgery, and Psychiatry* 67:66–72.

Becker, J.T., F. Boller, O.L. Lopez, et al. 1994. The natural history of Alzheimer's disease: Description of study cohort and accuracy of diagnosis. *Archives of Neurology* 51:585–94.

Becker, J.T., O.L. Lopez, and M.A. Butters. 1996. Episodic memory: Differential patterns of breakdown. In *The Cognitive Neuropsychology of Alzheimer-type Dementia*, edited by R.G. Morris. New York: Oxford University Press.

Becker, J.T., M.A. Mintun, K. Aleva, et al. 1996. Compensatory reallocation of brain resources supporting verbal episodic memory in Alzheimer's disease. *Neurology* 46 (3): 692–700.
Belleville, S., I. Peretz, and D. Malenfant. 1996. Examination of the working memory components in normal aging and in dementia of the Alzheimer type. *Neuropsychologia* 34 (3):195–207.
Berg, L. 1988. Clinical Dementia Rating (CDR). *Psychopharmacology Bulletin* 24:637–39.
Bigler, E.D., D.D. Blatter, C.V. Anderson, et al. 1997. Hippocampal volume in normal aging and traumatic brain injury. *American Journal of Neuroradiology* 18:11–23.
Birren, J.E. 1965. Age changes in speed of behavior: Its central nature and physiological correlates. In *Behavior, Aging, and the Nervous System*, edited by A. Welford and J.E. Birren. Springfield, Ill.: Charles Thomas, pp. 191–216.
Birren, J.E., and K.W. Schaie. 1990. *Handbook of the Psychology of Aging*, 3rd ed. San Diego: Academic Press.
Birren, J.E., A. Woods, and M.V. Williams. 1980. Behavioral slowing with age: Causes, organization, and consequences. In *Aging in the 1980s*, edited by L. Poon. Washington, D.C.: American Psychological Association, pp. 293–308.
Blessed, G., B.E. Tomlinson, and M. Roth. 1968. The associations between quantitative measures of dementia and of senile change in the cerebral grey matter of elderly subjects. *British Journal of Psychiatry* 114:797–811.
Bobinski, M., M.J. de Leon, A. Convit, et al. 1999. MRI of entorhinal cortex in mild Alzheimer's disease [letter]. *Lancet* 353 (9146):38–40.
Bookheimer, S.Y., M.H. Strojwas, M.S. Cohen, et al. 2000. Patterns of brain activation in people at risk for Alzheimer's disease. *New England Journal of Medicine* 343 (7): 450–60.
Bowen, J., L. Teri, W. Kukull, et al. 1997. Progression to dementia in patients with isolated memory loss. *Lancet* 349 (9054):763–65.
Braak, H., E. Braak, and J. Bohl. 1993. Staging of Alzheimer-related cortical destruction. *European Neurology* 33 (6):403–8.
Brewer, J.B., Z. Zhao, J.E. Desmond, et al. 1998. Making memories: Brain activity that predicts how well visual experience will be remembered. *Science* 281 (5380):1185–87.
Butters, M.A., D.P. Salmon, and N. Butters. 1994. Neuropsychological assessment of dementia. In *Neuropsychological Assessment of Dementia and Depression.*, edited by M. Storandt and G.R. VandenBos. Washington, D.C.: American Psychological Association.
Butters, N., E.L. Granholm, D.P. Salmon, et al. 1987. Episodic and semantic memory: A comparison of amnestic and demented patients. *Journal of Clinical and Experimental Neuropsychology* 9:479–97.
Carlesimo, G.A., and M. Oscar-Berman. 1992. Memory deficits in Alzheimer's patients: A comprehensive review. *Neuropsychology Review* 3 (2):119–69.
Celsis, P. 2000. Age-related cognitive decline, mild cognitive impairment or preclinical Alzheimer's disease? *Annals of Medicine* 32 (1):6–14.
Chen, P., G. Ratcliff, S.H. Belle, et al. 2001. Patterns of cognitive decline in presymptomatic Alzheimer's disease: A prospective community study. *Archives of General Psychiatry* 58:853–58.
Chertkow, H., and D. Bubb. 1990. Semantic memory loss in dementia of the Alzheimer type: What do various measures measure? *Brain* 113:397–417.

Chung, M.K., K.J. Worsley, T. Paus, et al. 2001. A unified statistical approach to deformation-based morphometry. *NeuroImage* 14:595–606.

Coleman, R.E. 2001. Positron emission tomography in the evaluation of dementia. Paper read at 48th Annual Meeting of the Society of Nuclear Medicine, http://psychiatry.medscape.com/Medscape/CNO/2001/SNM/Story.csm?story_id=2441.

Collette, F., E. Salmon, M. Van Der Linden, et al. 1997. Functional anatomy of verbal and visuospatial span tasks in Alzheimer's disease. *Human Brain Mapping* 5 (2):110–18.

Collie, A., and P. Maruff. 2000. The neuropsychology of preclinical Alzheimer's disease and mild cognitive impairment. *Neuroscience and Biobehavioral Reviews* 24 (3):365.

Collie, A., P. Maruff, R. Shafiq-Antonaci, et al. 2001. Memory decline in healthy older people: Implications for identifying mild cognitive impairment. *Neurology* 56:1533–38.

Convit, A., M.J. De Leon, C. Tarshish, et al. 1997. Specific hippocampal volume reductions in individuals at risk for Alzheimer's disease. *Neurobiology of Aging* 18 (2): 131–38.

Convit, A., J. de Asis, M.J. de Leon, et al. 2000. Atrophy of the medial occipitotemporal, inferior, and middle temporal gyri in non-demented elderly predict decline to Alzheimer's disease. *Neurobiology of Aging* 21 (1):19–26.

Craik, F.I.M., and J.D. Kester. 2000. Divided attention and memory: Impairment of processing or consolidation? In *Memory, Consciousness, and the Brain*, edited by E. Tulving. Philadelphia: Psychology Press.

Crook, T., R.T. Bartus, S.H. Ferris, et al. 1986. Age-associated memory impairment: Proposed diagnostic criteria and measures of clinical change: Report of a National Institute of Mental Health work group. *Developmental Neuropsychology* 2:261–76.

DeCarli, C., B.L. Miller, G.E. Swan, et al. 2001. Cerebrovascular and brain morphologic correlates of mild cognitive impairment in the National Heart, Lung, and Blood Institute Twin Study. *Archives of Neurology* 58 (4):643–47.

DeKosky, S.T., M.D. Ikonomovic, S.D. Styren, et al. 2002. Upregulation of choline acetyltransferase activity in hippocampus and frontal cortex of elderly subjects with mild cognitive impairment. *Annals of Neurology* 51:145–55.

de Leon, M.J., A.E. George, J. Golomb, et al. 1997. Frequency of hippocampal formation atrophy in normal aging and Alzheimer's disease. *Neurobiology of Aging* 18 (1):1–11.

Delis, D.C., J.H. Kramer, E. Kaplan, et al. 1987. *California Verbal Learning Test: Adult Version Manual.* San Antonio: Psychological Corporation.

DeSanti, S., M.J. deLeon, H. Rusinek, et al. 2001. Hippocampal formation glucose metabolism and volume losses in MCI and AD. *Neurobiology of Aging* 22:529–39.

Desmond, P.M., J.T. O'Brien, B.M. Tress, D.J. Ames, et al. 1994. Volumetric and visual assessment of the mesial temporal structures in Alzheimer's disease. *Australia and New Zealand Journal of Medicine* 24 (5):547–53.

D'Esposito, M., E. Zarahn, G.K. Aguirre, et al. 1997. The effect of pacing of experimental stimuli on observed functional MRI activity. *NeuroImage* 6 (2):113–21.

de Toledo-Morrell, L., M.P. Sullivan, F. Morrell, et al. 1997. Alzheimer's disease: In vivo detection of differential vulnerability of brain regions. *Neurobiology of Aging* 18 (5):463–68.

Devanand, D.P., M. Folz, M. Gorlyn, et al. 1997. Questionable dementia: Clinical course and predictors of outcome. *Journal of the American Geriatrics Society* 45:321–28.

Duckett, S. 1991. The normal aging human brain. In *The Pathology of the Aging Human Nervous System*, edited by S. Duckett. Philadelphia: Lea & Febiger.

Emery, V.O.B. 1985. Language and aging. *Experimental Aging Research Monographs* 11 (1):71–89.

Farah, M.J., M. D'Esposito, G.K. Aguirre, and S.L. Thompson Schill. 1997. Bold fMRI signal in left prefrontal cortex depends on specificity of semantic retrieval. *27th Annual Meeting of the Society for Neuroscience*, Part 23 (1–2):1054.

Farkas, E., and P.G. Luiten. 2001. Cerebral microvascular pathology in aging and Alzheimer's disease. *Progress in Neurobiology* 64 (6):575–611.

Fillenbaum, G.G., L.R. Landerman, and E.M. Simonsick. 1998. Equivalence of two screens of cognitive functioning: The Short Portable Mental Status Questionnaire and the Orientation-Memory-Concentration test. *Journal of the American Geriatrics Society* 46 (12):1512–18.

Flicker, C., S.H. Ferris, and B. Reisberg. 1991. Mild cognitive impairment in the elderly: Predictors of dementia. *Neurology* 41 (7):1006–9.

Folstein, M.F., S.E. Folstein, and P.R. McHugh. 1975. "Mini-Mental State": A practical method for grading the cognitive state of patients for the clinician. *Journal of Psychiatry Research* 12:189–98.

Fox, N.C., and M.N. Rossor. 1999. Diagnosis of early Alzheimer's disease. *Revue Neurologique (Paris)* 155 (Suppl 4):S33–37.

Fox, N.C., E.K. Warrington, and M.N. Rossor. 1999. Serial magnetic resonance imaging of cerebral atrophy in preclinical Alzheimer's disease [letter]. *Lancet* 353: 2125.

Fox, N.C., E.K. Warrington, J.M. Stevens, et al. 1996. Atrophy of the hippocampal formation in early familial Alzheimer's disease: A longitudinal MRI study of at-risk members of a family with an amyloid precursor protein 717Val-Gly mutation. *Annals of the New York Academy of Science* 777:226–32.

Friston, K.J., C.D. Frith, P.F. Liddle, et al. 1993. Functional connectivity: The principal-component analysis of large (PET) data sets. *Journal of Cerebral Blood Flow and Metabolism* 13 (1):5–14.

Gabrieli, J.D. 1998. Cognitive neuroscience of human memory [review]. *Annual Review of Psychology* 49:87–115.

Golomb, J., A. Kluger, M.J. deLeon, et al. 1994. Hippocampal formation size in normal human aging: A correlate of delayed secondary memory performance. *Learning and Memory* 1:45–54.

Grady, C.L., J.V. Haxby, M.B. Schapiro, et al. 1990. Subgroups in dementia of the Alzheimer type identified using positron emission tomography. *Journal of Neuropsychiatry and Clinical Neuroscience* 2 (4):373–84.

Gray, C., and S. Della Sala. 1996. Charting decline in dementia. In *The Cognitive Neuropsychology of Alzheimer-type Dementia*, edited by R. Morris. Oxford: Oxford University Press.

Grossman, M., F. Payer, K. Onishi, et al. 1997. Constraints on the cerebral basis for semantic processing from neuroimaging studies of Alzheimer's disease. *Journal of Neurology, Neurosurgery and Psychiatry* 63 (2):152–58.

Hachinski, V.C. 1990. The decline and resurgence of vascular dementia. *Canadian Medical Association Journal* 142 (2):107–11.

Haxby, J.V., C.L. Grady, E. Koss, et al. 1990. Longitudinal study of cerebral metabolic asymmetries and associated neuropsychological patterns in early dementia of the Alzheimer type. *Archives of Neurology* 47 (7):753–60.

Heaton, R.K., G.J. Chelune, J.L. Talley, et al. 1993. *Wisconsin Card Sorting Test Manual Revised and Expanded.* Odessa, Fla.: Psychological Assessment Resources.

Herholz, K. 1995. FDG PET and differential diagnosis of dementia. *Alzheimer Disease and Associated Disorders* 9 (1):6–16.

Herholz, K., A. Nordberg, E. Salmon, et al. 1999. Impairment of neocortical metabolism predicts progression in Alzheimer's disease. *Dementia and Geriatric Cognitive Disorders* 10:494–504.

Hickman, S.E., D.B. Howieson, A. Dame, et al. 2000. Longitudinal analysis of the effects of the aging process on neuropsychological test performance in the healthy young-old and oldest-old. *Developmental Neuropsychology* 17 (3):323–37.

Hodges, J.R., and K. Patterson. 1995. Is semantic memory consistently impaired early in the course of Alzheimer's disease? Neuroanatomical and diagnostic implications. *Neuropsychologia* 33 (4):441–59.

Hodges, J.R., D.P. Salmon, and N. Butters. 1991. The nature of the naming deficit in Alzheimer's and Huntington's disease. *Brain* 114 (Pt. 4):1547–58.

Horner, P.H., and F.H. Gage. 2000. Regenerating the damaged central nervous system. *Nature* 407:963–70.

Ishii, K., M. Sasaki, S. Yamaji, et al. 1998. Relatively preserved hippocampal glucose metabolism in mild Alzheimer's disease. *Dementia and Geriatric Cognitive Disorders* 9 (6): 317–22.

Iversen, L.L. 1987. Differences between early and late-onset Alzheimer's disease. *Neurobiology of Aging* 8:554–55.

Jack, C.R., Jr., R.C. Petersen, P.C. O' Brien, et al. 1992. MR-based hippocampal volumetry in the diagnosis of Alzheimer's disease. *Neurology* 42 (1):183–88.

Jack, C.R., Jr., R.C. Petersen, Y.C. Xu, et al. 1997. Medial temporal atrophy on MRI in normal aging and very mild Alzheimer's disease. *Neurology* 49 (3):786–94.

Jack, C.R., Jr., R.C. Petersen, Y. Xu, et al. 1998. Rate of medial temporal lobe atrophy in typical aging and Alzheimer's disease. *Neurology* 51 (4):993–99.

Jack, C.R., R.C. Petersen, Y.C. Xu, et al. 1999. Prediction of AD with MRI-based hippocampal volume in mild cognitive impairment. *Neurology* 52:1397–1403.

Jack, C.R., Jr., R.C. Petersen, Y. Xu, et al. 2000. Rates of hippocampal atrophy correlate with change in clinical status in aging and AD. *Neurology* 55 (4):484–89.

Johnson, M.K., and A.M. Hermann. 1995. Semantic relations and Alzheimer's disease: An early and disproportionate deficit in functional knowledge. *Journal of the International Neuropsychological Society* 1 (6):568–74.

Johnson, S.C., A.J. Saykin, L.A. Flashman, et al. 1998. Reduction of hippocampal formation in Alzheimer's disease and correlation with memory: A meta-analysis. *Journal of the International Neuropsychological Society* 4:22.

Johnson, S.C., A.J. Saykin, L.C. Baxter, et al. 2000. The relationship between fMRI activation and cerebral atrophy: Comparison of normal aging and Alzheimer disease. *NeuroImage* 11 (3):179–87.

Johnson, S.C., A.J. Saykin, L.A. Flashman, et al. 2001. Similarities and differences in semantic and phonological processing with age: Patterns of functional MRI activation. *Aging, Neuropsychology, and Cognition* 8 (4):307–30.

Jonker, C., M.I. Geerlings, and B. Schmand. 2000. Are memory complaints predictive for dementia?: A review of clinical and population-based studies. *International Journal of Geriatric Psychiatry* 15 (11):983–91.

Juottonen, K., M.P. Laakso, R. Insausti, et al. 1998. Volumes of the entorhinal and perirhinal cortices in Alzheimer's disease. *Neurobiology of Aging* 19 (1):15–22.

Juottonen, K., M.P. Laakso, K. Partanen, et al. 1999. Comparative MR analysis of the entorhinal cortex and hippocampus in diagnosing Alzheimer disease. *American Society of Neuroradiology* 20:139–44.

Kahn, R.L., A.E. Goldfarb, M. Pollock, et al. 1960. Brief objective measures for the determination of mental status in the elderly. *American Journal of Psychiatry* 117:326–28.

Kaszniak, A.W. 1986. The neuropsychology of dementia. In *Neuropsychological Assessment of Neuropsychiatric Disorders*, edited by I. Grant and K. Adams. New York: Oxford University Press.

Kato, T., D. Knopman, and H. Liu. 2001. Dissociation of regional activation in mild AD during visual encoding: A functional MRI study. *Neurology* 57:812–16.

Kempermann, G., and F.H. Gage. 1999. New nerve cells for the adult brain. *Scientific American* 280:48–53.

Killiany, R.J., M.B. Moss, M.S. Albert, et al. 1993. Temporal lobe regions on magnetic resonance imaging identify patients with early Alzheimer's disease. *Archives of Neurology* 50 (9):949–54.

Killiany, R.J., T. Gomez-Isla, M. Moss, et al. 2000. Use of structural magnetic resonance imaging to predict who will get Alzheimer's disease. *Annals of Neurology* 47:430–39.

Knopman, D.S., S.T. DeKosky, J.L. Cummings, et al. 2001. Practice parameter: Diagnosis of Dementia (an evidence-based review). Report of the Quality Standards Committee of the American Academy of Neurology. *Neurology* 56:1143–53.

Kohler, S., A.R. McIntosh, M. Moscovitch, et al. 1998. Functional interactions between the medial temporal lobes and posterior neocortex related to episodic memory retrieval. *Cerebral Cortex* 8 (5):451–61.

Kordower, J.H., Y. Chu, G.T. Stebbins, et al. 2001. Loss and atrophy of layer II entorhinal cortex neurons in elderly people with mild cognitive impairment. *Annals of Neurology* 49 (2):202–13.

Kral, V.A. 1958. Neuro-psychiatric observations in an old peoples home. *Journal of Gerontology* 13:169–76.

Kral, V.A. 1962. Senescent forgetfulness: Benign and malignant. *Canadian Medical Association Journal* 86:257–60.

Krasuski, J.S., G.E. Alexander, B. Horwitz, et al. 1998. Volumes of medial temporal lobe structures in patients with Alzheimer's disease and mild cognitive impairment (and in healthy controls). *Biological Psychiatry* 43 (1):60–68.

Kuhl, D.E., R.A. Koeppe, S. Minoshima, et al. 1999. In vivo mapping of cerebral acetylcholinesterase activity in aging and Alzheimer's disease. *Neurology* 52:691–99.

Laakso, M.P., H. Soininen, K. Partanen, et al. 1995. Volumes of hippocampus, amygdala and frontal lobes in the MRI-based diagnosis of early Alzheimer's disease: correlation with memory functions. *Journal of Neural Transmission, Parkinson Disease and Dementia Section* 9 (1):73–86.

Lange, K.W., B.J. Sahakian, N.P. Quinn, et al. 1995. Comparison of executive and visuospatial memory function in Huntington's disease and dementia of Alzheimer type matched for degree of dementia. *Journal of Neurology, Neurosurgery, and Psychiatry* 58 (5):598–606.

Lauter, H. 1985. What do we know about Alzheimer's disease today? *Danish Medical Bulletin* 32 (Suppl. 1):S1–21.

Levy, R. 1994. Aging-associated cognitive decline. Working party of the International Psychogeriatric Association in collaboration with the World Health Organization. *International Psychogeriatrics* 6 (1):63–68.

Mattis, S. 1988. *Dementia Rating Scale (DRS) Professional Manual.* Odessa, Fla.: Psychological Assessment Resources.

Morris, J.C. 1993. The Clinical Dementia Rating (CDR): Current version and scoring rules. *Neurology* 43:2412–14.

Morris, R., ed. 1996. *The Cognitive Neuropsychology of Alzheimer-type Dementia.* Oxford: Oxford University Press.

Morris, J.C., M. Storandt, J.P. Miller, et al. 2001. Mild cognitive impairment represents early-stage Alzheimer disease. *Archives of Neurology* 58 (3):397–405.

Moss, M.B., and M.S. Albert. 1988. Alzheimer's disease and other dementing disorders. In *Geriatric Neuropsychology*, edited by M.S. Albert and M.B. Moss. New York: Guilford Press.

Mountjoy, C.Q., M. Roth, N.J.R. Evans, et al. 1983. Cortical neuronal counts in normal elderly controls and demented patients. *Neurobiology of Aging* 4:1–11.

Nicolas, A.-S., S. Andrieu, F. Nourhashemi, et al. 2001. Successful aging and nutrition. *Nutrition Reviews* 59 (8):S88–92.

Parks, R.W., J.V. Haxby, and C.L. Grady. 1993. Positron emission tomography in Alzheimer's disease. In *Neuropsychology of Alzheimer's Disease and Other Dementias*, edited by R.W. Parks, R.F. Zec, and R.S. Wilson. Oxford: Oxford University Press.

Parnetti, L., D.T. Lowenthal, O. Presciutti, et al. 1996. 1H-MRS, MRI-based hippocampal volumetry, and 99mTc-HMPAO-SPECT in normal aging, age-associated memory impairment, and probable Alzheimer's disease. *Journal of the American Geriatrics Society* 44 (2):133–38.

Patterson, C., S. Gauthier, H. Bergman, et al. 2001. The recognition, assessment and management of dementing disorders: Conclusions from the Canadian Consensus Conference on Dementia. *Canadian Journal of Neurological Sciences* 28 (Suppl. 1): S3–16.

Pearlson, G.D., G.J. Harris, R.E. Powers, et al. 1992. Quantitative changes in mesial temporal volume, regional cerebral blood flow, and cognition in Alzheimer's disease. *Archives of General Psychiatry* 49 (5):402–8.

Perani, D., S. Bressi, S.F. Cappa, et al. 1993. Evidence of multiple memory systems in the human brain. A [18F]FDG PET metabolic study. *Brain* 116 (Pt. 4):903–19.

Petersen, R.C. 2000. Aging, mild cognitive impairment, and Alzheimer's disease. *Neurologic Clinics* 18 (4):789–806.

Petersen, R.C., G.E. Smith, R.J. Ivnik, et al. 1994. Memory function in very early Alzheimer's disease. *Neurology* 44 (5):867–72.

Petersen, R.C., G.E. Smith, R.J. Ivnik, et al. 1995. Apolipoprotein E status as a predictor of the development of Alzheimer's disease in memory-impaired individuals. *Journal of the American Medical Association* 273 (16):1274–78.

Petersen, R.C., G.E. Smith, S.C. Waring, et al. 1997. Aging, memory, and mild cognitive impairment. *International Psychogeriatrics* 9 (Suppl. 1):S65–69.

Petersen, R.C., G.E. Smith, S.C. Waring, et al. 1999. Mild cognitive impairment: Clinical characterization and outcome. *Archives of Neurology* 56 (3):303–8.

Petersen, R.C., J.C. Stevens, M. Ganguli, et al. 2001. Practice parameter: Early detection of dementia: Mild cognitive impairment (an evidence-based review). Report of the Quality Standards Subcommittee of the American Academy of Neurology. *Neurology* 56:1133–42.

Pfeiffer, E. 1975. A short portable mental status questionnaire for the assessment of organic brain deficit in elderly patients. *Journal of the American Geriatrics Society* 23 (10): 433–31.

Pietrini, P., G.E. Alexander, M.L. Furey, et al. 2000. The neurometabolic landscape of cognitive decline: In vivo studies with positron emission tomography in Alzheimer's disease. *International Journal of Psychophysiology* 37 (1):87–98.

Poon, L.W., et al. 1986. *Clinical Memory Assessment of Older Adults*, edited by T. Crook, K.L. Davis, C. Eisdorfer, et al. Washington, D.C.: American Psychological Association.

Practice parameter for diagnosis and evaluation of dementia [summary statement]. 1994. Report of the Quality Standards Subcommittee of the American Academy of Neurology. *Neurology* 44:2203–6.

Reuter-Lorenz, P.A., L. Stanczak, and A.C. Miller. 1999. Neural recruitment and cognitive aging: Two hemispheres are better than one, especially as you age. *Psychological Science* 10 (6):494–500.

Ritchie, K., S. Artero, and J. Touchon. 2001. Classification criteria for mild cognitive impairment: A population-based validation study. *Neurology* 56:37–42.

Rombouts, S.A., F. Barkhof, D.J. Veltman, et al. 2000. Functional MR imaging in Alzheimer's disease during memory encoding. *American Journal of Neuroradiology* 21: 1869–75.

Roses, A.D. 1997. Apolipoprotein E, a gene with complex biological interactions in the aging brain. *Neurobiology of Disease* 4:16–20.

Ross, M.H., D.A. Yurgelun-Todd, P.F. Renshaw, et al. 1997. Age-related reduction in functional MRI response to photic stimulation. *Neurology* 48 (1):173–76.

Rowe, J.W., and S. Wang. 1988. The biology and physiology of aging. In *Geriatric Medicine*, 2nd ed., edited by J.W. Rowe and R.W. Besdine. Boston: Little, Brown.

Salmon, D.P., W.C. Heindel, and K.L. Lange. 1999. Differential decline in word generation from phonemic and semantic categories during the course of Alzheimer's disease: Implications for the integrity of semantic memory. *Journal of the International Neuropsychological Society* 5:692–703.

Salthouse, T. 1985. Speed of behavior and its implications for cognition. In *Handbook of the Psychology of Aging*, edited by J.E. Birren and K.W. Schaie. New York: Van Nostrand, pp. 400–422.

Saykin, A.J., L.A. Flashman, S. Frutiger, et al. 1999. Neuroanatomic substrates of semantic memory impairment in Alzheimer's disease: Patterns of functional MRI activation. *Journal of the International Neuropsychological Society* 5:377–92.

Saykin, A., L. Flashman, S. Johnson, et al. 2000. Frontal and hippocampal memory circuitry in early Alzheimer's disease: Relation of structural and functional MRI changes. *NeuroImage* 11 (5):S123.

Schaie, K., and S. Willis. 1991. *Adult Development and Aging*. New York: HarperCollins.

Scheltens, P., D. Leys, F. Barkhof, et al. 1992. Atrophy of medial temporal lobes on MRI in "probable" Alzheimer's disease and normal ageing: Diagnostic value and neuropsychological correlates. *Journal of Neurology, Neurosurgery, and Psychiatry* 55 (10): 967–72.

Schroots, J.J.F., and J.E. Birren. 1993. Theoretical issues and basic questions in the planning of longitudinal studies of health and aging. In *Aging, Health and Competence: The Next Generation of Longitudinal Studies*, edited by J.J.F. Schroots. Amsterdam: Elsevier.

Schwamm, L.H., C. VanDyke, R.J. Kiernan, et al. 1987. The Neurobehavioral Cognitive Status Examination. *Annals of Internal Medicine* 107:486–91.

Shah, S., E.G. Tangalos, and R.C. Petersen. 2000. Mild cognitive impairment: When is it a precursor to Alzheimer's disease? *Geriatrics* 55 (9):62, 65–68.

Shihabuddin, L.S., P.H. Horner, J. Ray, et al. 2000. Adult spinal cord stem cells generate neurons after transplantation in the adult dentate gyrus. *Journal of Neuroscience* 20 (23):8727–35.

Shimamura, A.P. 1989. Disorders of memory: The cognitive science perspective. In *Handbook of Neuropsychology*, edited by F. Boller and J. Grafman. Amsterdam: Elsevier Science Publishers.

Shimamura, A.P. 1990. Aging and memory disorders: A neuropsychological analysis. In *Cognitive and Behavioral Performance Factors in Atypical Aging*, edited by M.L. Howe, M.J. Stones, and C.J. Brainerd. New York: Springer-Verlag.

Small, S.A., G.M. Perera, R. DeLaPaz, et al. 1999. Differential regional dysfunction of the hippocampal formation among elderly with memory decline and Alzheimer's disease. *Annals of Neurology* 45 (4):466–72.

Smith, C.D., A.H. Andersen, R.J. Kryscio, et al. 1999. Altered brain activation in cognitively intact individuals at high risk for Alzheimer's disease. *Neurology* 53:1391–96.

Smith, G., R.J. Ivnik, R.C. Petersen, et al. 1991. Age-associated memory impairment diagnoses: Problems of reliability and concerns for terminology. *Psychology and Aging* 6 (4):551–58.

Snowdon, D. 2001. *Aging with Grace.* New York: Bantam Books.

Soininen, H.S., K. Partanen, A. Pitkanen, et al. 1994. Volumetric MRI analysis of the amygdala and the hippocampus in subjects with age-associated memory impairment: Correlation to visual and verbal memory. *Neurology* 44 (9):1660–68.

Souder, E., A.J. Saykin, and A. Alavi. 1995. Multi-modal assessment in Alzheimer's disease. ADL in relation to PET, MRI and neuropsychology. *Journal of Gerontological Nursing* 21 (9):7–13.

Spirduso, W.W., and P.G. MacRae. 1990. Motor performance and aging. In *Handbook of the Psychology of Aging*, 3rd ed., edited by J.E. Birren and K.W. Schaie. San Diego: Academic Press.

Squire, L.R. 1992. Memory and the hippocampus: A synthesis from findings with rats, monkeys, and humans. *Psychological Review* 99 (2):195–231.

Terry, R.D., and P. Davies. 1983. Some morphologic and biochemical aspects of Alzheimer's disease. In *Aging of the Brain*, edited by D. Samuel. New York: Raven Press.

Tierney, M.C., J.P. Szalai, W.G. Snow, et al. 1996. Prediction of probable Alzheimer's disease in memory-impaired patients: A prospective longitudinal study. *Neurology* 46 (3):661–65.

Tomlinson, B.E. 1977. The neuropathology of dementia. In *Dementia*, edited by C.E. Wells. Philadelphia: F.A. Davis.

Troster, A.I. 1998. *Memory in Neurodegenerative Disease.* Cambridge: Cambridge University Press.

Tulving, E., and W. Donaldson. 1972. *The Organization of Memory.* New York: Academic Press.

Valenzuela, M.J., and P. Sachdev. 2001. Magnetic resonance spectroscopy in AD. *Neurology* 56 (5):592–98.

Wagner, A.D., D.L. Schacter, M. Rotte, et al. 1998. Building memories: Remembering and forgetting of verbal experiences as predicted by brain activity. *Science* 281 (5380): 1188–91.

Wechsler, D. 1987. *Wechsler Memory Scale-Revised (WMS-R)*. New York: Psychological Corporation.

Welsh, K., N. Butters, J. Hughes, et al. 1991. Detection of abnormal memory decline in mild cases of Alzheimer's disease using CERAD neuropsychological measures. *Archives of Neurology* 48 (3):278–81.

Welsh, K.A., N. Butters, J.P. Hughes, et al. 1992. Detection and staging of dementia in Alzheimer's disease: Use of the neuropsychological measures developed for the Consortium to Establish a Registry for Alzheimer's Disease. *Archives of Neurology* 49 (5): 448–52.

Wilson, R.S., M. Sullivan, L. deToledo-Morrell, et al. 1996. Association of memory and cognition in Alzheimer's disease with volumetric estimates of temporal lobe structures. *Neuropsychology* 10 (4):459–63.

Wolf, H., G.M. Ecke, S. Bettin, et al. 2000. Do white matter changes contribute to the subsequent development of dementia in patients with mild cognitive impairment?: A longitudinal study. *International Journal of Geriatric Psychiatry* 15 (9):803–12.

Woodard, J., S. Grafton, J. Votaw, et al. 1998. Compensatory recruitment of neural resources during overt rehearsal of word lists in Alzheimer's disease. *Neuropsychology* 12:491–504.

Xu, Y., C.R. Jack, Jr., P.C. O'Brien, et al. 2000. Usefulness of MRI measures of entorhinal cortex versus hippocampus in AD. *Neurology* 54 (9):1760–67.

CHAPTER TWO

The Spectrum of Dementias

Construct and Nosologic Validity

Thomas E. Oxman, M.D.

Questions about validity arise at multiple levels of the scientific enterprise. These questions concern the adequacy of *constructs* to "capture" the phenomena, the precision of operational procedures for *measuring* those constructs, and the correctness of *conclusions* about the inter-relationship of different constructs. Issues of scientific validity are approached primarily through improvement of the accuracy of current concepts, measures, and data by identifying and correcting factors that threaten validity, removing sources of error and bias.

In part, because of the rapid growth of the field, validity concerns abound in the science of Alzheimer disease (AD) and related dementias. Due to the preliminary state of our knowledge about the biology of most dementing diseases, concepts are continuously evolving to take account of newly reported findings. In this chapter, first discussed are validity concerns that arise at the level of conceptualizing the defining features of dementia. Central to this discussion is the notion of construct validity, which can best be viewed as a continuous process of refining our understanding of the meaning of a concept and the procedures by which it is operationally defined (Nunnally 1978). Next considered are issues in adequately measuring these definitional features, analyzing their interrelationships, and combining the measures into diagnostic judgments as to whether dementia is present as a syndrome. Finally, validity is examined as it relates to interpreting the results of studies of AD and related dementias along with the key questions for future research that this examination suggests.

Validity and the Defining Features of Dementia

Historically and semantically, *dementia* (from the root Latin phrase *de mens*) is a descriptive term, simply indicating that a person shows a pattern of observable abnormalities. The abnormalities are identified by a decline or loss of mental abilities. It was not until more recent times that the term took on an etiological dimension, becoming generally restricted to mental disturbances attributed to organic causes (Crook 1987). As a current scientific construct, dementia is operationalized by reference to one of several sets of consensus diagnostic criteria that are currently in use (see chap. 3). The main sets of criteria are those for primary degenerative dementia of the American Psychiatric Association's DSM-IV-TR (American Psychiatric Association 2000), and those for AD developed by a work group jointly sponsored by the National Institute of Neurological and Communicative Diseases and Stroke and the Alzheimer's Disease and Related Disorders Association (NINCDS-ADRDA) (McKhann et al. 1984).

Analysis of differing sets of diagnostic criteria reveals variability in specifics, but in essentials five features uniformly comprise the dementia construct. An adequate degree of theoretical or preoperational explication of these features is a prerequisite for construct validity. The central, or first-order, triad of features for dementia includes cognitive impairment, functional impairment, and neuropathology. Second-order modifiers describe the severity and the disease course of this triad; specifically, progression and deterioration. First the construct validity of measures for each of the component features defining this construct of dementia is presented, followed by their validity as a set of interrelated criteria for identifying dementia as a syndrome.

Cognitive Impairment and Its Assessment

Cognitive impairment is the sine qua non in the definition of dementia. Even if a person had known brain lesions and behavior that was socially aberrant in other ways, without evidence of cognitive impairment we would not say that the individual showed dementia. The impairment must be a global dysfunction affecting multiple areas of intellectual functioning, such as memory, abstraction, attention, visuospatial abilities, and language (see chap. 1).

The measurement of cognitive impairment depends on psychological testing procedures, which may range from brief mental status screening scales—suitable for bedside use and incorporation into home or office interviews—to extensive neuropsychological test batteries requiring a number of hours for administration (see chap. 3). Both the DSM-IV-TR and NINCDS-ADRDA criteria require impairment in memory and at least one other cognitive function and refer to the use of mental status measures to describe the impairment. The latter criteria require confirmation by neuropsychological tests for a diagnosis of probable AD. Reliance on these procedures emphasizes the need for adequate test validity and reliability.

A number of investigators have developed structured, brief mental status examinations. Among the most commonly used are the Mental Status Questionnaire (MSQ) (Kahn et al. 1960), Memory-Information-Concentration Test (Blessed, Tomlinson, and Ross 1968), Short Portable Mental Status Questionnaire (SPMSQ) (Pfeiffer 1975; Fillenbaum, Landerman, and Simonsyck 1998), and Mini-Mental State Examination (MMSE) (Folstein, Folstein, and McHugh 1975). Only in recent years are reliability and norms for an older population being established, and ethnic variations being examined (Valle et al. 1991; Clark et al. 1999). Standardized brief mental status examinations are best used cautiously, and primarily as screening devices. Because of these psychometric issues, new screening measures continue to be developed (Solomon and Pendlebury 1998; Scanlan and Borson 2001), but they have many of the same validity issues without the same familiarity and acceptance as older screening instruments (Gifford and Cummings 1999).

Numerous test batteries of intermediate length have also been developed for dementia (e.g., Mattis 1976; Storandt, Botwinick, and Danziger 1984; Eslinger et al. 1985). Scores on these tests correlate well with WAIS scores, and have high test-retest reliability, at least over short periods of time. However, all of these cognitive tests are best used as indicators for further investigation or longitudinally to monitor progressive deterioration rather than cross-sectionally for diagnosis.

Among the core validity concerns here is thus the challenge of extrapolating from a cross-sectional assessment of cognitive function to a judgment about whether a person has experienced a decline. Various psychometric strategies have been attempted in response to this challenge; none of them has proven entirely satisfactory. One of the most common has been reliance on a hypothesized pattern of divergence among the cognitive testing scores, with certain scores expected to be less affected by the disorder and therefore useful as an index of the person's premorbid level of function. Other approaches rely heavily on the individual's social and occupational history, and attempt to gauge the cognitive ability that he or she must have shown to engage in those activities. Only rarely are the results of earlier psychometric assessments available to serve as a comparison.

A corollary of this general difficulty in comparing present with earlier levels of cognitive function is that it is very difficult to take account of a person's initial ability or intelligence level, particularly when that level is lower than average. Among the mentally retarded, for example, establishing tests that are sensitive to further declines from an already limited cognitive repertoire has proven to be very difficult.

The approach usually substituted for being able to directly measure cognitive decline over time is to evaluate whether the individual's current performance deviates significantly from the normative level for individuals in the population who share similar demographic characteristics. Accordingly, another major validity issue is the adequacy of norms for the testing procedures being used. Even when age and gender are accounted for, the adequacy of the norms can be compromised by the unmeasured influence of other subject characteristics, such as educational level, socioeconomic status, and sociocultural, ethnic, and linguistic differences (Escobar et al. 1986; Bird et al. 1987; Unverzagt et al. 1996; Gurland et al. 2000).

Many memory and other cognitive tests (e.g., serial sevens) are strongly affected by education (Albert and Heaton 1988) and have not been established as highly valid for diagnosis (Oxman, Silberfarb, and Schnurr 1986). A number of studies suggest that the current cognitive screening procedures (particularly the MMSE) require a certain degree of education. Even when the norms are scaled downward, existing items on such instruments may not be sufficient to measure cognitive impairment accurately or yield accurate diagnoses among those of lower educational attainment (e.g., less than ninth-grade education). Rather, additional items may be necessary to tap into various dimensions of cognitive impairment among those with very limited or no formal education.

Populations in which a significant proportion of the individuals are poorly educated or illiterate demonstrate a higher prevalence of dementia of the Alzheimer type (Katzman et al. 1988; Hebert et al. 1995). Only further study will determine if education has a direct biological effect on the brain, if education-associated increased synaptic density is the result of unexplained environmental or socioeconomic factors, or if the finding is simply a measurement artifact (Advisory Panel on Alzheimer's Disease 1992).

The Epidemiologic Catchment Area (ECA) studies (Holzer et al. 1984), which administered a version of the Mini-Mental State Examination (Folstein et al. 1985), reported relatively high levels of cognitive impairment among adult African American and Hispanic populations, almost double the levels of cognitive impairment found in the general population. The work of Lopes-Aqueres et al. (1984) with a community sample of Hispanics also found higher than average levels of cognitive impairment. Although some studies have included certain ethnic subgroups, the absolute numbers of these subjects remain too limited to provide data adequate to generate reliable estimates (Farrer 2000).

There is still a need to develop relevant, culturally based expressions of cognition (Hall et al. 1996, 2000). For example, test items based on orientation to time may be less relevant for certain ethnic subpopulations. Rather, what may be more salient is an understanding of kinship terms or power relationships (as in the Chinese populations) or seasons (as in some Mexican and Mexican American groups) or knowledge of clans (as in some American Indian groups). A final key issue of the assessment of cognitive impairment is the "face validity" of testing procedures, so that they make sense and are accepted by those undergoing (and having to cooperate with) cognitive evaluation (Crook 1985). In this regard, sampling and testing of nonwhite populations has not been as representative because of lack of access to specialty clinics and distrust of academic medical centers (Farrer 2000).

Functional Impairment

As another key element in the dementia construct, functional impairment refers to difficulties with everyday behavior and changes in personality. Primary functional impairment is not merely a consequence of cognitive impairment, but has a different natural history, pathophysiology, and response to treatment (Mortimer et al. 1992; Levy et al. 1996; Sano et al. 1997). For example, early and predominant visual hallucinations are often a feature of dementia with Lewy bodies (DLB) as opposed to AD (McKeith et al. 1999). Functional impairment is not as precisely defined as cognitive impairment. Although subdomains are differentiated within this category, in the clinical and research settings in which elderly people are evaluated for dementia these have—not necessarily correctly—typically been lumped together. Thus, in this chapter, functional impairment encompasses all noncognitive aspects of behavior that may be affected in dementia. Noncognitive aspects include emotional and personality changes, psychiatric and behavioral symptoms, difficulties fulfilling occupational or social roles, and impaired performance of basic everyday tasks, or activities of daily living (ADLs).

As with cognitive function, a determination of whether an individual is experiencing functional impairment requires longitudinal knowledge of the person. This includes knowledge of the possibility that certain roles may have been occupationally overlearned while others remained unfamiliar, a matter of clinical judgment. This depends on information reported by patients themselves—or, more typically, by an informant—rather than behavior directly observed in the clinical setting (Hall et al. 1996, 2000). Informant reports can introduce both improvements in and additional threats to validity. The difference depends in part on the stage of dementia, where a person is residing, and the relationship of the informant to the person. Informant reports are less affected by education and premorbid intellectual function (Juva et al. 1997; Morales et al. 1997). In contrast, such reports are influenced by personality, affective state, and the relationship between the subject and the informant (Edwards and Danziger 1982; Heun, Meyer, and Muller 1997; Mackinnon and Mulligan 1998).

A comprehensive and standardized clinical instrument that includes functional assessment is the Cambridge Mental Disorders of the Elderly Examination (CAMDEX). Roth and colleagues (1986) developed the CAMDEX for multiple purposes, including to assist in diagnosing dementia, measuring cognitive impairment, and assessing behavior and adaptation in everyday life. Part of the CAMDEX consists of a standardized, structured interview with a relative or other caretaker concerning the patient's present state, past history, and family history. The CAMDEX relies as well on data from several other data collection approaches, including a patient interview, a cognitive examination, and interviewer observations. Three diagnostic scales—for Organicity, Multi-Infarct Dementia, and Depression—are included. After administering the CAMDEX to an American sample, Hendrie et al. (1988) reported high interrater reliabilities and good concurrent validity by correlations with cognitive impairment measures. Neri et al. (2001) reported similar results. Furthermore, the three diagnostic scales demonstrated the ability to discriminate between diagnostic subgroups within the sample. Hendrie et al. (2001) incorporated the CAMDEX-based informant assessment of function with a culturally sensitive screening instrument for comparative epidemiologic studies, the Community Screening Interview for Dementia (CSI "D").

Other potentially useful instruments for functional assessment include several variants of the Memory and Behavior Problem Checklist (Zarit, Reever, and Bach-Peterson 1980; Niederehe 1988b), the Behavioural and Mood Disturbance Scale (Greene et al. 1982), the Informant Questionnaire on Cognitive Decline in the Elderly (IQCODE) (Jorm and Jacomb 1989; Jorm et al. 2000), the Pleasant Events Schedule-AD (Teri and Logsdon 1991), the Dementia Questionnaire (Kawas et al. 1994), the Dementia Severity Rating Scale (Clark and Ewbank 1996), the Neuropsychiatric Inventory (Cummings 1997), the CERAD Behavior Rating Scale for Dementia (Mack et al. 1999), and the Clinical Dementia Rating (CDR) (Morris 1997; Waite et al. 1999). Research with such scales has indicated that the frequency of functional impairment is not a simple function of duration of illness or severity of the person's neuropsychological deficits (Zarit et al. 1980; Niederehe and Scott 1987; Tekin et al. 2001). Studies that lack detailed assessments of functional impairment are open to criticism for having neglected to give equal weight to one of the core features of dementia. Despite concerns about informant validity, inclusion of structured informant information with cognitive testing substantially improves discrimination and prediction of dementia, validating the position of function as a primary feature of dementia (Tierney et al. 1996; Mackinnon and Mulligan 1998; Hall et al. 2000; Tschanz et al. 2000).

Neuropathology

In addition to the notion of dementia as a behaviorally observable syndrome, the current scientific construct requires the presence, at least presumptively, of biological abnormalities in the central nervous system substrate for behavior. The postmortem neuropathological criteria for dementia of the Alzheimer type depend on the density and location of neuritic plaques and neurofibrillary tangles.

The various indices of neuropathological degeneration in this research domain tap into one or more pathophysiological processes at varying points in the disease progression. The pathogenic sequencing of, and the interrelationships between, these indices remain unclear. The various neuropathological parameters that can be quantified are overlapping and not unique to the disease categories that are currently defined. Thus, preoperational problems of defining discrete disease entities are a prominent obstacle to achieving construct validity.

The presence of neuropathological changes such as senile neuritic plaques, neurofibrillary tangles, and granulovacuolar degeneration at autopsy have long been thought to be the "gold standard" for the diagnosis of Alzheimer disease. However, just as with cognitive testing, there is a significant overlap between the neuropathology seen in usual aging and that seen in dementia. Senile plaques are evident in as many as 70% of those over age 65, occasionally—albeit rarely—in quantities comparable to those seen in AD (Crystal et al. 1988; Snowdon 1997). Neurofibrillary tangles, especially in the frontal cortex, are somewhat more specific in AD (Alafuzoff et al. 1987; Crystal et al. 1988; Molsa et al. 1987; Schmitt et al. 2000), and either absent or very scanty in the majority of cognitively normal older adults (Tomlinson 1977). Tangles are not specific to AD, having a presence in other disorders with varying etiologies, such as dementia pugilistica, head trauma, postencephalitic Parkinson disease, the Guam-Parkinson-dementia complex, and abnormal mineral intake (Katzman 1986; Mandybur 1990). The overlap of both plaques and tangles in usual aging and AD depends on the methods used to rate the lesions (Schmitt et al. 2000; Xuereb et al. 2000). For example, the National Institute on Aging and Reagan Institute (1997) criteria, which emphasize neurofibrillary tangles more than neuritic plaques, may be more sensitive in detecting incipient AD from the pool of presumed normals. It remains uncertain whether plaques or tangles is the primary lesion in AD or what the relationship between the two is. Recent research in transgenic mice suggests at least one connection in that abnormal forms of beta-amyloid can stimulate the formation of neurofibrillary tangles (Gotz et al. 2001; Lewis et al. 2001).

Similar to the situation with senile plaques and neurofibrillary tangles, there is a large overlap between the cognitively normal elderly persons and those diagnosed with a vascular dementia in the presence of small cerebral infarctions. Vascular dementia can result from several pathological conditions, including cerebral infarction, multiple emboli, lacunar disease, and Binswanger disease (see chaps. 8, 11, and 12). These conditions had been lumped together under the rubric of multiinfarct dementia (MID). Multiinfarct dementia is described as having a stepwise course and focal neurological signs, consistent with the sporadic occurrence of focal pathology. Hachinski and colleagues (1975) operationalized the MID construct in a clinical ischemia scale to aid in the differential diagnosis of MID versus AD. DSM-III-R included similar criteria. Most reviews found low reliability for the antemortem differentiation of AD and MID based on these criteria (see chap. 11 and Liston and LaRue1983; Wade et al. 1987; Zubenko et al. 1990; Chui et al. 1992). As many as 50% of people over age 65 without intellectual deterioration demonstrate at least small areas of infarction, usually less than 100 cc of brain softening (Tomlinson 1977). Also, as with plaques and tangles, the location of small infarcts is probably as important as the quantity.

Because of these problems the term *vascular dementia* (VaD) has replaced multiinfarct dementia and new criteria have been proposed (ICD-10, World Health Organization, 1993; DSM-IV, American Psychiatric Association, 1994; and those developed specifically as operationalized research criteria, such as the Alzheimer's Diseases Diagnostic and Treatment Centers [ADDTC] [Chui et al. 1992] and the National Institute of Neurological Disorders and Stroke–Association Internationale pour la Recherche et l'Enseignement en Neurosciences [NINDS-AIREN] [Roman et al. 1993]). Vascular dementia can occur from several different types of lesions, such as multiple infarcts, noninfarct vascular disease, and single key infarcts. The lesions and their locations coupled with the frequent overlap of AD and VaD result in considerable variability in the clinical presentation, making valid classification difficult (Liston and LaRue 1983). In addition to presenting as a separate type of dementia, cerebrovascular disease may also influence the onset and expression of AD (Looi and Sachdev 2000).

A similar problem occurs from the growing recognition of Lewy body pathology and the overlap between Parkinson disease (PD) and Alzheimer disease (Xuereb et al. 2000). At least 20% of persons with PD develop cognitive impairment (see chap. 9). Perry et al. (1990), among others, described a dementing syndrome with the neuropathological finding of diffuse Lewy bodies, normally associated subcortically with PD, but without marked movement disorder. Dementia with Lewy bodies does not appear to be just a severe form of PD (Gomez-Tortosa et al. 1999). Neither does it appear to be merely a variant of AD (Haroutunian et al. 2000). Neuropathological studies frequently find minimal evidence of AD in such patients. Conversely, 20–50% of persons with AD develop a movement disorder (Mayeux, Stern, and Spanton 1985; Ditter and Mirra 1987; Lennox et al. 1989) and tend to have more severe cognitive and functional impairment (Clark et al. 1997) or a more rapid progression (Lopez et al. 2000). The most common situation, however, is overlap between AD, PD, and VaD neuropathology. Thus, a major problem with neuropathological validity is determining which if any is the primary cause of dementia and its course.

As with cognitive testing, quantifiable criteria for neuropathology have been proposed, some with specification of numerical thresholds and anatomical locations, for Alzheimer disease (see chap. 4 and Khachaturian 1985; Alafuzoff et al. 1987; Ball et al. 1988; Braak and Braak 1991; Mirra et al. 1991), vascular dementia (Chui et al. 1992; Roman et al. 1993), and dementia with Lewy bodies (McKeith et al. 1996). However, application of the same criteria across studies can vary significantly due, in large part, to technical differences, variability in application, and, at times, modest interrater reliability (Duyckaerts et al. 1987; Lamy et al. 1989; Mirra et al. 1991; McKeith et al. 2000a; Xuereb et al. 2000).

Second-order Defining Features

Progression of Disease

The core triad of defining characteristics must fit several patterns before a judgment of a primary degenerative dementia such as Alzheimer disease is reached. Perhaps most important, there must be evidence that the syndrome is progressively worsening. Usually this progression will be gauged in terms of the cognitive and functional impairment, but conceivably could also be evidenced on measures of the degree of neuropathology. Degenerative dementia syndromes are those in which the progression is perceived to be gradual, slow, insidious. If the changes have occurred abruptly, the diagnostic tendency is to suspect instead a syndrome of delirium, or major structural damage from a large stroke or acute injury or toxicity.

Differential progression of cognitive and functional features is another important feature separating certain subtypes of dementia. For example, functional features such as stereotypic behavior in eating preferences, diminished social awareness, and disinhibition occur before comparable cognitive features in frontotemporal dementias in contrast to AD (Chow et al. 1999; Bozeat et al. 2000).

Dementias may develop as a result of many differing organic factors, some of them reversible, others not. In that subset of dementias caused by degenerative CNS diseases, including AD, a facet of the dementia progression feature is the notion of irreversibility. Not only does the disease course lie along a slope of decline, but this progression is considered inexorable and, thus far, neither preventable nor curable. Clinical evidence from the available cholinesterase inhibitors suggests the AD disease process may be temporarily slowed, but not reversed (see chap. 18). The treatability or reversibility of a dementia, however, is very much a moving target, premised on the current state of knowledge about normal aging (Kempermann and Gage 1999) as well as neuropathology. As we learn more about the pathogenesis of diseases like AD, PD, and stroke, we uncover new steps at which the cascade of neurobiological events might be blocked, if not reversed (e.g., a vaccine against the formation of neuritic plaques, the regeneration of nerve pathways via manipulation of nerve growth factors or via the implantation of healthy neuronal tissue).

Severity

Identification of dementia implicitly involves a judgment regarding the severity of impairment shown (in cognitive and noncognitive function) compared to the range of changes seen in normal aging. If an individual has identifiable neuropathology but still remains within normal limits cognitively and functionally, there may be debate on a semantic basis about whether this should be labeled "mild dementia" as opposed to some presymptomatic stage of disease. Dementia seems to imply surpassing a severity or threshold level for abnormality on at least one observable dimension (see chap. 1).

Most often, the severity of the disorder is documented by reference to the functional impairment dimension. Whereas ability levels can vary markedly on cognitive measures, coexisting impairment in everyday patterns of behavior is used as evidence that the cognitive impairment syndrome has reached proportions that go beyond the cognitive changes of normal aging.

Lack of control over heterogeneous levels of severity among research samples of persons with dementia is perhaps the most problematic confounding factor affecting construct validity in dementia research (Gifford and Cummings 1999). This is definitely the case for prevalence studies, in which the variability of rates for mild dementia is greater than that of rates for moderate to severe dementia: 0.5–20% for mild dementia versus 3–8% for severe dementia (Gurland and Cross 1986; Jorm, Korten, and Henderson 1987; Jorm and Jolley 1998). In part, such problems may stem from a relatively lower reliability and validity for the diagnosis of mild dementia, for which criteria vary and even careful examination in the clinical setting does not exclude misdiagnosis (Jorm and Jolley 1998; Tschanz et al. 2000). For example, in the Newcastle (Blessed et al. 1968) and Duke (Gianturco and Busse 1978) longitudinal studies, significant numbers of subjects were diagnosed as having mild dementia, but on follow-up two to three years later were judged not to have dementia (Lauter 1985). Such findings indicate the importance of independent and longitudinal assessment of both cognitive and functional impairment.

A central validity issue that involves both the disease progression and severity dimensions of dementia is that of validating measures to track changes over time and to locate the individual's current status within the overall continuum of the disease (so-called staging measures). Such measures must be shown to be sensitive to the changing status of persons with dementia (either naturalistically declining over time or temporarily improving as a result of current treatments), and must have a broad scale of measurement sufficient to reflect the range of expectable changes. A particular threat to valid measurement of change comes from instruments that cannot adequately reflect changes in later stages of dementia, due to floor effects.

Relationships among the Essential Features of Dementia

The validity of our knowledge about the interrelationships among the defining features of dementia depends on the construct validity of our measures for each feature, individually and on the statistical validity of comparisons between various features. In part, questions about the degree of interrelatedness are about how necessary various features are to the overall construct of dementia. Many pieces of research in the field of AD and related dementias have some bearing on the relations among the features of dementia. Some common ways of referring to these questions are characterized in figure 2.1.

Cognitive Impairment and Neuropathology

In many ways, analyses of this interrelationship are at the very core of dementia research. Depending on which feature is viewed as a criterion against which the other feature is evaluated, the analysis may be described somewhat differently. If, for instance, we begin with evidence of brain pathology and ask what it means in terms of cognition, we have the type of question about brain-behavior relationships that is characteristic of experimental research in neuropsychology. This might be termed *functional mapping* of affected brain regions.

If, however, we begin with a measure of cognitive impairment and ask to what degree it reflects particular types or extents of brain pathology, we have a question of construct validation as to whether mental status and neuropsychological tests can serve as valid indices of neuropathology. There has been a long research tradition of examining the correlation between cognitive measures and available neuropathological indices, such as counts of plaques and tangles from

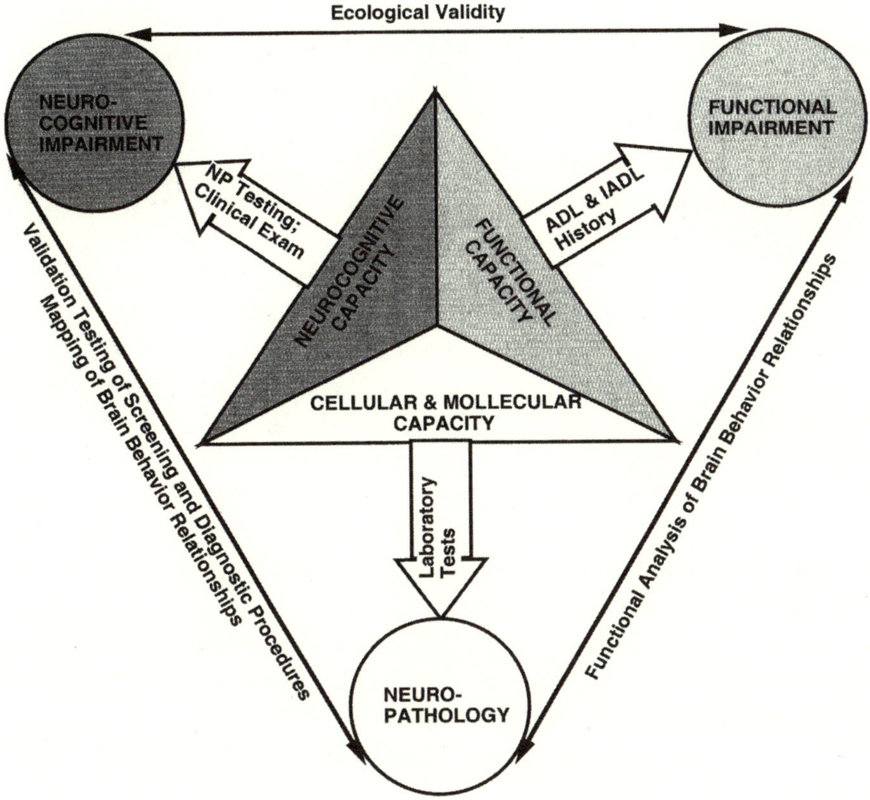

Figure 2.1. Interrelationships among the defining features of dementia

autopsied brain tissues, loss of synapses, or ratings of the degree of ventricular and sulcal enlargement visualized on CT or MRI brain scans. On the whole, the correlations have tended to be sufficient to suggest the validity, in gross terms, of cognitive measures with respect to such neuropathological criteria. However, the amount of disagreement between behavioral and neuropathological measures emphasizes that the relationship is not direct or precise. Other sources of substantial variance have to be considered.

Functional Impairment and Neuropathology

The same variety of validity questions arise regarding these interrelationships as discussed under the preceding section, except that here we are dealing with measures of activities of daily living and of psychiatric symptoms and "problem behaviors" (see chap. 18) in persons with dementia rather than cognitive impairment measures. Our knowledge of these interrelationships is more sparing because of relatively less evidence for the validity and reliability of functional impairment measures (McDowell and Newell 1996). As discussed previously, a root difficulty here is the lack of an adequate typology of what is being measured in the behavioral domain. The features that define what behaviors are problematic, for instance, may be attributes of the care context rather than having any inherent connection to the individual's degree or pattern of neuropathology.

One of the first efforts to systematize the collection of information about the everyday functioning of persons with dementia was conducted by the Newcastle group (Blessed et al. 1968). These researchers developed a Dementia Scale to measure the behavioral deterioration of elderly persons (Roth et al. 1986). Sums of the symptoms and behaviors indicated as present on this checklist (based on an interview with an informant) proved to be highly correlated with counts of plaques in patients' brain tissue (Blessed et al. 1968). This correlation accounted for more of the variance in plaque counts than did the correlation with cognitive scores. This Blessed (or Newcastle) Dementia Scale has subsequently been employed in numerous studies as a measure of the severity of the behavioral disturbance in dementia.

A central question is whether particular neuropathological features tend to be directly associated with specific emotional or behavioral symptoms, or other functional deficits (e.g., see chaps. 9 and 17). Some research suggests that persons who develop depressive symptoms as part of the dementia syndrome tend to have particularly evident neuropathological damage in certain brain structures (Zweig et al. 1988). As an alternative possibility, the type or degree of cognitive impairment might be an intervening variable that mediates the development of functional impairment. If this latter possibility is the case, functional impairments would be understood as sequela of becoming cognitively impaired, either because cognitive deficits leave one unable to carry out everyday tasks or because certain behavioral symptoms ensue from secondary emotional reactions to the experiencing of cognitive decline.

Cognitive impairment that occurs in some geriatric patients with depression has long been attributed to the severity of the depression. Several studies, however, have found that many elderly depressed patients seen in tertiary care medical centers manifest structural brain abnormalities, particularly white matter lesions, subcortical lesions, and disruption of striatofrontal pathways (see chaps. 14 and 15 and Coffey et al. 1990; Zubenko et al. 1990; Alexopoulos 2001). If this proves to be a replicable finding, another interpretation of these cases may be that both the cognitive impairment and the depression itself are manifestations of underlying neuropathology.

Cognitive Impairment and Functional Impairment

There has been relatively little research on this relationship. Neuropsychological measures are primarily validated to be informative about brain-behavior relationships rather than what might be called "behavior-behavior" relationships, that is, the implications of various cognitive deficits for real-world functioning (Niederehe and Scott 1987; Siegler and Poon 1989). The linkage of laboratory- or clinic-based measures to predicting behavior outside these settings is what some have termed the "ecological validity" of the measures. The availability of cholinesterase inhibitors has led to examination of change in both cognitive and noncognitive features of dementia (see chap. 18). Thus far, change in functional impairment appears to be less directly related to changes in cognition than might be anticipated. The weakness of this relationship is consistent with functional impairment being a primary feature of dementia (Mega et al. 1999; McKeith et al. 2000b).

The Validity of the Collective Essential Features in Diagnosing Dementia as a Syndrome

In addition to analyzing the cohesion among the defining features of dementia, we must consider as another validity question the degree to which applying a set of criteria based on these features leads to accurate diagnoses of dementia. There tends to be much semantic confusion on this topic. Several different questions are being asked, and we need to differentiate them by approaching the question of diagnostic accuracy at two levels.

Dementia versus Normal Changes of Aging

A logical first step in the diagnostic decision-making process is to determine whether any form of dementia is present. This is essentially a choice between normality (normal aging) and abnormality (mild cognitive impairment or some dementing disorder) (see chap. 1). The appropriate validity question here is quite generic: in cases in which a diagnosis of dementia is made—and only in those cases—on cross-checking will some evidence of neuropathology or disease progression be found that validates the accuracy of that decision? The specific type of neuropathology is not relevant to this question.

Some earlier autopsy studies suggested fairly high rates of mismatch between cognitive impairment data and plaque and tangle counts in brain tissue as the neuropathological criterion—roughly 30% for both false positive and false negative rates. In other words, some persons who were not assessed as being particularly impaired in function or cognition before death have shown elevated plaque and tangle counts (diagnostic false negatives), whereas others who appeared to have dementia have not had elevated counts (false positives) (Snowdon 1997).

To a large degree, the notion of pseudodementia arises in this context of imprecision in the link between the overtly observable features that may lead to a diagnosis of dementia and the presumed underlying etiological features. What is "pseudo" in these cases is not the judgment of cognitive and functional impairment. A person can be accurately labeled as having dementia in a purely descriptive sense if performing in an impaired fashion. The point of inaccuracy has been the clinical judgment that the individual is showing cognitive impairment due to a progressive and irreversible structural etiology. This error is typically uncovered by the subsequent course of the impairment, that is, if the individual improves and the dementia proves instead to be transient.

Differentiating Subtypes of Dementia

The second step in diagnostic decisions is differential diagnosis among the various subtypes of dementia (e.g., Alzheimer disease versus vascular dementia or dementia with Lewy bodies), generally based on whatever typology of biological factors is being used. The validity question here is whether an accurate subtyping of the neuropathological disease entity can be made based on the information available for clinical diagnosis, namely, assessments of cognitive and functional impairment, and whatever clinical and laboratory procedures are used to determine the likely status of the individual's CNS substrate. Typically, these procedures have mostly to do either with detecting or ruling out potentially reversible biological factors that may contribute to impaired cognition, or with evaluating gross morphological or functional changes that would be consistent with a degenerative process in the brain (e.g., MRI evidence of progressive brain atrophy, EEG recordings to document electrophysiological slowing, or PET data on reduced perfusion and metabolic activity of selective brain regions).

Research on this second diagnostic question has also depended on studies of patients for whom brain autopsies are obtained. Studies to date have tended to support the diagnostic accuracy of the consensus criteria for differentiating AD from other neuropathology. This support occurs under ideal conditions in tertiary research settings such as the federally funded Alzheimer disease research centers. In a series of 1139 patients with probable AD examined over seventeen years at one research center, sensitivity by autopsy data remained high at 94% to 98% and specificity improved from 52% to 88% (Lopez et al. 2000). The investigators suggest that the improved specificity is due to improvements in awareness and diagnosis of non-Alzheimer dementias.

A number of extraneous factors, however, may influence these findings, leaving it an open question whether comparable diagnostic accuracy would be achieved under less ideal conditions, such as in primary care settings, despite use of the same criteria. Other studies suggest that the relationship between clinical and neuropathological diagnosis is generally only modest (Alafuzoff et al. 1987; Xuereb et al. 2000). Not only may diagnostic expertise regarding dementia be less for clinicians in nonspecialized settings, but also complex selection factors may lead to differences in the types of patients seen in various settings (Xuereb et al. 2000) (see chap. 3).

An especially difficult problem that affects diagnostic validity is the issue of base rates of disorder in the patient samples undergoing diagnosis (Meehl and Rosen 1955). Basically, the accuracy of a diagnostic procedure is a delicate balance between sensitivity (the true positive rate of detecting a disorder when it is present) and selectivity (avoidance of misidentification of disorders in normal individuals). Increasing sensitivity often decreases selectivity, and vice versa, and both tend to be dependent on the proportion of cases in a clinical setting that actually have the disorder. If a high percentage, say 90%, of cases seen actually have dementia, the greatest diagnostic success will result from procedures with liberal criteria for identifying dementia. Because of selection factors, such high base rates would seemingly be more likely in specialized dementia research centers than in primary care or psychiatric settings where a greater mix of disorders may be found. The same procedures and criteria that yield highly accurate diagnoses in a high base rate situation will be much less accurate when the base rate is lower, yielding many more false positives.

Another important issue of subtyping is the possible difference between early- and late-onset forms of Alzheimer disease. While Alois Alzheimer's original pathological studies were of "presenile" dementia, numerous studies during the 1970s and 1980s suggested that there was no major difference between presenile and senile degenerative dementia (e.g., Sulkova 1983). However, a variety of subsequent studies caused a reevaluation of that conclusion. Whether or not the distinction proves to be age-related, these studies suggested the existence of two or more subtypes of AD. As summarized by Roth (1985) and Bondareff et al. (1987), type I AD appears in the middle of the eighth decade of life and has a less clear demarcation from normal aging. Neurochemical and neuropathological deficits are circumscribed. Type I is more common and considered "sporadic." Type II AD demonstrates more extensive neurochemical deficits, more marked frontotemporal cell loss, and loss of neurons in the nucleus locus ceruleus and nucleus basalis (see also chap. 6 and Iversen 1987). Type II is considered less common and usually inherited or "familial." More recently, the pendulum is moving back toward a unified version in which a majority of cases have similar genetic determinants or end points. Because of the limited human life span, proving this hypothesis for a disease with such a late onset is difficult. In either case, there may be more similarities than differences in the familial and sporadic forms of AD (Selkoe 2001).

The Validity of Findings about Dementia

Unresolved problems regarding the validity of measures of dementia obviously affect the research results that are obtained using those measures. We cannot have confidence that we have correctly interpreted a reported relationship unless we can trust that the measures used accurately represent what they are purported to mean. However, if measurement and construct validity issues have been adequately addressed, a number of other validity questions must be considered at the level of study results. Here we speak of statistical validity and internal and external validity. For the most part, the issues at this level concern the adequacy of the study methodology to support the conclusions we wish to draw from a study or experiment—in terms of the design features, controls over confounding variables, sampling techniques, and the like. The potential methodological pitfalls that can threaten the validity of findings are too many to enumerate here. Instead, one illustrative example is the impact of validity concerns on the "true" prevalence of dementia of the Alzheimer type (Larson 1989).

The factors discussed under diagnosis of dementia are straightforward in their application to procedures for screening and case identification in epidemiological research, which is after all a form of diagnosis. The set of criteria used and the accuracy of measures operationalizing each criterion may influence the rates at which cases are identified. The great variability in prevalence rates for

AD and dementia in general is unlikely to be due solely to variations in environmental or genetic risk factors among the populations studied.

Characteristics of the population to be sampled can strongly affect how generalizable the results of any study will be (external validity). Inclusion of a wide range of educational, cultural, and socioeconomic backgrounds is important. For example, one of the highest prevalence (and incidence) rates of dementia so far reported was 10.3 percent of those 65 years and older in the East Boston Study (Evans et al. 1989; Hebert et al. 1995). Among the validity issues of this study, however, were that it contained a high proportion of low-educated foreign-born subjects and was in a community with few institutional beds (raising the chance of more severe, detectable cases in the community).

With respect to examining subjects, the best method would be to assess all individuals in a defined population. For example, one of the strengths of the East Boston Study was that all individuals 65 years and older were identified and approached for participation in the study. For larger, more heterogeneous populations, the cost of such an approach is prohibitive. Random probability samples with multiple stages are an adequate alternative to improve generalizability. In a multistage study, a trained interviewer administers a screening procedure and a clinician evaluates those above a predetermined level and a selected (stratified) portion of those below that level, then sending subjects for laboratory investigations. Such a multistage procedure is employed in most community studies. However, as emphasized by Henderson and Jorm (1987), sample attrition in multistage assessment procedures can threaten statistical validity. Even if response rates are high at each stage (e.g., 80%), the cumulative effect by the time a subject undergoes laboratory screening in a three-stage design is substantial (80% × 80% × 80% = 51% response).

Ultimately of most concern, however, is not reducing methodological threats to validity so that there is a convergence of prevalence or incidence of disease around the world. True divergence of rates provides clues related to geographic, socioeconomic, or other population differences. The meta-analysis of prevalence and incidence studies by Jorm and colleagues (1987, 1998), the improved sensitivity to cultural and racial assessment shown by Hendrie et al. (2001), and the improved neuropathological-clinical diagnostic correlations described by Lopez et al. (2000) suggest that the variability in dementia types in different countries and cultures is not due just to methodological differences. This implies that we can learn about actual mechanisms of dementing diseases and potential disease modifications by studying biopsychosocial differences among peoples.

Discussion

Based on the issues discussed in this chapter, the following four areas may be especially salient for advancing the field of dementia research in terms of construct and experimental validity.

1. *The Relation of Dementia to Normal Aging Changes.* There needs to be continued attention at both the conceptual and empirical research levels on the spectrum of the changes seen in dementia and those characteristic of normal aging. Of particular consideration is whether qualitative distinctions are primary or whether dementia exceeds a threshold at the extreme end of a more quantitative continuum of changes. This principle needs clarification at both neuropathological and cognitive levels. In terms of cognitive changes, further exploration is necessary of differences between dementia syndromes and the construct of mild cognitive impairment (MCI), particularly whether MCI represents an early or, in some cases, arrested phase in the progression toward eventual dementia (see chap. 1).

   Measurement of reduced regional brain metabolism by positron emission tomography coupled with genetic risk factors and neuropsychological assessment promises to improve early detection (Small 2000). Development of radiotracers may soon allow confirmation of a clinical (cognitive and functional) diagnosis of AD in vivo. Radiotracer analogs of a dye used to stain postmortem amyloid are in development. These techniques could also be used to follow the course of illness in MCI along with the effects of therapeutic agents such as acetylcholinesterase inhibitors (Volkow et al. 2001).
2. *Attention to Confounding Variables.* From a validity perspective, another priority for dementia research should be to increase attention to "confounding" factors. The attention can now move beyond the statistical associations of confounding factors that may influence assessment, to the meaning of how these factors contribute to the expression of cognitive and functional impairment. This should include common comorbid medical and psychiatric conditions, such as depression (Meltzer et al. 1998) and, particularly, the role of cultural diversity, social class, and education (Friedland 1993). The cross-cultural work of Hendrie et al. (2001), for ex-

ample, suggests that there may be modifiable risk factors that interact with genetic predisposition (Farrer 2001).

3. *Functional Impairment and Quality of Life.* A core feature of dementia, functional impairment, including behavioral and emotional changes, has been relatively underresearched. A number of scales have appeared in recent years that improve research capacity to quantify adequately behavioral disturbances among the cognitively impaired, particularly for agitation, psychosis, and depression (Cohen-Mansfield 1986; Merriam et al. 1988; Swearer et al. 1988; Teri et al. 1988; Rosen et al. 1994; Cummings 1997; Kaufer et al. 2000). Despite the emphasis on examining this ecological validity of measures and treatments, a focus on problems encountered in patients' everyday life needs greater attention. Few research efforts have been directed toward developing and refining measures specifically for this purpose and the related assessment of quality of life.

   The difficult assessment of quality of life in persons with dementia is still at an exploratory stage. Progressive, severe cognitive and functional deficits limit the use of available measures and bias our judgment of patients' quality of life with dementia. Nevertheless, research strongly suggests that quality of life for persons with dementia can be reliably elicited from patient proxies (Albert et al. 1996). Measurement of both activity and positive affect suggests that even nonverbal institutionalized persons have positive quality of life aspects.

4. *Biological Markers in Dementia.* Dementia research will conquer its most basic validity issues only by continued investigation of the interrelations among the various neuropathological parameters that characterize dementing diseases, with an emphasis on clarifying cohesive disease entities.

   The most exciting research in this area is the exponential growth in genetic research, particularly in Alzheimer disease. Defects on four genes have been definitively connected to familial forms of AD. A corresponding physiological defect has been associated with each of these (chromosome 21, beta-amyloid precursor protein mutations; chromosome 19, ApoE4 polymorphism; chromosome 14, presenilin 1 mutations; chromosome 1, presenilin 2 mutations). Moreover, a variety of research suggests that each of these defects may have the common effect of altering the production or deposition of beta-amyloid in the brain (Selkoe 2001). There are also genetic conditions resulting in abnormal tau proteins leading to neurofibrillary tangles and dementia. A controversy has existed as to whether tau and neurofibrillary tangles or beta-amyloid and neuritic plaques are the primary pathology in AD (Lee 2001). Understanding the mechanism connecting these two types of lesions is more appropriate than such debates now and could offer new therapeutic options.

The finding that the prevalence of familial forms is low in comparison to sporadic forms has raised challenging issues to genetic research. To some this suggests the need for an expansive search for additional gene defects. Others believe that because of the late onset of AD at the end of the life span, the prevalence of familial genetic abnormalities is falsely low. Because the phenotypic presentation of familial and sporadic forms is so similar, attempts to alter the creation or deposition of toxic forms of beta-amyloid would now seem as important as the discovery of any additional gene defects.

Clinical Conclusions

There are three primary features of all dementing disorders: cognitive impairment, functional impairment, and neuropathology. Making a diagnosis of dementia requires identifying a progressive impairment in both cognition and function. In making a determination of cognitive function, there is no gold standard assessment tool. Greater validity of the determination of impairment is made not from selecting a particular tool but in serial use of the same tool, documenting a deterioration. Becoming familiar with one or two brief assessment tools, knowing their limitations, and using them systematically in a large number of patients should result in improved diagnostic accuracy. The cultural and educational background of a patient can alter the validity of most cognitive tests.

There is also no gold standard assessment of function. Longitudinal knowledge of the patient is required to make a determination in the early stages of dementia. This includes knowledge of the possibility that certain roles may have been occupationally overlearned while others remained unfamiliar. A closely related informant is highly valuable but not infallible.

As with cognition and function, no neuropathological lesion alone can make a diagnosis of dementia. A valid diagnosis includes all three primary features. There remains no reliable laboratory or genetic test. During life, the combined, systematic assessment of both cognition and function is recommended for all older persons. Discriminating among types of dementia, particularly in patients seen outside of specialty clinics, is difficult, but increasingly possible.

ACKNOWLEDGMENT

The author wishes to thank George Niederehe for his inspiration and ideas from the first edition version of this chapter.

REFERENCES

Advisory Panel on Alzheimer's Disease. 1991, 1992. *Third Report of the Advisory Panel on Alzheimer's Disease.* DHHS Publication No. (ADM) 92-1917. Washington, D.C.: U.S. Government Printing Office.

Alafuzoff, L.K., H. Iqbal, R. Friden, et al. 1987. Histopathological criteria for progressive dementia disorders: Clinical-pathological correlation and classification by multivariate data analysis. *Acta Neuropathologica* 74:209–25.

Albert, M.S., and R.K. Heaton. 1988. Intelligence testing. In *Geriatric Neuropsychology,* edited by M.S. Albert and M.B. Moss. New York: Guilford Press, pp. 13–32.

Albert, S.M., C. Castillo-Casteneda, M. Sano, et al. 1996. Quality of life in patients with Alzheimer's disease as reported by patient proxies. *Journal of the American Geriatrics Society* 44:1342–47.

Alexopoulos, G.S. 2001. The depression-executive dysfunction syndrome of late life: A specific target for D3 antagonists. *American Journal of Geriatric Psychiatry* 9:22–29.

American Psychiatric Association. 1994. *Diagnostic and Statistical Manual of Mental Disorders.* 4th ed. Washington, D.C.: American Psychiatric Association.

American Psychiatric Association. 2000. *Diagnostic and Statistical Manual of Mental Disorders.* 4th ed., text revision. Washington, D.C.: American Psychiatric Association.

Ball, M.J., S. Griffin-Brooks, J. MacGregor, et al. 1988. Neuropathological definition of Alzheimer disease: Multivariate analyses in the morphometric distinction between Alzheimer dementia and normal aging. *Alzheimer Disease and Associated Disorders* 2: 29–37.

Bird, H.R., G. Canino, M.R. Stipec, et al. 1987. Use of the Mini Mental State Examination in a probability sample of a Hispanic population. *Journal of Nervous and Mental Disorders* 175:731–37.

Blessed, G., B.E. Tomlinson, and M. Roth. 1968. The associations between quantitative measures of dementia and of senile change in the cerebral grey matter of elderly subjects. *British Journal of Psychiatry* 114:797–811.

Bondareff, W., C.G. Mountjoy, M. Roth, et al. 1987. Age and histopathologic heterogeneity in Alzheimer's disease. Evidence for subtypes. *Archives of General Psychiatry* 44:412–17.

Bozeat S., C.A. Gregory, M.A. Ralph, et al. 2000. Which neuropsychiatric and behavioural features distinguish frontal and temporal variants of frontotemporal dementia from Alzheimer's disease. *Journal of Neurology, Neurosurgery and Psychiatry* 69:178–86.

Braak, H., and E. Braak. 1991. Neuropathological staging of Alzheimer-related changes. *Acta Neuropathologica* 82:239–59.

Chow, T.W., B.L. Miller, V.N. Hayashi, et al. 1999. Inheritance of frontotemporal dementia. *Archives of Neurology* 56:817–22.

Chui, H.C., J.I. Victoroff, D. Margolin, et al. 1992. Criteria for the diagnosis of ischemic vascular dementia proposed by the state of California Alzheimer's Disease Diagnostic and Treatment Centers. *Neurology* 42:473–80.

Clark, C.M., and D.C. Ewbank. 1996. Performance of the Dementia Severity Rating Scale: A caregiver questionnaire for rating severity in Alzheimer disease. *Alzheimer Disease and Associated Disorders* 10:31–39.

Clark, C.M., D. Ewbank, A. Lerner, et al. 1997. The relationship between extrapyramidal signs and cognitive performance in patients with Alzheimer's disease enrolled in the CERAD study. *Neurology* 49:70–75.

Clark, C.M., L. Sheppard, G. Fillenbaum, et al. 1999. Variability in annual Mini-Mental State Examination score in patients with probable Alzheimer disease: A clinical perspective of data from the consortium to establish a registry for Alzheimer's disease. *Archives of Neurology* 56:857–62.

Coffey, C.E., G.S. Fiegel, W.T. Djang, et al. 1990. Subcortical hyperintensity on magnetic resonance imaging: A comparison of normal and depressed elderly subjects. *American Journal of Psychiatry* 147:187–89.

Cohen-Mansfield, J. 1986. Agitated behaviors in the elderly: II. Preliminary results in the cognitively deteriorated. *Journal of the American Geriatrics Society* 34:722–27.

Crook, T.H. 1985. Cognitive assessment in the year 2000. In *Aging 2000: Our Health Care Destiny*, vol. II: *Psychosocial and Policy Issues*, edited by C.M. Gaitz, G. Niederhe, and N.E. Wilson. New York: Springer Verlag, pp. 119–25.

Crook, T. 1987. Dementia. In *Handbook of Clinical Gerontology*, edited by L.L. Cartensen and B.A. Edelstein. New York: Pergamon, pp. 96–111.

Crystal, H., D. Dickson, P. Fuld, et al. 1988. Clinico-pathologic studies in dementia: Nondemented subjects with pathologically confirmed Alzheimer's disease. *Neurology* 38:1682–87.

Cummings, J.L. 1997. The Neuropsychiatric Inventory: Assessing psychopathology in dementia patients. *Neurology* 48 (Suppl. 5):S10–16.

Ditter, S.M., and S.S. Mirra. 1987. Neuropathological and clinical features of Parkinson's disease in Alzheimer's disease patients. *Neurology* 37:754–60.

Duyckaerts, C., J.P. Brion, J.J. Hauw, et al. 1987. Quantitative assessment of the density of neurofibrillary tangles and senile plaques in senile dementia of the Alzheimer type. Comparison of immunocytochemistry with aspecific antibody and Bodian's protargol method. *Acta Neuropathologica* 73 (2):167–70.

Edwards, D.F., and W.L. Danziger. 1982. Congruence between patients and collateral sources in interviews for dementia. *Gerontologist* 22 (5):147.

Escobar, J.I., A. Burnam, M. Karno, et al. 1986. Use of the Mini-Mental State Examination (MMSE) in a community population of mixed ethnicity: Cultural and linguistic artifacts. *Journal of Nervous and Mental Diseases* 174:607–14.

Eslinger, P.J., A.R. Damasio, A.L. Benton, et al. 1985. Neuropsychological detection of abnormal mental decline in older persons. *Journal of the American Medical Association.* 253:670–74.

Evans, D.A., H.H. Funkenstein, M.S. Albert, et al. 1989. Prevalence of Alzheimer's disease in a community population of older persons: Higher than previously reported. *Journal of the American Medical Association* 262:2551–56.

Farrer, L.A. 2000. Familial risk for Alzheimer disease in ethnic minorities: Nondiscriminating genes. *Archives of Neurology* 57:28–29.

Farrer, L.A. 2001. Intercontinental epidemiology of Alzheimer disease: A global approach to bad gene hunting. *Journal of the American Medical Association* 285:796–98.

Fillenbaum, G.G., L. R. Landerman, and E.M. Simonsick. 1998. Equivalence of two screens of cognitive functioning: The Short Portable Mental Status Questionnaire and the Orientation-Memory-Concentration test. *Journal of the American Geriatrics Society* 46:1512–18.

Folstein, M.F., S.A. Folstein, and P.R. McHugh. 1975. Mini-Mental State: A practical method for grading the cognitive state of patients for the clinician. *Journal of Psychiatric Research* 12:189–98.

Folstein, M.F., J.C. Anthony, I. Parhad, et al. 1985. The meaning of cognitive impairment in the elderly. *Journal of the American Geriatrics Society* 33:228–35.

Friedland, R.P. 1993. Epidemiology, education, and the ecology of Alzheimer's disease. *Neurology* 43:246–49.

Gianturco, D.T., and E.W. Busse. 1978. Psychiatric problems encountered during a long-term study of normal aging volunteers. In *Studies in Geriatric Psychiatry*, edited by A.D. Isaacs and F. Post. Chichester, New York, Brisbane: Wiley and Sons, pp. 1–16.

Gifford, D.R., and J.L. Cummings. 1999. Evaluating dementia screening tests: Methodologic standards to rate their performance. *Neurology* 52:224–27.

Gomez-Tortosa, E., K.M. Newell, M.C. Irizarry, et al. 1999. Clinical and quantitative pathologic correlates of dementia with Lewy bodies. *Neurology* 53:1284–91.

Gotz, J., F. Chen, J. van Dorpe, et al. 2001. Formation of neurofibrillary tangles in P301L tau transgenic mice induced by AB42 Fibrils. *Science* 293:1491–95.

Greene, J.G., R. Smith, M. Gardiner, et al. 1982. Measuring behavioral disturbance of elderly demented patients in the community and its effects on relatives: A factor analytic study. *Age and Ageing* 11:121–26.

Gurland, B.J., and Cross, P.S. 1986. Public health perspectives on clinical memory testing of Alzheimer's disease and related disorders. In *Handbook for Clinical Memory Assessment of Older Adults*, edited by L.W. Poon, T. Crook, K.L. Davis, et al. Washington, D.C.: American Psychological Association, pp. 11–20.

Gurland, B.J., D.E. Wilder, R. Lantigua, et al. 2000. Rates of dementia in three ethnoracial groups. *International Journal of Geriatric Psychiatry* 14:481–93.

Hachinski, V.C., L.D. Iliff, E. Zilhka, et al. 1975. Cerebral blood flow on dementia. *Archives of Neurology* 32:632–37.

Hall, K.S., A.O. Ogunniyi, H.C. Hendrie, et al. 1996. A cross-cultural community based study of dementias: Methods and performance of the survey instrument, Indianapolis, USA, and Ibadan, Nigeria. *International Journal of Methods for Psychiatry Research* 6:129–42.

Hall, K.S., S. Gao, C.L. Emsley, et al. 2000. Community Screening Interview for Dementia (CSI "D"): Performance in five disparate study sites. *International Journal of Geriatric Psychiatry* 15:521–31.

Haroutunian, V., M. Serby, D. Purohit, et al. 2000. Contribution of Lewy body inclusions to dementia in patients with and without Alzheimer disease neuropathological conditions. *Archives of Neurology* 57:1145–50.

Hebert, L.E., P.A. Scherr, L.A. Beckett, et al. 1995. Age-specific incidence of Alz-

heimer's disease in a community population. *Journal of the American Medical Association* 273:1354–59.
Henderson, A.S., and A.F. Jorm. 1987. Is case-ascertainment of Alzheimer's disease in field surveys practicable? *Psychological Medicine* 17:549–55.
Hendrie, H.C., K.S. Hall, H.M. Brittain, et al. 1988. The CAMDEX: A standardized instrument for the diagnosis of mental disorder in the elderly: A replication with a US sample. *Journal of the American Geriatric Society* 36:402–8.
Hendrie, H.C., A. Ogunniyi, K.S. Hall, et al. 2001. Incidence of dementia and Alzheimer disease in 2 communities: Yoruba residing in Ibadan, Nigeria, and African Americans residing in Indianapolis, Indiana. *Journal of the American Medical Association* 285:739–47.
Heun, R., W. Maier, and H. Muller. 1997. Subject and informant variables affecting family history diagnoses of depression and dementia. *Psychiatry Research* 71:175–80.
Holzer, C.E. III, G. L. Tischler, P.J. Leaf, et al. 1984. An epidemiologic assessment of cognitive impairment in a community population. In *Research in Community and Mental Health: A Research Annual,* vol. 4, edited by J.R. Greenly. Greenwich, Conn.: JAI Press, pp. 3–32.
Iseki, E., M. Matsushita, K. Kosaka, et al. 1989. Distribution and morphology of brain stem plaques in Alzheimer's disease. *Acta Neuropathologica* 78 (2):131–36.
Iversen, L.L. 1987. Differences between early- and late-onset Alzheimer's disease. *Neurobiology of Aging* 8:554–55.
Jorm, A.F., and P.A. Jacomb. 1989. The informant questionnaire on cognitive decline in the elderly (IQCODE); socio-demographic correlates, reliability, validity and some norms. *Psychological Medicine* 19:1015–22.
Jorm, A.F., and D. Jolley. 1998. The incidence of dementia: A meta-analysis. *Neurology* 51:728–33.
Jorm, A.F., A.E. Korten, and A.S. Henderson. 1987. The prevalence of dementia: A quantitative integration of the literature. *Acta Psychiatrica Scandinavica* 76:465–79.
Jorm, A.F., H. Christensen, A.E. Korten, et al. 2000. Informant ratings of cognitive decline in old age: Validation against change on cognitive tests over 7 to 8 years. *Psychological Medicine* 30:981–85.
Juva, K., M. Makela, T. Erkinjuntti, et al. 1997. Functional assessment scales in detecting dementia. *Age and Ageing* 26:393–400.
Kahn, R.L., A.E. Goldfarb, M. Pollock, et al. 1960. Brief objective measures for the determination of mental status in the elderly. *American Journal of Psychiatry* 117:326–28.
Katzman, R. 1986. Alzheimer's disease. *New England Journal of Medicine* 14:964–73.
Katzman, R., M. Zhang, Q.-Y. Qu, et al. 1988. A Chinese version of the Mini Mental State Examination: Impact of illiteracy in a Shanghai dementia survey. *Journal of Clinical Epidemiology* 41:971–78.
Kaufer, D.I., J.L. Cummings, P. Ketchel, et al. 2000. Validation of the NPI-Q, a brief clinical form of the Neuropsychiatric Inventory. *Journal of Neuropsychiatry and Clinical Neurosciences* 12:233–39.
Kawas, C., J. Segal, W.F. Stewart, et al. 1994. A validation study of the dementia questionnaire. *Archives of Neurology* 51:901–6.
Kempermann, G., and F.H. Gage. 1999. New nerve cells for the adult brain. *Scientific American* 280:48–53.
Khachaturian, Z.S. 1985. Diagnosis of Alzheimer's disease. *Archives of Neurology* 42: 1097–1105.

Lamy, C., C. Duyckaerts, P. Delaere, et al. 1989. Comparison of seven staining methods for senile plaques and neurofibrillary tangles in a prospective series of 15 elderly patients. *Neuropathology and Applied Neurobiology* 15 (6):563–78.

Larson, E.B. 1989. Alzheimer's disease in the community [editorial]. *Journal of the American Medical Association* 262:2591–92.

Lauter, H. 1985. What do we know about Alzheimer's disease today: An overview. *Danish Medical Bulletin.* 32 (Suppl. 1):S1–21.

Lee, V.M.-Y. 2001. Tauists and baptists united. *Science* 293:1446–47.

Lennox, G., J. Lowe, M. Landon, et al. 1989. Diffuse Lewy body disease: Correlative neuropathology using anti-ubiquitin immunocytochemistry. *Journal of Neurology, Neurosurgery, and Psychiatry* 52:1236–47.

Levy, M.L., J.L. Cummings, L.A. Fairbanks, et al. 1996. Longitudinal assessment of symptoms of depression, agitation, and psychosis in 181 patients with Alzheimer's disease. *American Journal of Psychiatry* 153:1438–43.

Lewis, J., D.W. Dickson, L. Wen-Lang, et al. 2001. Enhanced neurofibrillary degeneration in transgenic mice expressing mutant tau and APP. *Science* 293:1487–91.

Liston, E.H., and A. LaRue. 1983. Clinical differentiation of primary degenerative and multi-infarct dementia: A critical review of the evidence. Part I. Clinical studies. Part II. Pathological studies. *Biological Psychiatry* 18:1451–84.

Looi, J.C., and P.S. Sachdev. 2000. Vascular dementia as a frontal subcortical system dysfunction [editorial]. *Psychological Medicine* 30:997–1003.

Lopez-Aqueres, W., B. Kemp, M. Plopper, et al. 1984. Health needs of the Hispanic elderly. *Journal of the American Geriatrics Society* 32:191–98.

Lopez, O.L., S. Wisniewski, R.L. Hamilton, et al. 2000. Predictors of progression in patients with AD and Lewy bodies. *Neurology* 54:1774–79.

Mack, A.J.L., M.B. Patterson, and P.N. Tariot. 1999. Behavior Rating Scale for Dementia: Development of test scales and presentation of data for 555 individuals with Alzheimer's disease. *Journal of Geriatric Psychiatry and Neurology* 12:211–23.

Mackinnon, A., and R. Mulligan. 1998. Combining cognitive testing and informant report to increase accuracy in screening for dementia. *American Journal of Psychiatry* 155:1529–35.

Mandybur, T.I. 1990. The distribution of Alzheimer's neurofibrillary tangles and gliosis in chronic subacute sclerosing panencephalitis. *Acta Neuropathologica* 80:307–10.

Mattis, S. 1976. Mental status examination for organic mental syndrome in the elderly patient. In *Geriatric Psychiatry: A Handbook for Psychiatrists and Primary Care Physicians,* edited by L. Bellak and T.B. Karasu. New York: Grune and Stratton, pp. 77–121.

Mayeux, R., Y. Stern, and S. Spanton. 1985. Heterogeneity in dementia of the Alzheimer type: Evidence of subgroups. *Neurology* 35:453.

McDowell, I., and C. Newell. 1996. *Measuring Health: A Guide to Rating Scales and Questionnaires.* 2nd ed. New York: Oxford University Press.

McKeith, I.G., E.K. Perry, and R.H. Perry. 1999. Report of the second dementia with Lewy body international workshop: Diagnosis and treatment. Consortium on Dementia with Lewy Bodies. *Neurology* 53:902–5.

McKeith, I.G., D. Galasko, K. Kosaka, et al. 1996. Consensus guidelines for the clinical and pathologic diagnosis of dementia with Lewy bodies (DLB): Report of the Consortium on DLB international workshop. *Neurology* 47:1113–24.

McKeith, I.G., C.G. Ballard, R.H. Perry, et al. 2000a. Prospective validation of consensus criteria for the diagnosis of dementia with Lewy bodies. *Neurology* 54 (5):1050–58.

McKeith, I.G., J.B. Grace, Z. Walker, et al. 2000b. Rivastigmine in the treatment of Dementia with Lewy Bodies: Preliminary findings from an open trial. *International Journal of Geriatric Psychiatry* 15:387–92.

McKhann, G., D. Drachman, M. Folstein, et al. 1984. Clinical diagnosis of Alzheimer's disease: Report of the NINCDS-ADRDA Work Group under the auspices of Department of Health and Human Services Task Force on Alzheimer's disease. *Neurology* 35:453.

Meehl, P.E., and A. Rosen. 1955. Antecedent probability and the efficiency of psychometric signs, patterns or cutting scores. *Psychological Bulletin* 52:194–216.

Mega, M.S., D.M. Masterman, S.M. O'Connor, et al. 1999. The spectrum of behavioral responses to cholinesterase inhibitor therapy in Alzheimer disease. *Archives of Neurology* 56:1388–92.

Meltzer, C.C., G. Smith, S.T. DeKosky, et al. 1998. Serotonin in aging, late-life depression, and Alzheimer's disease: The emerging role of functional imaging. *Neuropsychopharmacology* 18:407–30.

Merriam, A.E., M.K. Aronson, P. Gaston, et al. 1988. The psychiatric symptoms of Alzheimer's disease. *Journal of the American Geriatrics Society* 36:7–12.

Mirra, S.S., A. Heyman, D. McKeel, et al. 1991. The Consortium to Establish a Registry for Alzheimer's Disease (CERAD), part II: Standardization of the neuropathologic assessment of Alzheimer's disease. *Neurology* 41:479–86.

Molsa, P.K., E. Sako, L. Paljarvi, et al. 1987. Alzheimer's disease: Neuropathological correlates of cognitive and motor disorders. *Acta Neurologica Scandinavica* 75: 376–84.

Morales, J.M., F. Bermejo, M. Romero, et al. 1997. Screening of dementia in community-dwelling elderly through informant report. *International Journal of Geriatric Psychiatry* 12:808.

Morris, J.C. 1997. Clinical dementia rating: A reliable and valid diagnostic and staging measure for dementia of the Alzheimer type. *International Psychogeriatrics* 9 (Suppl. 1): S173–76.

Mortimer, J.A., B. Ebbitt, S.P. Jun, et al. 1992. Predictors of cognitive and functional progression in patients with probable Alzheimer's disease. *Neurology* 42:1689–96.

National Institute on Aging and Regan Institute Working Group on Diagnostic Criteria for the Neuropathological Assessment of Alzheimer's Disease. 1997. Consensus recommendations for the postmortem diagnosis of Alzheimer's disease. *Neurobiology of Aging* 18 (Suppl. 4):S1–2.

Neri, M., M. Roth, S. Ruichi, et al. 2001. The validity of informant report for grading the severity of Alzheimer's dementia. *Aging* (Milano) 13:22–29.

Niederehe, G. 1988a. Assessment of the aged by relatives or significant others. *Psychopharmacology Bulletin* 24:595–600.

Niederehe, G. 1988b. TRIMS Behavioral Problem Checklist. *Psychopharmacology Bulletin* 24:771–78.

Niederehe, G., and J. Scott. 1987. Psychological and family factors influencing caregiver stress senile dementia. *The Southwestern: The Journal of Aging for the Southwest* 4:48–58.

Nunnally, J.C. 1978. *Psychometric Theory.* 2nd ed. New York: McGraw-Hill.

Oxman, T.E., P.M. Silberfarb, and P.P. Schnurr. 1986. Assessment of cognitive function in cancer patients. *Hospice Journal* 2:99–128.

Perry, R.H., D. Irving, G. Blessed, et al. 1990. Senile dementia of Lewy body type: A clinically and neuropathologically distinct form of Lewy body dementia in the elderly. *Journal of Neurological Science* 95:119–39.

Pfeiffer, E. 1975. A short portable mental status questionnaire for the assessment of organic brain deficit in elderly patients. *Journal of the American Geriatrics Society* 23 (10): 433–31.

Roman, G. C., T.K. Tatemichi, T. Erkinjuntti, et al. 1993. Vascular dementia: Diagnostic criteria for research studies: Report of the NINDS-AIREN International Workshop. *Neurology* 43:250–60.

Rosen, J., L.M. Burgio, M. Kollar, et al. 1994. The Pittsburgh Agitation Scale: A user-friendly instrument for rating agitation in dementia patients. *American Journal of Geriatric Psychiatry* 2:60–74.

Roth, M. 1985. Some strategies for tackling the problems of senile dementia and related disorders within the next decade. *Danish Medical Bulletin* 32 (Suppl. 1):S92–111.

Roth, M., E. Tym, C.Q. Mountjor, et al. 1986. CAMDEX: A standardized instrument for the diagnosis of mental disorders in the elderly with special reference to the early detection of dementia. *British Journal of Psychiatry* 149:698–709.

Sano, M., C. Ernesto, R.G. Thomas, et al. 1997. A controlled trial of selegiline, alpha-tocopherol, or both as treatment for Alzheimer's disease. The Alzheimer's Disease Cooperative Study. *New England Journal of Medicine* 336 (17):1216–22.

Scanlan, J., and S. Borson. 2001. The Mini-Cog: Receiver operating characteristics with expert and naïve raters. *International Journal of Geriatric Psychiatry* 16 (2):216–22.

Schmitt, F.A., D.G. Davis, D.R. Wekstein, et al. 2000. Preclinical AD revisited: Neuropathology of cognitively normal older adults. *Neurology* 55:37–376.

Selkoe, D.J. 2001. Alzheimer's disease: Genes, proteins, and therapy. *Physiological Reviews* 81:741–66.

Siegler, I.C., and L.W. Poon. 1989. The psychology of aging. In *Geriatric Psychiatry*, edited by E.W. Busse and D.G. Blazer. Washington, D.C.: American Psychiatric Press, pp. 163–202.

Small, G.W. 2000. Investigations into geriatric psychiatry. *American Journal of Geriatric Psychiatry* 8:276–83.

Snowdon, D.A. 1997. Aging and Alzheimer's disease: Lessons from the Nun Study. *The Gerontologist* 37:150–56.

Solomon, P.R., and W.W. Pendlebury. 1998. Recognition of Alzheimer's disease: The 7 Minute Screen. *Family Medicine* 30:265–71.

Storandt, M., J. Botwinick, W.L. Danziger, et al. 1984. Psychometric differentiation of mild senile dementia of the Alzheimer type. *Archives of Neurology* 41:497–99.

Sulkava, R. 1983. Accuracy of clinical diagnosis in primary degenerative dementia: Correlation with neuropathological findings. *Journal of Neurology, Neurosurgery, and Psychiatry* 46:9–13.

Sulkava, R., J. Wikstrom, A. Aromaa, et al. 1985. Prevalence of severe dementia in Finland. *Neurology* 35:1025–29.

Swearer, J.M., D.A. Drachman, B.F. O'Donnell, et al. 1988. Troublesome and disruptive behaviors in dementia: Relationships to diagnosis and disease severity. *Journal of the American Geriatrics Society* 36:1 6.

Tekin, S., L.A. Fairbanks, S. O'Connor, et al. 2001. Activities of daily living in Alzheimer's disease: Neuropsychiatric, cognitive, and medical illness influences. *American Journal of Geriatric Psychiatry* 9:81–86

Teri, L., and R.G. Logsdon. 1991. Identifying pleasant activities for Alzheimer's disease patients: The Pleasant Events Schedule-AD. *The Gerontologist* 31:124–27.

Teri, L., E.B. Larson, and B.V. Reifler. 1988. Behavioral disturbance in dementia of the Alzheimer's type. *Journal of the American Geriatrics Society* 36:1–6.

Tierney, M.C., J.P. Szalai, W.G. Snow, et al. 1996. The prediction of Alzheimer disease. The role of patient and informant perceptions of cognitive deficits. *Archives of Neurology* 53:423–27.

Tomlinson, B.E. 1977. The pathology of dementia. In *Dementia*, 2nd ed., edited by C.E. Wells. Philadelphia: F.A. Davis, pp. 113–53.

Tschanz, J.T., K.A. Welsh-Bohmer, I. Skook, et al. 2000. Dementia diagnoses from clinical and neuropsychological data compared: The Cache County study. *Neurology* 54: 1290–96.

Unverzagt, F.W., K.S. Hall, A.M. Torke, et al. 1996. Effect of age, education, and gender on CERAD neuropsychological test performance in an African-American sample. *Clinical Neuropsychology* 10:180–90.

U.S. Congress, Office of Technology Assessment. 1987. *Losing a Million Minds: Confronting the Tragedy of Alzheimer's Disease and Other Dementias.* OTA-BA-323. Washington, D.C.: U.S. Government Printing Office.

Valle, R., R. Hough, B. Kolody, et al. 1991. The Validation of the Blessed Mental Status Test and Mini-Mental Status Examination with an Hispanic Population. Final report submitted to the National Institute of Mental Health on research grant No. R01 MH43390, Hispanic Alzheimer's Research Project (HARP), San Diego State University.

Volkow, N.D., Y.S. Ding, J.S. Fowler, et al. 2001. Imaging brain cholinergic activity with positron emission tomography: Its role in the evaluation of cholinergic treatments in Alzheimer's dementia. *Biological Psychiatry* 49:211–20.

Wade, J.P.H., T.R. Mirsen, V.C. Hachinski, et al. 1987. The clinical diagnosis of Alzheimer's disease. *Archives of Neurology* 44:24–29.

Waite, L., D. Grayson, A.F. Jorm, et al. 1999. Informant-based staging of dementia using the clinical dementia rating. *Alzheimer Disease and Associated Disorders* 13:34–37.

World Health Organization. 1993. *The ICD-10 Classification of Mental and Behavioral Disorders: Diagnostic Criteria for Research.* Geneva: World Health Organization.

Xuereb, J.H., C. Brayne, C. Dufouil, et al. 2000. Neuropathological findings in the very old: Results from the first 101 brains of a population-based longitudinal study of dementing disorders. *Annals of the New York Academy of Sciences* 903:490–96.

Zarit, S., H., K.E. Reever, and J. Bach-Peterson. 1980. Relatives of the impaired elderly: Correlates of feelings of burden. *Gerontologist* 20:649–55.

Zubenko, G.S. 1990. Progression of illness in the differential diagnosis of primary dementia. *American Journal of Psychiatry* 147:435–38.

Zubenko, G.S., P. Sullivan, J.P. Nelson, et al. 1990. Brain imaging abnormalities in mental disorders of late life. *Archives of Neurology* 47:1107–11.

Zweig, R.M., C.A. Ross, J.C. Hedreen, et al. 1988. The neuropathology of aminergic nuclei in Alzheimer's disease. *Annals of Neurology* 24:233–42.

CHAPTER THREE

Diagnostic Procedures for Dementia

Christopher J. Patterson, M.D., FRCP(C), and A. Marc Clarfield, M.D., FCPC, FRCP

> The skillful doctor knows what is wrong by observing alone.
>
> CHANG CHUNG-CHING, C. 150 CE

> Diseases can be diagnosed from the specific character of the symptoms of each.
>
> GALEN, 130–200 CE

Making a diagnosis of dementia is the essential first step in the long and often difficult process of helping individuals and their caregivers to deal with the illness. There are several diagnostic systems for definitions of dementia. The DSM-IV criteria (American Psychiatric Association 1994) (tab. 3.1) have good to very good reliability (K 0.5 to 0.9) (Fratiglioni et al. 1992; Graham et al. 1996; Larson et al. 1996) and are widely accepted. Despite the advantage of precise, clearly defined, comprehensive criteria such as in DSM-IV, when clinicians are using different diagnostic criteria on the same population (in this case, the participants in the Canadian Study of Health and Aging), a striking difference in prevalence results (between 3.1% and 29%) (Erkinjuntti et al. 1997). Furthermore, most clinicians do not use formal diagnostic criteria. Only 25% of American physicians (Somerfield et al. 1991) and 11% of British consultants (Smith et al. 1992) surveyed used diagnostic criteria for dementia. Therefore, clinicians are likely to adopt a simpler rather than a more complex definition. We favor this simplified definition of dementia (Patterson et al. 2001):

- an acquired syndrome
- cognitive deficits (memory plus others)

Table 3.1. DSM-IV criteria for dementia

A. The development of multiple cognitive deficits manifested by both
   1. Memory impairment (impairment ability to learn new information or to recall previously learned information)
   2. One (or more) of the following cognitive disturbances:
      a. aphasia
      b. apraxia
      c. agnosia
      d. disturbances in executive functioning
B. The cognitive deficits in criteria A1 and A2 each cause significant impairment in social or occupational functioning and represent a significant decline from a previous level of functioning.
C. The deficits do not occur exclusively during the course of a delirium.
D. The disturbance is not better accounted for by another axis I disorder (e.g., major depressive disorder, schizophrenia).

Source: Adapted from DSM-IV.

- sufficient to interfere with social or occupational functioning
- deficits not due to clouding of consciousness or depression

Cultural differences can complicate the perception, definition, and diagnosis of dementia. For example, in some societies the very concept of dementia does not exist, as changes in cognition with increasing age may be attributed to normal aging (Herbert 2001).

Most clinicians use a Bayesian approach to make a diagnosis. This involves a conscious or unconscious appreciation of pretest probability and the application of a diagnostic test that results in a final or post-test probability of disease. In the general population, the pretest probability of dementia can be considered equal to the population prevalence. In specific populations (such as residents of long-term care facilities), the pretest probability equals the prevalence in that setting. The prevalence of dementia rises strikingly with age. Although 8–10% of individuals over age 65 have dementia, the syndrome is rare before the age of 65 and extremely common by the ninth decade. Based on a meta-analysis of population-based studies in the Western world (Ritchie, Kildea, and Robine 1992), figure 3.1 shows the age-related prevalence of dementia. For example, in Canada, the prevalence of dementia rises from 2.4% at ages 65–74 through 11.1% at ages 75–84 and reaches 34.5% by age 85 (Canadian Study of Health and Aging 1994). There are differences in prevalence among racial groups. For example, the prevalence in white North Americans is lower than that in black North Americans (Froelich, Bogardus, and Inouye 2001), and black Africans have a lower incidence and prevalence than African Americans (Hendrie et al. 1995, 2001). Within institutions, the prevalence is about 50% regardless of age (Canadian Study of Health and Aging 1994; Magaziner et al. 2000).

Knowledge of the pretest probability (or pretest odds) and the characteristics of the diagnostic test, specifically the likelihood ratio, enables one to establish the diagnostic probability (post-test probability or post-test odds) with considerable confidence (McGee 2001): pretest odds × likelihood ratio = post-test odds. For example, if a 75-year-old sighted person in otherwise good health is unable to draw an accurate clock face, the probability of dementia is calculated as follows: community prevalence of dementia at age 75 = 11% (odds ratio 1:9); the likelihood ratio of inability to draw an accurate clock face is 24 (Siu 1991). The post-test odds become 24:9, or about 2.7:1 (73%).

This simple test, therefore, raises the probability of dementia considerably. The same positive test when applied to a 65-year-old, however (prevalence 1–2%: odds ratio 1:100), is not helpful in establishing a diagnosis, as the post-test probability becomes only 24% (odds ratio 24:100). These examples illustrate a process that is frequently undertaken by clinicians without conscious deliberation. Table 3.2 shows some examples of likelihood ratios for specific tests.

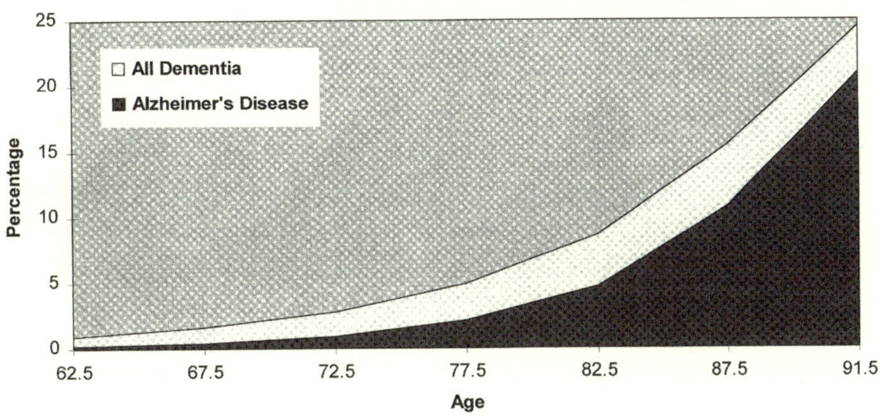

Figure 3.1. Community prevalence of dementia, based on a meta-analysis by Ritchie et al. 1992 (DSM-III criteria)

Table 3.2. Likelihood ratio of simple tests for dementia

Item	Likelihood Ratio If Abnormal	Likelihood Ratio If Normal
Orientation to month*	16	0.4
Orientation to year*	37	0.5
Clock drawing*	24	0.2
Recall of one or zero out of three objects*	3.1	
Recall of three out of three objects*		0.06
MMSE score		
20 or less**	14.5	
21–25**	2.2	
26 or more**	0.1	

*Siu 1991.
**McGee 2001.

Diagnosing Causes of Dementia

Unfortunately, there is no gold standard for the diagnosis of dementia. There are, however, gold standards for the diagnosis of certain causes of dementia, notably, specific neuropathological changes (e.g., for Alzheimer disease, vascular dementia, frontotemporal degeneration, and spongiform encephalopathy). The diagnostic accuracy of clinical criteria can therefore be validated against neuropathological examination.

Alzheimer Disease

Alzheimer disease (AD) is the most common etiology for dementia in the Western world, accounting for 60% or more of cases. It is characterized by a slowly progressive neurodegenerative process and is the archetype for dementia. In the typical case, initial symptoms usually involve loss of memory (especially short-term) and then language (usually retrieval of unfamiliar words and names). These cognitive changes are accompanied by progressive impairments in functional ability. Higher functions (e.g., instrumental activities, such as managing finances, driving, complex tasks), agnosias, apraxias, and sequencing abilities affect executive function and eventually lead to loss of functional autonomy. Loss of more basic activities such as bathing, dressing, and continence follows, often with behavioral abnormalities. These include apathy, aggression, and disinhibition. In the final stages of the disease, motor changes such as rigidity and flexion contractures often precede death. While it was commonly believed that the *average* duration of AD is in the region of six to ten years (Walsh,

Welch, and Lawson 1990), recent evidence suggests that it may be as short as three years (Wolfson et al. 2001). The onset of dementia may be preceded by mild cognitive deficits (see below) or affective changes (Schofield et al. 1997). Depressive symptoms occurring late in life are associated with a twofold risk of developing AD within the next three years (Berger et al. 1999).

Clinical criteria for dementia of the Alzheimer type (DSM-IIIR and DSM-IV) (American Psychiatric Association 1987, 1994) and the NINCDS-ADRDA criteria for probable Alzheimer disease (McKhann et al. 1984) have a sensitivity from 49% to 100% (average 81%) when compared with neuropathological confirmation. The specificity ranges from 47% to 100% (average 70%) (Galasko et al. 1994; Jobst, Barnetson, and Shepstone, 1998; Lim et al. 1999). This indicates that clinical criteria, especially in the setting of dementia clinics, are acceptably accurate for the diagnosis of AD.

Vascular Dementia

Vascular dementia (VaD) is commonly considered to be the second most prevalent type of dementia, and in some societies, such as China and Japan, the prevalence approaches that of Alzheimer disease (Fratiglioni, DeRonchi, and Agüero-Torres 1999). The diagnostic criteria for VaD must be considered in the context of recent evidence that challenges the paradigm of a sharp distinction between AD and VaD. Autopsy series from dementia clinics have revealed that "pure" VaD is extremely uncommon (Nolan et al. 1998). In one study, a cohort of Catholic nuns have been carefully followed over many years, with sequential cognitive testing and ultimately brain autopsy examination. Findings from this study have revealed that the distinction between AD and VaD is far from clear (Snowdon et al. 1997). To add to the complexity of the issue, many individuals who showed no signs of cognitive deterioration during life had definite neuropathological evidence of AD. The presence of even a single lacunar infarction increased the likelihood of clinical dementia by an odds ratio of 20 (Snowdon et al. 1997). Most authorities now consider "mixed" dementia (where AD and cerebrovascular disease coexist) to be the second most common etiology for dementia. "Pure" VaD is uncommon, with a community prevalence of 9–10% of dementia cases (Jobst, Barnetson, and Shepstone 1998; Lim et al. 1999).

Clinical diagnostic criteria for vascular dementia include the "California criteria" (Chui et al. 1992), the National Institute of Neurological Disease and Stroke and the Association Internationale pour la Recherche et l'Enseignement en Neurosciences (NINDS-AIREN) criteria (Roman, Tatemichi, Erkinjuntti et al. 1993), the Hachinski Ischemic Score (Hachinski, Lassen, and Marshall 1974; Rosen et al. 1980), and DSM-IV (American Psychiatric Association 1994). The NINDS-AIREN criteria have a sensitivity of 43% and specificity of 95% for VaD (Holmes et al. 1999). When compared with the other criteria, the Hachinski Ischemic Score, with a sensitivity and specificity both of 89%, appears to perform better than the other instruments (Moroney et al. 1997).

Dementia with Lewy Bodies

Dementia with Lewy bodies (DLB) is a dementing syndrome increasingly recognized in recent years. It is characterized by hallucinations and delusions occurring early (versus late in AD), marked day-to-day fluctuations, spontaneous Parkinsonism, and neuroleptic sensitivity (McKeith et al. 1996). In this condition, Lewy bodies, the pathological hallmark of Parkinson disease usually concentrated in the substantia nigra, are distributed throughout the cortices (Mega et al. 1996). The potential harm from prescribing neuroleptic drugs, and recent observations that cholinesterase inhibitors are beneficial (McKeith et al. 2000a), have driven clinicians to attempt identification of this syndrome more accurately. Unfortunately, the distinction between AD and DLB is often difficult, and pathological studies have revealed the presence of Lewy bodies in as many as 20% of AD cases coming to autopsy (Gearing et al. 1995). Recently published clinical criteria for DLB revealed that, when compared to neuropathological findings, the sensitivity was only 22% but specificity was 100% (Holmes et al. 1999). Revised criteria appear somewhat better (McKeith et al. 2000b). The presence of visual hallucinations and agnosia early in the course of a dementing illness appear to be the most helpful phenomena to distinguish DLB from AD.

Frontotemporal Dementia

Frontotemporal dementia (FTD) describes a spectrum of degenerative conditions that includes Pick disease and related conditions (Brun 1993). Characteristically, in contrast to both AD and VaD, individuals with FTD experience decline in executive functions *before* significant memory loss, and often experience language involvement affecting fluency, naming, and abstraction. The Lund-Manchester criteria (Lund and Manchester Groups 1994) and Consensus Diagnostic criteria for FTD (Neary et al. 1998) are the most well established criteria for FTD. While no clinical features reliably identify individuals with pathologically verified FTD, the Frontal Behavioral Inventory is a clinical tool that helps to distinguish FTD from AD (Kertesz, Davidson, and Fox 1997).

Creutzfeldt-Jakob Disease

Creutzfeldt-Jakob disease (CJD) is a rare, rapidly progressive neurological condition due to spongiform encephalopathy and related to "mad cow disease." Clinical criteria have been suggested based on the presence of abnormal movements, rapid clinical course, and characteristic EEG pattern (Brown et al. 1986). These criteria were accurate in 97% of neuropathologically proven cases (Poser et al. 1999). A cerebrospinal fluid protein 14-3-3 has high sensitivity and specificity for the diagnosis of CJD and is now recommended for confirmation of diagnosis (Knopman et al. 2001).

Important Conditions to Consider in the Differential Diagnosis of Dementia

Mild Cognitive Impairment

Epidemiological and longitudinal studies have confirmed that a prodromal stage of mild cognitive deficits precedes the onset of Alzheimer disease by several years (Ritchie et al. 1996). However, the presence of these mild deficits is not confined to those who are destined to develop dementia. It is important but often difficult to distinguish those who have what is increasingly designated mild cognitive impairment (MCI) (WHO 1993), with a 5–15% annual risk of developing AD, from those who have age-associated memory impairment (AAMI) (Crook et al. 1986), which is not considered to be progressive. The characteristics of MCI include memory complaints by the individual or observer, objective changes in memory but without evidence of diffuse cognitive impairments, and no significant decline in the ability to perform normal daily occupational or social function (Peterson et al. 1999). Distinguishing between this condition, normal aging, and dementia is a major challenge and an area of vigorous research. (See chap. 1.)

Depression

Depressive symptoms are extremely common in older individuals, and major affective disorder shares many features with dementia (Thorpe and Groulx 2001). While dementia and depression commonly coexist (see chaps. 14 and 15), an individual who is profoundly depressed may exhibit apathy, confusion, and complaints about memory and other cognitive functions. Daily functioning may be affected, and self-neglect may occur.

In the systematic review by Clarfield (1988), depression was one of the three main causes of "reversible" dementia. Clues to the presence of depression include prominent complaints about memory, "don't know" rather than "near miss" responses to mental status examination questions, flat affect, avoidance of eye contact, multiple somatic complaints, and pervasive anhedonia. Some older individuals will deny depression but admit to feeling despondent or downhearted. Instruments such as the Geriatric Depression Scale (Yesavage et al. 1982) and the Cornell Depression Scale (Alexopolous et al. 1998) are helpful in establishing a diagnosis of depression.

Metabolic Disturbances

The second group of disorders that may present with cognitive deficits resembling dementia are metabolic abnormalities. These include organ failure (cardiac, pulmonary, hepatic, and renal), single chemical abnormalities (e.g., hypercalcemia, hypothyroidism, malnutrition such as pellagra), and many others. These disorders can generally be detected by history, examination, and basic laboratory tests.

Side Effects of Medication

A wide variety of medications have been associated with central nervous system side effects, including cognitive deficits that can be mistaken for dementia. While not exhaustive, table 3.3 lists some of the medications that have commonly been associated with cognitive impairments. Withdrawal of the putative culprit drug(s) should be considered in an individual with a dementia syndrome.

Central Nervous System Infections

Overall, human immunodeficiency virus-acquired immune deficiency syndrome is still an uncommon cause of dementia, especially in older persons. However, the AIDS dementia complex does occur in 50–70% of people with clinical AIDS (McArthur 1987). Of these, up to 25% may have cognitive impairment or behavioral changes as the first manifestation of the disease. With the increasing incidence of AIDS in people without traditional risk factors, a high index of suspicion should be observed regarding individuals with a rapidly progressive cause, particularly those who are younger (Powell, Coyne, and Jen 1993). (See chap. 13.)

Table 3.3. Common medications that can cause cognitive impairment

Drug Group	Example
Anxiolytic-sedative-hypnotics	Benzodiazepines: diazepam, flurazepam, chlordiazepoxide, triazolam
Antidepressants	Amitriptyline, doxepin, desipramine, nortriptyline
	Tricyclic withdrawal
	Trazodone
	Monoamine oxidase inhibitors
	Selective serotonin reuptake inhibitors (esp. by syndrome of inappropriate antidiuretic hormone)
Antipsychotics	Phenothiazines
Lithium	Enhanced by diuretics
	Combined with loxapine
Antihypertensives	Reserpine, methyldopa, clonidine
Diuretics	Thiazides (esp. in hepatic cirrhosis or with digoxin)
	Acetozoleamide
Beta-adrenergic blockers	Propranalol
Calcium channel blockers	Diltiazem, verapamil
Digoxin	Digoxin excess; digoxin at therapeutic levels
Antiarrhythmics	Disopyramide, quinidine, procainamide, amiodarone
Anticonvulsants	Phenytoin, carbamazepine, phenobarbitone, Valproic acid
Anticholinergics	Antispasmodics (e.g., dicyclomine, oxybutinin)
	Antihistamines
Dopaminergics	Bromocriptine, amantadine, L-dopa, selegiline
Gastric motility enhancer	Metaclopamide
H-2 blocking agents	Cimetidine, ranitidine
Adrenergic agents	Salbutamol (oral)
Nonsteroidal anti-inflammatory drugs	Indomethacin, naproxen, ibuprofen, tiaprofenic acid
	COX-II inhibitors
Opiates	Pentazocine, meperidine
Corticosteroids	All
Antibiotics	Tetracycline, ciprofloxacin
Immunosuppressive	Cyclosporine, gold

Neurosyphilis remains a rare cause of dementia, but is increasingly prevalent in the immunosuppressed population. Early neurosyphilis may present with abnormal behaviors or an epileptic syndrome with memory loss. Late neurosyphilis, occurring ten to fifteen years after primary infection, is characterized by parenchymal involvement of the brain with progressive frontal lobe type dementia, personality changes, and ultimately general paralysis. The diagnosis is supported by abnormal pupillary reflexes and symptoms of tabes dorsalis. In the absence of neurological signs or a positive VDRL, lumbar puncture is unlikely to be helpful (Hammerstrom and Zimmer 1985).

Rare or opportunistic infections such as Whipple disease, Behçet, and various other fungal or parasitic meningitides occasionally present as dementia. They usually have features that are not typical of AD, which would trigger more extensive investigations even if the selective approach offered here is followed.

Clinical History and Examination

Clinical history, supported by collaborative information from family or caregivers, is the cornerstone of making a dementia diagnosis. In one series, the diagnosis of dementia was established by history in nearly 90% of cases (Larson et al. 1986). A caregiver's report that the patient's memory has declined within the past year is particularly helpful, although not conclusive (Morris 1993; Hogan and Ebly 2000). Features that should be explored include the onset, progression, and duration of symptoms. Cognitive changes (memory, word-finding difficulties, executive functioning, especially problems with instrumental activities of daily living), behavioral changes (especially social withdrawal, apathy, disinhibition, or aggression), and functional autonomy are areas to explore. Special attention should be paid to any history of executive dysfunction, with difficulties in areas such as ability to pay bills and management of financial affairs, planning meals, organizing shopping, driving, and the ability to perform manual tasks, hobbies, and other previously accomplished functions (Chertkow et al. 2001). The clinician should seek a history of risk factors for dementia, including alcohol excess, head injury, positive family history, hypertension, depression, and psychiatric symptoms such as hallucinations and delusions.

Physical Examination

The first purpose of physical examination is to discover any systemic disease that may aggravate, contribute to, or even cause cognitive dysfunction. The second purpose is to determine whether any such comorbid illness may be influencing the quality of life of the individual. The third purpose is to determine whether neurological signs can help refine the diagnosis.

Systemic illness such as cardiac failure, chronic liver disease, or hypothyroidism may contribute to cognitive dysfunction by impairing attention, concentration, and memory. While they are not considered "reversible" causes of dementia, their presence and severity may influence mental status, and treatment of the primary condition may improve cognitive function. Painful illnesses (e.g., arthritis) and conditions that disturb sleep (e.g., nocturia, fecal impaction, nocturnal dyspnea sleep apnea) may influence cognition, and quality of life may be improved by appropriate management.

Neurological examination should seek findings that point to specific diagnoses. For example, the presence of papilledema and focal signs may indicate tumor; extrapyramidal signs may point to DLB or Parkinson disease; prominent primitive reflexes (grasp, snout, palmar-mental) appearing early may indicate FTD; ataxia and proprioceptive loss suggest vitamin B_{12} deficiency; prominent increased lower limb tone, pathologically brisk reflexes, and apraxic gait may point to frontal pathology such as normal pressure hydrocephalus or periventricular vascular disease.

Neurological signs of Alzheimer disease may include impaired sense of smell, cortical sensory signs, rigidity, hesitant gait, and primitive reflexes. Unfortunately, these signs usually occur relatively late in the disease and lack the sensitivity and specificity to aid in diagnosis (Galasko et al. 1990; Franssen et al. 1991).

Mental Status Examination

Simple office-based mental status examination is enormously useful and an integral part of dementia assessment. Short screening instruments are widely used. The Mini-Mental State Examination (MMSE) has been most extensively studied (Folstein, Folstein, and McHugh 1975). Age- and culture-specific norms have been established (Crum et al. 1993; Grigoletto et al. 1999) and a standardized version offers improved reliability (Molloy, Alemayehu, and Roberts 1991). The MMSE contains thirty items and takes about ten minutes to complete. Although it examines immediate recall, orientation to time and place, attention/concentration, and some items of language and praxis, it is insensitive to changes in executive function or to psychotic or behavioral symptoms. These areas must be explored separately. Thus, while the overall sensitivity and specificity of the MMSE for diagnosing dementia are around 82% (Tombaugh and McIntyre 1992), individuals with early FTD and those with AD who have a high IQ and are well educated may score well into the "normal" range. The cut point at which sensitivity and specificity are optimal is 24/30. Other short instruments have been developed for brief mental status screening, but none is as well established as the MMSE.

The clock-drawing test is particularly interesting as it is quick, sensitive to changes in executive function, and often used together with the Mini-Mental State Examination. There are several different scoring systems, but for screening purposes a "normal" versus "abnormal" clock face is sufficient (Siu 1991). Other scoring methods allow for a much wider range of interpretations (Freedman et al. 1994).

When there is doubt about the diagnosis or when an individual is employed and occupational abilities need to be assessed, full neuropsychological testing is indicated. This is usually carried out by a trained psychologist or psychometrician. While full testing is valuable in specific cases, it is lengthy, expensive, and often exhausting to the recipient. Outside the research and academic setting, neuropsychological testing is best reserved for the specific indications noted above.

Laboratory Investigations

The focus of laboratory investigations has changed in recent years. The original intent was to rule out "reversible" causes of dementia. This was based on the belief that up to 20% of individuals with the clinical syndrome of dementia had reversible causes (Wells 1978). More recent evidence has changed this perception. A systematic review of published studies in 1988 (Clarfield 1988) revealed that only 3% of dementia cases in the world literature were fully reversible. More recent reviews and meta-analyses suggest that the true risk of fully reversible dementias may be even lower (Weytingh, Bossuyt, and van Crevel 1995). In no way does this limit the importance of searching for comorbid illnesses, as their treatment may improve quality of life, even if it does not reverse the cognitive deficits. For this reason, most evidence-based guidelines now recommend a limited number of laboratory tests for *all* individuals presenting with dementia (tab. 3.4) with other tests reserved for selected cases. However, not all authorities endorse this selective approach, and some consensus panels recommend a more comprehensive list of routine investigations.

One test for which controversy abounds is the serum vitamin B_{12} level. While vitamin B_{12} deficiency was once considered a cardinal example of reversible dementia, this is not borne out by the literature. Vitamin B_{12} deficiency is common in older people (Pennypacker et al. 1992), and persons with low levels of serum B_{12} have slightly lower cognitive scores than replete individuals (Bernard, Nakonezny, and Kashner 1998). However, evidence that replacement

Table 3.4. Selective approach to laboratory tests, to be used in all cases of suspected dementia

Laboratory Test	Comments
Complete blood count	Anemia, macrocytosis
Glucose	Diabetes; hyper/hypoglycemia
Electrolytes	Dehydration; hyponatremia (e.g., syndrome of inappropriate antidiuretic hormone)
	Hyper/hypokalemia
Thyroid-stimulating hormone	Hypothyroidism*
	Thyrotoxicosis
Calcium	Hypercalcemia (e.g., hyperparathyroidism, malignancy), hypocalcemia
B_{12}**	Deficiency as a cause for neurological/cognitive changes

*Only fair evidence that hypothyroidism causes reversible dementia (Clarnette and Patterson 1994).
**Recommended by some, but not all, authorities.

of vitamin B_{12} in individuals with dementia reverses or improves the dementia is limited (Healton et al. 1991; Martin et al. 1992; Cunha et al. 1995; Teunisse et al. 1996). The high prevalence of the condition, potential neurological sequelae of continued deficiency, and the presence of deficiency in the absence of hematological changes argue for the inclusion of this test in the routine laboratory screening panel. The next concern is the "normal" range of serum B_{12}. More sensitive measures of deficiency (e.g., methyl malonic acid, serum homocysteine levels) suggest that many individuals may have deficiency at the cellular level despite serum B_{12} levels that fall in the "normal" reference range. Some authorities would consider measurement of metabolites to investigate deficiency at serum levels below 250 pg/mL (Green and Kinsella 1995).

For Creutzfeldt-Jakob disease, an assay for the 14-3-3 protein (Moussavian, Potolicchio, and Jones 1997) in the cerebrospinal fluid appears highly sensitive (96%) and specific (99%) for the diagnosis (Hsich et al. 1996). False positives can occur with acute neurological conditions (e.g., stroke, viral encephalitis, paraneoplastic syndromes). This test is now recommended for confirming or rejecting the diagnosis of CJD when clinically suspected (Knopman et al. 2001).

A specific laboratory test for Alzheimer disease would be highly desirable. Reduced levels of the β-amyloid 1-42 fragment have been observed in the cerebrospinal fluid of individuals with AD when compared to normal controls (Andreasen et al. 1999a). In contrast, levels of tau are often elevated in the cerebrospinal fluid of individuals with AD (Galasko et al. 1997; Kurz et al. 1998; Andreasen et al. 1999b). The combination of reduced β-amyloid 1-42 and elevated levels of tau is particularly promising (Galasko et al. 1998; Hulstaert et al. 1999). While not recommended at this point for routine testing, absolute levels of these analytes or the ratio between them may in the future provide for more specific diagnostic testing for AD.

Genetic Testing

Individuals who have a first-degree relative with Alzheimer disease have two- to fourfold increase in their risk for the disease (Van Duijn, Clayton, and Chandra 1991; Blacker and Tanzi 1998). There are rare families in which an autosomal dominant transmission of AD occurs. These families possess one of several deterministic gene aberrations that lead to dementia occurring in middle age (Blacker and Tanzi 1998). By the age of 40, almost all individuals with Down syndrome have neuropathological changes typical of AD (Schupf et al. 1998). Individuals carrying the E4 allele of the apolipoprotein E (ApoE) gene on chromosome 19 have an increased risk of AD. There are three alleles: ApoE2, ApoE3, ApoE4. At a population level, the relative risk of AD for individuals over the age of 75 is 3.24 for those possessing the ApoE4 allele (Tilvis, Strandberg, and Juva 1998). Possession of a single ApoE4 allele increases the lifetime risk of AD by an odds ratio of 2.6 (95% CI, 1.6–4.0), but homozygotes for ApoE4 have an odds ratio of 14.9 (95% CI, 10.8–20.6) when compared to those with E2 or E3 (Farrer et al. 1997). However, the sensitivity (approximately 50%) and specificity (approximately 75% for one or more ApoE4 alleles) are not sufficiently high to aid in the diagnosis of the condition in an individual (Post et al. 1997). In a study involving more than 2000 patients from dementia clinics who came to autopsy, the sensitivity and specificity of *clinical* diagnosis were 93% and 55%, respectively. For ApoE4, sensitivity and specificity were 65% and 68%, respectively (Mayeux et al. 1998). Therefore, as a stand-alone test, diagnostic performance of ApoE4 was *inferior* to clinical assessment; however, when added to clinical assessment the combined specificity rose to 84%. Overall, the clinical role of ApoE genotype testing remains unclear, and it is not presently recommended for routine testing in individuals suspected of having AD (Knopman et al. 2001; Patterson et al. 2001).

In frontotemporal dementia various mutations on the tau gene have been observed in some populations (Wischik, Theuring, and Harrington 2001). At this point, however, such determinations remain a tool for the research setting and are not generally appropriate for clinical diagnosis.

Neuroimaging

As neuroimaging is the most resource-intensive of the investigations commonly used in dementia, its use should be carefully scrutinized. Universal neuroimaging would be justifiable if the prevalence of conditions whose treatment would influence prognosis or management was high, or if there were a significant risk of missing a potentially treatable condition. However, a systematic review revealed that potentially reversible structural causes of dementia were rare (Clarfield 1988). Normal pressure hydrocephalus was present in 1.6%, chronic subdural hematoma in 0.4%, and brain tumor in 1.5%.

Despite these figures, routine structural neuroimaging is recommended by the American Academy of Neurology (Rossor 1994; Cory-Bloom et al. 1995; Geldmacher and Whitehouse 1996; Knopman et al. 2001). In contrast, the Canadian Consensus Conference on Dementia (Clarfield 1991; Patterson et al. 2001) recommended that CT scanning be offered only when specific indications are present (tab. 3.5). A similar conclusion was reached by Chui and Zhang (1997). In support of this selective approach, CCCD criteria were applied retrospectively to a series of 200 patients attending a memory clinic in Montreal, all of whom had undergone neuroimaging and full assessment. Restriction of CT scanning to those fulfilling CCCD criteria would have reduced the number of CT scans by 60% and not a single "reversible" or potentially reversible condition would have been missed (Freter et al. 1998). However, one highly malignant tumor (whose treatment did not reverse the dementia or improve quality of life), would not have been detected. In the series of 119 dementia cases reported by Chui and Zhang (1997), one potentially treatable case of normal pressure hydrocephalus would have been missed using the selective approach.

In one study (Mendez et al. 1992) the use of computerized tomography scanning actually detracted from the correct final neuropathological diagnosis. This resulted from the frequent finding of periventricular white matter changes, which may exist in up to 12% of cognitively intact older individuals and are of uncertain significance (Amar et al. 1995). Furthermore, CT scanning may fail to detect pathologically proven strokes (Kurita et al. 1993).

Structural magnetic resonance imaging (MRI) scanning does not appear to

Table 3.5. Conditions suggesting referral for neuroimaging

History
1. Age less than 60 years
2. Use of anticoagulants or a history of bleeding disorder
3. Recent head trauma
4. Previous history of carcinoma (from sites that metastasize to brain, e.g., lung, breast)
5. Unexplained neurological symptoms (e.g., new-onset headaches, seizures)
6. Rapid unexplained decline (e.g., > one to two months) in cognition or functional status
7. "Short" duration of dementia (< two years)
8. History of urinary incontinence and gait disorder early in the course of dementia, suggestive of normal pressure hydrocephalus (in the later stages of Alzheimer disease, urinary incontinence and gait ataxia commonly occur)
9. Unusual or atypical cognitive, behavioral, or neuropsychological presentation

Physical
1. Localizing signs (e.g., hemiparesis, Babinski response)
2. Gait ataxia

Sources: Clarfield et al. 1991; Patterson et al. 1999.

offer any advantages in the routine assessment of individuals with dementia (Chertkow et al. 2001). In fact, the high prevalence of abnormalities seen in normal individuals (Schmidt et al. 1996; Roob et al. 1999) argues against routine use of MRI, as the findings are potentially misleading.

Another reason to consider structural neuroimaging is to confirm a diagnosis of Alzheimer disease. Quantitative imaging of the medial temporal lobes by CT or MRI scan distinguishes individuals with AD from normal controls. However, there is considerable overlap between these groups. Using pathological confirmation, one study revealed a 95% sensitivity, but a poor specificity of only 40% for the diagnosis of AD (Nagy et al. 1999).

For the individual who presents with clinically typical Alzheimer disease, selective computerized tomography scanning using criteria appears to be a reasonable approach. Where resources are available to justify the high incremental cost of detecting potentially remediable conditions, or a litigious environment exists, a stronger case could be made for universal neuroimaging.

Functional Imaging

Single-photon emission computerized tomography (SPECT) and positron emission tomography (PET) allow for the imaging of regional brain metabolism and was once thought to be valuable in the distinction between Alzheimer, frontotemporal, and vascular dementias (Read et al. 1995; Bonte et al. 1997; Pickut et al. 1997). While initial results were encouraging (Johnson et al. 1990), subsequent studies have shown that functional imaging is not superior to clinical criteria in distinguishing these conditions and is not presently recommended for clinical practice (Knopman et al. 2001). The role of these modalities in distinguishing individuals who are likely to progress to dementia from those who remain stable in the population with MCI is also unclear (Johnson et al. 1990). (See chap. 1.)

Functional magnetic resonance imaging is also being evaluated in this context (Bookheimer et al. 2000). Its place in clinical practice outside the research setting remains unclear at this time.

Follow-up

A vital part of the diagnosis of dementia is confirming the condition by appropriate follow-up. Particularly when the initial diagnosis is uncertain, regular review at intervals of three to six months will determine whether the individual is following the typical trajectory for one of the types of dementia, whether the course is atypical, or whether the deficits stabilize, as in many people with MCI.

Disclosure of Diagnosis

The case for informing an individual of the diagnosis rests on the patient's right to know (principle of autonomy). Knowledge of the diagnosis can allow for future planning (e.g., advance directives, power of attorney, and planning for future living arrangements). Disclosure allows for consent to treatment and participation in research. It also facilitates the dialogue between patient and caregiver, avoiding the conspiracy of silence that might otherwise exist. Arguments against disclosure include the risk of depression and, in rare instances, suicide; concern about diagnostic uncertainty; and the lack of effective disease-modifying treatments. In the North American context, most seniors and caregivers of AD state that they would wish to be told the diagnosis. Although each case should be weighed on its own merits, it is considered ethically preferable to inform persons with dementia of their diagnosis (Drickamer and Lachs 1992).

Table 3.6. Procedures recommended for all individuals suspected of having dementia

Procedure	Comments
History	Include corroborative information: explore onset, progression, pace of decline, function, past history of alcohol, head injury, hypertension, depression or psychiatric illness, neurological symptoms, incontinence Family history of dementia Consider age-specific prevalence of dementia (pretest probability)
Medication review	See table 3.3 for drugs that may affect cognition: inspect all drugs, both prescribed and over-the-counter medications
Physical examination	General examination for signs of systemic disease or organ failure
Neurological examination	Look for signs of raised intracranial pressure, focal abnormalities, primitive reflexes, extrapyramidal features, sensory changes, gait, balance, eyesight, hearing
Mental status examination	May use brief mental status instrument (e.g., MMSE and CDT); explore executive function Consider likelihood ratios (LRs) of mental status instruments to reach (post-test probability of) diagnosis
Follow-up	To assess trajectory of cognitive, functional, and behavioral features: response to treatment

Clinical Conclusions

Step 1: Establish Whether Dementia Is Present. Using DSM-IV criteria or its simplified version, clinical history (including corroborative information), and mental status examination should allow a clinician to determine whether the syndrome of dementia is present. In the event that the clinician cannot be sure whether the person has dementia or one of the differential diagnoses, further testing and follow-up are necessary. For example, if the choice lies between dementia and MCI, options include full neuropsychological testing or careful follow-up over time. A repeat interview in three to six months will usually determine whether the condition has progressed.

Step 2: Determine the Cause of Dementia. Once the diagnosis of dementia is established, further evaluation is necessary to determine its cause, and whether there are factors that may be aggravating or even causing the dementia syndrome. Bearing in mind the common types of dementia (AD, VaD, mixed, FTD, DLB) and considering the conditions that may simulate dementia (such as depression, metabolic disturbances, or medication side effects), physical examination, including careful scrutiny of all consumed medications, appropriate laboratory testing, and CT scanning where indicated will help to refine the diagnosis and determine if remedial factors may be present (see tab. 3.4).

Dementia is a common condition and one in which diagnosis should be within the reach of most physicians providing that a structured approach is followed.

REFERENCES

Alexopoulos, G.S., B.S. Meyers, R.C. Young, et al. 1993. The course of geriatric depression with "reversible dementia": A controlled study. *American Journal of Psychiatry* 150:1693–99.

Alexopolous, G., R. Abrams, R. Young, et al. 1998. Cornell scale for depression in dementia. *Biological Psychiatry* 232:271–84.

Amar, K., T. Lewis, G. Wilcock, M. Scott, et al. 1995. The relationship between white matter low attenuation on brain CT and vascular risk factors: A memory clinic study. *Age and Ageing* 24 (5):411–15.

American Psychiatric Association. 1987. *Diagnostic and Statistical Manual of Mental Disorders.* 3rd ed., revised. Washington, D.C.: American Psychiatric Association.

American Psychiatric Association. 1994. *Diagnostic and Statistical Manual of Mental Disorders.* 4th ed. Washington, D.C.: American Psychiatric Association.

Andreasen, N., C. Hesse, P. Davidsson, et al. 1999a. Cerebrospinal fluid beta-amyloid(1-42) in Alzheimer disease: Differences between early- and late-onset Alzheimer disease and stability during the course of disease. *Archives of Neurology* 56:673–80.

Andreasen, N., L. Minthon, A. Clarberg, et al. 1999b. Sensitivity, specificity, and stability of CSF-tau in AD in a community-based patient sample. *Neurology* 53:1488–94.

Berger, A.K., L. Fratiglioni, Y. Forsell, et al. 1999. The occurrence of depressive symptoms in the preclinical phase of AD: A population-based study. *Neurology* 53 (9):1998–2002.

Bernard, M.A., P.A. Nakonezny, and T.M. Kashner. 1998. The effect of vitamin B_{12} deficiency on older veterans and its relationship to health. *Journal of the American Geriatrics Society* 46:1199–1206.

Blacker, D., and R.E. Tanzi. 1998. The genetics of Alzheimer disease. *Archives of Neurology* 55:294–96.

Bonte, F.J., M.F. Weiner, E.H. Bigio, et al. 1997. Brain blood flow in the dementias: SPECT with histopathologic correlation in 54 patients. *Radiology* 202:793–97.

Bookheimer, S.Y., M.H. Strojwas, M.S. Cohen, et al. 2000. Patterns of brain activation in people at risk for Alzheimer's disease. *New England Journal of Medicine* 343:450–56.

Brown, P., F. Cathala, P. Castaigne, et al. 1986. Creutzfeldt-Jakob disease: Clinical analysis of a consecutive series of 230 neuropathologically verified cases. *Annals of Neurology* 20:597–602.

Brun, A. 1993. Frontal lobe degeneration of non-Alzheimer type revisited. *Dementia* 4: 126–31.

Burke, W.J., W.H. Roccaforte, and S.P. Wengel. 1991. The short form of the Geriatric Depression Scale: A comparison with the 30-item form. *Journal of Geriatric Psychiatry and Neurology* 4:173–78.

Canadian Study of Health and Aging. 1994. Study methods and prevalence of dementia. *Canadian Medical Association Journal* 150:899–913.

Chertkow, H., H. Bergman, H.M. Schipper, et al. 2001. Assessment of suspected dementia. *Canadian Journal of Neurological Sciences* 28 (Suppl. 1):S28–41.

Chui H.C., and Q. Zhang. 1997. Evaluation of dementia: A systematic study of the usefulness of the American Academy of Neurology's practice parameters. *Neurology* 49: 925–35.

Chui, H.C., J.I. Victoroff, D. Margolin, et al. 1992. Criteria for the diagnosis of ischemic vascular dementia proposed by the State of California Alzheimer's Disease Diagnostic and Treatment Centers. *Neurology* 42:473–80.

Clarfield, A.M. 1988. The reversible dementias: Do they reverse? *Annals of Internal Medicine* 109:476–86.

Clarfield, A.M. 1991. Assessing dementia: The Canadian Consensus. *Canadian Medical Association Journal* 144:851–53.

Clarnette, R.M., and Patterson, C.J. 1994. Hypothyroidism: Does treatment cure dementia? *Journal of Geriatric Psychiatry and Neurology* 7:23–27.

Corey-Bloom, J., L.J. Thal, D. Galasko, et al. 1995. Diagnosis and evaluation of dementia. *Neurology* 45 (2):211–18.

Crook, T., R..T. Bartus, and S.H. Ferris. 1986. Age-associated memory impairment: Proposed diagnostic criteria and measures of clinical change—report of a National Institute of Mental Health Work Group. *Developmental Neuropsychology* 2:261–76.

Crum, R.M., J.C. Anthony, S.S. Bassett, et al. 1993. Population-based norms for the Mini-Mental State Examination by age and educational level. *Journal of the American Medical Association* 269 (18):2386–91.

Cunha, U.G., Rocha, F.L., J.M. Peixoto, et al. 1995. Vitamin B_{12} deficiency and dementia. *International Psychogeriatrics* 7:85–88.

Drickamer, M.A., and M.S. Lachs. 1992. Should patients with Alzheimer's disease be told their diagnosis? *New England Journal of Medicine* 326:947–51.

Erkinjuntti, T., T. Ostbye, R. Steenhuis, et al. 1997. The effects of different diagnostic criteria on the prevalence of dementia. *New England Journal of Medicine* 337: 1667–74.

Farrer, L.A., L.A. Cupples, J.L. Haines, et al. 1997. Effects of age, sex and ethnicity on the association between apolipoprotein E genotype and Alzheimer disease. A meta-analysis. APOE and Alzheimer Disease Meta Analysis Consortium. *Journal of the American Medical Association* 278:1349–56.

Folstein, M., S. Folstein, and P. McHugh. 1975. Mini-Mental State: A practical method for grading the cognitive state of patients for the clinician. *Journal of Psychiatric Research* 12:189–98.

Franssen, E.H., B. Reisberg, A. Kluger, et al. 1991. Cognition-independent neurologic

symptoms in normal aging and probable Alzheimer's disease. *Archives of Neurology* 48: 148–54.
Fratiglioni, L., D. DeRonchi, and N. Agüero-Torres. 1999. Worldwide prevalence and incidence of dementia. *Drugs and Aging* 15:363–75.
Fratiglioni, L., M. Grut, Y. Forsell, et al. 1992. Clinical diagnosis of Alzheimer's disease and other dementias in a population survey: Agreement and causes of disagreement in applying Diagnostic and Statistical Manual of Mental Disorders, Revised Third Edition, Criteria. *Archives of Neurology* 49:927–32.
Freedman, M., L. Leach, E. Kaplan, et al. 1994. *Clock Drawing: A Neuropsychological Analysis*. New York: Oxford University Press.
Freter, S., H. Bergman, S. Gold, et al. 1998. Prevalence of potentially reversible dementias and actual reversibility in a memory clinic cohort. *Canadian Medical Association Journal* 159:657–62.
Froelich, T.E., S.T. Bogardus, and S.K. Inouye. 2001. Dementia and race: Are there differences between African Americans and Caucasians? *Journal of the American Geriatrics Society* 49:477–84.
Galasko, D., P.F. Kwo-on-Yuen, M.R. Klauber, et al. 1990. Neurological findings in Alzheimer's disease and normal aging. *Archives of Neurology* 47:625–27.
Galasko, D., L.A. Hansen, R. Katzman, et al. 1994. Clinical neuropathological correlations in Alzheimer's disease and related dementias. *Archives of Neurology* 51:888–95.
Galasko, D., C. Clark, L. Chang, et al. 1997. Assessment of CSF levels of tau protein in mildly demented patients with Alzheimer's disease. *Neurology* 48:632–35.
Galasko, D., L. Chang, R. Motter, et al. 1998. High cerebrospinal fluid tau and low amyloid beta42 levels in the clinical diagnosis of Alzheimer disease and relation to Apolipoprotein E genotype. *Archives of Neurology* 55:937–45.
Gearing, M., S.S. Mirra, J.C. Hedreen, et al. 1995. The Consortium to Establish a Registry for Alzheimer's Disease (CERAD). Part X. Neuropathology confirmation of the clinical diagnosis of Alzheimer's disease. *Neurology* 45:461–66.
Geldmacher, D.S., and P. Whitehouse. 1996. Evaluation of dementia. *New England Journal of Medicine* 335:330–36.
Graham, J.E., I. Rockwood, B.L. Beattie, et al. 1996. Standardization of the diagnosis of dementia in the Canadian Study of Health and Aging. *Neuroepidemiology* 15:246–56.
Green, R., and L.J. Kinsella. 1995. Current concepts in the diagnosis of cobalamin deficiency. *Neurology* 45:1435–40.
Grigoletto, F., G. Zappala, D.W. Anderson, et al. 1999. Norms for the Mini-Mental State Examination in a healthy population. *Neurology* 53 (2):315–20.
Hachinski, V.C., N.A. Lassen, and J. Marshall. 1974. Multi-infarct dementia: A cause of mental deterioration in the elderly. *Lancet* 2:207–10.
Hammerstrom, D.C., and B. Zimmer. 1985. The role of lumbar puncture in the evaluation of dementia: The University of Pittsburgh study. *Journal of the American Geriatrics Society* 33:397–400.
Healton, E.B., D. G. Savage, J.C. Brust, et al. 1991. Neurologic aspects of cobalamin deficiency. *Medicine* (Baltimore) 70:229–45.
Hendrie, H.C., B.O. Osuntokun, K.S. Hall, et al. 1995. Prevalence of Alzheimer's disease and dementia in two communities: Nigerian Africans and African Americans. *American Journal of Psychiatry* 152:1485–92.
Hendrie, H.C., A. Ogunniyi, K.S. Hall, et al. 2001. Incidence of dementia and Alzheimer

disease in two communities: Yoruba residing in Ibadan, Nigeria, and African Americans residing in Indianapolis, Indiana. *Journal of the American Medical Association* 285:739–47.

Herbert, C.P. 2001. Cultural aspects of dementia. *Canadian Journal of Neurological Sciences* 28 (Suppl. 1):S77–82.

Hogan, D.B., and E.M. Ebly. 2000. Predicting who will develop dementia in a cohort of Canadian seniors. *Canadian Journal of Neurological Sciences* 27:18–24.

Holmes, C., N. Cairns, P. Lantos, et al. 1999. Validity of current clinical criteria for Alzheimer's disease, vascular dementia and dementia with Lewy bodies. *British Journal of Psychiatry* 174:45–50.

Hsich, G., K. Kenney, C.J. Gibbs, et al. 1996. The 14-3-3 brain protein in cerebrospinal fluid as a marker for transmissible spongiform encephalopathies. *New England Journal of Medicine* 335:924–30.

Hulstaert, F., K. Blennow, A. Ivanoiu, et al. 1999. Improved discrimination of AD patients using beta-amyloid(1-42) and tau levels in CSF. *Neurology* 52:1555–62.

Jobst, K.A., L.P. Barnetson, and B. J. Shepstone. 1998. Accurate prediction of histologically confirmed Alzheimer's disease and the differential diagnosis of dementia: The use of NINCDS-ADRDA and DSMIII-R criteria, spect, X-ray CT, and apo E4 in medial temporal lobe dementias. Oxford Project to Investigate Memory and Aging. *International Psychogeriatrics* 10:271–302.

Johnson, K.A., B.L. Holman, T.J. Rosen, et al. 1990. Iofetamine I 123 single photon emission computed tomography is accurate in the diagnosis of Alzheimer's disease. *Archives of Internal Medicine* 150:752–56.

Kertesz, A., W. Davidson, and H. Fox. 1997. Frontal Behavioral Inventory: Diagnostic criteria for frontal lobe dementia. *Canadian Journal of Neurological Sciences* 24:29–36.

Knopman, D.S., S.T. DeKosky, J.L. Cummings, et al. 2001. Practice parameter: Diagnosis of dementia (an evidence-based review). Report of the Quality Standards Subcommittee of the American Academy of Neurology. *Neurology* 56:1143–53.

Kurita, A., R.S. Black, J.P. Blass, et al. 1993. Failure of CT scan to detect ischemic lesions in patients with dementia. *Journal of Geriatric Psychiatry and Neurology* 6:245–50.

Kurz, A., M. Riemenschneider, K. Buch, et al. 1998. Tau protein in cerebrospinal fluid is significantly increased at the earliest clinical stage of Alzheimer disease. *Alzheimer Disease and Associated Disorders* 12:372–77.

Larson, E.B., B.V. Reifler, S.M. Sumi, et al. 1986. Diagnostic tests in the evaluation of dementia. A prospective study of 200 elderly outpatients. *Archives of Internal Medicine* 146:1917–22.

Larson, E.B., J.K. Edwards, E. O'Meara, et al. 1996. Neuropathological diagnostic outcomes from a cohort of outpatients with suspected dementia. *Journals of Gerontology. Series A, Biological Sciences and Medical Sciences* 51:M313–18.

Lim, A., D. Tsuang, W. Kukull, et al. 1999. Clinico-neuropathological correlation of Alzheimer's disease in a community-based case series. *Journal of the American Geriatrics Society* 47:564–69.

Lund and Manchester Groups. 1994. Clinical and neuro-pathological criteria for frontotemporal dementia. *Journal of Neurology, Neurosurgery and Psychiatry* 57:416–18.

Magaziner, J., P. German, S.I. Zimmerman, et al. 2000. The prevalence of dementia in a statewide sample of new nursing home admissions aged 65 and older: Diagnosis by expert panel. Epidemiology of Dementia in Nursing Homes Research Group. *Gerontologist* 40:663–72.

Martin, D.C., J. Francis, J. Protetch, et al. 1992. Time dependency of cognitive recovery with cobalamin replacement: Report of a pilot study. *Journal of the American Geriatrics Society* 40:168–72.

Mayeux, R., A.M. Saunders, S. Shea, et al. 1998. Utility of the apolipoprotein E genotype in the diagnosis of Alzheimer's disease. Alzheimer's Disease Centers Consortium on Apolipoprotein E and Alzheimer's Disease. *New England Journal of Medicine* 338:506–11.

McArthur, J.C. 1987. Neurological manifestations of AIDS. *Medicine* 66:407–37.

McGee, S. 2001. *Evidence-Based Physical Diagnosis.* Philadelphia: W.B. Saunders Co., pp. 3–22, 55.

McKeith, I.G., D. Galasko, K. Kosaka, et al. 1996. Consensus guidelines for the clinical and pathologic diagnosis of dementia with Lewy bodies (DLB): Report of the consortium on DLB international workshop. *Neurology* 47:1113–24.

McKeith, I.G., T. Del Ser, S. PierFranco, et al. 2000a. Efficacy of rivastigmine in dementia with Lewy bodies: A randomised, double-blind, placebo-controlled international study. *Lancet* 356:2031–36.

McKeith, I.G., C.G. Ballard, R.H. Perry, et al. 2000b. Prospective validation of Consensus criteria for the diagnosis of dementia with Lewy bodies. *Neurology* 54:1050–58.

McKhann, G., D. Drachman, M. Folstein, et al. 1984. Clinical diagnosis of Alzheimer's disease: Report of the NINCDS-ADRDA Work Group under the auspices of Department of Health and Human Service Task Force on Alzheimer's Disease. *Neurology* 34:939–44.

Mega, M.S., D.L. Masterman, D.F. Benson, et al. 1996. Dementia with Lewy bodies: Reliability and validity of clinical and pathologic criteria. *Neurology* 47:1403–9.

Mendez, M.F., A.R. Mastri, B.A. Zander, et al. 1992. A clinicopathological study of CT scans in Alzheimer's disease. *Journal of the American Geriatrics Society* 40:476–78.

Mielke, R., and W.D. Heiss. 1998. Positron emission tomography for diagnosis of Alzheimer's disease and vascular dementia. *Journal of Neural Transmission* 53 (Suppl.): S237–50.

Molloy, D., E. Alemayehu, and R. Roberts. 1991. Reliability of a standardized Mini-Mental State Examination. *American Journal of Psychiatry* 148:102–5.

Moroney, J.T., E. Bagiella, D.W.I. Desmond, et al. 1997. Meta-analysis of the Hachinski Ischemic Score in pathologically verified dementias. *Neurology* 49:1096–1105.

Morris, J.C. 1993. The Clinical Dementia Rating (CDR): Current version and scoring rules. *Neurology* 43:2412–14.

Moussavian, M., S. Potolicchio, and R. Jones. 1997. The 14-3-3 brain protein and transmissible spongiform encephalopathy. *New England Journal of Medicine* 336:873–75.

Nagy, Z., N.J. Hindley, H. Braak, et al. 1999. Relationship between clinical and radiological diagnostic criteria for Alzheimer's disease and the extent of neuropathology as reflected by 'stages': A prospective study. *Dementia and Geriatric Cognitive Disorders* 10:109–14.

Neary, D., J.S. Snowden, L. Gustafson, et al. 1998. Frontotemporal lobar degeneration: A consensus on clinical diagnostic criteria. *Neurology* 51:1546–54.

Nolan, K.A., M.M. Lino, A.W. Seligmann, et al. 1998. Absence of vascular dementia in an autopsy series from a dementia clinic. *Journal of the American Geriatrics Society* 46: 597–604.

Patterson, C., S. Gauthier, H. Bergman, et al. 2001. The recognition, assessment and management of dementing disorders: Conclusions from the Canadian Consensus Conference on Dementia. *Canadian Journal of Neurological Sciences* 28 (Suppl. 1): S3–16.

Pennypacker, L.C., R.H. Allen, J.P. Kelly, et al. 1992. High prevalence of cobalamin deficiency in elderly outpatients. *Journal of the American Geriatrics Society* 40:1197–1204.

Petersen, R.C., G.E. Smith, S.C. Waring, et al. 1999. Mild cognitive impairment: Clinical characterization and outcome. *Archives of Neurology* 56:303–8.

Pickut, B.A., J. Saerens, P. Marien, et al. 1997. Discriminative use of SPECT in frontal lobe-type dementia versus (senile) dementia of the Alzheimer's type. *Journal of Nuclear Medicine* 38:929–34.

Poser, S., B. Mollenhauer, A. Kraubeta, et al. 1999. How to improve the clinical diagnosis of Creutzfeldt-Jakob disease. *Brain* 122:2346–51.

Post, S.G., P.J. Whitehouse, R.H. Binstock, et al. 1997. Consensus statement: The clinical introduction of genetic testing for Alzheimer's disease. *Journal of the American Medical Association* 277:832–36.

Powell, A.L., A.C. Coyne, and L. Jen. 1993. A retrospective study of syphilis seropositivity in a cohort of demented patients. *Alzheimer Disease and Associated Disorders* 7: 33–38.

Read, S.L., B.L. Miller, I. Mena, et al. 1995. SPECT in dementia: Clinical and pathological correlation. *Journal of the American Geriatrics Society* 43:1243–47.

Ritchie, K., D. Kildea, and J.M. Robine. 1992. The relationship between age and the prevalence of senile dementia: A meta-analysis of recent data. *International Journal of Epidemiology* 21:763–69.

Ritchie, K., D. Leibovici, B. Ledésert, et al. 1996. A typology of subclinical senescent cognitive disorder. *British Journal of Psychiatry* 168:470–76.

Roman, G.C., T.K. Tatemichi, T. Erkinjuntti, et al. 1993. Vascular dementia: Diagnostic criteria for research studies. Report of the NINDS-AIREN International Workshop. *Neurology* 43:250–60.

Roob, G., R. Schmidt, P. Kapeller, et al. 1999. MRI evidence of past cerebral microbleeds in a healthy elderly population. *Neurology* 52:991–94.

Rosen, W.G., R.D. Terry, P.A. Fuld, et al. 1980. Pathological verification of ischemic score in differentiation of dementias. *Annals of Neurology* 7:486–88.

Rossor, N.B. 1994. Management of neurological disorders: Dementia. *Journal of Neurology, Neurosurgery and Psychiatry* 57:1451–56.

Schmidt, R., M. Hayn, F. Fazekas, et al. 1996. Magnetic resonance imaging white matter hyperintensities in clinically normal elderly individuals: Correlations with plasma concentrations of naturally occurring antioxidants. *Stroke* 27:2043–47.

Schofield, P.W., K. Marder, G. Dooneief, et al. 1997. Association of subjective memory complaints with subsequent cognitive decline in community-dwelling elderly individuals with baseline cognitive impairment. *American Journal of Psychiatry* 154:609–15.

Schupf, N., D. Kapell, B. Nightingale, et al. 1998. Earlier onset of Alzheimer disease in men with Down's syndrome. *Neurology* 50:991–95.

Siu, A.L. 1991. Screening for dementia and investigating its causes. *Annals of Internal Medicine* 115:122–32.

Smith, C.W., E.J. Byrne, T. Arie, et al. 1992. Diagnosis of dementia II—Diagnostic methods: A survey of current consultant practice and review of the literature. *International Journal of Geriatric Psychiatry* 7:323–29.

Snowdon, D.A., L.H. Greiner, J.A. Mortimer, et al. 1997. Brain infarction and the clinical expression of Alzheimer's disease: The nun study. *Journal of the American Medical Association* 277:813–17.

Somerfield, M.R., C.S. Wiesman, W. Ury, et al. 1991. Physicians' practices in the diagnosis of dementing disorders. *Journal of the American Geriatrics Society* 39:172–75.

Teunisse, S., A.E. Bollen, W.A. van Gool, et al. 1996. Dementia and subnormal levels of vitamin B_{12}: Effects of replacement therapy on dementia. *Journal of Neurology* 243: 522–29.

Thorpe, L., and B. Groulx. 2001. Depressive syndromes in dementia. *Canadian Journal of Neurological Sciences* 28 (Suppl. 1):S83–95.

Tilvis, R.S., T.E. Strandberg, and K. Juva. 1998. Apolipoprotein E phenotypes, dementia and mortality in a prospective population sample. *Journal of the American Geriatrics Society* 46:712–15.

Tombaugh, T.N., and N.J. McIntyre. 1992. The Mini-Mental State Examination: A comprehensive review. *Journal of the American Geriatrics Society* 40:922–35.

Van Duijn, D.M., D. Clayton, and V. Chandra. 1991. Familial aggregation of Alzheimer's disease and related disorder: A collaborative re-analysis of case-control studies. *International Journal of Epidemiology* 20:S12–20.

Walsh, J.S., H.G. Welch, and E.B. Larson. 1990. Survival of outpatients with Alzheimer-type dementia. *Annals of Internal Medicine* 113:429–34.

Wells, C. 1978. Chronic brain disease: An overview. *American Journal of Psychiatry* 135: 1–12.

Weytingh, M.D., P.M. Bossuyt, and H. van Crevel. 1995. Reversible dementia: More than 10% or less than 1%?: A quantitative review. *Journal of Neurology* 242:466–71.

Wischik, C.M., F. Theuring, and C.R. Harrington. 2001. The molecular basis of tau protein pathology in Alzheimer's disease and related neurodegenerative dementias. In *Neurobiology of Alzheimer's Disease (Molecular and Cellular Neurobiology)*, edited by D. Dawbarn and S.J. Allen. New York: Oxford University Press, pp. 103–206.

Wolfson, C., D.B. Wolfson, M. Asgharian, et al. 2001. A reevaluation of the duration of survival after the onset of dementia. *New England Journal of Medicine* 344:1111–16.

World Health Organization. 1993. *The ICD-10 Classification of Mental and Behavioural Disorders: Diagnostic Criteria for Research.* Geneva: World Health Organization.

Yesavage, J.A., T.L. Brink, T.L. Rose, et al. 1982. Development and validation of a geriatric depression screening scale: A preliminary report. *Journal of Psychiatric Research* 3 (17):37–49.

Part II / Alzheimer Dementias

CHAPTER FOUR

The Neuropathology of Alzheimer Dementia

Jerzy Wegiel, V.D.M., Ph.D.,
Thomas Wisniewski, M.D., Ph.D.,
Barry Reisberg, M.D., Ph.D.,
and Wayne Silverman, Ph.D.

Alzheimer disease (AD) is a neurodegenerative disorder characterized by progressive dementia associated with widespread encephalopathy. Clinical symptoms include memory loss, decline in ability to perform routine tasks, impairment of judgment, disorientation, personality change, difficulty in learning, and eventually loss of language and self-care skills (Folstein, Folstein, and McHugh 1975; McKhann et al. 1984; Reisberg et al. 1982, 2000; Katzman 1986; Reisberg 1988). Although the validity of clinically made diagnosis has increased substantially in recent years, the clinical diagnosis of AD is made with limited certainty and requires confirmation in postmortem examination (Reisberg et al. 1997; Small et al. 1997). Brain pathology in AD is characterized by a broad spectrum of changes that includes accumulation of fibrillar amyloid-β (Aβ) protein in plaques and vessels, neurofibrillary degeneration, and synaptic and neuronal loss. β-amyloidosis and neurofibrillary changes are such consistent features that postmortem neuropathologic diagnosis of AD is based on semiquantitative assessment of fibrillar plaques and neurofibrillary tangles (Mirra et al. 1991; Mirra, Hart, and Terry 1993).

Neuropathologic Diagnostic Criteria for Alzheimer Disease

Semiquantitative diagnostic criteria for Alzheimer disease were introduced by Tomlinson and Henderson (1975), who referred to the presence of numerous neocortical plaques and tangles and granulovacuolar degeneration in the hippocampus. Ball et al. (1985) proposed criteria that focused on hippocampal pathology, including the number of neurons with tangles and granulovacuolar degeneration, and neuronal loss.

Diagnostic criteria were also proposed by an expert panel representing the National Institute of Aging, the American Association of Retired Persons, the National Institute of Neurological and Communicative Disorders and Stroke, and the National Institute of Mental Health (Khatchaturian 1985). Diagnosis required examination of the frontal, temporal, and parietal cortices, hippocampus, amygdala, basal ganglia, substantia nigra, cerebellar cortex, and spinal cord. Diagnosis was based on the number of senile plaques (per 200× field) stained with Bielschowsky silver technique, the thioflavin S method with ultraviolet illumination, or the Congo red technique. These criteria were: for subjects less than 50 years of age, > 2–5 neuritic plaques; 50–65 years of age, 8 or more plaques; 66–75 years of age, 10 or more plaques; and over 75 years of age, 15 or more plaques. According to these criteria, the diagnosis of AD was possible in the absence of a clinical history of dementia and without the presence of neurofibrillary tangles.

Diagnostic criteria recommended by the Consortium to Establish a Registry for Alzheimer's Disease (CERAD) required the semiquantitation of neuritic plaques and included a description of preferred evaluation methods. Bielschowsky staining was suggested (alternative methods also were mentioned), diffuse plaques were to be ignored, a history of dementia was necessary, and the certainty of the diagnosis was to be indicated (i.e., possible, probable, or definite AD). Diagnostic samples comprised middle frontal gyrus, superior and middle temporal gyrus, inferior parietal lobule, anterior cingulate gyrus, hippocampus, entorhinal cortex, amygdala, and midbrain including substantia nigra (Mirra et al. 1991; Mirra, Hart, and Terry 1993).

More recently, diagnostic criteria for the neuropathologic assessment of Alzheimer disease were recommended by the National Institute on Aging and Reagan Institute Working Group (1997). These recommendations were: (a) to use the semiquantitative methods outlined by CERAD (Mirra, Hart, and Terry

1993) to assess neuritic plaques and neurofibrillary tangles; (b) to examine the hippocampal formation and neocortex for the presence of neurofibrillary tangles; and (c) to establish the extent of neurofibrillary changes following the topographic staging proposed by Braak and Braak (1991). The CERAD protocols were recommended for tissue fixation, processing, sectioning, and staining with modified Bielschowsky, Gallyas, or thioflavine S methods judged to be appropriate. To evaluate Alzheimer disease and to rule out potentially confounding disorders, microscopic examination of the following brain structures was recommended: (a) areas of neocortex, including superior temporal gyrus, inferior parietal lobe, midfrontal cortex, occipital cortex including primary visual cortex and association cortex; (b) hippocampal formation at the level of lateral geniculate body; (c) hippocampal formation including entorhinal cortex at the level of the uncus; and (d) substantia nigra and locus ceruleus. In addition to classical Alzheimer disease lesions, the diagnostic protocol included the assessment of major coexisting lesions (e.g., Lewy bodies and vascular lesions).

Pathogenesis and Pathomechanisms of Alzheimer Disease

The pathogenesis of Alzheimer disease is complex, and the common clinical and neuropathological features can arise from several different genetic causes. In the majority of cases, AD is classified as sporadic AD with late onset (after 65 years of age) and without a clear link to any genetic markers. Approximately 5–10% of cases of AD appear to be transmitted as a pure autosomal dominant trait with high age-dependent penetrance (Nishimura, Yu, and St. George-Hyslop 1999). More than 50% of early-onset familial AD is related to mutations in the presenilin 1 (PS1) gene on chromosome 14, with a small percentage being related to mutations in presenilin 2 (PS2) gene on chromosome 1 and the amyloid precursor protein (APP) gene on chromosome 21 (Goate et al. 1991; Levy-Lahad et al. 1995; Rogaev et al. 1995; Sherrington et al. 1995). Inheritance of ApoE-ε4 allele encoded by a gene on chromosome 19 (Pericak-Vance et al. 1991) increases risk for late-onset AD (Corder et al. 1993).

Processing of Amyloid Precursor Protein

Amyloid precursor protein consists of 695 to 770 amino acids, depending on the size of the inserts (Goldgaber et al. 1987; Kang et al. 1987). It is produced in the endoplasmic reticulum and transits to the Golgi, where it is post-translationally modified via N- and O-linked glycosylation and tyrosine sulfation and transported to the cell membrane. In neurons, APP is present in vesicles in the cell body, axon, and dendrites and at synaptic sites (Weideman et al. 1989).

Amyloid-β (Aβ) peptides are the product of proteolytic cleavage of amyloid precursor protein. The 42-43 amino acid (aa) portion of APP corresponding to Aβ lies in the junction of the ectodomain and transmembrane domain, with 14 to 15 residues embedded in the membrane and 28 residues outside of the membrane. Aβ1-40 aa and 1-42 aa are the products of intracellular processing of APP with β- and γ-secretases in the endoplasmic reticulum, trans-Golgi network, and endosomal-lysosomal system (Cook et al. 1997; Hartmann et al. 1997; Wild-Bode et al. 1997; Xu et al. 1997; Greenfield et al. 1999). In neurons, Aβ42 is produced almost exclusively in the endoplasmic reticulum/intermediate compartment, whereas the trans-Golgi network is the main site of Aβ40 production (Hartmann et al. 1997; Greenfield et al. 1999). In contrast to Aβ40, which is the main secreted Aβ species, most Aβ42 is not destined for secretion. The ratio of Aβ42 to 40 in secreted Aβ is 1:10, whereas the ratio of Aβ42 to 40 in intracellular Aβ is 1:3 (Turner et al. 1996; Cook et al. 1997; Tienari et al. 1997; Wild-Bode et al. 1997; Skovronsky, Doms, and Lee 1998). Despite the relative paucity of Aβ42 production, Aβ42 is the predominant species in fibrillar plaques (Iwatsubo et al. 1994). Amyloid precursor protein is also cleaved by α-secretase between amino acids 16 and 17 of the Aβ domain precluding Aβ formation, with the intracellular carboxy-terminal domain of APP generated by α-secretase subsequently cleaved by γ-secretase within the transmembrane domain to generate a nonamyloidogenic 22-24 residue (3kD) fragment termed p3 (Sisodia et al. 1990).

Intracellular Accumulation of Aβ Peptides

Aβ42 accumulates in the perikaryon of pyramidal neurons as discrete granules that are cathepsin D-positive, which suggests that they may represent lysosomes or lysosome-derived structures (Gouras et al. 2000; D'Andrea et al. 2001; Gyure et al. 2001). These deposits precede plaque formation by decades (Gyure et al. 2001). It was generally hypothesized that Aβ had to be assembled into highly insoluble extracellular amyloid fibrils to exert a cytotoxic effect (Pike et al. 1991, 1993; Lorenzo and Yankner 1994; Iverson et al. 1995), but recent studies have indicated that prefibrillar, diffusible assemblies of Aβ are also deleterious (Chui et al. 1999; Hsia et al. 1999) and that the pathogenically critical process of oligomerization of Aβ begins intraneuronally (Walsh et al. 2000).

Aβ peptide contains several amino acids, particularly aspartate and asparagine at positions 1, 7, 23, and 27, which are vulnerable to racemization, isomerization, and deamidation and represent sites of major potential spontaneous chemical damage (Geiger and Clark 1987; Stephenson and Clark 1989). These age-related post-translational amino acid modifications may interfere with the normal function of intracellular Aβ (Azizeh et al. 2000). The presence of altered aspartyl residues in the form of L-isoAsp and D-Asp in intracellular neurofibrillary tangles (Shapira, Austin, and Mirra 1988; Payan et al. 1992) may indicate that racemized Aβ peptides are involved in neurofibrillary degeneration (Murphy et al. 1994). Death of neurons, a prominent feature of AD, results in the release of oligomerized intracellular Aβ42 into the surrounding milieu. This product of neuron degradation may stimulate production of amyloidogenic fragments of APP and amplify the levels of intracellular Aβ in neighboring cells (Bahr et al. 1998), acting as a nidus for deposition of secreted Aβ40 and contributing to fibrillar plaque formation (Wilson, Doms, and Lee 1999). In fact, overexpression of APP, overproduction of Aβ, and early intracellular accumulation of Aβ, going back to early childhood in some cases (Lemere et al. 1996), could be the precondition for both early onset of amyloidosis β (Gyure et al. 2001) and neurofibrillary degeneration in adults with Down syndrome (DS) (Wilson, Doms, and Lee 1999).

Extracellular Fibrillar Amyloid Deposition

In the human brain, fibrillar Aβ accumulates in plaques within extracellular spaces in gray matter, in the wall of leptomeningeal and parenchymal arteries and veins, and in the basal lamina of capillaries. This pattern of amyloid deposition suggests more than one source of Aβ. It has been proposed that the deposition of fibrillar Aβ in plaques is associated with neurons (Cork et al. 1990; Probst et al. 1991; Wisniewski, Wegiel, and Kotula 1996; Wisniewski et al. 1998; Price et al. 1998; Wegiel and Wisniewski 1999) or microglial cells (Wisniewski et al. 1989; Wegiel and Wisniewski 1990), in the walls of capillaries with perivascular cells of monocyte-macrophage-microglial lineage (Wisniewski et al. 1992; Wisniewski and Wegiel 1993), and in the walls of brain arteries and veins with smooth muscle cells (Wisniewski and Wegiel 1994). Neuronal dystrophy in the fibrillar plaque perimeter (Wisniewski et al. 1989), smooth muscle cell degeneration and death in the wall of amyloid-positive arteries and veins (Wisniewski and Wegiel 1994), and endothelial cell degeneration with capillary lumen obliteration in amyloid-positive capillaries (Wisniewski et al.

1992) are evidence of toxicity of fibrillar Aβ or amyloid-associated factors. Accumulation of paired helical filaments in swollen dystrophic neurites in the perimeter of plaques indicates that extracellular fibrillar Aβ contributes to local enhancement of tau pathology, but only in neurons already affected by neurofibrillary degeneration (Wegiel et al. 2001b).

Fibrillar plaques consist of an amyloid core surrounded by several microglial cells, dystrophic neurites, and amyloid wisps dispersed between astrocytic processes penetrating the periphery (Terry and Wisniewski 1972; Wisniewski et al. 1989; Wegiel and Wisniewski 1990; Wegiel et al. 2000, 2001c). Computer-aided three-dimensional reconstruction of plaques and microvessels in APP_{sw} transgenic mice shows perivascular development of cored plaques. The perivascular location of almost all examined plaques and the infiltration of the interface between vessels and plaques with cells of monocyte/microglia lineage indicate that plaques are formed by inflammatory cells of blood origin. The increase in the number of microglial cells, from one or two in an early plaque to more than 100 in a several-month-old plaque, is associated with amyloid core growth and the progression of neuronal degeneration. It suggests that rather than arresting plaque formation, recruitment of inflammatory cells of blood origin sustains plaque growth.

Fibrillar Amyloid Degradation and Removal

Poor correlation or lack of correlation between the number of senile plaques and clinical progression, especially in the late stages of Alzheimer disease (Arriagada et al. 1992; Hyman, Marzloff, and Arriagada 1993; Nagy et al. 1995; Crystal et al. 1988), suggests a balance between plaque formation and degradation (Hyman, Marzloff, and Arriagada 1993). Morphometry of neocortical plaques in subjects without dementia and those with severe dementia shows a shift from fibrillar to nonfibrillar plaques during the course of AD (Wegiel et al. 2001a). This shift is associated with degradation of classical and primitive plaques into residual plaques that contain a declining amount of fibrillar Aβ or are free of fibrils. The decrease in the volume of Aβ in amygdala during the late stages of AD from 230 mm^3 to 50 mm^3 indicates that even in severely atrophic brains, effective mechanisms of fibrillar amyloid degradation and removal operate (Wegiel et al. 1999b). Further, the decrease in the total number of neurons free of neurofibrillary tangles that is associated with the reduction of the volume of amyloid suggests that factor(s) of neuronal origin control amyloid deposition, and that the loss of neurons inhibits amyloid accumulation. The absence of a correlation between the total number of neurons with neurofibrillary changes and the total volume of amyloid suggests that neurons affected by neurofibrillary pathology do not contribute to amyloid deposition. The arrest of plaque formation in amygdala during the late stages of AD results in the disappearance of Aβ deposits about 2.2 years after the loss of neurons (Wegiel et al. 1999b).

Diffuse Aβ Deposition

Diffuse amorphous nonfibrillar Aβ deposits, also called amorphous plaques (Rozemuller et al. 1989), preplaques (Mann and Esiri 1989), or preamyloid (Lalowski et al. 1996), are considered to be of neuronal origin (Cork et al. 1990; Probst et al. 1991; Wisniewski, Wegiel, and Kotula 1996; Price et al. 1998; Wisniewski H. et al. 1998; Wegiel and Wisniewski 1999). Some studies suggest periterminal neuronal Aβ release (Price et al. 1998). The absence of fibrillar amyloid, dystrophic neurites, activated microglial cells and astrocytes, and chaperone proteins suggests that some diffuse Aβ deposits may correspond to intracellular Aβ accumulation in nerve terminals (Wegiel and Wisniewski 1999). Different properties of diffuse deposits in the molecular layer of the human cerebellum (Snow et al. 1994; Wegiel et al. 1999a), the molecular layer of human and animal dentate gyrus (Wegiel and Wisniewski 1999), the human parvopyramidal layer of the presubiculum (Wisniewski H. et al. 1998), the human caudate nucleus (Gearing et al. 1993; Kida, Wisniewski, and Wisniewski 1995; Gearing, Levey, and Mirra 1997), the internal layers of the entorhinal cortex (Thal et al. 1999) and neocortex (Funato et al. 1998), and plaquelike parenchymal deposits of APP after ischemia (Lin et al. 1999) suggest that diffuse deposits are heterogeneous and represent several types of Aβ deposits with topographically specific differences in the amount, distribution, and properties of APP and nonfibrillar products of APP processing. Some authors suggest that early plaques may be composed primarily of Aβ peptides with truncated N-termini (Gowing at al. 1994; Saido et al. 1995). It was proposed that Aβ17-42 and other prevalent Aβ x-42 peptides may initiate or accelerate plaque formation, perhaps by acting as nucleating centers that seed the subsequent deposition of relatively less amyloidogenic but apparently more abundant full-length Aβ (Pike, Overman, and Cotman 1995). However, the fact that diffuse plaques in the parvopyramidal layer in the presubiculum, caudate nucleus, and the molecular layer of the cerebellar cortex do not fibrillize opposes the hypothesis that diffuse plaques are a precondition for fibrillar plaque formation (Gearing et al. 1993; Gearing, Levey, and Mirra 1997; Wisniewski H. et al. 1998; Wegiel et al. 1999a).

Neurofibrillary Degeneration

Tau is a phosphoprotein that promotes the assembly of tubulin into microtubules, which are essential for neurite outgrowth and axonal transport. Human tau exists in six isoforms, which are all products of a single gene and the result of alternate splicing of its messenger RNA. The isoforms differ by the presence of three or four microtubule binding repeats of thirty-one amino acids each, and by having none, one, or two amino-terminal inserts of twenty-nine amino acids each (Goedert et al. 1989).

The degree of phosphorylation regulates the function of tau protein in neurons. Phosphorylation increases from 2–3 mol of phosphate per mol of tau protein in optimally active tau within normal brain to 5–9 mol of phosphate per mol of tau protein in AD (Köpke et al. 1993). Tau in paired helical filaments, the main component of neurofibrillary tangles, is phosphorylated in at least twenty-one sites (Iqbal and Grundke-Iqbal 1995; Morishima-Kawashima et al. 1995). Hyperphosphorylation of tau may be the result of either higher activities of protein kinases (microtubule-associated protein kinases, glycogen synthase kinase, and other proline directed kinases) or lower activities of protein phosphatases (protein phosphatase 2A and 2B; for references, see Matsuo et al. 1994). The accumulation of abnormally phosphorylated tau in fibrillar form is associated with reduction of normal microtubules, failure of axoplasmic transport and all functions that depend on an intact cytoskeleton, and retrograde degeneration resulting in loss of synapses. In the early "pretangle" stage of changes, soluble hyperphosphorylated tau appears in the body, processes, and synapses of neurons (Bancher et al. 1989). Abnormally phosphorylated tau self-associates via its microtubule-binding domain and forms paired helical filaments (Grundke-Iqbal et al. 1986). The progress of cell degeneration is associated with a slow accumulation of bundles of paired helical filaments around cell nuclei (neurofibrillary tangles) and in dendrites (neurofibrillary threads). In neurons in the late stage of accumulation of paired helical filaments, normal neurofilaments and neurotubules are virtually absent. Severely affected neurons die and eventually the only trace of the affected cell is a ghost tangle. The process of pyramidal neuron degeneration in the hippocampus of people with sporadic AD takes about 3.4–5.4 years from the pretangle stage to cell death

(Bobinski et al. 1998b), after which the residues of cell organelles are degraded relatively quickly. Bundles of fibrils of ghost tangles are penetrated and separated by processes of activated astrocytes. The complete degradation of ghost tangles, consisting of the loss of immunocytochemical characteristics and helical morphology and transformation into amorphous material dispersed between astrocytic processes, takes another several years (Bancher et al. 1989; Wisniewski and Wegiel 1991).

Staging of Neurofibrillary Changes

The numerical density of neurons with neurofibrillary tangles has been found to display a strong relationship with the presence and severity of dementia (Braak and Braak 1991, 1995; Arriagada et al. 1992; Bancher et al. 1993, 1996; Bierer et al. 1995; Gomez-Isla et al. 1996; Thal et al. 2000). Neurofibrillary degeneration is the major cause of neuronal loss in AD and both neurofibrillary degeneration and neuronal loss exhibit consistent and characteristic region-specific, lamina-specific, and cell-type-specific patterns. The steady progression of functional decline seen clinically reflects the gradual expansion of Alzheimer pathology, which begins in the transentorhinal/entorhinal cortex, and then spreads in a predictable pattern across the amygdala, hippocampus, neocortex, and subcortical nuclei. Stage I is associated with the appearance of the first neurofibrillary tangles in transentorhinal cortex, and stage II is associated with neurofibrillary degeneration of neurons in entorhinal cortex and Ammons horn (transentorhinal stages). At this time, stages I and II do not seem to be associated with any obvious memory deficit and are interpreted as corresponding to a clinically silent period of AD. Severe neurofibrillary degeneration and neuronal loss in the entorhinal cortex, amygdala, and hippocampus is seen in stages III and IV (limbic stages). This is associated with destruction of the limbic loop responsible for signal transfer from the neocortex to the hippocampal formation and vice versa. In stage IV neurofibrillary changes expand into the adjoining association areas of the temporal neocortex. These changes are associated with mild impairment of cognitive functions. In stage V severe neurofibrillary degeneration and neuronal loss occur in association neocortical areas, and in stage VI sensory cortex is also affected (neocortical stages). Individuals in stages V and VI display a broad spectrum of clinical symptoms characteristic of progressive dementia (Braak and Braak 1991, 1995).

Clinicopathological Correlations in Alzheimer Disease

Sporadic Alzheimer Disease

General Markers of Brain Atrophy

The appearance of the brain in the early stages of Alzheimer disease does not show macroscopically detectable features. In the later stages of AD, the expansion of ventricles, particularly the temporal horns of the lateral ventricles, atrophy of the entorhinal cortex, hippocampal formation and amygdala, and atrophy of neocortex are all detectable, both in magnetic resonance imaging (MRI) and in postmortem examination. The onset and progression of atrophic changes vary across different brain subdivisions in people with sporadic AD, indicating that some brain structures show higher vulnerability to AD pathology than others.

The overall weight of the brain decreases in advanced Alzheimer disease by 19%; however, the volume of the amygdala decreases by 45% (Scott, DeKosky, and Scheff 1991) and the basal nucleus of Meynert complex by 69% (Dziewiatkowski, Wegiel, and Wisniewski 1994). In comparison to controls, the volume of the hippocampal formation decreases by 36% for incipient nonverbal and ambulatory patients and by 60% once AD has progressed to the point that patients become immobile. Over the duration of clinically manifest AD, from Global Deterioration Scale (GDS) and Functional Assessment Staging (FAST) stage 3 until demise, the projected decrease in the volume of the hippocampal formation is 60%. The projected decreases in the volumes of the cornu Ammonis, subicular complex, and entorhinal cortex over the duration of AD are 64%, 70%, and 51%, respectively. In the final substages of AD, significant atrophy will be present in the cornu Ammonis and all of its sectors and layers except CA4, the subicular complex and all of its parts, and the entorhinal cortex (Bobinski et al. 1995).

Memory System

Neurofibrillary pathology is considered the major cause of neuronal loss and atrophy of the hippocampal formation (Ball 1977; Hyman et al. 1984; Bobinski et al. 1996, 1997), and neuronal loss in the entorhinal cortex and hippocampal formation appears to be a major contributor to the memory impairment seen in Alzheimer disease (Hyman et al. 1984; Bobinski et al. 1998a, b). Neurofibrillary degeneration and the loss of projection neurons are responsible for the impairment of the majority of afferent and efferent connections, producing a functional isolation of the hippocampal formation from other parts of the memory system. A strong correlation between the decrease in the volume of the hippocampal formation subdivisions and the decrease in the total number of neurons has been observed and suggests a causative role of neuronal loss in hippocampal formation volumetric loss. The correlation between the relative decrease in the total number of neurons and the relative increase in the total number of neurofibrillary tangles provides strong support for the argument that neurofibrillary pathology is a leading factor in neuronal and volumetric loss in the hippocampal formation of persons with AD (Bobinski et al. 1996, 1997, 1998a, b).

Atrophy of the hippocampal formation is a function of the duration of neurofibrillary pathology in hippocampal subdivisions. Structures with the earliest onset of neurofibrillary changes, especially the entorhinal cortex and the CA1 sector of the cornu Ammonis, exhibit the most severe atrophy at the time of demise in the end stage of AD (67% and 68%, respectively). The structures affected later in the course of AD, such as subiculum, sectors CA2 and CA3, and presubiculum, are slightly less atrophic (62%, 63%, 55%, and 57%, respectively). The dentate gyrus, which is affected much later than are other structures of the hippocampal formation, is the least atrophic part of the hippocampal formation (Bobinski et al. 1995).

Changes in the memory system are accompanied by neuronal (Gomez-Isla et al. 1997) and synaptic loss in association neocortex (Masliah et al. 1989). These changes are related to clinical presentation as indicated by findings that the numerical density of synaptic terminals correlates with Mini-Mental State Examination (MMSE) scores (DeKosky and Scheff 1990; Terry et al. 1991).

Nigrostriatal System

Rigidity, bradykinesia, and akinesia are clinical features of Parkinson disease (PD) (American Psychiatric Association 1994). However, they are also seen in persons with AD (Franssen et al. 1991, 1993). Gait is significantly compromised at the end of the sixth stage of AD as assessed with the GDS and FAST procedure. Evident rigidity on examination of the passive range of motion of major joints is present in the great majority of patients throughout the course of GDS stage 7. Rigidity appears to be a precursor to the appearance of contractures in multiple joints in nearly all AD patients in FAST substages 7d to 7f.

Our recent morphometric studies have revealed the likely anatomic substrate of parkinsonianlike symptoms (e.g., bradykinesia, rigidity, gait disturbance) seen in sporadic Alzheimer disease and in persons with Down syndrome/Alzheimer disease (Reisberg et al. 2000). A severe loss of pigmented neurons in pars compacta occurs not only in PD/AD (51%), but also in DS/AD (47%) and sporadic AD (39%), although an extremely severe neuronal loss (from 78% to 82%) in dorsolateral rostral nuclei (medial, internal, and lateral) distinguishes cases with PD from those with DS and AD. The large neurons of the caudate and putamen showed a significant loss related to neurofibrillary pathology (35% in sporadic AD, 56% in accelerated aging combined with early-onset AD in the cohort with DS, and 33% in aged people with PD and Alzheimer-type pathology). The small striatal neurons appeared to be resistant to AD- or PD-related pathology, showing no significant loss (Badmaev et al. 2000).

Cerebellum

The pattern of Alzheimer disease cerebellar pathology has unique features. Usually the cerebellum is free of neurofibrillary changes with only a few subjects in the late stages of AD showing neurofibrillary degeneration in the dentate nucleus. Amyloid angiopathy of the leptomeningeal and cortical vessels is seen in both normal aged individuals and persons with AD, with both groups having almost the same numerical density of affected vessels. In cases of AD, plaques appear in the molecular layer of the cerebellar cortex, but only in the diffuse form free of fibrillar amyloid and dystrophic neurites. However, in spite of the absence of fibrillar amyloidosis and neurofibrillary degeneration, the volume of the molecular layer of the cerebellum is reduced by 24% and of the cerebellar cortex granular layer by 22% in AD at the time of demise of persons in GDS/FAST stage 7 in comparison with controls. A decrease in the total number of Purkinje cells correlates with atrophy of the molecular layer. By the end stage of disease, at the time of demise, 32% of these cells appear to be lost, whereas a 30% reduction in the total number of granule cells is associated with the atrophy of the molecular and granular layers.

This pattern of Alzheimer disease pathology suggests that cerebellar atrophy might be secondary to neuronal loss in cerebral structures connected with the cerebellum or the effects of accumulating nonfibrillar, possibly intraneuronal Aβ. The correlation between the duration of AD and both the decrease in the total number of granule cells and the volumetric loss of the molecular and granular layers of the cerebellar cortex indicates that cerebellar atrophy is related in some yet unspecified way to the basic pathologic process of AD. The correlation between the atrophy of the cerebellar cortex and FAST staging of clinical severity at the time of demise, as well as with the duration of AD, indicates that cerebellar pathology progresses in association with clinical changes throughout the course of AD (Wegiel et al. 1999a).

Alzheimer Disease in People with Trisomy of Chromosome 21

Significantly improved survival and extended life expectancy—from about 9 years of age early in the twentieth century to more than 50 years of age currently (Baird and Sadownick 1987; Eyman, Call, and White 1991; Strauss and Eyman 1996)—has attracted increased attention to the age-associated changes exhibited by adults with Down syndrome. Accelerated aging (Roth et al. 1996; Lott and Head 2001) and the presence of an extra copy of the gene encoding APP associated with trisomy 21 increase the risk of AD in this population (Epstein 1986). Adults with DS invariably develop amyloidosis β, neurofibrillary degeneration, and, in many but certainly not all cases, cognitive declines characteristic of AD after reaching 40–50 years of age (Wisniewski, Wisniewski, and Wen 1985; Coyle, Oster-Granite, and Gearhart 1986; Mann et al. 1989, 1992; Armstrong and Smith 1994; Wisniewski et al. 1994; Hof et al. 1995; Hyman et al. 1995).

In Down syndrome, Alzheimer-type pathology is superimposed on a neural substrate having preexisting developmental abnormalities. Therefore, dementia must be assessed against a baseline of lifelong mental retardation, and neuropathology must be assessed against developmental abnormalities that include prenatal defects of neurogenesis, synaptogenesis, and lamination. Gross brain pathology is not detected in utero in individuals with DS but emerges during early postnatal development (Zellweger 1977; Wisniewski, Laure-Kamionowska, and Wisniewski 1984; Wisniewski 1990; Kemper 1991; Golden and Hyman 1994). Smaller cerebral and cerebellar hemispheres, hippocampus, ventral pons, and mammillary bodies (Raz et al. 1995) are associated with reduced populations of neurons and synapses as well as an impoverished development of dendritic networks (Colon 1971; Purpura 1975; Ross, Galaburda, and Kemper 1984; Wisniewski, Wisniewski, and Wen 1985; Becker, Armstrong, and Chang 1986).

Dementia among Adults with Down Syndrome

The first symptoms of clinically significant functional deterioration are seen at a mean age of 56 years, but there is a substantial range around this mean. The estimated prevalence of dementia increases with age from 8% at ages 35–49, to 55% in the age group from 50 to 59 years, to 75% in subjects over the age of 60 (Lai and Williams 1989). Earlier signs of deterioration have been identified as loss of social interaction, decrease in motivation, personality changes, and early signs of dyspraxia and disorientation. Deterioration in the ability to perform coordinated movements is progressive, and affected individuals eventually can no longer walk, show severe signs of disorientation, lose daily-life skills, become incontinent, and, in the end stages of AD, are entirely dependent on nursing care. Ninety-eight percent of persons with both DS and AD who showed severe deterioration developed seizures (Hauser et al. 1986; Zigman, Seltzer, and Silverman 1994).

Neuropathological Changes in Adults with Down Syndrome

People with Down syndrome, who have three copies of the amyloid precursor protein gene due to their trisomy 21, are affected by accelerated aging and develop Alzheimer-type neuropathology by about 40 years of age (Wisniewski et al. 1994). In contrast to earlier postmortem studies suggesting a similar course of Alzheimer-type pathology in the general and DS populations (Mann and Esiri 1989), numerous studies have indicated that Alzheimer disease-related pathology associated with DS is qualitatively and quantitatively distinct (Allsop et al. 1989; Wisniewski et al. 1994; Muketova-Ladinska et al. 1995; Teller et al. 1996). The fact that virtually all people with DS who survive until 40 years of age are affected suggests that the extra copy of the chromosome encoding APP results in overproduction of Aβ and extracellular deposition of fibrillar amyloid in cored plaques and vascular walls (Rumble et al. 1989). Differences in APP processing associated with DS are even detectable in embryonic life. Soluble Aβ42 appears in the brains of individuals with DS from gestational week 21 but is absent in age-matched controls, suggesting that DS-related overexpression of APP leads specifically to an increase in Aβ42 (Teller et al. 1996). The deposition of Aβ in diffuse plaques may begin as early as 8 years of age (Leverenz and Raskind 1998), with approximately 50% of individuals with DS under age 30 showing Aβ deposition (Wisniewski, Wisniewski, and Wen 1985; Mann et al. 1989; Wisniewski et al. 1994; Lemere et al. 1996). Taken together, these results indicate that there is a period of about twenty-five years during which numerous but almost exclusively diffuse, nonfibrillized amyloid deposits are formed without neurofibrillary changes (Allsop et al. 1989; Wisniewski et al. 1994). The impact of these early plaques on neurons appears to be undetectable, and the clinical consequences of these deposits in young and middle-age individuals with DS seem to be negligible. The leading features of the next step of pathological changes include the accumulation of fibrillar plaques, neurofibrillary degeneration, progressive neuronal loss, and functional deterioration, and it is during this stage of progression that diagnoses of clinical dementia are usually made.

The Alzheimer-type functional impairment observed in persons with Down syndrome, occurring sometime in their 50s, appears to be related to neurofibrillary degeneration and the development of neuritic, fibrillized, thioflavin S-positive plaques that are associated with neuropil degeneration (Wisniewski et al. 1994; Wegiel et al. 1996; Sadowski et al. 1999). Our morphometric studies of the entorhinal cortex, hippocampal formation with cornu Ammonis, dentate gyrus and subicular complex, and amygdaloid body in the brains of 13 control people ranging from 32 to 83 years of age at the time of their demise and 15 cases with DS from 38 to 67 years of age at death indicated that neuronal loss in the majority of the memory system subdivisions of people with DS was correlated with age and that neurofibrillary pathology was the major correlate of neuronal degeneration and death. Between 38 and 54 years of age, individuals with DS lost almost all stellate neurons in the second layer of the entorhinal cortex. The estimated rate of loss was 6 neurons per hour. Between the ages of 41 and 68, people with DS lost about 16 neurons per hour in the amygdala and subiculum proper, and the estimated rate of loss in the CA1 sector was about 44 pyramidal neurons per hour. These results suggest that a smaller neuronal "reserve" due to developmental deficits may contribute to the increased risk of dementia in this population (Kuchna et al. 2001).

Familial Alzheimer Disease: Mutations in the Amyloid Precursor Protein Gene

Seven different mutations within or near the Aβ domain of the amyloid precursor protein gene have been found in approximately twenty familial Alzheimer disease kindreds (Lys670Asn/Met671Leu, Ala692Gly, Ile716Val, Val717Ile, Val717Gly, and Val717Phe) (Levy et al. 1990; Chartier-Harlin et al. 1991; Goate et al. 1991; Murrell et al. 1991; Hendriks et al. 1992). Alzheimer disease is associated with a double mutation at codon 670/671 (Lys-Met-Asn-Leu substitution) in a Swedish family. Cells transfected with the Swedish double mutation secrete more soluble Aβ peptides than cells expressing wild type constructs (Citron et al. 1992, 1994). Three different mutations at codon 717 (Val-Ile in two English and two Japanese families, Val-Phe in one American family, and Val-Gly in one English family) are also associated with an AD phenotype. Persons with mutations in the APP gene at codon 717 have more severe pathology than persons with sporadic AD, but share the same pattern and distribution of pathologic features (Karlinksy et al. 1992; Mann et al. 1992). Cells expressing mutations at codon 717 produce more fibrillogenic Aβ42 (Suzuki et al. 1944). Two other APP gene mutations are associated with extensive Aβ angiopathy. A mutation at codon 693 causing E693Q substitution leads to hereditary cerebral hemorrhage with amyloidosis of the Dutch type (HCHWA-D) without the deposition of mature neuritic plaques (Levy et al. 1990), although this mutation increases fibrillization of Aβ peptides (Wisniewski, Ghiso, and Frangione 1991). A mutation at the neighboring codon 692 causing A692G substitution leads to HCHWA of the Flemmish type (Hendriks et al. 1992), in which senile plaques with amyloid cores and dystrophic neurites are present (Cras et al. 1998).

Familial Alzheimer Disease: Mutations in Presenilin 1 and Presenilin 2 Genes

About 50–60% of familial Alzheimer disease is linked to mutations of the presenilin 1 and presenilin 2 genes. So far, more than seventy disease-causing mutations in the PS1 gene have been identified (see register at www.alzforum.org/members/resources/presflmutations/ps1/press1table.html). The abnormalities in the PS2 gene are rare, and only two mutations, Asn141Ile and Met239Val, have been reported in seven related Volga-German families and in one Italian pedigree (Levy-Lahad et al. 1995; Rogaev et al. 1995).

The mRNA of both presenilin 1 and presenilin 2 has been found in many cell types, including neurons. Presenilins are preferentially concentrated in the endoplasmic reticulum and Golgi complex (Kovacs et al. 1996). The physiologic function of presenilins has not yet been determined, although functional analogies suggest that PS1 is involved in: (a) trafficking of cellular proteins including C-terminal fragments of APP, (b) regulation of signal transduction during development, and (c) apoptosis (Nishimura, Yu, and St. George-Hyslop 1999). How presenilins are involved in the pathogenesis of AD is still not known, but PS1 may be a critical cofactor for γ-secretase activity or may even be γ-secretase itself (Wolfe et al. 1999). Presenilin mutations are associated with increased production of the more amyloidogenic Aβ1-42 in human brain, in transfected cells, and in transgenic mice (Borchelt et al. 1996; Duff et al. 1996;

Citron et al. 1997). The link between PS1 and glycogen synthase kinase 3β (GSK-3β), its substrate tau, and β-catenin may indicate that PS1 mutations affect tau phosphorylation and contribute to neurofibrillary degeneration (Murayama et al. 1998; Takashima et al. 1998).

Presenilin 1 mutations are associated with a broad spectrum of both clinical and neuropathological changes. This suggests that even subtle differences in amino acid substitution at any one codon might translate into alterations in the topology of the PS1 protein, γ-secretase activity, and cellular and extracellular pathology (Mann et al. 2001). Variation in age of onset, duration of disease, and clinical features of the disease, as well as amyloid load, rates of neurofibrillary tangles, and neuronal loss among individuals who share the same PS1 mutation and identical ApoE status suggests that as yet unidentified individual or pedigree-specific genetic or epigenetic factors modify the phenotypic consequences of PS1 mutation (Gomez-Isla et al. 1999; Mann 2001 et al.).

Clinical Features of Alzheimer Disease in Subjects with Presenilin Mutations

The age of onset, duration of disease, profile of clinical symptoms, and pattern of neuropathological changes can vary substantially among subjects with different presenilin 1 mutations, as well as among family members with an identical presenilin 1 mutation. Presenilin mutations are associated with the early onset of dementia, but age of onset may vary by thirty years. The earliest symptoms of dementia, at 23 years, were found in a Polish pedigree with familial AD associated with the PS1 mutation P117L (Wisniewski T. et al. 1998). Individual differences in one pedigree, with the age of onset ranging from 27 to 35 years and duration of disease ranging from six to twenty-nine years, suggest that factors in addition to the simple presence of the mutation contribute to the clinical course of the disease (Devi et al. 2000; Mann et al. 2001). Other features of AD that vary substantially among persons with PS1 mutations include the association of cognitive deficits with violent behavior, mood swings, depression, apathy, visual and auditory hallucinations, Parkinson disease, paraparesis, myoclonus, or seizures (Devi et al. 2000).

Neuropathological Changes in Subjects with Presenilin Mutations

Presenilin mutations are associated with deposition of more amyloid than in sporadic Alzheimer disease and severe amyloid angiopathy with accentuation of parenchymal and vascular amyloidosis in cerebellum (Lemere et al. 1996; Wegiel et al. 1998). The study of cortex in ten different PS1 and PS2 mutations (thirty cases) revealed consistent and significant increases in total Aβ and Aβx-42/43 but an unchanged amount of Aβx-40 in senile plaques when compared with sporadic AD cases (Gomez-Isla et al. 1999). The number of cortical neurofibrillary tangles correlated with the duration of illness. Some of the PS1 mutations (M139V, I143F, G209V, R269H, E280A) were associated with faster rates of formation of neurofibrillary tangles and about 2.5-fold higher rates of neuronal loss when compared with sporadic AD cases and PS2 mutations (Gomez-Isla et al. 1999). The presence of Lewy bodies in the amygdala in 61% of the cases with PS1 mutations but in only 17% of the cases with sporadic AD suggests that PS1 mutations increase the risk of neuronal degeneration with Lewy body formation, which in turn could contribute additionally to neuronal loss and possibly an accelerated/modified clinical course (Lippa et al. 1998). A severe involvement of the cerebellum in PS1 AD mutations has been noted in respect to particular mutations (E280A, I143T, M139V, G209V, P117L) (Wegiel et al. 1998; Mann et al. 2001).

The study of fifty-four cases of early-onset familial Alzheimer disease encompassing twenty-five presenilin 1 gene mutations suggested two distinct histopathological profiles that result from the location of the particular mutation. The type 1 histological profile was generally seen in cases with mutations between codon 1 and codon 200. These cases were characterized by many diffuse plaques in isocortex, few cored plaques, and mild or moderate amyloid angiopathy. In contrast, the type 2 histological profile was associated with mutations occurring after codon 200. It also showed many diffuse plaques, but the number and size of cored plaques increased and these were often clustered around blood vessels severely affected by amyloid angiopathy. The extent of amyloid angiopathy was related to mutational position and might involve a PS1-mediated dysfunction of Notch signaling. Mutations of the PS1 gene may therefore alter the topology of the PS1 protein in favor of Aβ formation and deposition and contribute to amyloid angiopathy, particularly in cases in which the mutation lies beyond codon 200 (Mann et al. 2001).

The deletion of exon 9 in the presenilin 1 gene seems to present a separate clinical and histological subtype of Alzheimer disease. Persons with exon 9 deletion often present with spastic paraparesis. Histologically they are distinguishable by the presence of very large, rounded plaques (known as "cotton wool" plaques) composed of mainly Aβ42(43), relatively free from neuritic changes and glial components, and usually devoid of a compact amyloid core (Crook et al. 1998; Mann et al. 2001; Verkkoniemi et al. 2001).

Polymorphism of the Apolipoprotein E Gene

Linkage analysis in families with late-onset Alzheimer disease led to the discovery of an association between late-onset familial and sporadic Alzheimer disease and the apolipoprotein E gene encoded on chromosome 19q (Pericak-Vance et al. 1991; Saunders et al. 1993). There are three alleles of ApoE, which are designated ApoE-ε2, ApoE-ε3, and ApoE-ε4. ApoE-ε3 is the most common form and comprises about 78% of all alleles, whereas the prevalence of ApoE-ε4 is about 14% and ApoE-ε2 about 8%, although these proportions may vary in populations with different ethnic background. ApoE-ε4 homozygotes are at greater risk for AD at slightly earlier age than individuals with other ApoE genotypes (Corder et al. 1993). The presence of ApoE-ε4 allele also influences the age at onset of dementia in individuals with DS (Schupf et al. 1996). Inheritance of the ApoE-ε4 allele correlates with increased deposition of Aβ in vascular walls and plaques (Rebeck et al. 1993; Schmechel et al. 1993). The recognition that inheritance of ApoE-ε4 predisposes to AD provided the first genetic risk factor for the common, late-onset form of AD.

To explain the association between ApoE-ε4 and Alzheimer disease, apolipoprotein E-isoform-specific interactions with microtubule-associated protein 2c and differences in binding with Aβ have been proposed (Strittmatter and Roses 1995). ApoE-ε4 produces a greater acceleration in amyloid fibril formation than either ApoE-ε3 or ApoE-ε2 (Ma et al. 1994). The effect of ApoE-ε4 is significantly more pronounced on Aβ1-42(43) than on Aβ1-40 (Younkin 1995). In persons with the ApoE-ε4 allele, formation of soluble Aβ-ApoE complexes can lead to a reduced clearance of Aβ peptides as well as a direct amyloid fibril-promoting effect of ApoE-ε4 (Wisniewski et al. 1994).

Clinical Conclusions

The characteristic course of dementia associated with sporadic Alzheimer disease can be followed using the Functional Assessment Staging procedure, which can document progressive declines over approximately twice the temporal interval of Alzheimer disease as the Mini-Mental State Examination (Reisberg at al. 2000). The MMSE and other cognitive tests that have been traditionally used to assess dementia are of limited utility once cognitive declines have progressed to a point corresponding to the end of FAST stage 6. Functional Assessment Staging stage 7, with six identifiable functional substages, effectively documents deterioration during the second half of the potential temporal duration of AD. In the latter portion of the FAST, when traditional dementia assessment measures are subject to floor effects, morphometry of the hippocampal formation has revealed a correlation between FAST 7 substages and markers of neurofibrillary degeneration, neuronal loss, and atrophy of the hippocampus (Bobinski et al. 1995, 1997).

Neuropathologically, Alzheimer disease is characterized by a slowly progressive encephalopathy that clearly involves fibrillar amyloid β deposition in plaques and vessels, and region-specific neurofibrillary degeneration and neuronal loss that begins in the transentorhinal/entorhinal cortex and spreads over time to the amygdala and hippocampus, temporal neocortex, association and sensory cortex, and finally cerebellum (Braak and Braak 1991; Bobinski et al. 1995, 1997, 1998a, b; Wegiel et al. 1999, 2001a, b).

Familial Alzheimer disease associated with amyloid precursor protein, presenilin 1, or presenilin 2 gene mutations shows a broad spectrum of clinical features that can vary substantially across cohorts with different mutations and across individuals with the same mutation. This variability includes age of onset, duration, and progression of specific symptoms associated with dementia. Variation in the patterns of neuropathological changes modified in familial AD and in trisomy of chromosome 21 includes the amount, morphology, immunoproperties of parenchymal and vascular amyloid, rate of neurofibrillary changes, and patterns of neuronal loss. The characteristics of familial AD demonstrate that clinical and neuropathological changes are related to the particular genes affected and to mutational position. However, individual and pedigree-specific genetic and epigenetic factors appear to modify the phenotypic consequences of mutations and broaden the spectrum of observed clinical and neuropathological changes.

None of the existing therapeutic strategies arrests or modifies neurofibrillary degeneration. Therefore, we currently cannot block or impede the progressive neurofibrillary degeneration-associated neuronal loss and the resulting degradation of the neuronal network that underlies the devastating dementia. However, the successful treatment of amyloidosis β in transgenic mice, such as with a recent vaccination approach (Schenk et al. 1999; Sigurdsson et al. 2001), permits the development of new strategies for the treatment of AD.

ACKNOWLEDGMENTS

This work was supported in part by funds from the New York State Office of Mental Retardation and Developmental Disabilities, grants from the National Institute of Health (including National Institute of Child Health and Human Development grant PO1-HD35897 and National Institute of Aging grants AG03051 and AG08051), and funds from the American Parkinson Disease Association, Inc.

REFERENCES

Allsop, D., S.-I. Haga, C. Haga, et al. 1989. Early senile plaques in Down's syndrome brains show a close relationship with cell bodies of neurons. *Neuropathology and Applied Neurobiology* 15:531–42.

American Psychiatric Association. 1994. *Diagnostic and Statistical Manual of Mental Disorders.* 4th ed. Washington, D.C.: American Psychiatric Association.

Armstrong, R.A., and C.U.M. Smith. 1994. β-Amyloid (β/A4) deposition in the medial temporal lobe in Down's syndrome: Effects of brain region and patient age. *Neurobiology of Disease* 1:139–44.

Arriagada, P.V., J.H. Growdon, E.T. Hedley-Whyte, et al. 1992. Neurofibrillary tangles but not senile plaques parallel duration and severity of Alzheimer's disease. *Neurology* 42:631–39.

Azizeh, B.Y., E. Head, M.A. Ibrahim, et al. 2000. Molecular dating of senile plaques in the brains of individuals with Down syndrome and in aged dogs. *Experimental Neurology* 163:111–22.

Badmaev, E., J. Wegiel, K. Nowicki, et al. 2000. Neuronal degeneration and loss in nigro-striatal system in Alzheimer disease, Down syndrome, and Parkinson disease. *Journal of Neuropathology and Experimental Neurology* 60:545.

Bahr, B.A., K.B. Hoffman, A.J. Yang, et al. 1998. Amyloid β-protein is internalized selectively by hippocampal field CA1 and neurons to accumulate amyloidogenic carboxyterminal fragments of the amyloid precursor protein. *Journal of Comparative Neurology* 397:139–47.

Baird, P.A., and A.D. Sadownick. 1987. Life expectancy in Down's syndrome. *Journal of Pediatrics* 110:849–54.

Ball, M.J. 1977. Neuronal loss, neurofibrillary tangles and granulovacuolar degeneration in the hippocampus with ageing and dementia. *Acta Neuropathologica* 37:111–18.

Ball, M.J., M. Fishman, V. Hachinski, et al. 1985. A new definition of Alzheimer's disease: A hippocampal dementia. *Lancet* 1:14–16.

Bancher, C., C. Brunner, H. Lassmann, et al. 1989. Accumulation of abnormally phosphorylated tau precedes the formation of neurofibrillary tangles in Alzheimer's disease. *Brain Research* 477:90–99.

Bancher, C., H. Braak, P. Fischer, et al. 1993. Neuropathological staging of Alzheimer lesions and intellectual status in Alzheimer's and Parkinson's disease patients. *Neuroscience Letters* 162:179–82.

Bancher, C., K. Jellinger, H. Lassmann, et al. 1996. Correlation between mental state and quantitative neuropathology in the Vienna longitudinal study of dementia. *European Archive of Psychiatry and Clinical Neurosciences* 246:137–46.

Becker, L.E., D.L. Armstrong, and F. Chan. 1986. Dendritic atrophy in children with Down's syndrome. *Annals of Neurology* 20:520–26.

Bierer, L.M., P.R. Hof, D.P. Purohit, et al. 1995. Neocortical neurofibrillary tangles correlate with dementia severity in Alzheimer's disease. *Archive of Neurology* 52: 81–88.

Bobinski, M., J. Wegiel, H.M. Wisniewski, et al. 1995. Atrophy of the hippocampal formation subdivisions correlates with stage and duration of Alzheimer disease. *Dementia* 6:205–10.

Bobinski, M., J. Wegiel, H.M. Wisniewski, et al. 1996. Neurofibrillary pathology: Correlation with hippocampal formation atrophy in Alzheimer disease. *Neurobiology of Aging* 17:909–19.

Bobinski, M, J. Wegiel, M. Tarnawski, et al. 1997. Relationships between regional neuronal loss and neurofibrillary changes in the hippocampal formation and duration and severity of Alzheimer disease. *Journal of Neuropathology and Experimental Neurology* 56: 414–20.

Bobinski, M, M.J. de Leon, M. Tarnawski, et al. 1998a. Neuronal and volume loss in CA1 of the hippocampal formation uniquely predicts duration and severity of Alzheimer disease. *Brain Research* 805:267–69.

Bobinski, M., J. Wegiel, M. Tarnawski, et al. 1998b. Duration of neurofibrillary changes in the hippocampal pyramidal neurons. *Brain Research* 799:156–58.

Borchelt, D.R., G. Thinakaran, C.B. Eckman, et al. 1996. Familial Alzheimer's disease-linked presenilin 1 variants elevate Aβ1-42/1-40 ratio in vitro and in vivo. *Neuron* 17: 1005–13.

Braak, H., and E. Braak. 1991. Neuropathological staging of Alzheimer-related changes. *Acta Neuropathologica* 82:239–69.

Braak, H., and E. Braak. 1995. Staging of Alzheimer's disease-related neurofibrillary changes. *Neurobiology of Aging* 16:271–84.

Chartier-Harlin, M-C., F. Crawford, H. Houlden, et al. 1991. Early-onset Alzheimer's disease caused by mutations at codon 717 of the β-amyloid gene. *Nature* 353:844–46.

Chui, D.-H., H. Tanahashi, K. Ozawa, et al. 1999. Transgenic mice with Alzheimer presenilin 1 mutations show accelerated neurodegeneration without plaque formation. *Nature Medicine* 5:560–64.

Citron, M., T. Oltersdorf, C. Haass, et al. 1992. Mutation of the beta-amyloid precursor protein in familial Alzheimer's disease increases beta-protein production. *Nature* 360:672–74.

Citron, M., C. Vigo-Pelfrey, D.B. Teplow, et al. 1994. Excessive production of amyloid-β protein by peripheral cells of symptomatic and presymptomatic patients carrying the Swedish familial Alzheimer disease mutation. *Proceedings of the National Academy of Sciences USA* 91:11993–97.

Citron, M., D. Westaway, W.M. Xia, et al. 1997. Mutant presenilins of Alzheimer's disease increase production of 42-residue amyloid β-protein in both transfected cells and transgenic mice. *Nature Medicine* 3:67–72.

Colon, E.J. 1997. Quantitative cytoarchitectonics of the human cerebral cortex. *Psychiatria Neurologia Neurochirurgia* 74:291–302.

Cook, D.G., M.S. Forman, J.C. Sung, et al. 1997. Alzheimer's Aβ(1-42) is generated in the endoplasmic reticulum/intermediate compartments on NT2N cells. *Nature Medicine* 3:1021–23.

Corder, E.H., A.M. Saunders, W.J. Strittmatter, et al. 1993. Gene dose of apolipoprotein E type 4 allele and the risk of Alzheimer's disease in late onset families. *Science* 261:921–23.

Cork, L.C., C. Masters, K. Beyreuther, et al. 1990. Development of senile plaques. Relationships of neuronal abnormalities and amyloid deposits. *American Journal of Pathology* 137:1383–92.

Coyle, J.T., M.L. Oster-Granite, and J.D. Gearhart. 1986. The neurobiologic consequences of Down syndrome. *Brain Research Bulletin* 16:773–87.

Cras, P., F. van Harskamp, L. Hendriks, et al. 1998. Presenile Alzheimer dementia characterized by amyloid angiopathy and large amyloid core type senile plaques in the APP 692 Ala→Gly mutation. *Acta Neuropathologica* 96:253–60.

Crook, R., A.Verkoniemi, J. Perez-Tur, et al. 1998. A variant of Alzheimer's disease with spastic paraparesis and unusual plaques due to deletion of exon 9 of presenilin 1. *Nature Medicine* 4:452–55.

Crystal, H., D. Dickson, P. Fuld, et al. 1988. Clinico-pathologic studies in dementia: Nondemented subjects with pathologically confirmed Alzheimer's disease. *Neurology* 38:1682–87.

D'Andrea, M.R., R.G. Nagele, H.-Y. Wang, et al. 2001. Evidence that neurons accumulating amyloid can undergo lysis to form amyloid plaques in Alzheimer's disease. *Histopathology* 38:120–34.

De Kosky, S.T., and S.W. Scheff. 1990. Synapse loss in frontal cortex biopsies in Alzheimer's disease: Correlation with cognitive severity. *Annals of Neurology* 27:457–64.

Devi, G., A. Fotiou, D. Jyrinji, B. Tycko, et al. 2000. Novel presenilin1 mutations associated with early onset of dementia in a family with both early-onset and late-onset alzheimer disease. *Archives of Neurology* 57:1454–56.

Duff, K., C. Eckman, C. Zehr, et al. 1996. Increased amyloid β42(43) in brains of mice expressing mutant presenilin 1. *Nature* 383:710–13.

Dziewiatkowski, J., J. Wegiel, and H.M. Wisniewski. 1994. Atrophy of the nucleus basalis Meynerti complex (NBMC) in end-stage of Alzheimer's disease. *Neurobiology of Aging* 15 (Suppl. 1):S111.

Epstein, C.J. 1986. Trisomy 21 and the nervous system: From cause to cure. In *The Neurobiology of Down Syndrome*, edited by C.J. Epstein. New York: Raven Press, pp. 1–15.

Eyman, R., T. Call, and J. White. 1991. Life expectancy of persons with Down syndrome. *American Journal of Mental Retardation* 95:603–12.

Folstein, M.F., S.E. Folstein, and P.R. McHugh. 1975. Mini-Mental State: A practical method for grading the cognitive state of patients for the clinician. *Journal of Psychiatric Research* 12:189–98.

Franssen, E.H., B. Reisberg, A. Kluger, et al. 1991. Cognition independent neurologic symptoms in normal aging and probable Alzheimer's disease. *Archives of Neurology* 48: 148–54.

Franssen, E.H., A. Kluger, C.L. Torossian, et al. 1993. The neurologic syndrome of severe Alzheimer's disease. Relationships to functional decline. *Archives of Neurology* 50: 1029–39.

Funato, H., M. Yoshimura, T. Yamazaki, et al. 1998. Astrocytes containing amyloid β-protein (Aβ)-positive granules are associated with Aβ40-positive diffuse plaques in the aged human brain. *American Journal of Pathology* 152:983–92.

Gearing, M., A.I. Levey, and S.S. Mirra. 1997. Diffuse plaques in the striatum in Alzheimer disease (AD): Relationship to the striatal mosaic and selected neuropeptide markers. *Journal of Neuropathology and Experimental Neurology* 56:1363–70.

Gearing, M., R.W. Wilson, E.R. Unger, et al. 1993. Amyloid precursor protein (APP) in the striatum in Alzheimer's disease: An immunohistochemical study. *Journal of Neuropathology and Experimental Neurology* 52:22–30.

Geiger, T., and D. Clark. 1987. Deamidation, isomerization, and racemization at asparaginyl and aspartyl residues in peptides. *Journal of Biological Chemistry* 262:785–94.

Geula, C., C.-K. Wu, D. Saroff, et al. 1998. Aging renders the brain vulnerable to amyloid β-protein neurotoxicity. *Nature Medicine* 4:827–31.

Goate, A., M.C. Chartier-Harlin, M. Mullan, et al. 1991. Segregation of a missense mutation in the amyloid precursor protein gene with familial Alzheimer's disease. *Nature* 349:704–6.

Goedert, M., M.G. Spillantini, R. Jakes, et al. 1989. Multiple isoforms of human microtubule associated protein tau: Sequences and localization in neurofibrillary tangles of Alzheimer's disease. *Neuron* 3:519–26.

Golden, J.A., and B.T. Hyman. 1994. Development of the superior temporal neocortex is anomalous in trisomy 21. *Journal of Neuropathology and Experimental Neurology* 53: 513–20.

Goldgaber, D., M.I. Lerman, O.W. McBride, et al. 1987. Characterization and chromosomal localization of a cDNA encoding brain amyloid of Alzheimer's disease. *Science* 235:877–80.

Gomez-Isla, T., J.L. Price, D.W. McKeel, Jr., et al. 1996. Profound loss of layer II entorhinal cortex neurons occurs in very mild Alzheimer's disease. *Journal of Neuroscience* 16:4491–4500.

Gomez-Isla, T., R. Hollister, M. West, et al. 1997. Neuronal loss correlates with but exceeds neurofibrillary tangles in Alzheimer's disease. *Annals of Neurology* 41:17–24.

Gomez-Isla, T., W.B. Growdon, M.J. McNamara, et al. 1999. The impact of different presenilin 1 and presenilin 2 mutations on amyloid deposition, neurofibrillary changes and neuronal loss in the familial Alzheimer's disease brain: Evidence for other phenotype-modifying factors. *Brain* 122:1709–19.

Gouras, G.K., J. Tsai, J. Naslund, et al. 2000. Intraneuronal Aβ42 accumulation in human brain. *American Journal of Pathology* 156:15–20.

Gowing, E., A.E. Roher, A.S. Woods, et al. 1994. Chemical characterization of Aβ17-42 peptide, a component of diffuse amyloid deposits of Alzheimer disease. *Journal of Biological Chemistry* 269:10987–90.

Greenfield, J.P., J. Tsai, G.K. Gouras, et al. 1999. Endoplasmic reticulum and trans-Golgi network generate distinct populations of Alzheimer β-amyloid peptides. *Proceedings of the National Academy of Sciences USA* 96:742–47.

Grundke-Iqbal, I., K. Iqbal, Y.C. Tung, et al. 1986. Abnormal phosphorylation of the microtubule associated protein τ (tau) in Alzheimer cytoskeletal pathology. *Proceedings of the National Academy of Sciences USA* 83:4913–17.

Gyure, K.A., R. Durham, W.F. Stewart, et al. 2001. Intraneuronal Aβ-amyloid precedes development of amyloid plaques in Down syndrome. *Archives of Pathology and Laboratory Medicine* 125:489–92.

Hartmann, T., S.C. Bieger, B. Bruhl, et al. 1997. Distinct sites of intracellular production for Alzheimer's disease Aβ 40/42 amyloid peptides. *Nature Medicine* 3:1016–20.

Hauser, W.A., M.L. Morris, I.L. Heston, et al. 1986. Seizures and myoclonus in patients with Alzheimer's disease. *Neurology* 36:1226–30.

Hendriks, L., C.M. van Duijn, P. Cras, et al. 1992. Presenile dementia and cerebral haemorrhage linked to a mutation at codon 692 of the β-amyloid precursor gene. *Nature Genetics* 1:218–21.

Hof, P.R., C. Bouras, D.P. Perl, et al. 1995. Age-related distribution of neuropathologic changes in the cerebral cortex of patients with Down's syndrome. *Archives of Neurology* 52:379–91.

Hsia, A.Y., E. Masliah, L. McConlogue, et al. 1999. Plaque-independent disruption of neural circuits in Alzheimer's disease mouse models. *Proceedings of the National Academy of Sciences USA* 96:3228–33.

Hyman, B.T., K. Marzloff, and P.V. Arriagada. 1993. The lack of accumulation of senile plaques or amyloid burden in Alzheimer's disease suggests a dynamic balance between amyloid deposition and resolution. *Journal of Neuropathology and Experimental Neurology* 53:594–600.

Hyman, B.T., G.W. Van Hoesen, A.R. Damasio, et al. 1984. Alzheimer's disease: Cell-specific pathology isolates the hippocampal formation. *Science* 225:1168–70.

Hyman, B.T., H.L. West, G.W. Rebeck, et al. 1995. Neuropathological changes in Down's syndrome hippocampal formation. Effect of age and apolipoprotein E genotype. *Archives of Neurology* 52:373–78.

Iqbal, K., and I. Grundke-Iqbal. 1995. Alzheimer abnormally phosphorylated tau is more hyperphosphorylated than the fetal tau and causes the disruption of microtubules. *Neurobiology of Aging* 16:375–79.

Iverson, L.L., R.J. Mortishire-Smith, S.J. Pollack, et al. 1995. The toxicity in vitro of β-amyloid protein. *Biochemistry* 311:1–16.

Iwatsubo, T., A. Okada, N. Suzuki, et al. 1994. Visualization of Aβ42(43) and Aβ40 in senile plaques with specific monoclonals: Evidence that the initially deposited species is Aβ42(43). *Neuron* 13:45–53.

Kang, J., H.G. Lemaire, A. Unterback, et al. 1987. The precursor of Alzheimer's disease amyloid A4 protein resembles a cell-surface receptor. *Nature* 325:733–36.

Karlinsky, H., G. Vaula, J.L. Haines, et al. 1992. Molecular and prospective phenotypic characterization of a pedigree with familial Alzheimer's disease and a missense mutation in codon 717 of the β-amyloid precursor protein gene. *Neurology* 42:1445–53.

Katzman, R. 1986. Alzheimer's disease. *New England Journal of Medicine* 314:964–73.

Kemper, T.L. 1991. Down syndrome. In *Cerebral Cortex*, edited by A. Peters and E. Jones. New York: Plenum Press, vol. 9, pp. 511–26.

Khatchaturian, Z.S. 1985. Diagnosis of Alzheimer's disease. *Archives of Neurology* 42: 1097–1105.

Kida, E., K.E. Wisniewski, and H.M. Wisniewski. 1995. Early amyloid-β deposits show different immunoreactivity to the amino- and carboxy-terminal regions of β-peptide in Alzheimer's disease and Down's syndrome brain. *Neuroscience Letters* 193:105–8.

Köpke, E., Y.-C. Tung, S. Sheikh, et al. 1993. Microtubule associated protein tau: Abnormal phosphorylation of a non-paired helical filament pool in Alzheimer disease. *Journal of Biological Chemistry* 268:24374–83.

Kovacs, D.M., H.J. Fausett, K.J. Page, et al. 1996. Alzheimer associated presenilin 1 and 2: Neuronal expression in brain and localization to intracellular membranes in mammalian cells. *Nature Medicine* 2:224–29.

Kuchna, I., J. Wegiel, M. Tarnawski, et al. 2001. Alzheimer type pathology in the memory system of people with Down syndrome. *Journal of Neuropathology and Experimental Neurology* 60:545.

Lai, F., and M.D. Williams. 1989. A prospective study of Alzheimer disease in Down syndrome. *Archives of Neurology* 46:849.

Lalowski, M., A.A. Golabek, C.A. Lemere, et al. 1996. The "non-amyloidogenic" p3 fragment (Aβ17-42) is a major constituent of Down syndrome cerebellar preamyloid. *Journal of Biological Chemistry* 271:33623–31.

Lemere, C.A., F. Lopera, K.S. Kosik, et al. 1996. The E280A presenilin 1 Alzheimer mutation produced Aβ42 deposition and severe cerebellar pathology. *Nature Medicine* 2: 1146–50.

Leverenz, J.B., and M.A. Raskind 1998. Early amyloid deposition in the medial temporal lobe of young Down syndrome patients: A regional quantitative analysis. *Experimental Neurology* 150:296–304.

Levy, E., M.D. Carman, I. Fernandez-Madrid, et al. 1990. Mutation of the Alzheimer's disease amyloid gene in hereditary cerebral hemorrhage, Dutch type. *Science* 248: 1124–26.

Levy-Lahad, E., W. Wasco, P. Poorkaj, et al. 1995. Candidate gene for the chromosome 1 familial Alzheimer's disease locus. *Science* 269:973–97.

Lin, B., R. Schmidt-Kastner, R. Busto, et al. 1999. Progressive parenchymal deposition of β-amyloid precursor protein in rat brain following global cerebral ischemia. *Acta Neuropathologica* 97:359–68.

Lippa, C.F., H. Fujiwara, D.M.A. Mann, et al. 1998. Lewy bodies contain altered α-synuclein in brains of many familial Alzheimer's disease patients with mutations in presenilin and amyloid precursor protein genes. *American Journal of Pathology* 135: 1365–70.

Lorenzo, A., and B.A. Yankner. 1994. β-amyloid neurotoxicity requires fibril formation and is inhibited by Congo red. *Proceedings of the National Academy of Sciences USA* 91: 12243–47.

Lott, I.T., and E. Head. 2001. Down syndrome and Alzheimer's disease: A link between development and aging. *Mental Retardation Developmental Disabilities Research Review* 7:172–78.

Ma, J., A. Yee, Jr., H.B. Brewer, et al. 1994. Amyloid associated proteins a1-antichymotrypsin and apolipoprotein E promote assembly of Alzheimer β protein into filaments. *Nature* 372:92–94.

Mann, D.M.A., and M.M. Esiri. 1989. The pattern of acquisition of plaques and tangles in the brains of patients under fifty years of age with Down's syndrome. *Journal of Neurological Sciences* 89:169–79.

Mann, D.M.A., A. Brown, D. Prinja, et al. 1989. An analysis of the morphology of senile plaques in Down's syndrome patients of different ages using immunocytochemical and lectin histochemical methods. *Neuropathology and Applied Neurobiology* 15: 317–29.

Mann, D.M.A., D. Jones, J.S. Snowden, et al. 1992. Pathological changes in the brain of a patient with familial Alzheimer's disease having a missense mutation at codon 717 in the amyloid precursor protein gene. *Neuroscience Letters* 137:225–28.

Mann, D.M.A., S.M. Pickering-Brown, A. Takeuchi, et al. 2001. Amyloid angiopathy and variability in amyloid β deposition is determined by mutation position in presenilin-1-linked Alzheimer's disease. *American Journal of Pathology* 158:2165–75.

Masliah, E., R.D. Terry, R.M. DeTeresa, et al. 1989. Immunohistochemical quantification of the synapse-related protein synaptophysin in Alzheimer disease. *Neuroscience Letters* 103:234–39.

Matsuo, E.S., R.-W. Shin, M.L. Billingsley, et al. 1994. Biopsy derived adult human brain tau is phosphorylated at many of the same sites as an Alzheimer's disease paired helical filament tau. *Neuron* 13:989–1002.

McKhann, G., D. Drachman, M. Folstein, et al. 1984. Clinical diagnosis of Alzheimer's disease. *Neurology* 34:939–44.

Mirra, S.S., A. Heyman, D. McKeel, et al. 1991. The Consortium to Establish a Registry for Alzheimer's Disease (CERAD). Part II: Standardization of the neuropathologic assessment of Alzheimer disease. *Neurology* 41:479–86.

Mirra, S.S., M.N. Hart, and R.D. Terry. 1993. Making the diagnosis of Alzheimer's disease: A primer for practicing pathologist. *Archives of Pathology and Laboratory Medicine* 117:132–44.

Morishima-Kawashima, M., M. Hasegawa, K. Takio, et al. 1995. Hyperphosphorylation of tau in PHF. *Neurobiology of Aging* 16:365–80.

Muketova-Ladinska, E.B., C.R. Harrington, M. Roth, et al. 1995. Distribution of tau protein in Down's syndrome: Quantitative differences from Alzheimer's disease. *Developmental Brain Dysfunction* 7:311–29.

Murayama, M., S. Tanaka, J. Palatino, et al. 1998. Direct association of presenilin-1 with β-catenin. *FEBS Letters* 433:73–77.

Murphy, G.M., F.S. Forno, L. Higgins, et al. 1994. Development of monoclonal antibody specific for the COOH-terminal of Aβ-amyloid 1-42 and its immunohistochemical reactivity in Alzheimer's disease and related disorders. *American Journal of Pathology* 144:1082–88.

Murrell, J., M. Farlow, B. Ghetti, et al. 1991. A mutation in the amyloid precursor protein associated with hereditary Alzheimer's disease. *Science* 254:97–99.

Nagy, Z., M.M. Esiri, K.A. Jobst, et al. 1995. Relative roles of plaques and tangles in the dementia of Alzheimer's disease: Correlations using three sets of neuropathological criteria. *Dementia* 6:21–31.

National Institute on Aging and Reagan Institute Working Group on Diagnostic Criteria for the Neuropathological Assessment of Alzheimer's Disease. 1997. Consensus recommendations for the postmortem diagnosis of Alzheimer's disease. *Neurobiology of Aging* 18 (Suppl. 4):S1–2.

Nishimura, M., G. Yu, and P.H. St. George-Hyslop. 1999. Biology of presenilins as causative molecules for Alzheimer disease. *Clinical Genetics* 55:219–25.

Payan, I.L., S.-J. Chou, G.H. Fisher, et al. 1992. Altered aspartate in Alzheimer neurofibrillary tangles. *Neurochemical Research* 17:187–91.

Pericak-Vance, M.A., J.L. Bebout, P.C. Gaskell, et al. 1991. Linkage studies in familial Alzheimer disease: Evidence for chromosome 19 linkage. *American Journal of Human Genetics* 48:1034–50.

Pike, C.J., A.J. Walencewicz, C.G. Glabe, et al. 1991. In vitro aging of β-amyloid protein causes peptide aggregation and neurotoxicity. *Brain Research* 563:311–14.
Pike, C.J., D. Burdick, A.J. Walencewicz, et al. 1993. Neurodegeneration induced by β-amyloid peptides in vitro: The role of peptide assembly state. *Journal of Neuroscience* 13:1676–87.
Pike, C.J., M.J. Overman, and C.W. Cotman. 1995. Amino-terminal deletions enhance aggregation of β-amyloid peptides in vitro. *Journal of Biological Chemistry* 270: 23895–98.
Price, L.P., G. Thinkaran, D.R. Borchelt, et al. 1998. Neuropathology of Alzheimer's disease and animal models. In *Neuropathology of Dementing Disorders*, edited by W.R. Markesbery. London: Arnold, pp. 121–41.
Probst, A., D. Langui, S. Ipsen, et al. 1991. Deposition of beta/A4 protein along neuronal plasma membranes in diffuse senile plaques. *Acta Neuropathologica* 83:21–29.
Purpura, D.P. 1975. Normal and aberrant neuronal development in the cerebral cortex of human fetus and young infants. In *Brain Mechanisms in Mental Retardation*, edited by N.A. Buchwald and M.A.B. Brazier. New York: Academic Press, pp. 141–69.
Raz, N., I.J. Torres, S.D. Briggs, et al. 1995. Selective neuroanatomic abnormalities in Down's syndrome and their cognitive correlates: Evidence from MRI morphometry. *Neurology* 45:356–66.
Rebeck, G.W., J.S. Reiter, D.K. Strickland, et al. 1993. Apolipoprotein E in sporadic Alzheimer's disease: Allelic variation and receptor interactions. *Neuron* 11:575–80.
Reisberg, B. 1988. Functional Assessment Staging (FAST). *Psychopharmacology Bulletin* 24:653–59.
Reisberg, B., S.H. Ferris, M.J. de Leon, et al. 1982. The Global Deterioration Scale for assessment of primary degenerative dementia. *American Journal of Psychiatry* 139: 1136–39.
Reisberg, B., A. Burns, H. Brodaty, et al. 1997. Diagnosis of Alzheimer's disease: Report of an International Psychogeriatric Association Work Group under the cosponsorship of the Alzheimer's Disease International, the European Federation of Neurological Societies, the World Health Organization, and the World Psychiatric Association. *International Psychogeriatrics* 9 (Suppl. 1):S11–38.
Reisberg, B., E. Franssen, M.A. Shah, et al. 2000. Clinical diagnosis of dementia: A review. In *Dementia*, edited by M. Maj and N. Sartorius. Chichester: John Wiley & Sons, Ltd., pp. 69–115.
Rogaev, E.I., R. Sherrington, E.A. Rogaeva, et al. 1995. Familial Alzheimer's disease in kindreds with missense mutation in a gene on chromosome 1 related to the Alzheimer's disease type 3 gene. *Nature* 376:775–78.
Ross, M.H., A.M. Galaburda, and T.L. Kemper. 1984. Down's syndrome: Is there a decreased population of neurons? *Neurology* 34:909–16.
Roth, G.M., B. Sun, F.S. Greensite, et al. 1996. Premature aging in persons with Down syndrome: MR findings. *American Journal of Neuroradiology* 17:1283–89.
Rozemuller, J.M., P. Eikelenboom, F.C. Stam, et al. 1989. A4 protein in Alzheimer's disease: Primary and secondary cellular events in extracellular amyloid deposition. *Journal of Neuropathology and Experimental Neurology* 48:674–91.
Rumble, B., R. Retallack, C. Hilbich, et al. 1989. Amyloid A4 protein and its precursor in Down's syndrome and Alzheimer's disease. *New England Journal of Medicine* 320: 1446–52.

Sadowski, M., H.M. Wisniewski, M. Tarnawski, et al. 1999. Entorhinal cortex of aged subjects with Down's syndrome shows severe neuronal loss caused by neurofibrillary pathology. *Acta Neuropathologica* 97:156–64.

Saido, T.C., T. Iwatsubo, D.M.A. Mann, et al. 1995. Dominant and differential deposition of distinct β-amyloid peptide species, AβN3(pE), in senile plaques. *Neuron* 14: 457–66.

Saunders, A.M., W.J. Strittmatter, D. Schmechel, et al. 1993. Association of apolipoprotein E allele β4 with late-onset familial and sporadic Alzheimer's disease. *Neurology* 43:1467–72.

Schenk, D., R. Barbour, W. Dunn, et al. 1999. Immunization with amyloid-β attenuates Alzheimer disease-like pathology in the PDAPP mice. *Nature* 400:173–77.

Schmechel, D.E.A., A.M. Saunders, W.J. Strittmatter, et al. 1993. Increased amyloid β-peptide deposition in cerebral cortex as a consequence of apolipoprotein E genotypes in late-onset Alzheimer's disease. *Proceedings of the National Academy of Sciences USA* 90:9649–53.

Schupf, N., D. Kapell, J.H. Lee, et al. 1996. Onset of dementia is associated with apolipoprotein E-ε4 in Down's syndrome. *Annals of Neurology* 40:799–801.

Scott, S.A., S.T. DeKosky, and S.W. Scheff. 1991. Volumetric atrophy of the amygdala in Alzheimer's disease: Quantitative serial reconstruction. *Neurology* 41:351–56.

Shapira, R., G. E. Austin, and S.S. Mirra. 1988. Neuritic plaque amyloid is highly racemized. *Journal of Neurochemistry* 50:69–74.

Sherrington, R., E.I. Rogaev, Y. Liang, et al. 1995. Cloning of a gene bearing missense mutations in early-onset familial Alzheimer's disease. *Nature* 374:754–60.

Sigurdsson, E.M., H. Scholzowa, P. Mehta, et al. 2001. Immunization with a non-toxic/non-fibrillar amyloid-β homologous peptide reduces Alzheimer's disease associated pathology in trangenic mice. *American Journal of Pathology* 159:439–47.

Sisodia, S.S., E.H. Koo, K. Beyreuther, et al. 1990. Evidence that β-amyloid protein in Alzheimer's disease is not derived by normal processing. *Science* 248:492–95.

Skovronsky, D.M., R.W. Doms, and V.M.-Y. Lee. 1998. Detection of a novel intraneuronal pool of insoluble amyloid β-protein that accumulates with time in culture. *Journal of Cell Biology* 141:1031–39.

Small, G.W., P.V. Rabins, P.P. Barry, et al. 1997. Diagnosis and treatment of Alzheimer disease and related disorders. Consensus statement of the American Association for Geriatric Psychiatry, the Alzheimer's Association, and the American Geriatrics Society. *Journal of the American Medical Association* 278:1363–71.

Snow, A.D., R.T. Sekiguchi, D. Nochlin, et al. 1994. Heparan sulfate proteoglycan in diffuse plaques of hippocampus but not of cerebellum in Alzheimer's disease brain. *American Journal of Pathology* 144:337–47.

Stephenson, R.C., and S. Clark. 1989. Succinimide formation from aspartyl and asparaginyl peptides as a model for the spontaneous degradation of proteins. *Journal of Biological Chemistry* 264:6164–70.

Strauss, D., and R. Eyman. 1996. Mortality of people with mental retardation in California with and without Down syndrome. *American Journal of Mental Retardation* 100: 643–53.

Strittmatter, W.J., and A.D. Roses. 1995. Apolipoprotein E and Alzheimer disease. *Proceedings of the National Academy of Sciences USA* 92:4725–27.

Suzuki, N., T.T. Cheung, X.D. Cai, et al. 1994. An increased percentage of long amyloid β protein secreted by familial amyloid β protein precursor (βAPP717) mutants. *Science* 264:1336–40.

Takashima, A., M. Murayama, O. Murayama, et al. 1998. Presenilin 1 associates with glycogen synthase kinase-3β and its substrate tau. *Proceedings of the National Academy of Sciences USA* 95:9637–41.

Teller, J.K., C. Russo, L.M. DeBusk, et al. 1996. Presence of soluble amyloid β-peptide precedes amyloid plaque formation in Down's syndrome. *Nature Medicine* 2:93–95.

Terry, R.D., and H.M. Wisniewski 1972. Ultrastructure of senile dementia and of experimental analogues. In *Aging and the Brain*, edited by C.M. Gaitz. New York: Plenum, pp. 89–116.

Terry, R.D., E. Masliah, D.P. Salmon, et al. 1991. Physical basis of cognitive alterations in Alzheimer's disease; synapse loss is the major correlate of cognitive impairment. *Annals of Neurology* 30:572–80.

Thal, D.R., I. Sassin, C. Schultz, et al. 1999. Fleecy amyloid deposits in the internal layers of the human entorhinal cortex are comprised of N-terminal truncated fragments of Aβ. *Journal of Neuropathologic and Experimental Neurology* 58:210–16.

Thal, D.R., M. Holzer, U. Rüb, et al. 2000. Alzheimer-related τ-pathology in the perforant path target zone and in the hippocampal stratum oriens and radiatum correlates with onset and degree of dementia. *Experimental Neurology* 163:98–110.

Tienari, P.J., N. Ida, E. Ikonen, et al. 1997. Intracellular and secreted Alzheimer β-amyloid species are generated by distinct mechanisms in cultured hippocampal neurons. *Proceedings of the National Academy of Sciences USA* 94:4125–30.

Tomlinson, B.E., and G. Henderson. 1975. Some quantitative cerebral findings in normal and demented old people. In *Neurobiology of Aging*, edited by R. Terry and S. Gershon. New York: Raven Press, pp. 183–204.

Turner, R.S., N. Suzuki, A.S.C. Chyung, et al. 1996. Amyloid β 40 and β 42 are generated intracellularly in human neurons and their secretion increases with maturation. *Journal of Biological Chemistry* 271:8966–77.

Verkkoniemi, A. H. Kalimo, A. Paetau, et al. 2001. Variant Alzheimer disease with spastic paraparesis: Neuropathological phenotype. *Journal of Neuropathology and Experimental Neurology* 60:483–92.

Walsh, D.M., B.P. Tseng, R.E. Rydel, et al. 2000. The oligomerization of amyloid β-protein begins intracellularly in cells derived from human brain. *Biochemistry* 39: 10832–39.

Wegiel, J., and H.M. Wisniewski. 1990. The complex of microglial cells and amyloid star in three-dimensional reconstruction. *Acta Neuropathologica* 81:116–24.

Wegiel, J., and H.M. Wisniewski. 1999. Projections of neurons in neuritic plaques formation. *Neuroscience News* 2:34–39.

Wegiel, J., H.M. Wisniewski, J. Dziewiatkowski, et al. 1996. Differential susceptibility to neurofibrillary pathology among patients with Down syndrome. *Dementia* 7: 135–41.

Wegiel, J., H.M. Wisniewski, I. Kuchna, et al. 1998. Cell-type specific enhancement of amyloid-β deposition in a novel presenilin-1 mutation (P117L). *Journal of Neuropathology and Experimental Neurology* 57:831–38.

Wegiel, J., H.M. Wisniewski, J. Dziewiatkowski, et al. 1999a. Cerebellar atrophy in Alzheimer disease: Clinicopathological correlations. *Brain Research* 818:41–50.

Wegiel, J., H.M. Wisniewski, J. Morys, et al. 1999b. Neuronal loss and amyloid-β removal in the amygdala of people with Down syndrome. *Neurobiology of Aging* 20: 259–69.

Wegiel, J., K-C.Wang, M. Tarnawski, et al. 2000. Microglial cells are the driving force in fibrillar plaque formation whereas astrocytes are a leading factor in plaque degradation. *Acta Neuropathologica* 100:356–64.

Wegiel J, M. Bobinski, M. Tarnawski, et al. 2001a. Shift from fibrillar to nonfibrillar Aβ deposits in the neocortex of subjects with Alzheimer disease. *Journal of Alzheimer's Disease* 3:49–57.

Wegiel, J., M. Bobinski, M. Tarnawski, et al. 2001b. Fibrillar amyloid-β affects neurofibrillary changes but only in neurons already involved in neurofibrillary degeneration. *Acta Neuropathologica* 101:585–90.

Wegiel, J., K.-C. Wang, H. Imaki, et al. 2001c. The role of microglial cells and astrocytes in fibrillar plaques evolution in transgenic APP_{sw} mice. *Neurobiology of Aging* 22: 49–61.

Weidemann, A., G. Koenig, D. Bunke, et al. 1989. Identification, biogenesis, and localization of precursors of Alzheimer disease A4 amyloid protein. *Cell* 57:115–26.

Wild-Bode, C., T. Yamazaki, A. Capell, et al. 1997. Intracellular generation and accumulation of amyloid β-peptide terminating at amino acid 42. *Journal of Biological Chemistry* 272:16085–88.

Wilson, C.A., R.W. Doms, and V.M.-Y. Lee. 1999. Intracellular APP processing and Aβ production in Alzheimer disease. *Journal of Neuropathology and Experimental Neurology* 58:787–94.

Wisniewski, H.M., and J. Wegiel. 1991. Spatial relationships between astrocytes and classical plaque components. *Neurobiology of Aging* 12:593–600.

Wisniewski, H.M., and J. Wegiel. 1993. Migration of perivascular cells into the neuropil and their involvement in β-amyloid plaque formation. *Acta Neuropathologica* 85: 586–95.

Wisniewski, H.M., and J. Wegiel. 1994. β-amyloid formation by myocytes of leptomeningeal vessels. *Acta Neuropathologica* 87:233–41.

Wisniewski, H.M., J. Wegiel, and L. Kotula. 1996. Some neuropathological aspects of Alzheimer's disease and its relevance to other disciplines. *Neuropathology and Applied Neurobiology* 22:3–11.

Wisniewski, H.M., J. Wegiel, and E.R. Popovitch. 1994. Age-associated development of diffuse and thioflavine-S-positive plaques in Down syndrome. *Developmental Brain Dysfunction* 7:330–39.

Wisniewski, H.M., J. Wegiel, K.-C. Wang, et al. 1989. Ultrastructural studies of the cells forming amyloid fibers in classical plaques. *Canadian Journal of Neurological Sciences* 16:535–42.

Wisniewski, H.M., J. Wegiel, K.-C. Wang, et al. 1992. Ultrastructural studies of the cells forming amyloid in the vessel wall in Alzheimer disease. *Acta Neuropathologica* 84:117–27.

Wisniewski, H.M., M. Sadowski, K. Jakubowska-Sadowska, et al. 1998. Diffuse, lake-like amyloid-β deposits in the parvopyramidal layer of the presubiculum in Alzheimer disease. *Journal of Neuropathology and Experimental Neurology* 57:674–83.

Wisniewski, K.E. 1990. Down syndrome children often have brain with maturation delay, retardation of growth and cortical dysgenesis. *American Journal of Medical Genetics* 7 (Suppl.):S274–81.

Wisniewski, K.E., M. Laure-Kamionowska, and H.M. Wisniewski. 1984. Evidence of arrest of neurogenesis and synaptogenesis in brains of patients with Down's syndrome. *New England Journal of Medicine* 311:1187–88.

Wisniewski, K.E., H.M. Wisniewski, and G.Y. Wen. 1985. Occurrence of neuropathological changes and dementia of Alzheimer's disease in Down's syndrome. *Annals of Neurology* 17:278–82.

Wisniewski, T., J. Ghiso, and B. Frangione. 1991. Peptides homologous to the amyloid protein of Alzheimer's disease containing a glutamine for glutamic acid substitution have accelerated amyloid fibril formation. *Biochemical and Biophysical Research Communications* 179:1247–54.

Wisniewski, T., E.M. Castano, A.A. Golabek, et al. 1994. Acceleration of Alzheimer's fibril formation by apolipoprotein E in vitro. *American Journal of Pathology* 145: 1030–35.

Wisniewski, T., W.K. Dowjat, J.D. Buxbaum, et al. 1998. A novel Polish presenilin-1 mutation (P117L) is associated with familial Alzheimer's disease and leads to death as early as the age of 28 years. *Neuroreport* 9:217–21.

Wolfe, M.S., W. Xia, B.H. Ostaszewski, et al. 1999. Two transmembrane aspartates in presenilin-1 required for presenilin endoproteolysis and γ-secretase activity. *Nature* 398:513–17.

Xu, H., D. Sweeney, R. Wang, et al. 1997. Generation of Alzheimer's β-amyloid protein in the trans-Golgi in the apparent absence of vesicle formation. *Proceedings of the National Academy of Sciences USA* 94:3748–52.

Younkin, S.G. 1995. Evidence that Aβ42 is the real culprit in Alzheimer's disease. *Annals of Neurology* 37:287–88.

Zellweger, H. 1977. Down syndrome. In *Handbook of Clinical Neurology*, vol. 31, edited by P.J. Vinken and G.W. Bruyn. New York: Elsevier, pp. 367–469.

Zigman, W.B., G.B. Seltzer, and W.P. Silverman. 1994. Behavioral and mental health changes associated with aging in adults with mental retardation with or without Down syndrome. In *Life Course Perspectives on Adulthood and Old Age*, edited by M.M. Seltzer, M.W. Krauss, and M.P. Janicki. Washington, D.C.: American Association on Mental Retardation, pp. 67–94.

CHAPTER FIVE

Neural Inflammatory Mechanisms in Alzheimer Syndrome

Edith G. McGeer, Ph.D., OC, and
Patrick L. McGeer, M.D., Ph.D., FRCP(C), OC

Postmortem studies have revealed a state of chronic inflammation in affected regions of the brain in Alzheimer disease (AD). Chronic inflammation can be damaging to host cells, and the brain may be particularly vulnerable because neurons, once lost, are not replaced. There is good evidence that the inflammation is killing neurons in brain with AD, suggesting that anti-inflammatory agents might slow the process of the disease. More than twenty epidemiological studies have shown that persons taking nonsteroidal anti-inflammatory drugs (NSAIDs) or who have diseases for which these drugs are routinely used have a greatly reduced incidence of AD. In one small clinical trial, the NSAID indomethacin appeared to halt the progression of memory loss in patients with AD. The NSAIDs inhibit the synthesis of prostaglandins, which are relatively weak stimulators of inflammation. If agents were identified that would block the more powerful stimulators, such as activated complement components and inflammatory cytokines, they might have important therapeutic benefits in AD as well as a range of other disorders in which inflammation plays a deleterious role.

Immunohistochemical studies have revealed that many inflammatory markers newly appear or are upregulated in affected regions of brain with Alzheimer

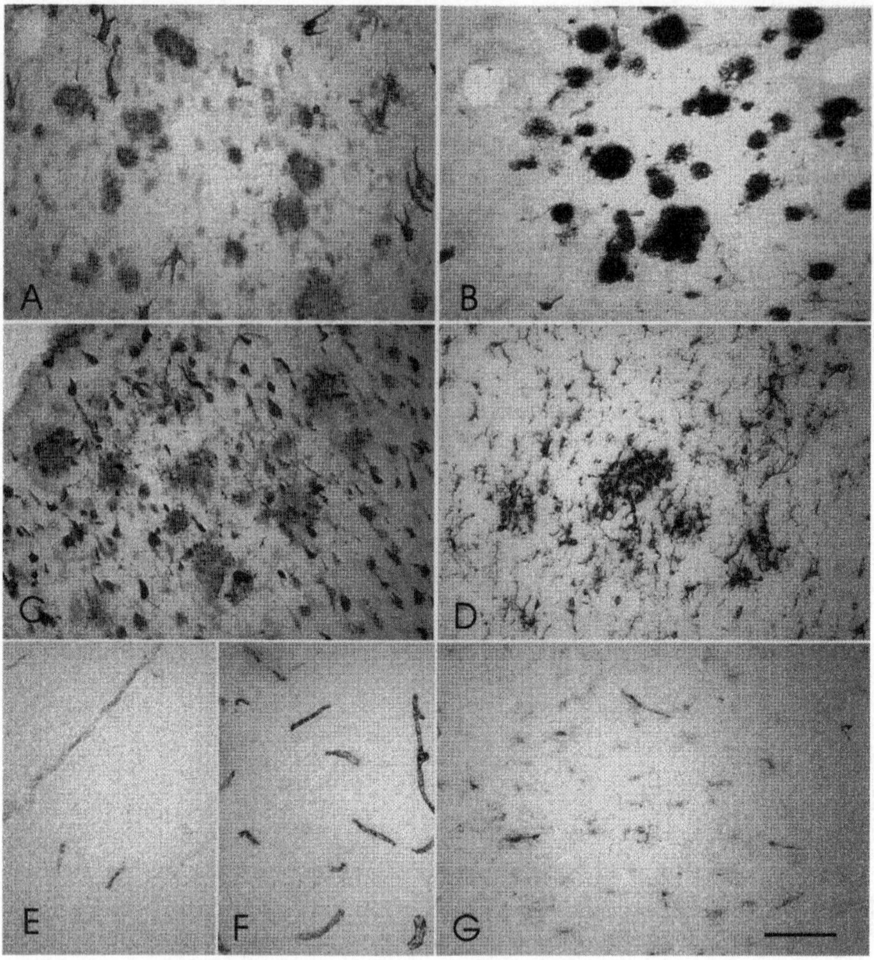

Figure 5.1. Immunohistochemistry in Alzheimer (*A, B, C, D*) and control (*E, F, G*) cortical regions. Staining with antibodies to the complement fragments C3d (*A*), C4d (*B, E*), amyloid P (*C, F*), and HLA-DR, a marker of reactive microglia (*D, G*). Both plaques and tangles in AD are stained for C3d and C4d, the opsonizing components of complement. Antibodies to amyloid P stain tangles and plaques in AD as well as some capillaries; faint staining of some capillaries is seen in controls. Antibodies to HLA-DR stain reactive microglia, mainly clustered on plaques in AD. Calibration bar in *G* applies to all and = 100 mm.

disease. A few of the more important of these are activated complement proteins, including the membrane attack complex; the pentraxins, C-reactive protein and amyloid P; the complement receptors and HLA-DR on activated microglia; the inflammatory cytokines, such as interleukin-1α (IL-1α), IL-1β, IL-6, and tumor necrosis factor-α (TNF-α); and other influencing factors, such as α2-macroglobulin and α1-antichymotrypsin. These are discussed briefly in this chapter, and the immunohistochemical appearance of some in brain with AD is illustrated in figure 5.1. Details on these and others may be found in any of the many reviews that have now appeared on inflammation in AD (McGeer and McGeer 1996; Neuroinflammation Working Group 2000).

The Complement System

The complement system consists of nine major components (C1–C9) that become serially activated in a cascade (fig. 5.2). What sets it off is dissociation of the C1 complex when the C1q component binds to a target. C1r acts on C1s, which acts on C2 and C4. C3 then become activated in the cascade process where the enzymatic action of each component amplifies the next in line. The fragments C4b and C3b form covalent bonds with their targets, irreversibly attaching to them in a process called opsonization. This permits macrophages expressing high levels of complement receptor to lock onto the opsonized targets and clean up the labeled debris. If the complement system is chronically activated, it proceeds to assemble the terminal components in a dangerous macromolecule known as the membrane attack complex. This inserts only into viable cells, making holes in them and causing death. Meanwhile, the small fragments C3a, C4a, and C5a, known as anaphylotoxins, stimulate inflammation. So the overall cascade identifies, opsonizes, and destroys its target, while dispatching messengers to seek help.

The tangles and plaques of Alzheimer disease are clearly marked with the opsonizing complement components, C4d and C3d (fig. 5.1A and B) (Ishii and Haga 1984; Eikelenboom et al. 1989; McGeer et al. 1989). Little or no such staining is seen in control brain (fig. 5.1E). Dystrophic neurites in brain with AD are immunostained for the membrane attack complex (Itagaki et al. 1994; Webster et al. 1997a, b). Again, such staining is not seen in control brains. This lytic molecule is designed to destroy foreign bacteria and viruses, and there are protective mechanisms that defend host cells. However, if the concentration of

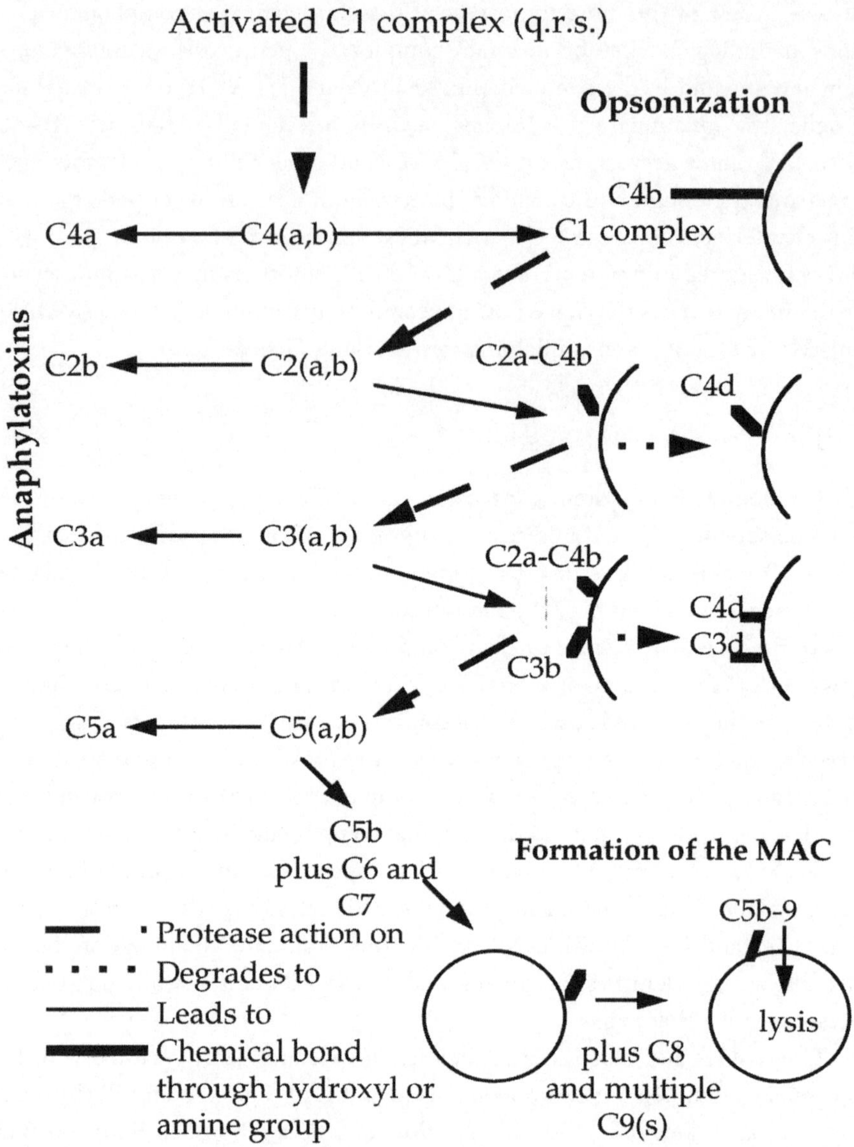

Figure 5.2. Schematic diagram of the complement cascade

the membrane attack complex exceeds the defensive ability of host tissue, then self-attack can occur in a process called bystander lysis. It is the smoking gun of autodestruction in AD, as the neurites are progressively eliminated by self-attack.

What Activates the Complement Cascade in Alzheimer Disease?

Complement is generally thought of as being part of the adaptive immune system, where T and B cells are cloned and antibodies made to foreign proteins, antibodies that bind to C1q to activate the complement system. But the complement system is phylogenetically much older than the adaptive immune system that evolved with higher vertebrates. The complement system exists in primitive organisms and plays a major role in the innate immune system. The innate immune system is less sophisticated than the adaptive immune system and may more readily confuse friend and foe. The innate immune system appears to be playing a major role in AD. We use the term *autotoxicity* to describe self-attack by the innate immune system, to distinguish it from *autoimmunity*, which is self-attack by the adaptive immune system (McGeer and McGeer 2000).

Recently it was established that some nonantibody materials can bind to C1q and activate the complement cascade. Among these molecules are several found to be elevated in brain with AD and deposited in senile plaques; these include C-reactive protein (Jiang et al. 1992), amyloid P (Akiyama et al. 1991; Hicks et al. 1992), and the beta-amyloid peptide (Aβ) (Rogers et al. 1992; Watson et al. 1997), which is a major component of the senile plaques. All three may play important roles in the chronic activation of complement seen in regions of brain affected by AD.

C-reactive protein, amyloid P, and Aβ all activate the complement cascade by binding to the collagen tail of C1q while antibodies bind to the globular head (Jiang, Robey, and Gewerz 1992; Ying et al. 1993; Webster, Bonnell, and Rogers 1997a). The result is the same, but the mechanism of activation is quite different. Potentially exciting from a therapeutic point of view is that the autodestructive action of complement might be prohibited by preventing binding to its collagen tail, while leaving its globular head free for adaptive functioning through antibodies.

Activated Microglia Surround the Lesions of Alzheimer Disease

The resident phagocytes of the central nervous system are the microglia. Phagocytes were discovered initially by Eli Metchnikoff in his great work of 1892. He impaled starfish larvae with rose thorns and noticed the gathering around of mesodermal cells, which he named phagocytes. He believed that tissue phagocytes were the main line of defense of the body. In 1919, Del Rio Hortega (1919) solved the puzzle of "el tercer elemento" in brain. The problem had baffled the great neuroanatomist Ramon y Cajal, who recognized only neurons and astrocytes. Del Rio Hortega found that this third element was composed of two cell types. One he named oligodendroglia and the other microglia. He recognized that microglia could become activated and were phagocytic. The fact that microglia were the brain's representatives of the phagocytic system was challenged in the 1990s, but immunohistochemical studies on brain with AD and experiments with microglia in culture have shown them to have all the characteristics of phagocytes. When activated, they upregulate a large number of proteins. These include complement receptors because they are the cells that respond to the complement system's call for the phagocytosis of opsonized targets (Rozemuller et al. 1989; Akiyama and McGeer 1990).

Microglia are always present in brain, but generally rest in a quiescent state. Their activation can be revealed by immunostaining for some of the markers upregulated on activation. Such immunostaining reveals the presence of activated microglia in brain tissue with AD and their virtual absence in normal brain tissue (McGeer et al. 1987; Rogers et al. 1988). The microglia appear in clumps on senile plaques (fig. 5.1D), as well as elsewhere in affected AD tissue. They seem to be unable to phagocytose the senile plaques and tangles of AD and thus remain chronically activated. In this state they produce massive amounts of oxygen radicals and other materials which may, in themselves, be toxic to host cells. Many experiments in tissue culture have shown that the secretions of activated microglia can kill neurons (Giulian et al. 1996; Klegeris and McGeer 2000). Thus, the activated microglia, like the membrane attack complex of complement, probably contribute to the rapid and progressive neuronal loss in brain with AD.

That activation of microglia may not always be harmful in Alzheimer disease is suggested by the surprising finding that vaccination of the PDAPP transgenic mouse strain (which overexpresses human Aβ with the 717 valine to phenylalanine mutation) with Aβ reduces the Aβ burden. In mice vaccinated at 6 weeks of age, there was prevention of Aβ deposition, and in mice vaccinated at 11 months of age, there was a marked reduction of deposition (Schenk et al. 1999). High serum titers against Aβ were generated. One interpretation is that antibodies reach the brain and in doing so promote clearance of secreted Aβ and assist in the phagocytosis of deposited Aβ. A further interpretation is that antigen-antibody complexes promote phagocytosis by directly stimulating microglial Fc receptors and possibly also by activating complement with subsequent stimulation of microglial complement receptors. If this is the true explanation, it represents an example of the adaptive immune system coming to the rescue by raising the phagocytic level of microglia above the threshold necessary to maintain Aβ clearance. An alternative interpretation recently put forward (DeMattos et al. 2001) is that the anti-Aβ antibody binds to plasma Aβ, changing the plasma-brain gradient to such an extent that soluble Aβ leaves the brain. Whether such a strategy can be useful in AD needs to be tested. Human vaccination trials are now under way. Success may not be easily accomplished since AD plaques are more highly insoluble compared with transgenic mouse amyloid deposits (Kuo et al. 2001), suggesting that there may be greater resistance to phagocytosis in vivo or to the amount of soluble Aβ that can be drawn out of the brain.

Nonspecific Inflammatory Mediators

The inflammatory cytokines, interleukin-1α (IL-1α), IL-1β, IL-6, and TNF-α, and the two acute phase proteins, α2-macroglobulin (A2M) and α1-antichymotrypsin (ACT), are relatively nonspecific mediators, but the possibility that they also play a role in inflammation in brain with Alzheimer disease was initially suggested by the reports that they are all upregulated in Alzheimer disease tissue and are prominently associated with Alzheimer disease lesions (Griffin et al. 1989; Dickson et al. 1993; Wood et al. 1993; Cacebelos et al. 1994). The inflammatory cytokines IL-1, IL-6, and TNF-α are products of both activated microglia and activated astrocytes and powerfully stimulate their activity. Localization of these cytokines to such activated cells has been demonstrated in AD by immunohistochemistry (Lieberman et al. 1989; Sharif et al. 1993; Yamabe et al. 1994; Walker, Kim, and McGeer 1995). ACT is a product of activated astrocytes that is localized to senile plaques in brain with AD (Abraham, Shirahama, and Potter 1990). A2M is a potent, broad-spectrum protease inhibitor, thought to have evolved as a primitive host defense mechanism. A2M is detected immunohistochemically in association with neurofibrillary tangles and senile plaques in brain with AD (Bauer et al. 1991).

Several reports have appeared indicating that the risk of Alzheimer disease is substantially influenced by a total of ten polymorphisms in these inflammatory agents (Kamboh et al. 1997; Blacker et al. 1998; Papassotiropoulos et al. 1999; Collins et al. 2000; Du et al. 2000; Grimaldi et al. 2000; Licastro et al. 2000a, b; Nicoll et al. 2000; Rebeck 2000; McCusker 2001). The polymorphisms are in promoter regions, and those alleles that favor increased production of the inflammatory mediators are more common in AD than in controls. The polymorphisms are, however, all fairly common ones in the general population, so there is a strong likelihood that any given individual will inherit one or more of the high-risk alleles. The odds ratio for a single one of these polymorphisms is, understandably, much lower than that for polymorphisms in apolipoprotein E, where inheritance of the ApoE4 allele substantially increases the risk of AD (Strittmatter et al. 1993). However, McCusker (2001) showed that carrying the high-risk allele of TNFA substantially increases the risk of AD in carriers of the ApoE4 allele. And it has also already been reported that the odds ratio is greatly increased if an individual carries two of the high-risk alleles in the inflammatory mediators. For example, Nicoll et al. (2000) found that simultaneous inheritance of the high-risk alleles for IL1A-889 and IL1B+3953 increased the odds ratio for developing AD to 10.8 (i.e., the prevalence of AD in persons carrying these isoforms is almost 11 times as great as in persons of the same age carrying neither of these isoforms). The overall chances of an individual's developing AD might be profoundly affected by a "susceptibility profile" reflecting the combined influence of inheriting multiple high-risk alleles (McGeer and McGeer 2001). Identification of such profiles could lead to strategies for therapeutic intervention in the very early stages of the disorder.

Local Production of Inflammatory Components

For many years it was generally believed that the complement proteins, C-reactive protein and amyloid P, were produced in the liver and carried in the circulation to other organs. The presence of amyloid P in the brain in AD was even taken as an indication of leakage in the blood-brain barrier (Kalaria and Grahovac 1990). Application of molecular genetic techniques has made it possible to demonstrate that all these components, as well as the nonspecific inflammatory mediators, are produced locally in brain and that their production is upregulated in affected regions in brain with AD (Yasojima et al. 1999, 2000). This is possible because the relative levels of the mRNA can be reliably measured in postmortem tissue by application of the reverse transcriptase-polymerase chain reaction technique. In this technique, total RNA is extracted from tissue and converted into cDNA by reverse transcriptase and chosen primers used in the polymerase chain reaction technique to amplify selected genes. These can be separated on gels and visualized by staining with ethidium bromide, with relative levels determined densitometrically. The type of data obtained in the midtemporal gyrus of AD and control cases is illustrated in figure 5.3A for the complement proteins C1q and C9, C-reactive protein, amyloid P, HLA-DR, and the complement receptor CD11b. This upregulation is generally limited to areas of brain pathologically affected in AD and is not seen peripherally in organs such as the liver (fig. 5.3B).

Similar work in other tissues such as heart, artery, and joints has revealed the presence of the complement and pentraxin mRNAs in these tissues as well, and their upregulation in infarcted heart, atherosclerotic artery, and osteoarthritic joints (Yasojima et al. 1998, 2001). Thus, a local innate immune reaction may be a common feature in many chronic degenerative diseases.

Intensity of the Inflammatory Reaction in Alzheimer Disease Brain

The degree of upregulation of mRNA levels in inflamed tissue may be an indicator of the level of involvement of the innate immune system. Figure 5.4 compares the upregulation of the mRNAs for C1q and C9 in AD hippocampus, infarcted heart, atherosclerotic plaques, and osteoarthritic joints. It can be seen that the highest upregulation is in AD hippocampus. Thus, the inflammatory reaction is probably very intense, although the process is silent because the brain has no pain fibers and is prevented from swelling by the blood-brain barrier.

The initial causes of pathology in these diseases are quite different—plaques and tangles in Alzheimer disease, anoxia in heart disease, too much fat in atherosclerosis, and mechanical grinding in osteoarthritis. But the secondary process is common to all. The innate immune system may be playing a role in all of these conditions, and the effectiveness of NSAIDs in preventing heart disease and stroke (Arnau and Agusti 1997; Bath 1997) may involve interactions with the innate immune system as well as effects on platelet fluidity.

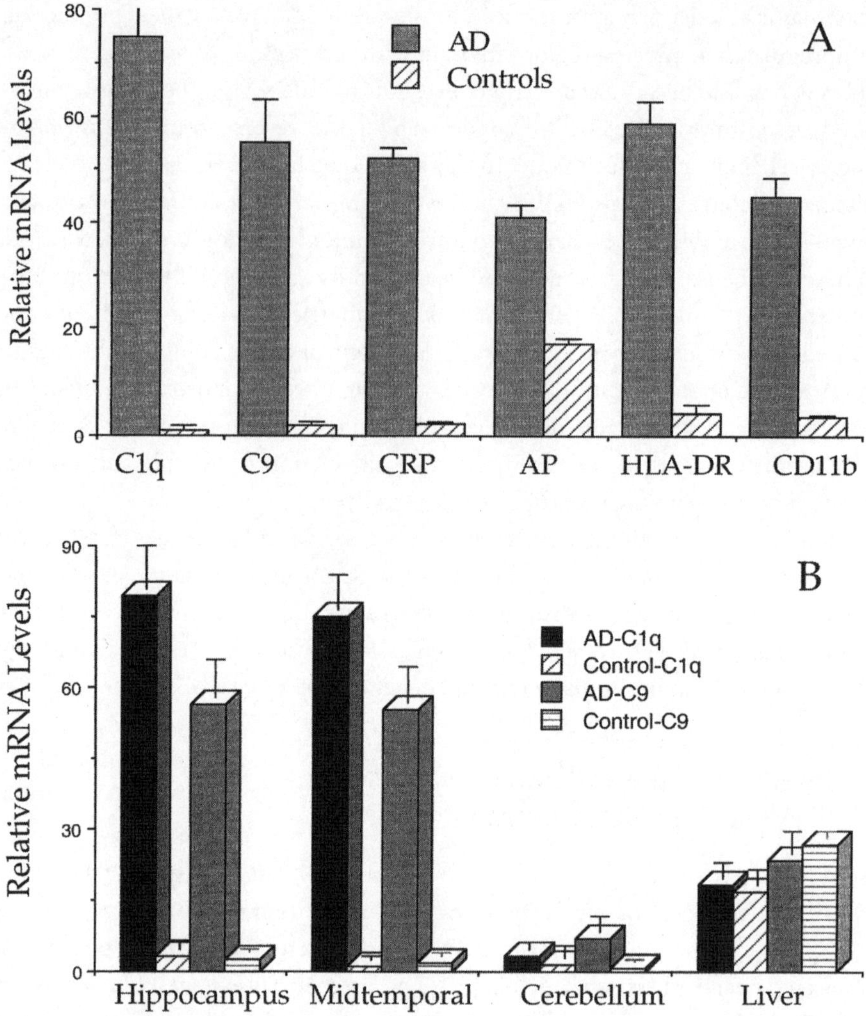

Figure 5.3. A: Relative levels in AD and control midtemporal gyrus of the mRNAs for the complement proteins C1q and C9, C-reactive protein, amyloid P, HLA-DR, and the complement receptor CD11b. *B*: The upregulation is generally limited to pathologically affected areas of brain such as the hippocampus and midtemporal gyrus and is not seen in unaffected regions such as the cerebellum or in peripheral organs such as the liver.

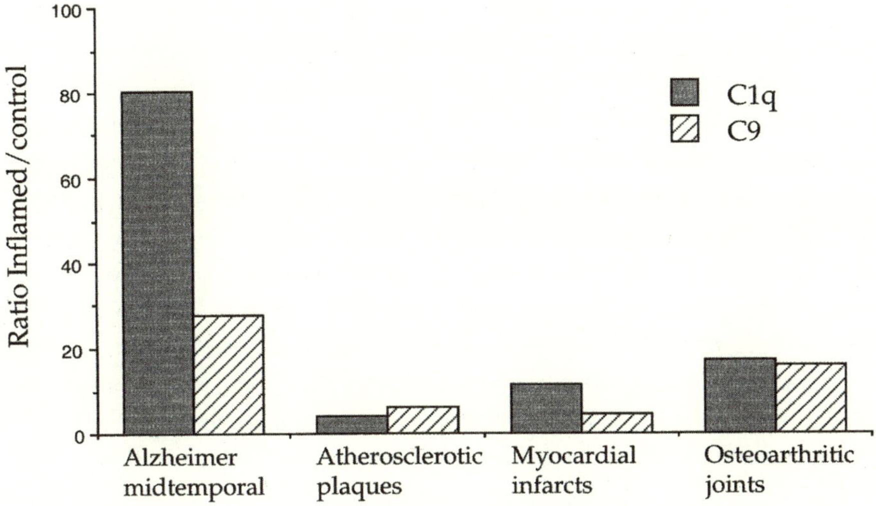

Figure 5.4. A comparison of the upregulation of the levels of the mRNAs for C1q and C9 in AD midtemporal gyrus, infarcted heart, atherosclerotic plaques, and osteoarthritic joints. In each case, the figure plotted is the ratio of the level found in the diseased tissue to that in normal tissue of the same type.

Studies of the levels of the mRNAs for various inflammatory mediators may also indicate which are the most promising targets for therapeutic intervention. The immunohistochemical studies of brain with AD have been useful in revealing the presence of many inflammatory mediators in pathologically affected regions, but such studies are only qualitative. More quantitative biochemical studies are clearly needed, and the measurement of relative mRNA levels, such as illustrated in figures 5.3 and 5.4, may provide one useful approach.

Epidemiological and Clinical Evidence that Inflammation Plays a Role in the Pathology of Alzheimer Disease

If inflammation is playing a major role in converting Alzheimer disease from a relatively benign pathology into a malignant inflammatory condition, people taking anti-inflammatory medications for other purposes might be inadvertently protecting themselves against the autotoxic effects of Alzheimer disease. There are now more than twenty published epidemiological studies that show that people known to be taking anti-inflammatory agents or who have arthritis generally, or rheumatoid arthritis in particular, for which anti-inflammatory agents are routinely used, had considerably reduced odds of developing AD (McGeer, Schulzer, and McGeer 1996; Stewart et al. 1997; Broe et al. 2000; Veld et al. 2000). A revealing study was conducted by Stewart and colleagues in Baltimore (1997). More than 2000 patients were enrolled in early middle age and followed for long periods of time to assess the factors contributing to later onset of disease. The Stewart group therefore had records they could check regarding AD and drugs. They found for those using NSAIDs for two years or less, the risk was reduced by about one-third. For those using NSAIDs for more than two years, the risk was reduced by 60%. An even greater reduction for chronic use of NSAIDs was recently reported by Veld et al. (2000) from a study in Rotterdam. The reduction of 78% they found was close to that of 79% previously reported from studies of rheumatoid arthritics (McGeer, Schulzer, and McGeer 1996).

Will NSAIDs work clinically in Alzheimer disease? One small trial was led by Joe Rogers in Sun City on the effects of indomethacin (Rogers et al. 1993). In this six-month, double-blind clinical trial, indomethacin appeared to arrest progression in the AD cases, while the placebo group deteriorated at the expected rate. NSAIDs inhibit cyclo-oxygenase (COX) and thereby interfere with the production of prostaglandins. There are two forms of COX: COX-1 and COX-2. Traditional NSAIDs, such as aspirin or indomethacin, are generally COX-1 inhibitors, but recent emphasis has been on the development of COX-2 inhibitors with fewer gastrointestinal side effects. There has been another trial reported from Australia in which diclofenac, a mixed COX-1/COX-2 inhibitor, slowed the progression of AD, although, due to the small numbers, statistical significance was marginal (Scharf et al. 1999). Trials have been done with COX-2 inhibitors, with reportedly poor results (Sainati et al. 2000). But there may be a reason for this. COX-2 is concentrated in neurons, and several studies have shown that it is involved in synaptic transmission. The objective here is to handcuff overaggressive microglia, but not to hammer AD-affected neurons that are struggling to survive.

Drug Targets for Future Development

As noted above, NSAIDs inhibit the synthesis of prostaglandins. Prostaglandins are known to be inflammatory mediators, although far from the most powerful ones. NSAIDs therefore strike at fringe players in this whole autotoxic and inflammatory scheme. Nevertheless, they are off-the-shelf medications and form a good starting point. The epidemiological and clinical evidence concerning NSAIDs and AD should whet the appetite of investigators for the potential of agents directed at core activities such as the complement system or activated microglia.

It is important to realize that this therapeutic approach is very different from attempts to replace the lost cholinergic activity in Alzheimer disease with drugs such as Aricept or to stimulate metabolism. Such pharmacological approaches are not aimed at slowing the continued destruction of neurons that is almost certainly the main cause of the deterioration. The suggestion is that anti-inflammatory treatment may inhibit such neuronal death.

Agents capable of blocking the chronic inflammation fueled by the innate immune system should have wide application since such inflammation may be a major driving force in the most important diseases of our time: Alzheimer disease, heart attack, and stroke. We need to learn much more about the innate immune system, how it recognizes targets, and ways to inhibit autoattack by this system and by the inflammatory mediators that are stimulated as part of the reaction.

Further study of the brain's innate immune system and the factors that regulate its activity may also shed new light on primary inflammatory processes relatively uncomplicated by blood-borne elements. In one sense, the brain provides a model system with some similarities to the simple organisms in which Metchnikoff identified macrophages as playing a key role in inflammation.

Clinical Conclusions

The evidence seems strong that chronic inflammation and autotoxicity are playing a major role in the clinical progression of Alzheimer disease, but only large clinical trials of effective anti-inflammatory agents in very early Alzheimer disease can prove the validity of this approach. Clinicians have been reluctant to prescribe NSAIDs, particularly for elderly patients, because of the possibility of gastrointestinal side effects. But AD is such a devastating disease that the risk seems worthwhile. Another approach might be to test the nitric oxide-releasing NSAIDs, since they are apparently much less apt to cause gastrointestinal injury (Wallace, Pittman, and Cirino 1995). The innate immune system offers many points of attack, so combinations of drugs may well be additive or even synergistic and allow each to be used at a nontoxic level. Thus, a relatively low dose of an

NSAID might be used in combination with dapsone, an anti-inflammatory agent of a different type which has also been reported to reduce the risk of AD (McGeer et al. 1992). Steroids are anti-inflammatory drugs that should not be used because they can have deleterious effects on hippocampal neurons.

A second possibility that may have future clinical application is that combinations of certain polymorphisms in inflammatory mediators may be sufficiently strong risk factors that genotyping can be used to identify susceptible individuals so that preventative therapy can be undertaken. This may strengthen the present approach of using ApoE genotyping to identify individuals at risk.

ACKNOWLEDGMENTS

Our research has been supported by grants from the Jack Brown and Family AD Research Fund and the Alzheimer Society of Canada, as well as donations from the Friends of UBC and individual British Columbians. We thank Dr. Claudia Schwab for providing the photomicrographs.

REFERENCES

Abraham, C.R., T. Shirahama, and H. Potter. 1990. α1-Antichymotrypsin is associated solely with amyloid deposits containing the β-protein: Amyloid and cell localization of α1-antichymotrypsin. *Neurobiology of Aging* 11:123–29.

Akiyama, H., and P.L. McGeer. 1990. Brain microglia constitutively express β2 integrins. *Journal of Neuroimmunology* 30:81–93.

Akiyama, H., T. Yamada, T. Kawamata, et al. 1991. Association of amyloid P component with complement proteins in neurologically diseased tissue. *Brain Research* 548: 349–52.

Arnau, J.M., and A. Agusti. 1997. Is aspirin underused in myocardial infarction? *Pharmacoeconomics* 12:524–32.

Bath, P.M.W. 1997. The medical management of stroke. *International Journal of Clinical Practice* 51:504–10.

Bauer, J., S. Strauss, U. Schreiter-Gasser, et al. 1991. Interleukin-6 and α2-macroglobulin indicate an acute-phase state in Alzheimer's disease cortex. *FEBS Letters* 285: 111–14.

Blacker, D., M.A. Wilcox, N.M. Laird, et al. 1998. Alpha-2-macroglobulin is genetically associated with Alzheimer disease. *Nature Genetics* 19:357–60.

Broe, G.A., D.A. Grayson, H.M. Creassey, et al. 2000. Anti-inflammatory drugs protect against Alzheimer disease at low doses. *Archives of Neurology* 57:1586–91.

Cacebelos, R., X.A. Alvarez, I. Fernandez-Novoa, et al. 1994. Brain interleukin-1 beta in Alzheimer's disease and vascular dementia. *Methods and Findings in Experimental and Clinical Pharmacology* 16:141–45.

Collins, J.S., R.T. Perry, B. Watson Jr., et al. 2000. Association of a haplotype for tumor necrosis factor in siblings with late-onset Alzheimer disease: The NIMH Alzheimer disease genetics initiative. *American Journal of Medical Genetics* 96:823–30.

Del Rio Hortega, P. 1919. El "tercer elemento" de los centros nerviosos. Poder fagocitario y movilidad de la microglia. *Boletín de la Sociedad Española de Biología* ix:154–66.

DeMattos, R.B., K.R. Nales, D.J. Cummins, et al. 2001. Peripheral anti-A beta antibody alters CNS and plasma A beta clearance and decreases brain A beta burden in a mouse model of Alzheimer's disease. *Proceedings of the National Academy of Sciences USA* 98: 8850–55.

Dickson, D.W., S.C. Lee, L.A. Mattiace, et al. 1993. Microglia and cytokines in neurological disease, with special reference to AIDS and Alzheimer disease. *Glia* 7:75–83.

Du, Y., R.C. Dodel, B.J. Eastwood, et al. 2000. Association of an interleukin 1 alpha polymorphism with Alzheimer's disease. *Neurology* 55:480–83.

Eikelenboom, P., C.E. Hack, J.M. Rozemuller, et al. 1989. Complement activation in amyloid plaques in Alzheimer's dementia. *Virchows Archives of Cell Pathology* 56: 259–62.

Giulian, D., L.J. Haverkamp, J.H. Yu, et al. 1996. Specific domains of beta-amyloid from Alzheimer plaque elicit neuron killing in human microglia. *Journal of Neuroscience* 16: 6021–37.

Griffin, W.S.T., L.C. Stanley, C. Ling, et al. 1989. Brain interleukin 1 and S-100 immunoreactivity are elevated in Down syndrome and Alzheimer's disease. *Proceedings of the National Academy of Sciences USA* 86:7611–15.

Grimaldi, L.M., V.M. Casadei, C. Ferri, et al. 2000. Association of early-onset Alzheimer's disease with an interleukin-1a gene polymorphism. *Annals of Neurology* 47: 361–65.

Hicks, P.S., L. Saunero-Nazia, T.W. Duclos, et al. 1992. Serum amyloid P component binds to histones and activates the classical complement pathway. *Journal of Immunology* 149:3689–94.

Ishii, T., and S. Haga. 1984. Immuno-electron-microscopic localization of complements in amyloid fibrils of senile plaques. *Acta Neuropathology (Berlin)* 63:296–300.

Itagaki, S., H. Akiyama, H. Saito, et al. 1994. Ultrastructural localization of complement membrane attack complex (MAC)-like immunoreactivity in brains of patients with Alzheimer's disease. *Brain Research* 645:78–84.

Jiang, H., F. Robey, and H. Gewurz. 1992. Localization of sites through which C-reactive protein binds to and activates complement to residues 14-26 and 76-92 of the human C1q A chain. *Journal of Experimental Medicine* 175:1373–79.

Kalaria, R.N., and I. Grahovac. 1990. Serum amyloid P immunoreactivity in hippocampal tangles, plaques and vessels: Implications for leakage across the blood-brain barrier in Alzheimer's disease. *Brain Research* 516:349–53.

Kamboh, M.I., C.E. Aston, R.E. Ferrell, et al. 1997. Genetic effect of alpha-1-antichymotrypsin on the risk of Alzheimer disease. *Genomics* 40:382–84.

Klegeris, A., and P.L. McGeer. 2000. Interaction of various intracellular signaling mechanisms involved in mononuclear phagocyte toxicity toward neuronal cells. *Journal of Leukocyte Biology* 67:127–33.

Kuo, Y.-M., T.A. Kokjohn, T.G. Beach, et al. 2001. Comparative analysis of Aβ chemical structure and amyloid plaque morphology of transgenic mice and Alzheimer disease brains. *Journal of Biological Chemistry* 276:12991–98.

Licastro, F., S. Pedrini, M. Bonafe, et al. 2000a. Polymorphisms of the IL-6 gene increase the risk for late onset Alzheimer's disease and affect IL-6 plasma levels. *Neurobiology of Aging* 21 (Suppl. 1):S38.

Licastro, F., S. Pedrini, C. Ferri, et al. 2000b. Gene polymorphism affecting α1-antichymotrypsin and interleukin-1 plasma levels increases Alzheimer's disease risk. *Annals of Neurology* 48:388–91.

Lieberman, A.P., P.M. Pitha, H.S. Shin, et al. 1989. Production of tumor necrosis factor and other cytokines by astrocytes stimulated with lipopolysaccharide or a neurotropic virus. *Proceedings of the National Academy of Sciences USA* 86:6348–52.

McCusker, S.M. 2001. Association between polymorphism in regulatory region of gene encoding tumour necrosis factor A and risk of Alzheimer's disease and vascular dementia: A case-control study. *Lancet* 357:436–39.

McGeer, P.L., and E.G. McGeer. 2000. Autotoxicity and Alzheimer disease. *Archives of Neurology* 57:789–90.

McGeer, P.L., and E.G. McGeer. In press. Polymorphisms in inflammatory genes enhance the risk of Alzheimer disease. *Archives of Neurology.*

McGeer, P.L., M. Schulzer, and E.G. McGeer. 1996. Arthritis and antiinflammatory agents as possible protective factors for Alzheimer's disease: A review of 17 epidemiological studies. *Neurology* 47:425–32.

McGeer, P.L., S. Itagaki, H. Tago, et al. 1987. Reactive microglia in patients with senile dementia of the Alzheimer type are positive for the histocompatibility glycoprotein HLA-DR. *Neuroscience Letters* 79:195–200.

McGeer, P.L., H. Akiyama, S. Itagaki, et al. 1989. Immune system response in Alzheimer's disease. *Canadian Journal of Neurological Science* 16:516–27.

McGeer, P.L., N. Harada, H. Kimura, et al. 1992. Prevalence of dementia amongst elderly Japanese with leprosy: Apparent effect of chronic drug therapy. *Dementia* 3: 146–49.

Metchnikoff, E. 1892. *Lecons sur la pathologie comparée de l'inflammation.* Paris: Masson.

Neuroinflammation Working Group. 2000. Inflammation and Alzheimer's disease. *Neurobiology of Aging* 21:383–421.

Nicoll, J.A.R., R.E. Mrak, D. Graham, et al. 2000. Association of interleukin-1 gene polymorphisms with Alzheimer's disease. *Annals of Neurology* 47:365–68.

Papassotiropoulos, A., M. Bagli, F. Jessen, et al. 1999. A genetic variation of the inflammatory cytokine interleukin-6 delays the initial onset and reduces the risk for sporadic Alzheimer's disease. *Annals of Neurology* 45:666–68.

Rebeck, G.W. 2000. Confirmation of the genetic association of interleukin-1A with early onset sporadic Alzheimer's disease. *Neuroscience Letters* 293:75–77.

Rogers, J., J. Luber-Narod, C.D. Styren, et al. 1988. Expression of immune system-associated antigens by cells of the human central nervous system: Relationship to the pathology of Alzheimer's disease. *Neurobiology of Aging* 9:339–49.

Rogers, J., N.R. Cooper, S. Webster, et al. 1992. Complement activation by β-amyloid in Alzheimer disease. *Proceedings of the National Academy of Sciences USA* 89:10016–20.

Rogers, J., L.C. Kirby, S.R. Hempelman, et al. 1993. Clinical trial of indomethacin in Alzheimer's disease. *Neurology* 43:1609–11.

Rozemuller, J.M., P. Eikelenboom, S.T. Pals, et al. 1989. Microglial cells around amyloid plaques in Alzheimer's disease express leucocyte adhesion molecules of the LFA-1 family. *Neuroscience Letters* 101:288–92.

Sainati, S.M., D.M. Ingram, S. Talwalker, et al. 2000. Results of a double-blind, placebo-controlled study of Celebrid for the progression of Alzheimer's disease. *Sixth International Stockholm-Springfield Symposium of Advances in Alzheimer Therapy*, p. 180.

Scharf, S., A. Mander, A. Ugoni, et al. 1999. A double-blind, placebo-controlled trial of diclofenac misoprostol in Alzheimer's disease. *Neurology* 53:197–201.

Schenk, D., R. Barbour, W. Dunn, et al. 1999. Immunization with amyloid-beta attenuates Alzheimer-disease-like pathology in the PDAPP mouse. *Nature* 400:173–77.

Sharif, S.F., R.J. Hariri, V.A. Chang, et al. 1993. Human astrocyte production of tumour necrosis factor-alpha, interleukin-1 beta, and interleukin-6 following exposure to lipopolysaccharide endotoxin. *Neurological Research* 15:109–12.

Stewart, W.F., C. Kawas, M. Corrada, et al. 1997. Risk of Alzheimer's disease and duration of NSAID use. *Neurology* 48:626–32.

Strittmatter, W.J., A. Saunders, D. Schmechel, et al. 1993. Apolipoprotein E: High avidity binding to β-amyloid and increased frequency of type 4 allele in late-onset familial Alzheimer disease. *Proceedings of the National Academy of Sciences USA* 90:1977–81.

Veld, B.A.I., A. Ruitenberg, L.J. Launer, et al. 2000. Duration of non-steroidal antiinflammatory drug use and risk of Alzheimer's disease: The Rotterdam study. *Neurobiology of Aging* 21 (Suppl. 1):S204.

Walker, D.G., S.U. Kim, and P.L. McGeer. 1995. Complement and cytokine gene expression in cultured microglia derived from postmortem human brains. *Journal of Neuroscience Research* 40:478–93.

Wallace, J.L., Q.J. Pittman, and G. Cirino. 1995. Nitric oxide-releasing NSAIDs: A novel class of GI-sparing anti-inflammatory drugs. *Agents and Actions—Supplement* 46:121–29.

Watson, M.D., A.E. Roher, K.S. Kim, et al. 1997. Complement interactions with amyloid β 1-42: A nidus for inflammation in AD brains. *Amyloid* 4:147–56.

Webster, S., B. Bonnell, and J. Rogers. 1997a. Charge-based binding of complement component C1q to the Alzheimer amyloid beta-peptide. *American Journal of Pathology* 150:1531–36.

Webster, S., L.F. Lue, L. Brachova, et al. 1997b. Molecular and cellular characterization of the membrane attack complex, C5b-9, in Alzheimer's disease. *Neurobiology of Aging* 18:415–21.

Wood, J.A., P.L. Wood, R. Ryan, et al. 1993. Cytokine indices in Alzheimer's temporal cortex: No change in mature IL beta or IL-1RA but increases in the associated acute phase proteins IL-6, alpha 2-macroglobulin and C-reactive protein. *Brain Research* 629:245–52.

Yamabe, T., G. Dhir, E.P. Cowan, et al. 1994. Cytokine-gene expression in measles-infected adult human glial cells. *Journal of Neuroimmunology* 49:171–79.

Yasojima, K., K.C. Schwab, E.G. McGeer, et al. 1998. Human heart generates complement proteins that are upregulated and activated after myocardial infarction. *Circulation Research* 83:860–69.

Yasojima, K., K.C. Schwab, E.G. McGeer, et al. 1999. Upregulated production and activation of the complement system in Alzheimer disease brain. *American Journal of Pathology* 154:927–36.

Yasojima, K., K.C. Schwab, E.G. McGeer, et al. 2000. Human neurons generate C-reactive protein and amyloid P: Upregulation in Alzheimer's disease. *Brain Research* 887:80–89.

Yasojima, K., K. C. Schwab, E.G. McGeer, et al. 2001. Generation of C-reactive protein and complement components in atherosclerotic plaques. *American Journal of Pathology* 158:1039–51.

Ying, S.C., A.T. Gewurz, H. Jiang, et al. 1993. Human serum amyloid P component oligomers bind and activate the classical complement pathway via residues 14-26 and 76-92 of the A chain collagen-like region of C1q. *Journal of Immunology* 150:169–76.

CHAPTER SIX

Clinical Subgroups of Alzheimer Disease

Magnus Sjögren, M.D., Ph.D.,
Anders Wallin, M.D., Ph.D.,
and Kaj Blennow, M.D., Ph.D.

The diagnostic criteria for Alzheimer disease (AD) may give the impression that Alzheimer disease is a relatively homogeneous disorder (McKhann et al. 1984). Historically, AD has, in fact, been regarded as one disease entity (Raskind, Carta, and Bravi 1995). However, evidence from longitudinal clinical studies, as well as pathological and genetic investigations, has revealed great heterogeneity. One evident example is familial AD, in which the age at onset, the duration of disease, and the phenomenology vary. Even greater heterogeneity is found in sporadic AD, especially when the onset is at a late age. This heterogeneity makes diagnosis difficult and creates a need for disease markers. However, the heterogeneity itself obstructs the identification of positive disease markers. A practicable way is to try to find markers that are specific for subgroups of persons with AD rather than for the whole AD population. Furthermore, studies have suggested that the available treatments for cognitive symptoms in AD, cholinesterase inhibitors, are more effective in some but not all persons with AD (Minthon et al. 1993; Byrne and Arie 1994). Therefore, the identification of subgroups of AD is an urgent task. This chapter describes some of the clinical subgroups of AD that have been identified so far.

Subgroups of Sporadic Alzheimer Disease Identified in Clinical Studies

Originally, Alzheimer disease was considered an uncommon disorder presenting with a severe decline in cognitive functions and a presenile onset (Alzheimer 1987 [1907]). Cognitive deterioration in the senium ("senile dementia") was considered to be a variant of normal human aging, and at least partly a result of cerebrovascular insufficiency (Raskind, Carta, and Bravi 1995). This notion seems to have prevailed for more than sixty years after the publication of Alzheimer's original work. However, clinicopathological work by Blessed, Tomlinson, and Roth (1968) demonstrated similar neuropathological changes in patients with senile dementia and in those with AD. A shift in paradigm took place. In subsequent studies, both types of patients were sampled as one group whose members were considered to suffer from the same disorder, AD (Raskind, Carta, and Bravi 1995). Despite this, some researchers persisted in acknowledging AD as two disorders, one with an early age and the other with a late age at onset. In fact, the senior author of the paper by Blessed et al. continued to emphasize the importance of preserving the division of AD into one group with an early onset and another with a late onset (Roth 1981, 1986).

In clinical studies of Alzheimer disease, differences between persons with an early onset and those with a late onset were repeatedly found. For example, Seltzer and Sherwin (1983), who investigated the clinical characteristics of sixty-five patients with AD, found that early AD more often presented with impairment in spontaneous speech, verbal comprehension, object naming, and writing. A tendency toward a higher frequency of apraxia in the early AD group was also found, but the difference was not significant. Chui et al. (1985) examined 146 patients with AD using clinical measures and rating scales with language variables derived from the Mini-Mental State Examination (MMSE) (Folstein, Folstein, and McHugh 1975). They found that an early age at onset was associated with a larger number of language disturbances. This result was in part replicated by Sevush, Leve, and Brickman (1993), who found that impairment in spontaneous speech, repetition, comprehension, reading, and writing was more common in persons with early AD than in those with late AD. These findings were supported by clinical studies by Becker et al. (1988), Filley, Kelly, and Heaton (1986), and Imamura and colleagues (1998). Mayeux, Stern, and Spanton (1985) also reported on differences in language functions between persons with early-onset and those with late-onset disease. However, it is possible that some of the patients included in their study had Lewy body dementia, not AD. Other investigators could not identify any differences in language functions between persons with early AD and those with late AD (Grosse, Gilley, and Wilson 1991). One investigator even reported that language impairments were more frequent in late AD (Bayles 1991).

The rate of decline in cognitive functions has been reported to be increased and the relative rate of survival to be decreased in early Alzheimer disease compared to late Alzheimer disease. Heyman studied ninety-two patients with early AD and found that particularly those with severe dysphasia had higher rates of institutionalization and death and that these patients often were younger than the other patients with early AD. These differences could not be explained by the degree of cognitive impairment (Heyman et al. 1987). Shorter survival times in early AD than in late AD were found by Seltzer and Sherwin (1983) and by Barclay and colleagues (1985). On the other hand, Go and colleagues (1978) found significantly longer survival times in early AD than in late AD. However, Lucca and colleagues (1993) followed fifty-six patients with AD and found that the rate of decline in cognitive functions was faster in early AD than in late AD. Several other studies have supported and replicated the finding that early AD is associated with a more rapid cognitive decline than late AD (Dastoor and Martin 1988; Mortimer et al. 1992). There are, however, also reports suggesting that the age at onset has no influence on the rate of cognitive decline in AD (Haupt, Kurz, and Pollmann 1992).

The subdivision of Alzheimer disease into early Alzheimer disease and late Alzheimer disease has gained support from neurochemical studies. Bird and colleagues (1983) found that, in early AD, choline acetyltransferase activity was significantly lower in several cortical areas and in the hippocampus and cerebellum compared to normal controls, whereas, in late AD, this activity was decreased in only the hippocampus. Rossor and colleagues (1984) also found more widespread neurochemical abnormalities in early AD compared to late AD. These findings were supported by Bondareff and colleagues (1987a), who observed a greater loss of noradrenergic locus ceruleus neurons in early AD than in late AD. More recent neurochemical studies have found differences in structural proteins measured in the cerebrospinal fluid. Sjögren and colleagues (2000a) found that the cerebrospinal fluid level of light neurofilament protein, one of the proteins that is a major constituent of the intermediate filaments in neurons, is highly increased in late AD but at normal levels in early AD. However, studies of other structural proteins in the cerebrospinal fluid, such as tau and the 42 amino acid β-amyloid (Aβ 42), did not reveal any differences (Sjögren et al. 2000b). Some histopathological studies have also suggested quantitative differences in the density of senile plaques and neurofibrillary tangles between early AD and late AD, with higher density in early AD (Mann, Yates, and Marcyniuk 1984; Nochlin et al. 1993).

Some brain imaging studies (for instance, positron emission tomography [PET] studies of cerebral glucose metabolic patterns) have also revealed differences between early Alzheimer disease and late Alzheimer disease. An asymmetric impairment of cortical glucose metabolism was found to be more frequent in early AD than in late AD (Koss et al. 1985) and significantly lower left parietal metabolic ratios were found in early AD than in late AD (Small et al. 1989). A higher degree of parietal metabolic dysfunction in early AD than in late AD has also been reported (Grady et al. 1987; Mielke et al. 1991).

These differences between early Alzheimer disease and late Alzheimer disease have been suggested to be merely quantitative (Bondareff et al. 1987b; Raskind, Carta, and Bravi 1995). However, certain phenomenological features are seldom reported in late AD and, therefore, some investigators conclude that there are no qualitative differences between subgroups of persons with AD. One of the most recurrent findings, especially in earlier reports, is that parietal symptoms (apraxia, visual agnosia, sensory dysphasia) are found only in some persons with AD. These patients most often have had an early onset of the disease (Lauter 1970; Constantinidis 1978; Seltzer and Sherwin 1983; Chui et al. 1985; Faber-Langendoen et al. 1988; Blennow, Wallin, and Gottfries 1991; Blennow and Wallin 1992). Some investigators even reserve the term *AD* for the variant with a presenile onset of symptoms (early AD), as did Alzheimer himself (Alzheimer 11987 [1907]), and divide late AD into two clinical forms: senile dementia (characterized by memory disturbances, disorientation, and simplified language but no parietal symptoms) and Alzheimer (alzheimerized) dementia (characterized by a clinical picture similar to that of early AD, with marked parietal symptoms superimposed on the clinical picture of senile dementia) (Sourander and Sjögren 1970; Constantinidis and Richard 1985; Blennow, Wallin, and Gottfries 1991).

Blennow and colleagues suggested that, based on predominant symptomatology, two subgroups can be delineated. One group, AD type I, is characterized by memory disturbances and predominant parietal symptoms, a relatively early age at onset, low frequency of vascular factors, normal blood-brain barrier function, and a low frequency of white matter changes on computerized tomography (CT) of the brain (Blennow, Wallin, and Gottfries 1991; Blennow et al. 1991). Alzheimer disease type II is characterized by memory disturbances and a decline in global cognitive functions, no or mild parietal symptoms, a high frequency of episodes of confusion, a relatively older age at onset, a relatively high frequency of vascular factors, mildly impaired blood-brain barrier function, and a high frequency of white matter changes on CT of the brain. They are of the opinion that AD type I matches the classical description of AD, or "pure" AD, that is, a disease with degeneration of the neurons in the cerebral cortex but without vascular changes or lesions in the white matter (Sjögren 1950; Tomlinson and Corsellis 1984; Constantinidis and Richard 1985; Gustafson 1985; Terry 1985; Blennow, Wallin, and Gottfries 1991; Blennow et al. 1991; Cummings and Benson 1992; Wallin, Blennow, and Scheltens 1994). In AD type II, age-related and vascular changes (small blood vessel disease with white matter changes) are part of the pathogenesis of dementia (i.e., the production of dementia symptoms). Blennow and colleagues (1991) believe that this subdivision may be relevant to the prognoses and outcomes in clinical trials.

Qualitative differences were also described by Helkala and colleagues (1996). Two subgroups of AD with phenomenological and neurophysiological differences were identified: one group ($n = 12$) had impaired memory and executive functions but relatively intact verbal and visuospatial functions, whereas the other subgroup ($n = 23$) presented with more global impairment. On EEG examination, the latter group had higher theta amplitude in the temporo-occipital, centroparietal, and frontal derivation and a lower peak and mean frequency than the former group and controls. The investigators suggested that the difference was due to more widespread damage in ascending activating systems in the latter group, but that damage to the hippocampus was of equal extent in both groups. The groups did not differ in degree of dementia or age.

Phenomenological patterns and subgroups may be more easily identified when neuropsychological measures are used. Based on results of extensive neuropsychological testing, some investigators have tried to identify phenomenological subgroups of AD. The reasoning in these works is mostly in terms of qualitative differences. One of the first attempts was made by McDonald in 1969. From cluster analysis of neuropsychological test results, he concluded that older persons with AD had preserved parietal functions. Furthermore, persons with disturbed parietal functions had a poorer prognosis.

In 1986, Martin and colleagues performed a factor analysis of neuropsychological data obtained from testing of forty-two patients with Alzheimer disease. This revealed two relatively independent factors, one comprising semantic variables and the other visuospatial skills. More than 70% of the variance could be assigned to these two factors. Further analysis of the data suggested three subgroups: (a) AD with relatively equal impairment of both semantic knowledge and visuospatial skills, (b) AD with impaired semantic knowledge but relatively spared visuospatial functioning, and (c) AD with relatively intact semantic knowledge but impaired visuospatial skills. Positron emission tomography scan suggested that these different subgroup characteristics were accompanied by specific patterns of metabolic disturbances: (a) deficits in both cognitive domains were accompanied by bilateral hypometabolism of the temporal and parietal lobes, (b) disturbances in the semantic domain by significantly greater hypometabolism in the left temporal region, and (c) deficits in visuospatial skills by hypometabolism in the right parietal region. A follow-up study of the patients from the first investigation suggested distinct patterns of deterioration based on subgroup membership. In those who presented with deficits in both cognitive domains (a) this general cognitive decline continued, but those in the semantic subgroup (b) and the visuospatial subgroup (c) showed deterioration primarily in the cognitive domain that had initially been affected (Martin 1990). In a larger study performed by Becker and colleagues (1988), Martin's (1986) initial findings were replicated. In this study, the same three subgroups were identified, each with its specific neuropsychological deficits.

Using various cluster analysis methods on the CERAD data, which include a large group of patients with Alzheimer disease ($n = 960$), Fisher, Rourke, and Bieliauskas (1999) identified subgroups with neuropsychological differences similar to those reported by Martin (1990). Three clinical subgroups of AD emerged. Subgroup 1 was characterized by severe naming impairment but borderline to normal figure copying skills. As the lesions in this group were supposed to be in the left hemisphere, this group was named left-hemisphere AD. Subgroup 2 presented with an average naming ability but moderately impaired figure copying performance, suggesting right hemisphere lesions. This group was named right-hemisphere AD. Subgroup 3 presented with profound anomia and constructional dyspraxia. This group was supposed to have more global lesions and was consequently named global AD. This extensive study followed the patients for ten years. The influence of cofactors, such as degree of dementia, was insignificant, but patients in the group with left-hemisphere AD were older and less educated than the patients in the other subgroups. The initial patterns of neuropsychological performance remained discernible (stable) across time in the groups with left-hemisphere AD and global AD but were less consistent in the group with right-hemisphere AD (Fisher et al. 1997; Fisher, Rourke, and Bieliauskas 1999).

Others who have used analogous methods (Naugle et al. 1985) have found similar results. Several reports have described a subtype of AD characterized by severe atrophy of the posterior cortical areas of the brain, especially the occipital lobe. The term *posterior cortical atrophy* has been used for this group, which is clinically characterized by disturbances of higher visual functions, including object agnosia, prosopagnosia, alexia, environmental agnosia, and Balint syndrome (Pantel and Schroder 1996). Other cognitive functions, including language and memory and frontal lobe functions (e.g., insight and judgment), remain relatively preserved until late in the course of disease. Brain CT and MRI usually reveal focal bilateral parietal and occipital atrophy. The underlying pathological change varies, but most cases of posterior cortical atrophy investigated postmortem have had Alzheimer encephalopathy. Until 1996, fifty-eight cases of posterior cortical atrophy had been described, the first one by Arnold Pick in 1902. Posterior cortical atrophy has been suggested to be a subgroup of AD (Hof et al. 1993; Pantel and Schroder 1996). Furthermore, occipital lobe pathology associated with constructional apraxia may predict a faster cognitive decline in AD (Smith et al. 2001).

In a study on patients with Alzheimer disease ($n = 32$), the term *posterior cortical atrophy* was not used, but a subgroup was described that was characterized by prevailing visuospatial deficits with associated decreases in cerebral blood flow in the parietal and occipital cortical regions, including the primary visual cortex. In contrast, other patients with AD had more generalized reductions in cerebral blood flow and more predominant memory disturbances and global signs (Pietrini et al. 1996).

Some researchers believe that the heterogeneity of Alzheimer disease reflects different stages of the disease, thereby implying that the phenomenology of Alzheimer disease is homogeneous. They agree that there are variations in the phenomenology, but do not believe that these reflect possible subgroups. Instead, they are thought to be attributable to specific stages of the disease progression, which follows a strict timetable (Constantinidis 1978; Reisberg, Ferris, and Crook 1982; Hom 1992). This reasoning has been criticized by Fisher and colleagues, who put forward several arguments against the "stage model" (Fisher et al. 1996): (1) Several different stage models have been presented, but there seems to be no consensus on which one should be applied. (2) Autopsy-confirmed cases of AD contradict the notion of a homogeneous deterioration of cognitive functions. (3) There are several reports of AD cases with an initially circumscribed cognitive impairment that continues to be salient as the disease progresses. (4) Several autopsy-confirmed cases of AD do not follow a specific schedule by which cognitive functions decline and behavioral symptoms and neurological signs appear.

Subgroups of Alzheimer Disease Identified in Familial Alzheimer Disease

Studies of families with inherited diseases offer a great opportunity to better understand the clinical expressions and pathophysiological mechanisms of a disease. The delineation of what are primary and secondary features or comorbidity is likely to be revealed in these studies. Several familial forms of AD have been described and the corresponding mutations have been identified. Clinical heterogeneity has been found both within and between families, but the identification of clinical subgroups within one family with inherited AD (a mutation) has seldom been suggested. Familial AD accounts for only a small part, a few percent, of all cases of AD. Nevertheless, identified familial AD genes may also play some part in sporadic nonfamilial AD. Polymorphism in one or more of these genes may involve a mechanism of action that, in concert with other mechanisms, will lead to the development of dementia. In the long run, knowledge gathered from investigations on familial AD may also increase our understanding of sporadic AD. Below are some reports on clinical heterogeneity in familial AD.

One study of 180 individuals with dementia from 24 families with familial Alzheimer disease revealed phenotypic heterogeneity (Bird et al. 1989). Five families had an early age at onset (mean 42 years; range 30–51 years), and 8 families had a relatively late age at onset (mean 68 years; range 59–78 years). One family presented with an almost schizophrenialike onset of disease and was neuropathologically characterized by neurofibrillary tangles and granulovacuolar change but no amyloid plaques. In another family with a late age at onset, there was clinical as well as pathological evidence of anterior horn cell disease. Clinical heterogeneity, and consequently subgroups, was more evident between the families than within them.

Lopez-Alberola and colleagues (1997) studied phenomenological aspects of familial Alzheimer disease and found indications of heterogeneity. Forty-two families with familial AD were investigated. In all of them, a late age at onset of disease was common. A high degree of phenotypic heterogeneity occurred independent of gender, ethnicity, and apolipoprotein E (ApoE) genotype. The degree of phenotypic heterogeneity was comparable within and between the family groups with the exception that the phenotypic heterogeneity in age at onset and rate of decline was greater between the families than within them. A similar trend was found for severity of cortical atrophy. The investigators suggested that strong nongenetic factors may have an influence on the degree of phenotypic heterogeneity in late-onset familial AD.

In a study of a large family, Hannequin and colleagues (1995) delineated the clinical features of early-onset familial Alzheimer disease linked to chromosome 14. These clinical features and those reported in eight traditional chromosome 14-linked families with familial AD were compared with the clinical features reported in six families with a mutation in the amyloid precursor protein (APP) gene on chromosome 21. The age at onset in the chromosome 14-linked families with familial AD was lower and the duration shorter than in the family with the APP mutation. This study revealed a phenotypic heterogeneity between the families in that seizures, myoclonus, and extrapyramidal signs were more frequent in cases with chromosome 14-linked familial AD. No differences were found in neuropsychological performance either at onset of the disease or with the progression of dementia. However, Lampe and colleagues (1994) reported that progressive aphasia was more frequent in chromosome 14-linked familial AD than in chromosome 21-linked familial AD.

The genetic influence on phenotype in Alzheimer disease was investigated by Tunstall and colleagues (2000). They studied sibling pairs affected with AD for a range of cognitive and noncognitive symptoms and found significant familial (genetic) effects on age at onset and mood state, and a relatively high effect on agitation. The influence of ApoE locus was found to account for 4% of the variation in age at onset. The conclusion was drawn that there was a substantial influence from the genotype on the phenotypic variation in AD. This notion is supported in a review by Lippa (1999). Differences in age at onset and age at death were found between AD caused by presenilin 1 or presenilin 2 mutations and AD caused by APP mutations or sporadic AD. Some hereditary forms of AD are associated with considerable β-amyloid deposition in the brain and yet others have morphologically distinct β-amyloid deposits or other unique histopathological features.

Taken together, clinical heterogeneity is found in familial Alzheimer disease in age at onset as well as in symptoms and neurological signs. Based on age at onset and phenomenology, two subgroups can be delineated: one with an early age at onset represented by persons with chromosome 1-, 14-, and 21-linked familial AD; and another with a later age at onset, represented by several kindreds of Volga German ancestry with the same chromosome 1 gene mutation as in early AD (Bird et al. 1996). Several families with chromosome 21-related APP mutations have an older age at onset compared to most families with chromosome 1- and 14-related mutations. Language disturbances and neurological signs also seem to be more frequent in chromosome 14-related familial AD (Lampe et al. 1994). This suggests an influence of nongenetic environmental factors. Such factors may be susceptible to therapeutic efforts.

The Influence of the Apolipoprotein E Genotype on the Clinical Expression of Alzheimer Disease

Apolipoprotein E is a plasma protein that participates in the transportation of cholesterol and other lipids from and to various cells in the body (Mahley 1988). Apolipoprotein E is also involved in the repair response to tissue injury (Poirier 1994), the maintenance and repair of nerve cell membranes (Mahley 1988), the growth of neurites, dendrite remodeling, and synaptogenesis (Poirier 1994). Apolipoprotein E is encoded by the ApoE gene alleles, which exist in the population in three types: ε2, ε3, and ε4. The most common allele is ε3, which has a prevalence of about 78% in the normal healthy population. Second most common is the ε4 allele (15%), followed by the ε2 allele (7%) (Roses 1996).

Inheritance of apolipoprotein E ε4 (ApoE4) has been associated with familial late-onset Alzheimer disease and sporadic Alzheimer disease (Corder et al. 1993; Poirier et al. 1993; Saunders et al. 1993; Strittmatter et al. 1993). The influence of ApoE genotype inheritance on the phenomenology of AD has been investigated in some studies. Some investigators have reported that inheritance of ApoE4 is associated with an earlier age at onset (Corder et al. 1993; Lehtovirta et al. 1996). Some reports suggest an association between ApoE4 inheritance and depressive (Ramachandran et al. 1996; Cacabelos et al. 1997) and psychotic (Harwood et al. 1999) symptoms, but several investigators have found no relationship between symptoms and ApoE allele inheritance (Mahieux et al. 1995; Class et al. 1997; Lopez et al. 1997). Cacabelos et al. (1997) found an association, although not significant, between ApoE ε3 inheritance and behavioral dysfunction, anxiety, and psychosis and between ApoE4 inheritance and disorientation, agitation, and motor disorders. Furthermore, some studies have indicated that inheritance of the ApoE4 genotype is associated with decreased choline acetyltransferase activity, reduced number of nicotine receptor binding sites in the brain, and consequently an inferior response to treatment with cholinesterase inhibitors compared to other persons with AD (Poirier et al. 1995; Poirier 1999).

Methodological Issues

The methods used, the number of patients included, and the aims vary in the presented studies. This implies that the studies are not fully comparable. For example, earlier studies often included a small number of patients or presented the subgroups in case reports, whereas later studies more often have included larger groups of patients. A shortcoming in earlier studies was that multivariate statistical methods were not used. Thus, the effects of age, gender, and educational level were sometimes not taken into account. The variation in neuropsychological measures and methods used for analyzing symptoms and signs is great. While some investigators have used a battery of neuropsychological tests, specifically designed to measure cognition in persons with dementia, others have relied on simple psychometric instruments, such as the MMSE. Some investigations have been made before the introduction of the criteria for Lewy body dementia (McKeith et al. 1996), some studies have used old-fashioned criteria for the diagnosis of AD, and most studies have not included neuropathological verification of the clinical diagnosis. These aspects should be taken into consideration when the issue about the presence of clinical subgroups of AD is addressed. The investigations that have included a large number of thoroughly diagnosed persons with AD and have used modern neuropsychological tests are the most likely to have high validity. However, pilot and smaller studies may give clues to identifying subgroups. It is also important to underscore that, to yield valid results, the neuropsychological test batteries used should cover as many aspects of cognition as is possible or relevant, not only a few of them.

Summary and Clinical Conclusions

As judged from the clinical and pathological diagnostic criteria of Alzheimer disease (McKhann et al. 1984), the disorder would seem to be relatively homogeneous. However, much speaks in favor of AD being a heterogeneous disorder (for instance, evidence from clinical, neurochemical, brain imaging, and pathological studies). This heterogeneity has led to a search for subgroups of AD. There are several reasons for this. First, there may be diagnostic markers that are viable only in particular subgroups of AD. Second, as shown in some studies (Minthon et al. 1993; Byrne and Arie 1994), drugs may be selectively effective (that is, they may improve cognition in some but not all subgroups of AD). Third, as subgroups may have certain characteristics, such as a specific rate of progression, the identification of these subpopulations may improve and individualize treatment and care.

Based on clinical studies of sporadic Alzheimer disease, it has been suggested that Alzheimer disease be divided into subgroups by (1) age at onset, (2) symptomatology, and (3) underlying genetic change. The most recognized division of AD is probably that into one group with an early onset (before or at the age of 65) and another with a later onset. Several studies have found clinical, neurochemical, and brain imaging differences between early and late AD; early AD has a more aggressive course, shorter survival time, more language disturbances, more widespread neurochemical changes, and more metabolic disturbances in the left parietal region than late AD. Another suggested division, based on neuropsychological performance by persons with AD, is into three groups, one with left hemisphere engagement, one with right hemisphere engagement, and one with more global affliction. With regard to familial AD, chromosome 1-linked familial AD seems to be associated with more language disturbances and neurological signs than chromosome 21-linked familial AD (with an APP gene mutation). Furthermore, inheritance of the ApoE4 genotype has been suggested to be associated with a lower age at onset, decreased cholinergic activity in the brain, and an inferior response to treatment with cholinesterase inhibitors than inheritance of other ApoE genotypes. For the clinician, symptomatological heterogeneity is to be expected. This will most probably influence the choice of treatment and the prognosis. However, today, it is too early to suggest guidelines for treatment of specific subgroups of Alzheimer disease.

REFERENCES

Alzheimer, A. 1987 [1907]. About a peculiar disease of the cerebral cortex (1907 article translated by L. Jarvik and H. Greensome). *Alzheimer Disease and Associated Disorders* 1:7–8.

Barclay, L.L., A. Zemcov, J.P. Blass, et al. 1985. Factors associated with duration of survival in Alzheimer's disease. *Biological Psychiatry* 20:86–93.
Bayles, K.A. 1991. Age at onset of Alzheimer's disease: Relation to language dysfunction. *Archives of Neurology* 48:155–59.
Becker, J.T., F.J. Huff, R.D. Nebes, et al. 1988. Neuropsychological function in Alzheimer's disease. Pattern of impairment and rates of progression. *Archives of Neurology* 45:263–68.
Bird, T.D., S. Stranahan, S.M. Sumi, et al. 1983. Alzheimer's disease: Choline acetyltransferase activity in brain tissue from clinical and pathophysiological subgroups. *Annals of Neurology* 14:284–93.
Bird, T.D., G.D. Schellenberg, E.M. Wijsman, et al. 1989. Evidence for etiologic heterogeneity in Alzheimer's disease. *Neurobiology of Aging* 10:432–34; discussion, 446–38.
Bird, T.D., E. Levy-Lahad, P. Poorkaj, et al. 1996. Wide range in age of onset for chromosome 1-related familial Alzheimer's disease. *Annals of Neurology* 40:932–36.
Blennow, K., and A. Wallin. 1992. Clinical heterogeneity of probable Alzheimer's disease. *Journal of Geriatric Psychiatry and Neurology* 5:106–13.
Blennow, K., A. Wallin, and C.G. Gottfries. 1991. Presence of parieto-temporal symptomatology distinguishing early and late onset Alzheimer's disease. *International Journal of Geriatric Psychiatry* 6:147–54.
Blennow, K., A. Wallin, C.G. Gottfries, et al. 1991. Significance of decreased lumbar CSF levels of HVA and 5-HIAA in Alzheimer's disease. *Neurobiology of Aging* 13:107–13.
Blessed, G., B.E. Tomlinson, and M. Roth. 1968. The association between quantitative measures of dementia and of senile change in the cerebral grey matter of elderly subjects. *British Journal of Psychiatry* 114:797–811.
Bondareff, W., C.Q. Mountjoy, M. Roth, et al. 1987a. Neuronal degeneration in locus ceruleus and cortical correlates of Alzheimer disease. *Alzheimer Disease and Associated Disorders* 1:256–62.
Bondareff, W., C.Q. Mountjoy, M. Roth, et al. 1987b. Age and histopathologic heterogeneity in Alzheimer's disease. Evidence for subtypes. *Archives of General Psychiatry* 44:412–17.
Byrne, E.J., and T. Arie. 1994. Tetrahydroaminoacridine and Alzheimer's disease. *British Medical Journal* 308:868–69.
Cacabelos, R., B. Rodriguez, C. Carrera, et al. 1997. Behavioral changes associated with different apolipoprotein E genotypes in dementia. *Alzheimer Disease and Associated Disorders* 11 (Suppl. 3):S27–34.
Chui, H.C., E.L. Teng, V.W. Henderson, et al. 1985. Clinical subtypes of dementia of the Alzheimer type. *Neurology* 35:1544–50.
Class, C.A., F.W. Unverzagt, S. Gao, et al. 1997. The association between Apo E genotype and depressive symptoms in elderly African-American subjects. *American Journal of Geriatric Psychiatry* 5:339–43.
Constantinidis, J. 1978. Is Alzheimer's disease a major form of senile dementia?: Clinical, anatomical and genetic data. In *Alzheimer's Disease: Senile Dementia and Related Disorders*, edited by R. Katzman, R. D. Terry, and K.L. Bick. New York: Raven Press, pp. 15–25.
Constantinidis, J., and J. Richard. 1985. Alzheimer's disease. In *Handbook of Clinical Neurology*, edited by J.A.M. Fredriks. Amsterdam: Elsevier, pp. 247–82.

Corder, E.H., A.M. Saunders, W.J. Strittmatter, et al. 1993. Gene dose of apolipoprotein E type 4 allele and the risk of Alzheimer's disease in late onset families. *Science* 261:921–23.

Cummings, J.L., and D.F. Benson. 1992. *Dementia: A Clinical Approach.* Boston: Butterworth-Heinemann.

Dastoor, D.P., and G.C. Martin. 1988. Age-related patterns of decline in dementia as measured by the hierarchic dementia scale. *American Journal of Alzheimer's Care and Related Disorders Research* 3:29–35.

Faber-Langendoen, K., J.C. Morris, J.W. Knesevich, et al. 1988. Aphasia in senile dementia of the Alzheimer type. *Annals of Neurology* 23:365–70.

Filley, C.M., J. Kelly, and R.K. Heaton. 1986. Neuropsychologic features of early- and late-onset Alzheimer's disease. *Archives of Neurology* 43:574–76.

Fisher, N.J., B.P. Rourke, and L.A. Bieliauskas. 1999. Neuropsychological subgroups of patients with Alzheimer's disease: An examination of the first 10 years of CERAD data. *Journal of Clinical and Experimental Neuropsychology* 21:488–518.

Fisher, N.J., B.P. Rourke, L.A. Bieliauskas, et al. 1996. Neuropsychological subgroups of patients with Alzheimer's disease. *Journal of Clinical and Experimental Neuropsychology* 18:349–70.

Fisher, N.J., B.P. Rourke, L.A. Bieliauskas, et al. 1997. Unmasking the heterogeneity of Alzheimer's disease: Case studies of individuals from distinct neuropsychological subgroups. *Journal of Clinical and Experimental Neuropsychology* 19:713–54.

Folstein, M., S. Folstein, and P. McHugh. 1975. "Mini-Mental State": A practical method for grading the cognitive state of patients for the clinician. *Journal of Psychiatric Research* 12:189–98.

Go, R.C.P., A.B. Todorov, R.C. Elston, et al. 1978. The malignancy of dementias. *Annals of Neurology* 3:559–61.

Grady, C.L., J.V. Haxby, B. Horwitz, et al. 1987. Neuro-psychological and cerebral metabolic function in early vs. late onset dementia of the Alzheimer type. *Neuropsychologia* 25:807–16.

Grosse, D.A., D.W. Gilley, and R.S. Wilson. 1991. Episodic and semantic memory in early versus late onset Alzheimer's disease. *Brain and Language* 41:531–37.

Gustafson, L. 1985. Differential diagnosis with special reference to treatable dementias and pseudodementia conditions. *Danish Medical Bulletin* 32 (Suppl. 1):S55–60.

Hannequin, D., D. Campion, S. Tardieu, et al. 1995. Phenotype of familial forms of early-onset Alzheimer's disease linked to chromosome 14: Clinical and neuropsychological characteristics of a large group. *Revue Neurologique* (Paris) 151:682–90.

Harwood, D.G., W.W. Barker, R.L. Ownby, et al. 1999. Apolipoprotein-E (APO-E) genotype and symptoms of psychosis in Alzheimer's disease. *American Journal of Geriatric Psychiatry* 7:119–23.

Haupt, M., A. Kurz, and S. Pollmann. 1992. Severity of symptoms and rate of progression in Alzheimer's disease: A comparison of cases with early and late onset. *Dementia* 3:21–24.

Helkala, E.L., T. Hanninen, M. Hallikainen, et al. 1996. Slow-wave activity in the spectral analysis of the electroencephalogram and volumes of hippocampus in subgroups of Alzheimer's disease patients. *Behavioral Neuroscience* 110:1235–43.

Heyman, A., W.E. Wilkinson, B.J. Hurwitz, et al. 1987. Early-onset Alzheimer's disease: Clinical predictors of institutionalization and death. *Neurology* 37:980–84.

Hof, P.R., N. Archin, A.P. Osmand, et al. 1993. Posterior cortical atrophy in Alzheimer's disease: Analysis of a new case and re-evaluation of a historical report. *Acta Neuropathologica* 84:215–23.
Hom, J. 1992. General and specific cognitive dysfunctions in patients with Alzheimer's disease. *Archives of Clinical Neuropsychology* 7:121–33.
Imamura, T., Y. Takatsuki, M. Fujimori, et al. 1998. Age at onset and language disturbances in Alzheimer's disease. *Neuropsychologia* 36:945–49.
Koss, E., R. P. Friedland, B.A. Ober, et al. 1985. Differences in lateral hemispheric asymmetries of glucose utilization between early- and late-onset Alzheimer-type dementia. *American Journal of Psychiatry* 142:638–40.
Lampe, T.H., T.D. Bird, D. Nochlin, et al. 1994. Phenotype of chromosome 14-linked familial Alzheimer's disease in a large kindred. *Annals of Neurology* 36:368–78.
Lauter, H. 1970. Uber Spätformen der Alzheimerischen Krankheit und ihre Beziehungzur senilen Demenz. *Psychiatry Clinics* 3:169–89.
Lehtovirta, M., H. Soininen, S. Helisalmi, et al. 1996. Clinical and neuropsychological characteristics in familial and sporadic Alzheimer's disease: Relation to apolipoprotein E polymorphism. *Neurology* 46:413–19.
Lippa, C.F. 1999. Familial Alzheimer's disease: Genetic influences on the disease process [review]. *International Journal of Molecular Medicine* 4:529–36.
Lopez, O.L., M.I. Kamboh, J.T. Becker, et al. 1997. The apolipoprotein E epsilon 4 allele is not associated with psychiatric symptoms or extrapyramidal signs in probable Alzheimer's disease. *Neurology* 49:794–97.
Lopez-Alberola, R.F., W.W. Barker, D.G. Harwood, et al. 1997. Interfamilial and intrafamilial phenotypic heterogeneity in familial Alzheimer's disease. *Journal of Geriatric Psychiatry and Neurology* 10:1–6.
Lucca, U., M. Comelli, M. Tettamanti, et al. 1993. Rate of progression and prognostic factors in Alzheimer's disease: A prospective study. *Journal of the American Geriatrics Society* 41:45–49.
Mahieux, F., R. Couderc, A. Moulignier, et al. 1995. Isoform 4 of apolipoprotein E and Alzheimer disease. Specificity and clinical study. *Revue Neurologique* (Paris) 151: 231–39.
Mahley, R.W. 1988. Apolipoprotein E: Cholesterol transport protein with expanding role in cell biology. *Science* 240:622–30.
Mann, D.M., P.O. Yates, and B. Marcyniuk. 1984. Alzheimer's presenile dementia, senile dementia of Alzheimer type and Down's syndrome in middle age form an age related continuum of pathological changes. *Neuropathology and Applied Neurobiology* 10: 185–207.
Martin, A. 1990. Neuropsychology of Alzheimer's disease: The case for subgroups. In *Modular Deficits in Alzheimer-type Dementia*, edited by M.F. Schwarts. Cambridge, Mass.: MIT Press, pp. 144–75.
Martin, A., P. Brouwers, F. Lalonde, et al. 1986. Towards a behavioral typology of Alzheimer's patients. *Journal of Clinical and Experimental Neuropsychology* 8:594–610.
Mayeux, R., Y. Stern, and S. Spanton. 1985. Heterogeneity in dementia of the Alzheimer type: Evidence of subgroups. *Neurology* 35:453–61.
McDonald, C. 1969. Clinical heterogeneity in senile dementia. *British Journal of Psychiatry* 115:267–71.
McKeith, I.G., D. Galasko, K. Kosaka, et al. 1996. Consensus guidelines for the clinical

and pathologic diagnosis of dementia with Lewy bodies (DLB): Report of the consortium on DLB international workshop. *Neurology* 47:1113–24.
McKhann, G., D. Drachman, M. Folstein, et al. 1984. Clinical diagnosis of Alzheimer's disease: Report on the NINCDS-ADRDA work group under the auspices of Department of Health and Human Services task force on Alzheimer's disease. *Neurology* 34:939–44.
Mielke, R., K. Herholz, M. Grond, et al. 1991. Differences of regional glucose metabolism between presenile and senile dementia of Alzheimer type. *Neurobiology of Aging* 13:93–98.
Minthon, L., L. Gustafson, G. Dalfelt, et al. 1993. Oral tetrahydroaminoacridine treatment of Alzheimer's disease evaluated clinically and by regional cerebral blood flow and EEG. *Dementia* 4:32–42.
Mortimer, J.A., B. Ebbitt, S.P. Jun, et al. 1992. Predictors of cognitive and functional progression in patients with probable Alzheimer's disease. *Neurology* 42:1689–96.
Naugle, R.I., C.M. Cullum, E.D. Bigler, et al. 1985. Neuropsychological and computerized axial tomography volume characteristics of empirically derived dementia subgroups. *Journal of Nervous and Mental Disorders* 173:596–604.
Nochlin, D., G. van Belle, T.D. Bird, et al. 1993. Comparison of the severity of neuropathologic changes in familial and sporadic Alzheimer's disease. *Alzheimer Disease and Associated Disorders* 7:212–22.
Pantel, J., and J. Schroder. 1996. Posterior cortical atrophy: A new dementia syndrome or a form of Alzheimer's disease? *Fortschritte der Neurologie Psychiatrie* 64:492–508.
Pietrini, P., M.L. Furey, N. Graff-Radford, et al. 1996. Preferential metabolic involvement of visual cortical areas in a subtype of Alzheimer's disease: Clinical implications. *American Journal of Psychiatry* 153:1261–68.
Poirier, J. 1994. Apolipoprotein E in animal models of CNS injury and in Alzheimer's disease. *Trends in Neuroscience* 17:525–30.
Poirier, J. 1999. Apolipoprotein E: A pharmacogenetic target for the treatment of Alzheimer's disease. *Molecular Diagnosis* 4:335–41.
Poirier, J., J. Davignon, D. Bouthillier, et al. 1993. Apolipoprotein E polymorphism and Alzheimer's disease. *Lancet* 1342:697–99.
Poirier, J., M.C. Delisle, R. Quirion, et al. 1995. Apolipoprotein E4 allele as a predictor of cholinergic deficits and treatment outcome in Alzheimer disease. *Proceedings of the National Academy of Sciences USA* 92:12260–64.
Ramachandran, G., K. Marder, M. Tang, et al. 1996. A preliminary study of apolipoprotein E genotype and psychiatric manifestations of Alzheimer's disease. *Neurology* 47: 256–59.
Raskind, M.A., A. Carta, and D. Bravi. 1995. Is early-onset Alzheimer's disease a distinct subgroup within the Alzheimer population? *Alzheimer Disease and Associated Disorders* (Suppl. 1):S2–6.
Reisberg, B., S.H. Ferris, and T. Crook. 1982. Signs, symptoms, and course of age-associated cognitive decline. In *Alzheimer's Disease: A Report of Progress in Research*, edited by S. Corkin, K.L. Davis, J.H. Growdon, et al. New York: Raven Press, pp. 177–81.
Roses, A.D. 1996. Apolipoprotein E alleles as risk factors in Alzheimer's disease. *Annual Review of Medicine* 47:387–400.
Rossor, M.N., L.L. Iversen, G.P. Reynolds, et al. 1984. Neurochemical characteristics

of early and late onset types of Alzheimer's disease. *British Medical Journal* 288: 961–64.

Roth, M. 1981. The diagnosis of dementia in late and middle life. In *The Epidemiology of Dementia*, edited by J.A. Mortimer and L.M. Schumann. New York: Oxford University Press, pp. 124–61.

Roth, M. 1986. The association of clinical and neurological findings and its bearing on the classification and aetiology of Alzheimer's disease. *British Medical Bulletin* 42: 42–50.

Saunders, A.M., W.J. Strittmatter, D. Schmechel, et al. 1993. Association of apolipoprotein E allele epsilon 4 with late-onset familial and sporadic Alzheimer's disease. *Neurology* 43:1467–72.

Seltzer, B., and I. Sherwin. 1983. A comparison of clinical features in early- and late-onset primary degenerative dementia. One entity or two? *Archives of Neurology* 40: 143–46.

Sevush, S., N. Leve, and A. Brickman. 1993. Age at disease onset and pattern of cognitive impairment in probable Alzheimer's disease. *Journal of Neuropsychiatry and Clinical Neuroscience* 5:66–72.

Sjögren, H. 1950. Twenty-four cases of Alzheimer's disease. *Acta Medica Scandinavica* 245:225–33.

Sjögren, M., L. Rosengren, L. Minthon, et al. 2000a. Cytoskeleton proteins in CSF distinguish frontotemporal dementia from AD. *Neurology* 54:1960–64.

Sjögren, M., L. Minthon, P. Davidsson, et al. 2000b. CSF levels of tau, beta-amyloid (1-42) and GAP-43 in frontotemporal dementia, other types of dementia and normal aging. *Journal of Neural Transmission* 107:563–79.

Small, G.W., D.E. Kuhl, W.H. Reige, et al. 1989. Cerebral glucose metabolic patterns in Alzheimer's disease: Synapse loss is the major correlate of cognitive impairment. *Archives of General Psychiatry* 46:527–32.

Smith, M.Z., M.M. Esiri, L. Barnetson, et al. 2001. Constructional apraxia in Alzheimer's disease: Association with occipital lobe pathology and accelerated cognitive decline. *Dementia and Geriatric Cognitive Disorders* 12:281–88.

Sourander, P., and H. Sjögren. 1970. The concept of Alzheimer's disease and its clinical implications. In *Alzheimer's Disease*, edited by G.E.W. Wolstenholme and M. O'-Connors. London: Ciba Foundation Symposium, pp. 11–36.

Strittmatter, W.J., A.M. Saunders, D. Schmechel, et al. 1993. Apolipoprotein E: High-avidity binding to beta-amyloid and increased frequency of type 4 allele in late-onset familial Alzheimer disease. *Proceedings of the National Academy of Sciences USA* 90: 1977–81.

Terry, R.D. 1985. Some unanswered questions about the mechanisms and etiology of Alzheimer's disease. *Danish Medical Bulletin* 32 (Suppl. 1):S22–24.

Tomlinson, B.E., and J.A.N. Corsellis. 1984. Ageing and the dementias. In *Greenfield's Neuropathology*, edited by J. Hume Adams, J.A.N. Corsellis, and L.W. Duchen. London: Edward Arnold, pp. 951–1025.

Tunstall, N., M.J. Owen, J. Williams, et al. 2000. Familial influence on variation in age of onset and behavioural phenotype in Alzheimer's disease. *British Journal of Psychiatry* 176:156–59.

Wallin, A., K. Blennow, and P. Scheltens. 1994. Research criteria for clinical diagnosis of "pure" Alzheimer's disease. *Drugs Today* 30:265–73.

CHAPTER SEVEN

Progressive Aphasia, Frontotemporal Dementia, and Other "Focal Dementias"

Howard S. Kirshner, M.D.

Dementia and related neurodegenerative diseases are clinically varied, with individual differences in the mode of presentation, the presence of associated deficits, and the rate of progression. The diagnosis of dementia and of the specific disease process depends on the clinical documentation of a pattern of multiple deficits in memory, other cognitive processes, and behavior in excess of the effects of normal aging (see chap. 1). Dementias, especially Alzheimer disease (AD), are considered to be diffuse or generalized, in that they affect neurons in topographically widespread areas of both cerebral hemispheres. Vascular dementias, too, usually involve infarctions in multiple areas of the brain (multiinfarct dementia). Such diffuse or multifocal patterns of brain disease contrast with focal brain disorders such as single strokes and brain tumors, which produce symptoms by causing dysfunction in a single area of the brain.

The distinction between focal and diffuse diseases, however, is not absolute. Even diffuse dementias such as AD are selective in the areas of cortex they involve; association cortices in the frontal, temporal, and parietal lobes, and specific deep gray matter areas, are zones of predilection and bear the brunt of the degeneration, whereas primary motor and sensory cortices are relatively spared. Focal lesions are likewise not purely localized; they disrupt the functions of other brain areas by edema, diaschisis (reduced metabolic activity of distant but synaptically connected areas of the brain), and disruption of cortical connections. Focal lesions such as strokes that occur in strategic areas of aged brains may precipitate a seemingly diffuse encephalopathy or dementia.

This chapter is devoted to unusual patterns of neurodegenerative disease that mimic focal brain disorders. By their symptomatic focality, these syndromes are atypical of diffuse dementing illnesses such as AD. The emphasis is on language, the best-studied higher cortical function in such diseases, with briefer consideration of other apparently focal neurologic syndromes.

Language in Alzheimer Disease

Alzheimer's seminal case report (1907) contains a description of a fluent aphasia. Compared with language changes in normal aging, studies of persons with dementia using standard aphasia test batteries have shown nearly universal impairment of language, although with marked variability from case to case (Appell, Kertesz, and Fisman 1982; Cummings et al. 1985; Murdoch et al. 1987; Faber-Langendoen et al. 1988; Price et al. 1993; Emery 1999, 2000). This subject is also discussed in chapters 6 and 8. Language has not been emphasized as a major aspect of the early cognitive deficit of dementia. Memory difficulty and deficits of higher-level reasoning rather than language disorders are typically the presenting features of dementing diseases (Liston 1979; McKhann et al. 1984; American Psychiatric Association 2000).

The pattern of language in persons with Alzheimer disease is usually fluent, with little or no difficulty in articulation or flow of speech during early stages. Phonology and rote, simple syntactic aspects of language appear relatively preserved, whereas semantics deteriorate. The content of language is deficient, with word-finding pauses, circumlocutions, and a paucity of abstract content (Snowdon 2001). Naming is virtually always affected as well, especially recall of proper names. Naming deficits are easily measurable in early to middle-stage AD (Williams, Mack, and Henderson 1989). Later in the disease, even names of common objects become lost. Persons with dementia may use a general category or a nonspecific word such as "thing" to denote a specific member of that category (Schwartz, Marin, and Saffran 1979; Emery 1985, 2000). In confrontational naming tasks, misperception of the item to be named may account for some of the deficit (Rochford 1971; Kirshner, Webb, and Kelly 1984; Shuttleworth and Huber 1988). Persons with dementia also have special difficulty with series naming, as in naming as many animals as possible in a minute (Miller and Hague 1975; Emery 1996, 2000). Naming in AD is often more impaired for verbs than for nouns, and for natural objects than for artifacts (Garrard et al. 1998). Receptive vocabulary and auditory comprehension are less affected, but complex comprehension tasks become impaired in later stages. Repetition is usually maintained at relatively normal levels late into the disease.

Reading comprehension and writing are generally affected more than are auditory comprehension and speech, although reading aloud may appear surprisingly normal. Much of the inability to comprehend printed sentences in persons with AD can be attributed to working memory deficits (Kempler et al. 1998). Horner et al. (1988) found that impairment of narrative writing correlates well with the severity of dementia. Rapcsak and colleagues (1989) reported that the agraphia of AD involves poor spelling of irregular words, while spelling and writing of regular words and nonwords is relatively preserved. This pattern is referred to as "lexical agraphia." Hughes and colleagues (1997) also found that patients performed better in writing high-frequency than low-frequency words. Errors tended to be phonologically acceptable (e.g., "waid" for "wade"). Some persons with early AD had normal writing; others showed a pattern of "surface dysgraphia," or a tendency to write phonetically, with correct spellings of phonologically simple words but errors on more complex or nonphonetic words.

On aphasia testing batteries, such as the Western Aphasia Battery (Appell, Kertesz, and Fisman 1982; Price et al. 1993), persons with early Alzheimer disease often exhibit the language profile of anomic aphasia. Later in the course of the disease, the pattern resembles transcortical sensory aphasia (Appell, Kertesz, and Fisman 1982; Cummings et al. 1985; Murdoch et al. 1987) or Wernicke aphasia (Appell, Kertesz, and Fisman 1982), both syndromes involving preserved fluency with abnormal language content and impaired comprehension. Only preserved repetition distinguishes transcortical sensory aphasia from Wernicke aphasia, in which repetition is impaired. Nonfluent aphasia syndromes such as Broca and transcortical motor aphasia are rarely encountered in AD (Price et al. 1993). In advanced stages, speech output becomes reduced, often limited mainly to the expressions of immediate biologic need. Muteness or echolalia may be seen in the terminal stages of AD (Appell, Kertesz, and Fisman 1982). Bayles and colleagues (2000) investigated the language function of forty-nine patients with late-stage dementia and found that loss of language expression correlated with loss of independent ambulation and bowel and bladder control. Even these patients with very advanced dementia could produce meaningful words, although their ability to name and to comprehend questions and commands was severely limited.

Language deterioration has been found in epidemiologic studies to be an important predictor of prognosis in dementia. Further, Folstein and Breitner (1981) found that deficient language performance on the Mini-Mental State Examination (MMSE) by persons with dementia was associated with a family history of presumed AD. Language tests distinguish persons with AD from normal, aged control subjects better than other cognitive tasks (Bayles and Boone 1982; Emery 1985, 1999). Kaszniak and colleagues (1978) found that language impairment in persons with AD predicted early mortality.

A controversial question has been whether persons with early or presenile onset of Alzheimer disease have disproportionately more language deficit than persons with later or senile onset. Several studies have reported that presenile cases are more likely to manifest aphasia than are late-onset cases (Seltzer and Sherwin 1983; Berg et al. 1984; Chui et al. 1985; Filley, Kelly, and Heaton 1986) (see chap. 6). Faber-Langendoen et al. (1988) found that language disorder correlated not only with the early onset of dementia but also with its rapid progression. Other studies (Cummings et al. 1985; Selnes et al. 1988; Bayles 1991), however, failed to confirm an association between age of onset and language impairment. In the latter two studies, there was a clear correlation between the severity of dementia and the severity of language disorder. Once the factor of dementia severity was controlled, however, there was no correlation between age of onset and the degree of language involvement. The implication is that persons with presenile AD have more severe overall cognitive deficits at the time of presentation than do persons with the senile form.

Primary Progressive Aphasia

In contrast to the pattern of gradual language dissolution in Alzheimer disease, syndromes have been reported in which language deterioration is the presenting feature of a degenerative disorder. The report by Mesulam (1982) crystallized interest in such cases. Mesulam described six patients in whom a fluent or nonfluent aphasia progressed over a period of years, while right hemisphere functions, memory, social graces, reasoning, and comportment remained intact. Such patients often continue working, pursuing hobbies, and even begin artistic expression (Edwards-Lee et al. 1997; Mesulam 2001). Computerized tomography (CT) scanning and electroencephalography yielded evidence of focal left hemisphere dysfunction in some cases. A single patient underwent biopsy of the left superior temporal gyrus, and the sections showed lipofuscin staining in neurons but provided no definite findings of neuronal loss, gliosis, neuritic plaques, neurofibrillary tangles, or intraneuronal Pick inclusion bodies. Mesulam postulated that these cases represented a selective degenerative disease with a predilection for specific neurons in the left perisylvian language cortex. Since then, numerous reports have appeared documenting the clinical entity of primary progressive aphasia (Heath, Kennedy, and Kapur 1983; Kirshner et al. 1984; Chawluk et al. 1986; Sapin, Anderson, and Pulaski 1989; Kempler et al. 1990; Scheltens et al. 1990; Tyrrell et al. 1990; Mesulam 2001). The pattern is variable, with some cases of fluent and some of nonfluent aphasia, but nonfluent aphasia is considered a more reliable marker for the disorder of primary progressive aphasia (Weintraub, Rubin, and Mesulam 1990). The aphasia progresses over a period of years, without the development of signs of generalized dementia in most cases. Mesulam (1987) later defined primary progressive aphasia as a syndrome of progressive aphasia, without other cognitive deficits over a period of at least two years.

Computerized tomography and magnetic resonance imaging scans reveal either focal left perisylvian or generalized atrophy; electroencephalography shows variable slowing, and tests of spinal fluid and blood are unremarkable. With the advent of positron emission tomography (PET), areas of focal hypometabolism have been described in cases of this syndrome (Chawluk et al. 1986; Kempler et al. 1990; Tyrrell et al. 1990, 1991). Tyrrell and colleagues (1990) found that early cases had isolated areas of reduced cerebral blood flow in the left temporal lobe, while more advanced cases had involvement of the frontal and parietal as well as the temporal lobes. This suggests that the disease process begins in the dominant temporal lobe, then spreads to adjacent cortical areas. Recently, the same authors (Tyrrell et al. 1991) reported three cases with progressive dysarthria and orofacial dyspraxia, followed by other cognitive deficits, in whom the changes on PET images were predominantly frontal. The PET changes in all of these cases are distinct from those reported with AD, in which bilateral temporoparietal areas of reduced blood flow and metabolism are characteristic (Frackowiak et al. 1981). Foster and colleagues (1983) reported PET studies of patients with presumed AD in which either aphasic or visuospatial deficits predominated. These small groups of cases showed contrasting patterns of cerebral glucose metabolism: patients with aphasia had more left hemisphere hypometabolism, patients with visuospatial deficits had more right hemisphere hypometabolism, and those with predominantly memory loss had no consistent metabolic asymmetry.

Many persons with presumed Alzheimer disease present with language disorders or exhibit disproportionate aphasia in comparison to other cognitive deficits, yet a more generalized dementia can be diagnosed either at presentation or over time (Foster and Chase 1983; Gordon and Selnes 1984; Kirshner et al. 1984; Poeck and Luzzatti 1988). Some of these authors (Foster and Chase 1983; Gordon and Selnes 1984; Poeck and Luzzatti 1988) have questioned whether progressive aphasia is a true syndrome or merely a point in the spectrum of typical dementing diseases, in which the pathologic changes first become evident in a relatively localized area of the brain. Mesulam (1987, 2001) has continued to define progressive aphasia as a syndrome of differing underlying pathologies distinct from AD.

Two clinical variants of primary progressive aphasia have also been reported. The first, progressive anarthria or dysarthria, has been described primarily in association with corticobasal degeneration (Kertesz et al. 1994; Chapman et al. 1997). Tyrell and colleagues (1991) described three such cases, all with evidence of bilateral frontal lobe hypometabolism on PET scanning. The second variant, primary progressive apraxia, has been described in several case reports (Azouvi et al. 1993; Rapcsak et al. 1995) and in an autopsy-proved case of Pick disease (Fukui et al. 1996).

Neuropathology of Progressive Aphasia

Neuropathologic studies in well-documented cases of progressive aphasia have been few, but the available studies support the concept that several different pathologic substrates can produce the syndrome of progressive aphasia. The first disease documented to cause progressive aphasia was Pick disease. Pick's original case report (1892) involved a patient in whom a prominent language deterioration accompanied a dementia. Pick anticipated contemporary studies by noting that the aphasia was similar to the syndrome of transcortical sensory aphasia, which had been described several years earlier by Wernicke and Lichtheim in patients with focal brain lesions.

Pick also addressed the issue of focal versus diffuse disease, stating that "simple progressive brain atrophy can lead to symptoms of local disturbance through local accentuation of the diffuse process" (1892, p. 166). The neuropathology of Pick disease involves a focal, lobar atrophy affecting the frontal and temporal lobes of one or both hemispheres. Surviving cortical neurons may have large, silver-staining cytoplasmic inclusions called Pick bodies. In the current era, cases of pathologically confirmed Pick disease have been reported in which aphasia was the presenting symptom. Wechsler's patient (1977) presented with isolated, progressive, fluent aphasia but developed more clear dementia over the ensuing two years. At postmortem examination, definite lobar atrophy and microscopic Pick inclusion bodies were found (Wechsler et al. 1982). The patient of Holland and colleagues (1985) had a twelve-year history of progressive language deficits involving predominantly pure word deafness. He was able to write notes to his family, keep his own financial records, and take public transportation to his appointments. Late in the course of the disease, behavioral disturbances supervened. Graff-Radford and colleagues (1990) reported an autopsy-proved case of Pick disease in which a profound anomia was the presenting symptom. These authors postulated that the localized degeneration of the left inferior and middle temporal gyri produced a relatively pure anomia, whereas later degeneration of the remainder of the left temporal lobe, and later both frontal lobes and the right temporal lobe, resulted in the progressive aphasia and dementia.

Closely related to Pick disease is the familial disorder reported by Morris and colleagues from St. Louis (1984), termed *hereditary dysphasic dementia.* Ten cases were reported from three generations of a single family, four with autopsy confirmation, suggesting an autosomal dominant inheritance pattern. These patients presented with anomia and fluent aphasia as well as generalized dementia. The pathology included frontal and temporal lobe atrophy, but Pick bodies were not seen. The affected cortex contained some senile plaques, gliosis, spongiform change, and loss of neurons. Neuronal loss was also present in the substantia nigra of the midbrain. The authors considered the pathology to be intermediate between Alzheimer and Pick diseases. Apart from the lack of Pick bodies, however, the cases would seem closest to a familial Pick disease. This kindred has more recently been found to have a tau mutation (see below under "Frontotemporal Dementia"). A patient with progressive aphasia has also been reported in whom autopsy showed a focal left frontotemporal atrophy, neuronal loss, and gliosis without Pick bodies (Caplan and Richardson 1986).

Two cases of progressive aphasia, previously reported in a clinical series (Kirshner et al. 1984), came to autopsy in our hospital (Kirshner et al. 1987). These patients had quite different clinical presentations. The first had a ten-year history of progressive word deafness and deterioration of expressive speech. Symptoms began with word deafness and a pattern of prefixing and suffixing extra syllables to words (logoclonia), which later gave way to complete jargon aphasia. Reading and writing as well as comportment and memory remained intact for at least five years into the illness. In late stages the patient became mute, able to write only single words, and less responsive to printed messages. He also began having temper outbursts with his family, once seizing the steering wheel while his wife was driving. He was institutionalized and became completely noncommunicative before he died, a full ten years after onset of the aphasia. The second patient had a mixed aphasia with anomia and paraphasic errors, more rapidly progressive than the first case. About two years after initial examination, and three to four years after onset of the aphasia, this patient presented with widespread muscle atrophy and fasciculations, suggesting motor neuron disease. He died soon after of respiratory failure. At autopsy, both patients had focal atrophy of the left frontal and temporal lobes. Microscopically, both had a spongiform change, or vacuolation, of the neuropil, principally affecting the second cortical layer, along with neuronal loss and gliosis. Senile plaques, neurofibrillary tangles, and Pick bodies were absent. In summary, these patients had neuropathological changes consistent with "dementia without specific findings" (Kim et al. 1981; Knopman et al. 1990). The localized nature of the changes in the left frontotemporal cortex in our cases confirmed Mesulam's postulate (1982) of a focal degeneration of neurons in the left hemisphere perisylvian language cortex. Similar cases of primary progressive aphasia were reported by Green and colleagues (1990), Kempler et al. (1990), and Kertesz et al. (1994).

Another neuropathologic entity underlying primary progressive aphasia is corticobasal degeneration, a progressive syndrome of Parkinsonism, motor deficits of one arm of apraxic nature, and dementia (Gibb, Luthert, and Marsden 1990). Several recent reports, however, have demonstrated language, cognitive, and behavioral syndromes in this disorder. Lippa and colleagues (1991) reported a patient who presented with a progressive syndrome of transcortical motor aphasia and subtle right-sided motor deficits. At autopsy, the patient had a focal, left frontal degeneration with ballooned, achromatic neurons. This was the first case of corticobasal degeneration in which the initial symptoms were a progressive aphasia. Other authors (Bergeron et al. 1996; Litvan, Cummings, and Mega 1998) emphasized behavioral and cognitive symptoms such as disinhibition, hypersexuality, irritability, and frank dementia. Clearly, corticobasal degeneration and primary progressive aphasia overlap both clinically and pathologically (Mathuranath et al. 2000).

Kertesz and colleagues (2000) postulated that Pick disease, primary progressive aphasia with nonspecific neuropathological findings, and corticobasal degeneration all share the features of focal onset in the frontal or temporal lobes, neuronal loss, gliosis, and absence of senile plaques and neurofibrillary tangles characteristic of Alzheimer disease. Kertesz and colleagues (2000) proposed the term *Pick complex* to include all of these disorders. The valid diagnosis of etiologically distinct causes of dementia increasingly involves molecular biology and genetics, with discovery of specific protein abnormalities underlying dementing syndromes and diseases. We shall return to this discussion after consideration of frontotemporal dementia, below.

Another neurodegenerative disease associated with progressive aphasia is Creutzfeldt-Jakob disease (CJD). Usually, this disease manifests with mood and personality changes, rapidly progressive dementia, myoclonus, often with exaggerated or myoclonic responses to startle, and epileptic seizures (Prusiner 2001). Most cases progress to death within several months. Mandell, Alexander, and Carpenter (1989) reported a case of pathologically proved CJD in which fluent aphasia was the sole presenting complaint and only major deficit over an eight-month period. By eleven months after onset, however, progressive dementia had developed, and death from status epilepticus occurred at thirteen months. Kirk and Ang (1994) also reported a case of CJD presenting with Broca aphasia, but progressing to global aphasia within four weeks and to death in seven weeks. In comparison with cases of progressive aphasia, the progression to dementia in CJD tends to be much faster, and the clinical features of myoclonus, exaggerated startle, and a characteristically abnormal electroencephalogram should aid in diagnosis. The pathology also differs from that of the two cases of Kirshner et al. (1987) with progressive aphasia, in that the spongy change is seen in all six layers of the cortex and throughout both hemispheres (Masters and Richardson 1978) in CJD, but only in the superficial cortical layers in primary progressive aphasia. The vacuoles in CJD are typically intracellular, while those in our cases were both intra-and extracellular.

Perhaps the most relevant issue in the area of progressive aphasia is whether Alzheimer disease is the cause of at least some syndromes of this type. Alzheimer disease is the most common disease producing dementia. Alzheimer's original case report (1907) documented aphasic disturbances of a fluent nature, along with behavioral and cognitive deficits. As yet, however, only three cases of pathologically proven AD have been reported in which aphasia was an isolated presenting symptom (Green et al. 1990; Kempler et al. 1990). Green and colleagues (1990) reported eight cases of progressive aphasia ascertained from a large dementia study, of which two came to postmortem examination. The first showed a spongiform change with neuronal loss similar to that described by Kirshner et al. (1987). The second had pathologically proved AD. At autopsy, the changes of neuritic plaques and neurofibrillary tangles were widespread throughout the brain. Green et al. (1990) and Kempler et al. (1990) predicted that most cases of progressive aphasia will prove to have AD, because this is by such a large margin the most common cause of dementia. From subsequent literature, however, it appears that the presentation of a nonfluent aphasia without generalized dementia generally predicts a non-Alzheimer pathology. The neuronal loss of AD may begin focally, but the areas most likely to be involved in the early months and years are the association cortices of the parietal and posterior temporal lobes, and also the hippocampus and deep frontal structures. Hence, the presentation of AD with nonfluent aphasia must be extremely rare. Presentations involving fluent aphasia and anomia, however, may be more common. Hodges and colleagues (1992) presented a syndrome of "semantic dementia" in which naming is the most prominent early deficit; further progression involves a fluent aphasia. The neuropathology of semantic dementia is less specific than that of nonfluent primary progressive aphasia, involving AD in some cases.

Other Atypical Presentations of Alzheimer Disease

A number of publications have dealt with the clinical heterogeneity of Alzheimer disease, a subject discussed in chapter 6. A controversy has surrounded the clinical dictum that early-onset cases of AD are more likely to manifest focal deficits such as aphasia, apraxia, and agnosia than the senile cases (Seltzer and Sherwin 1983; Chui et al. 1985; Filley, Kelly, and Heaton 1986). Studies by Selnes et al. (1988) and Bayles (1991) failed to confirm this association, finding only that degree of language disorder correlates with severity of dementia. The presence of clinically obvious aphasia may be used to identify a subgroup of persons with AD, but the significance of this finding for prognosis or rate of progression remains uncertain.

Another subgroup of Alzheimer disease with focal onset involves persons who present with visuospatial deficits ordinarily associated with right hemisphere dysfunction. The best documented case is that reported by Crystal and colleagues (1982). This patient presented with difficulty feeling where her left hand was in space. Examination showed left-sided sensory extinction, astereognosis, and pseudoathetosis of the left arm. Over the next two years, signs of a progressive dementia developed. Computerized tomography scanning showed only cerebral atrophy, somewhat more marked in the right hemisphere than the left, and biopsy of the right frontal cortex showed numerous plaques and tangles. This case presents a right hemisphere counterpart to the syndrome of progressive aphasia.

We examined a 46-year-old woman with progressive difficulty in recognizing family members and friends (prosopagnosia, or failure to recognize faces), together with mild deficits of memory and topographic orientation. This patient underwent a PET study that showed focal hypometabolism of the right temporal lobe. This finding also mirrors the focal left temporal hypometabolism seen in PET studies of persons with progressive aphasia (Tyrrell et al. 1990). As stated earlier, Foster et al. (1983) reported patients with presumed AD and disproportionate visuospatial deficits had predominantly right hemisphere hypometabolism on PET. In general, right hemisphere presentations of dementing illness are much less common than left hemisphere syndromes, although the reasons for this discrepancy are not clear.

Another subgroup of Alzheimer disease involves persons with myoclonus or extrapyramidal signs. In the study of Chui and colleagues (1985), either of these signs was associated with severe dementia. Mayeux, Stern, and Spanton (1985) divided cases of presumed AD into four groups: (1) typical, (2) extrapyramidal, (3) myoclonic, and (4) benign (a subgroup that progressed little over years of follow-up). The extrapyramidal group had features of Parkinson disease, either related or unrelated to drug therapy, and tended to progress rapidly. While some such cases have AD pathology (Boller et al. 1980; Chui et al. 1986), others have diffuse Lewy body disease (Forno, Barbour, and Norville 1978; Gibb, Esiri, and Lees 1987; Perry et al. 1990). The subject of dementia associated with Parkinson disease and other subcortical dementias is discussed in chapter 9. The myoclonic group likewise progressed rapidly, often to a mute state, and the four groups did not differ significantly in age except that the myoclonic group had an earlier onset. A single case has also been reported in which a progressive left hemiparesis with hyperreflexia and spasticity was the initial symptom of a progressive dementia, which was proven at autopsy to represent AD.

A last association with dementia in this group is motor neuron disease. Most cases of pathologically studied motor neuron disease with dementia have not had changes of AD, but rather of atypical dementia. We recently saw a patient with dementia and signs of motor neuron disease who had changes of AD disease at autopsy. Dementia and motor neuron disease is discussed later under atypical presentations.

Frontotemporal Dementia

At the same time U.S. authors were describing primary progressive aphasia, British and European authors were describing a complementary group of focal dementing illnesses, under the term *frontotemporal dementia* (FTD). These case descriptions have included focal aphasias when the disease process affected the left frontal or temporal lobe, but other behavioral presentations are also common and may predate the language disturbance. These include loss of memory and attention and frontal lobe behavioral changes such as disinhibition, impulsivity, impersistence, abulia or lack of spontaneity, loss of social awareness, neglect of hygiene, inflexibility, hyperorality, ritualized behaviors, and inappropriate sexual interest (Neary and Snowden 1996). Neary and colleagues (1998) presented diagnostic criteria for FTD. The incidence of this disease is unknown but has been as high as 8% in the Lund-Manchester series; a Dutch study found a definite increase in familial dementia in persons with FTD, and the age of onset was younger in familial cases than in typical senile dementia (Stevens et al. 1998). Clearly, the diagnoses of primary progressive aphasia and FTD overlap, with primary progressive aphasia representing one mode of presentation of FTD.

Within the spectrum of frontotemporal dementia, some patients present with predominantly frontal lobe signs, whereas others present with predominantly temporal lobe signs. The frontal variant of FTD involves the progressive development of a frontal lobe syndrome (frontal lobe dementia). Personality changes rather than cognitive or memory loss may predominate in the presenting clinical picture of these patients. Apathy, pathologic unconcern, jocularity and disinhibition, obsessive traits, and loss of social empathy and awareness, as well as distractibility and poor attention characterize these patients (Neary et al. 1988). Similar presentations with behavioral or personality changes rather than cognitive or memory changes have been described also in Pick disease (Munoz-Garcia and Ludwin 1984). As mentioned earlier, Tyrrell et al. (1991) reported three patients with frontal hypometabolism on PET scans who had a distinctive syndrome of dysarthria, orofacial apraxia, and later development of more widespread cognitive deficits. One patient had associated signs of motor neuron disease. No autopsy confirmation was available, but these cases may be considered to represent a frontal variant of the progressive aphasia syndrome. The temporal variant of FTD is perhaps less clearly demarcated, but patients have been reported with increased artistic expression (Edwards-Lee et al. 1997). Primary progressive aphasia, of course, can occur with predominantly left frontal or temporal degeneration.

The neuropathology underlying frontotemporal dementia is essentially identical to that of primary progressive aphasia and is generally distinct from Alzheimer disease. In particular, a nonspecific pathology with neuronal loss, gliosis, and spongiform change has been characteristic. Neary and Snowden (1996) divided the pathology into three subgroups: (1) frontal lobe microvacuolation with neuronal loss; (2) predominantly gliosis without vacuolation; and (3) FTD associated with motor neuron disease. Recently, families with FTD have been reported with a genetic link to chromosome 17q21-q22, providing the first neurobiological correlate of this behaviorally defined syndrome (Heutink et al. 1997). In the words of an editorial writer, this linkage places behavioral neurology "on the [gene] map" (Wilhelmsen 1997, p. 140). The defective gene appears to affect tau protein, leading to the new term *tauopathies* for these conditions (Bird 1998). Among the cases of FTD associated with the chromosome 17 tau gene defect are cases previously reported by Morris and colleagues (1984) under the name *hereditary dysphasic dementia* (Lendon et al. 1998). Recently, a separate gene locus has been discovered on chromosome 9q for familial amyotrophic lateral sclerosis associated with FTD. One other biological marker that distinguishes FTD (or progressive aphasia) from AD is the increased frequency of apolipoprotein E4 in AD, which was not found in a series of patients with progressive aphasia reported by Mesulam (1997). In the future, advances in molecular biology and genetics are likely to lead to more specific diagnostic disease categories, and perhaps eventually to treatments for these uniformly progressive disorders.

Atypical Presentations of Pick Disease and Atypical Dementias

As mentioned earlier, Pick disease is a lobar degeneration involving the frontal or temporal lobes on one or both sides. Microscopically, lobar atrophy is accompanied by loss of neurons, gliosis, and silver-staining intraneuronal inclusions called Pick bodies, as well as swollen, chromatolytic neurons (Munoz-Garcia and Ludwin 1984). Investigators have differed as to whether Pick disease is clinically distinguishable from AD by either brain-imaging studies or neuropsychological test profiles. Knopman and colleagues (1989) reported that five of six autopsy-proved cases of Pick disease had focal atrophy of the frontal or temporal poles by CT scan, while none of seven from a matched group of patients with AD had such findings. On neuropsychological testing, relative preservation of recent memory and relative impairment of verbal fluency characterized performance of patients with Pick disease as compared to those with AD. These differences, however, did not appear to hold up over time; the groups were less distinguishable at later stages. The double dissociation between greater impairment of immediate as compared to short-term memory in left hemisphere focal degenerative disorders versus greater impairment of short-term as compared to immediate memory in AD has also been emphasized in primary progressive aphasia (Grossman et al. 1996). Gustafson and Nilsson (1982) described several clinical features that distinguished patients with Pick disease from those with AD: logorrhea, reduced spontaneous speech output, and echolalia. Positron emission tomography scanning can also be useful in distinguishing Pick disease and FTD from AD. Kamo and colleagues (1987) reported prominent frontal lobe hypometabolism on PET scanning in a pathologically proved case of Pick disease; in AD, PET findings are typically more posterior, involving the parietal lobes.

A number of other presentations have been reported in pathologically proved Pick disease. During the later stages, persons with Pick disease may develop the Kluver-Bucy syndrome, including hyperorality, hypersexuality, and visual agnosia (Cummings and Duchen 1981; Gustafson and Nilsson 1982). The Kluver-Bucy syndrome generally reflects bilateral temporal lobe damage.

A final issue is the association of dementia and motor neuron disease. Motor neuron disease (or amyotrophic lateral sclerosis) is usually characterized by progressive weakness and muscle wasting, fasciculations, and upper motor neuron signs such as spasticity. Most cases have no associated mental or cognitive change, but motor neuron disease can be associated with dementia (Wikstrom et al. 1982; Horoupian et al. 1984), with FTD (Neary et al. 1990; Neary and Snowden 1996), and with primary progressive aphasia (Kirshner et al. 1987; Tyrrell et al. 1991). The neuropathology in all of these cases involved neuronal loss and gliosis and spongiform change in superficial cortical layers, without neurofibrillary tangles, senile plaques, or Pick inclusion bodies. As discussed earlier, these changes have been referred to as "atypical dementia" or "dementia lacking specific histological features" (Kim et al. 1981; Masse, Mokol, and Brion 1981; Knopman et al. 1990). In the series of Knopman and colleagues (1990), these cases were as common as Pick disease. The atypical pathological changes are also similar to those of hereditary dysphasic dementia (Morris et al. 1984), dialysis encephalopathy (Windelman and Ricanti 1986), and the Parkinsonian-dementia complex of Guam, which can also feature motor neuron degeneration (Tan et al. 1981).

Clinical Conclusions

This chapter has reviewed the various syndromes of progressive, focal clinical deficits seen in dementing and neurodegenerative diseases. It should be clear that the study of these atypical cases is in its infancy, and the distinctions between focal and generalized disease are blurred at best. Careful examination of the patient and documentation of language and cognitive difficulties, as well as the rest of the neurological examination, is crucial in the proper recognition and clinical diagnosis of these syndromes. A family history and the age of onset, as well as the rate of progression, should be sought. Emerging brain-imaging modalities such as PET scanning and continued clinical-pathologic correlation with autopsy studies should add dramatically to our knowledge of these interesting syndromes in the coming years. Most important, molecular markers such as abnormal tau proteins in FTD and abnormal ApoE isoforms will be increasingly helpful in the diagnosis of specific neurobehavioral syndromes. Once the diagnostic categories are secure, investigation of the molecular basis of these disorders can proceed. It is likely that specific treatments will emerge as the biochemical defects are discovered, just as they have in Alzheimer disease.

REFERENCES

Alzheimer, A. 1907. Uber eine eigenartige Erkrankung der Hirnrinde. *Allgemeine Zeitschrift für Psychiatrie und Psychisch-Gerichliche Medizin* 64:146–48.

American Psychiatric Association. 2000. *Diagnostic and Statistical Manual.* 4th ed., text revision. Washington, D.C.: American Psychiatric Association.

Appell, I., A. Kertesz, and M. Fisman. 1982. A study of language functioning in Alzheimer patients. *Brain and Language* 17:73–91.

Azouvi, P., C. Bergego, L. Robel, et al. 1993. Slowly progressive apraxia: Two case studies. *Journal of Neurology* 240:347–50.

Bayles, K.A. 1991. Age at onset of Alzheimer's disease: Relation to language dysfunction. *Archives of Neurology* 48:155–59.

Bayles, K.A., and D.R. Boone. 1982. The potential of language tasks for identifying senile dementia. *Journal of Speech and Hearing Disorders* 47:210–17.

Bayles, K.A., C.K. Tomoeda, R.F. Cruz, et al. 2000. Communication abilities of individuals with late-stage Alzheimer disease. *Alzheimer Disease and Associated Disorders* 14:176–81.

Berg, L., W.L. Danzinger, M. Storandt, et al. 1984. Predictive features in mild senile dementia of the Alzheimer type. *Neurology* 34:563–69.

Bergeron, C., M.S. Pollanen, L. Weyer, et al. 1996. Unusual clinical presentations of cortical-basal ganglionic degeneration. *Annals of Neurology* 40:893–900.

Bird, T.D. 1998. Genotypes, phenotypes, and frontotemporal dementia. *Neurology* 50: 1526–27.

Boller, F., T. Mizutani, U. Roessmann, et al. 1979. Parkinson disease, dementia, and Alzheimer disease: Clinicopathological correlations. *Annals of Neurology* 7:329–35.

Burke, D.M., and D.G. McKay. 1997. Memory, language, and aging. *Philosophical Transactions of the Royal Society of London,* Series B 352:1845–56.

Caplan, L.R., and E.P. Richardson. 1986. Case records of the Massachusetts General Hospital. *New England Journal of Medicine* 314:1101–11.

Chapman, S.B., R.N Rosenberg, M.F. Weiner, et al. 1997. Autosomal-dominant progressive syndrome of motor-speech loss without dementia. *Neurology* 49:1298–1306.

Chawluk, J.B., M.M. Mesulam, H. Hurtig, et al. 1986. Slowly progressive aphasia without generalized dementia: Studies with positron emission tomography. *Annals of Neurology* 19:68–74.

Chui, H.C., E.L. Teng, V.W. Henderson, et al. 1985. Clinical subtypes of dementia of the Alzheimer type. *Neurology* 35:1544–50.

Chui, H.C., J.A. Mortimer, U. Slager, et al. 1986. Pathologic correlates of dementia in Parkinson's disease. *Archives of Neurology* 43:991–95.

Crystal, H.A., D.S. Horoupian, R. Katzman, et al. 1982. Biopsy-proven Alzheimer disease presenting as a right parietal lobe syndrome. *Annals of Neurology* 12:186–88.

Cummings, J.L., and L.W. Duchen. 1981. Kluver-Bucy syndrome in Pick disease: Clinical and pathological correlations. *Neurology* 31:1415–22.

Cummings, J.L., D.F. Benson, M.A. Hill, et al. 1985. Aphasia in dementia of the Alzheimer type. *Neurology* 35:394–97.

Edwards-Lee, T., B.L. Miller, D.F. Benson, et al. 1997. The temporal variant of frontotemporal dementia. *Brain* 120:1027–40.

Emery, V.O.B. 1985. Language and aging. *Experimental Aging Research* 11:3–62.

Emery, V.O.B. 1996. Language functioning. In *The Cognitive Neuropsychology of Alzheimer-type Dementia,* edited by R.G. Morris. Oxford: Oxford University Press, pp. 166–93.

Emery, V.O.B. 1999. On the relationship between memory and language in the dementia spectrum of depression, Alzheimer syndrome, and normal aging. In *Language and Communication in Old Age: Multidisciplinary Perspectives,* edited by H. Hamilton. New York: Garland Publishing, pp. 25–62.

Emery, V.O.B. 2000. Language impairment in dementia of the Alzheimer type: A hierarchical decline? *International Journal of Psychiatry in Medicine* 30:145–64.

Faber-Langendoen, K., J.C. Morris, J.W. Knesevich, et al. 1988. Aphasia in senile dementia of the Alzheimer type. *Annals of Neurology* 23:365–70.

Filley, C.M., J. Kelly, and R.K. Heaton. 1986. Neuropsychologic features of early- and late-onset Alzheimer's disease. *Archives of Neurology* 43:574–76.

Folstein, M.F., and J.C.S. Breitner. 1981. Language disorder predicts familial Alzheimer's disease. *Johns Hopkins Medical Journal* 149:145–47.

Forno, L.S., P.J. Barbour, and R.L. Norville. 1978. Presenile dementia with Lewy bodies and neurofibrillary tangles. *Archives of Neurology* 35:818–22.

Foster, N.L., and T.N. Chase. 1983. Diffuse involvement in progressive aphasia. *Annals of Neurology* 13:224–25.

Foster, N.L., T.N. Chase, P. Fedio, et al. 1983. Alzheimer's disease: Focal cortical changes shown by positron emission tomography. *Neurology* 33:961–65.

Frackowiak, R.S.J., C. Pozzilli, N.J. Legg, et al. 1981. Regional cerebral oxygen supply and utilization in dementia: A clinical and physiological study with oxygen-15 and positron tomography. *Brain* 104:753–78.

Fukui, T., K. Sugita, M. Kawamura, et al. 1996. Primary progressive apraxia in Pick's disease: A clinicopathologic study. *Neurology* 47:467–73.

Garrard, P., K. Patterson, P.C. Watson, et al. 1998. Category specific semantic loss in dementia of Alzheimer's type: Functional-anatomical correlations from cross-sectional analyses. *Brain* 121:633–46.

Gibb, W.R.G., P.J. Luthert, and C.D. Marsden. 1990. Corticobasal degeneration. *Brain* 112:1171–92.

Gibb, W.R.G., M.M. Esiri, and A.J. Lees. 1987. Clinical and pathological features of diffuse cortical Lewy body disease (Lewy body dementia). *Brain* 110:1131–53.

Gordon, B., and O. Selnes. 1984. Progressive aphasia "without dementia": Evidence of more widespread involvement. *Neurology* 34 (Suppl.):S102.

Graff-Radford, N.R. , A.R. Damasio, B. T. Hyman, et al. 1990. Progressive aphasia in a patient with Pick's disease: A neuropsychological, radiologic, and anatomic study. *Neurology* 40:620–26.

Green, J., J.C. Morris, J. Sandson, et al. 1990. Progressive aphasia: A precursor of global dementia? *Neurology* 40:423–29.

Grossman, M., J. Mickanin, K. Onishi, et al. 1996. Progressive nonfluent aphasia: Language, cognitive, and PET measures contrasted with probable Alzheimer's disease. *Journal of Cognitive Neuroscience* 8:135–54.

Gustafson, L., and L. Nilsson. 1982. Differential diagnosis of presenile dementia on clinical grounds. *Acta Psychiatrica Scandinavia* 65:194–209.

Heath, P.D., P. Kennedy, and N. Kapur. 1983. Slowly progressive aphasia without generalized dementia. *Annals of Neurology* 13:687–88.

Heutink, P., M. Stevens, P. Rizzu, et al. 1997. Hereditary frontotemporal dementia is linked to Chromosome 17q21-q22: A genetic and clinicopathological study of three Dutch families. *Annals of Neurology* 41:150–59.

Hodges, J.R., K. Patterson, S. Oxbury, et al. 1992. Semantic dementia: Progressive fluent aphasia with temporal lobe atrophy. *Brain* 115:1783–1806.

Holland, A.L., D.H. McBurney, J. Moossy, et al. 1985. The dissolution of language in Pick's disease with neurofibrillary tangles: A case study. *Brain and Language* 24:36–58.

Horner, J., A. Heyman, D. Dawson, et al. 1988. The relationship of agraphia to the severity of dementia in Alzheimer's disease. *Archives of Neurology* 45:760–63.

Horoupian, D.S., L. Thal, R. Katzman, et al. 1984. Dementia and motor neuron disease: Morphometric, biochemical, and Golgi studies. *Annals of Neurology* 16:305–13.

Hosler, B.A. 2000. Linkage of familial amyotrophic lateral sclerosis with frontotemporal dementia to chromosome 9q21-q22. *Journal of the American Medical Association* 284:1664–69.

Hughes, J.C, N. Graham, K. Patterson, et al. 1997. Dysgraphia in mild dementia of Alzheimer's type. *Neuropsychologia* 35:533–45.

Kamo, H., P.L. McGeer, R. Harrop, et al. 1987. Positron emission tomography and histopathology in Pick's disease. *Neurology* 37:439–45.

Kaszniak, A.W., J. Fox, D.L. Gardell, et al. 1978. Predictors of mortality in presenile and senile dementia. *Annals of Neurology* 3:246–52.

Kempler, D., E.J. Metter, W.H. Riege, et al. 1990. Slowly progressive aphasia: Three cases with language, memory, CT and PET data. *Journal of Neurology, Neurosurgery and Psychiatry* 53:987–93.

Kempler, D., A. Lamor, L.K. Tyler, et al. 1998. Sentence comprehension deficits in Alzheimer's disease: A comparison of off-line vs. on-line sentence processing. *Brain and Language* 64:297–316.

Kertesz, A., L. Hudson, I.R.A. MacKenzie, et al. 1994. The pathology and nosology of primary progressive aphasia. *Neurology* 44:2065–72.

Kertesz, A., P. Martinez-Lage, W. Davidson, et al. 2000. The corticobasal degeneration syndrome overlaps progressive aphasia and frontotemporal dementia. *Neurology* 55: 1368–75.

Kim, R.C., G.H. Collins, J.E. Parisi, et al. 1981. Familial dementia of adult onset with pathological findings of a "non-specific" nature. *Brain* 104:61–68.

Kirk, A., and L.C. Ang. 1994. Unilateral Creutzfeldt-Jakob disease presenting as rapidly progressive aphasia. *Canadian Journal of Neurological Sciences* 21:350–52.

Kirshner, H.S., W.G. Webb, and M.P. Kelly. 1984. The naming disorder of dementia. *Neuropsychologia* 22:23–30.

Kirshner, H.S., W.G. Webb, M.P. Kelly, et al. 1984. Language disturbance: An initial symptom of cortical degenerations and dementia. *Archives of Neurology* 41:491–96.

Kirshner, H.S., P. Tanridag, L. Thurman, et al. 1987. Progressive aphasia without dementia: Two cases with focal spongiform degeneration. *Annals of Neurology* 22:527–32.

Knopman, D.S., K.J. Christensen, L.J. Schut, et al. 1989. The spectrum of imaging and neuropsychological findings in Pick's disease. *Neurology* 39:362–68.

Knopman, D.S., A.R. Mastri, W.H. Frey II, et al. 1990. Dementia lacking distinctive histologic features: A common non-Alzheimer degenerative dementia. *Neurology* 40: 251–56.

Lendon, C.L., T. Lynch, J. Norton, et al. 1998. Hereditary dysphasic dementia: A frontotemporal dementia linked to 17q21-22. *Neurology* 50:1546–55.

Lippa, C.F., R. Cohen, T.W. Smith, et al. 1991. Primary progressive aphasia with focal neuronal achromasia. *Neurology* 41:882–86.

Liston, E.H. 1979. The clinical phenomenology of presenile dementia: A critical review of the literature. *Journal of Nervous and Mental Disorders* 167:329–36.

Litvan, I., J.L. Cummings, and M. Mega. 1998. Neuropsychiatric features of corticobasal degeneration. *Journal of Neurology, Neurosurgery and Psychiatry* 65:717–21.

Mandell, A.M., M.P. Alexander, and S. Carpenter. 1989. Creutzfeldt-Jakob disease presenting as isolated aphasia. *Neurology* 39:55–58.
Masse, G., J. Mokol, and S. Brion. 1981. Atypical presenile dementia. Report of an anatomo-clinical case and review of the literature. *Journal of Neurological Science* 52: 245–67.
Masters, C.L., and E.P. Richardson, Jr. 1978. Subacute spongiform encephalopathy (Creutzfeldt-Jakob disease). The nature and progression of spongiform change. *Brain* 101:333–44.
Mathuranath, P.S., J.H. Xuereb, T. Bak, et al. 2000. Corticobasal ganglionic degeneration and/or frontotemporal dementia? A report of two overlap cases and review of the literature. *Journal of Neurology, Neurosurgery and Psychiatry* 68:304–12.
Mayeux, R., Y. Stern, and S. Spanton. 1985. Heterogeneity in dementia of the Alzheimer type: Evidence of subgroups. *Neurology* 35:453–61.
McKhann, G., D. Drachman, M. Folstein, et al. 1984. Clinical diagnosis of Alzheimer's disease. *Neurology* 34:939–44.
Mesulam, M.-M. 1982. Slowly progressive aphasia without generalized dementia. *Annals of Neurology* 11:592–98.
Mesulam, M.-M. 1987. Primary progressive aphasia—differentiation from Alzheimer's disease. *Annals of Neurology* 22:533–34.
Mesulam, M.-M. 2001. Primary progressive aphasia. *Annals of Neurology* 49:425–32.
Mesulam M.-M., N. Johnson, Z. Grujic, et al. 1997. Apolipoprotein E genotypes in primary progressive aphasia. *Neurology* 49:51–55.
Miller, E., and F. Hague. 1975. Some characteristics of verbal behaviour in presenile dementia. *Psychological Medicine* 5:255–59.
Morris, J.C., M. Cole, B.Q. Banker, et al. 1984. Hereditary dysphasic dementia and the Pick-Alzheimer spectrum. *Annals of Neurology* 16:455–66.
Munoz-Garcia, D., and S.K. Ludwin. 1984. Classic and generalized variants of Pick's disease: A clinicopathological, ultrastructural, and immunocytochemical comparative study. *Annals of Neurology* 16:467–80.
Murdoch, B.E., H.J. Chenery, V. Wilks, et al. 1987. Language disorders in dementia of the Alzheimer type. *Brain and Language* 31:122–37.
Neary, D., and J. Snowden. 1996. Fronto-temporal dementia: Nosology, neuropsychology, and neuropathology. *Brain and Cognition* 31:176–87.
Neary, D., J.S. Snowden, B. Northen, et al. 1988. Dementia of frontal-lobe type. *Journal of Neurology, Neurosurgery and Psychiatry* 51:353–61.
Neary, D., J.S. Snowden, D.M.A. Mann, et al. 1990. Frontal lobe dementia and motor neuron disease. *Journal of Neurology, Neurosurgery and Psychiatry* 53:23–32.
Neary, D., J.S. Snowden, L. Gustafson, et al. 1998. Frontotemporal lobar degeneration: A consensus on clinical diagnostic criteria. *Neurology* 51:1546–54.
Perry, R.H., D. Irving, G. Blessed, et al. 1990. Senile dementia of Lewy body type: A clinically and neuropathologically distinct form of Lewy body dementia in the elderly. *Journal of Neurological Science* 95:119–39.
Pick, A. 1892. Uber die Beziehungen der Senilen Hirnatrophie zur Aphasie. *Prager Medicinische Wochenschrift* 17:165–67.
Poeck, K., and C. Luzzatti. 1988. Slowly progressive aphasia in three patients. *Brain* 111: 151–68.
Price, B.H., H. Gurvit, S. Weintraub, et al. 1993. Neuropsychological patterns and lan-

guage deficits in 20 consecutive cases of autopsy-confirmed Alzheimer's disease. *Archives of Neurology* 50:931–37.

Prusiner, S.B. 2001. Shattuck lecture: Neurodegenerative diseases and prions. *New England Journal of Medicine* 344:1516–26.

Rapcsak, S.Z., S.A. Arthur, D.A. Bliklen, et al. 1989. Lexical agraphia in Alzheimer's disease. *Archives of Neurology* 46:65–68.

Rapcsak, S.Z, C. Ochipa, K. C. Anderson, et al. 1995. Progressive ideomotor apraxia: Evidence for a selective impairment of the action production system. *Brain and Cognition* 27:213–36.

Rochford, G. 1971. A study of naming errors in dysphasic and demented patients. *Neuropsychologia* 9:437–43.

Sapin, L.R., F.H. Anderson, and P.D. Pulaski. 1989. Progressive aphasia without dementia: Further documentation. *Annals of Neurology* 25:411–13.

Scheltens, P., G.I. Hazenberg, I. Lindeboom, et al. 1990. A case of progressive aphasia without dementia: "Temporal" Pick's disease. *Journal of Neurology, Neurosurgery and Psychiatry* 53:79–80.

Schwartz, M.F., O.M. Marin, and E.M. Saffran. 1979. Dissociations of language function in dementia: A case study. *Brain and Language* 7:277–306.

Selnes, O.A., K. Carson, B. Rovner, et al. 1988. Language dysfunction in early- and late-onset possible Alzheimer's disease. *Neurology* 38:1053–56.

Seltzer, B., and I. Sherwin. 1983. A comparison of clinical features in early- and late-onset primary degenerative dementia: One entity or two? *Archives of Neurology* 40:143–46.

Shuttleworth, E.C., and S.I. Huber. 1988. The naming disorder of dementia of Alzheimer type. *Brain and Language* 34:222–34.

Snowdon, D. 2001. *Aging with Grace.* New York: Bantam Books.

Stevens, M., C.M van Duijn, W. Kamphorst, et al. 1998. Familial aggregation in frontotemporal dementia. *Neurology* 50:1541–45.

Tan, N.T., B.A. Kakulas, C.L. Masters, et al. 1981. Neuropathology of the cortical lesions of the Parkinsonian dementia (PD) complex of Guam. *Clinical Experimental Neurology* 17:227–34.

Tyrrell, P., E.K. Warrington, R.S.J. Frackowiak, et al. 1990. Heterogeneity in progressive aphasia due to focal cortical atrophy. *Brain* 113:1321–36.

Tyrrell, P., L.D. Kartsounis, R.S.J. Frackowiak, et al. 1991. Progressive loss of speech output and orofacial dyspraxia associated with frontal lobe hypo-metabolism. *Journal of Neurology, Neurosurgery, and Psychiatry* 54:351–57.

Wechsler, A.F. 1977. Presenile dementia presenting as aphasia. *Journal of Neurology, Neurosurgery and Psychiatry* 40:303–5.

Wechsler, A.F., A. Verity, S. Rosenschein, et al. 1982. Pick's disease. A clinical, computed tomographic, and histologic study with Golgi impregnation observations. *Archives of Neurology* 39:287–90.

Weintraub, S., N.P. Rubin, and M.-M. Mesulam. 1990. Primary progressive aphasia: Longitudinal course, neuropsychological profile, and language features. *Archives of Neurology* 47:1329–35.

Westbury, C., and D. Bub. 1997. Primary progressive aphasia: A review of 112 cases. *Brain and Language* 60:381–406.

Wikstrom, J., A. Paetau, J. Palo, et al. 1982. Classic amyotrophic lateral sclerosis with dementia. *Archives of Neurology* 39:681–83.

Wilhelmsen, K.C. 1997. Frontotemporal dementia is on the MAP. *Annals of Neurology* 41:139–40.
Williams, B.W., W. Mack, and V.W. Henderson. 1989. Boston Naming Test in Alzheimer's disease. *Neuropsychologia* 27:1073–79.
Williams, R.S., and S. Pogacar. 1984. Alzheimer's disease presenting as slowly progressive aphasia. *Rhode Island Medical Journal* 67:181–85.
Windelman, M.D., and E.S. Ricanati. 1986. Dialysis encephalopathy: Neuro-pathological aspects. *Human Pathology* 17:823–33.

CHAPTER EIGHT

"Retrophylogenesis" of Memory in Dementia of the Alzheimer Type

A New Evolutionary Memory Framework

V. Olga B. Emery, Ph.D.

This chapter is a theoretical and empirical discussion of the memory deficit of dementia of the Alzheimer type (DAT). Data are presented suggesting DAT involves a process of what I will term "retrophylogenesis" because memory structures last to evolve in phylogenesis deteriorate first in this dementia. A new three-tiered evolutionary memory framework is introduced, each tier originating in a different period in phylogenetic history: motor memory, emotional memory, and neocortical memory. The concept of "retroontogenesis" is introduced in the context of neocortical memory in DAT.

Memory loss is among the most apparent early symptoms of DAT of both onset subtypes and has a progressive deteriorating course (see chaps. 3 and 6). No matter which classification system one references, memory impairment is a necessary although not sufficient diagnostic criterion for DAT (Reisberg et al. 1997). Knowledge about the ways in which memory is affected in DAT not only advances our thinking about the relation between brain structures and memory processing, but is also critical for early differential diagnosis and contributes to rationally based clinical and pharmacologic intervention (Bergener 1994). Despite universal agreement that memory deterioration is a cardinal feature of

DAT, the next level of explanation, which pertains to the nature and pattern of memory loss, is less clear-cut. Because they are too narrowly conceived, and for other reasons to be discussed, there appears to be a lack of fit between memory frameworks in use and data relating to memory loss in DAT; this in turn confounds and obscures our understanding of this dementia syndrome (Morris 1996; Emery 1999). As part of the discussion, first memory will be defined; then insufficiencies of current memory paradigms as they relate to DAT will be discussed; finally, a reconceptualized memory framework as it pertains to DAT will be introduced.

Memory Defined

Memory is the term for the capacity to keep, reproduce, and bring into the present information about external and internal environments, including past experiences, happenings, and learning, the actual constituents of which are no longer materially present to the senses. The term *memory* refers to internal "re-presentations." Memory is a construct and is not directly observable, but is inferred from some behavior, change in level of performance, or other indicator. Although memory is usually defined as a higher-order cognitive process (Howe 2000) and will be dealt with as such throughout most of this discussion, it is important to note here that the capacity for memory is not limited to the brain. For example, by definition and of necessity, the process of immunization depends on a form of memory as part of the immune system (Lanzavecchia and Sallusto 2000). And as a second example of memory in the broader systems of organisms, much of behavior in animals is based on "genetic memory" (Udalova and Karas 1996).

Human memory appears to be the result of integrated neurocognitive or psychochemical systems. The basic functions of memory are encoding, storage, and retrieval, all of which involve neuronal processes (Howe 2000). Pragmatically, then, memory is the ability to encode and then retrieve and use information previously encoded, processed, and stored. Formation of memories involves the making of new synaptic connections between neurons (Squire 1987; Black and Greenough 1998). Memory involves a persistent change in the relationship between neurons through structural modifications and biochemical events within neurons that change the way in which neighboring neurons communicate (Squire 1987). A word that stays in your head as an electrochemical signal for only a few seconds can leave a trace that will last for decades; the brain stores words and images not directly but as electrochemical signals or traces (Neath 1998). Synapses change according to previous experience; thus, formation of memories creates synaptic change (Black and Greenough 1998; Gluck and Myers 1998). Memory can be viewed as a specific form of a more general biological process called neural plasticity; plasticity refers to the idea that a neuron can change structurally or functionally in a way that is long-lasting (Hochner and Kandel 1986; Squire 1987; Gluck and Myers 1998; Neath 1998; Almkvist 2000).

Phylogenetic Context of Memory

Memory is a critical adaptational tool enabling an organism to retain information so that every minute of existence won't require a de novo response to the same or similar challenges. Thus, memory has survival value. As such, memory is a phylogenetically evolved structural and functional system, enabling organisms to interact more efficiently and flexibly in physical and social environments. Phylogenetically, human memory appears to be a product of modified old brain parts and newer brain parts working together, having evolved over millions of years (Luria 1973; Damasio 1999; MacLean 2001). For example, the hippocampus, one of a number of brain areas critical for memory, has evolved and shifted location over human phylogenetic history (Luria 1973; MacLean 2001). Accordingly, investigations of memory based on static, nondiachronic, simple localizationist assumptions are doomed to failure. The long, complex phylogenetic history of memory would suggest that memory is a multitiered, multidimensional, hierarchically organized tool or "organ" of adaptation laid down in many places of the organism, with redundancy and superimposition as features reflective of phylogenetics.

One model of the brain (and by inclusion of memory) that incorporates and builds on human evolutionary history is that of the triune brain, comprised of the evolved three tiers of reptilian brain, paleomammalian brain, and neomammalian brain (MacLean 2001). MacLean (2001) states that these three separate but interconnected "brains" reflect our phylogenetic relation to reptiles, early mammals, and later mammals. By extension, then, human memory can be viewed as having evolved through reptilian, paleomammalian, and neomammalian phases, with evolved neocortical memory structures and functions not completely isolated or cut off from more primitive memory remnants, instincts, and organization. In the triune brain formulation, the primitive reptilian brain is an expansion of upper brain stem; within the reptilian complex are neural mechanisms responsible for species preservation and self-preservation (Dobzhansky 1964; Udalova and Karas 1996; MacLean 2001). Experiments with animals as diverse as squirrel monkeys and turkeys have found that the reptilian complex contains programs responsible for hunting, homing, mating, fighting, and establishing territory (MacLean 2001); all of these activities involve, among other things, genetic memory (Udalova and Karas 1996). The second tier, or paleomammalian brain, is responsible for the fundamental emotions of fear, rage, lust, and primitive jealousy, which underlie much behavior and represent rudiments of emotional memory associated with a complex of brain areas, including the amygdala (Kesner 1998; Damasio 1999; MacLean 2001). Finally, the third "brain," or neomammalian formation, which is the most developed in humans, is described as a problem-solving, memorizing device that aids the two older formations through neocortical capacities of reasoning, symbolization, language, insight, foresight, judgment, planning, decision making, and ability to look back into the past and forward to contemplate the future (MacLean 2001); none of these is possible without memory. The triune brain formulation has been described here not so we accept every detail or particular, but as a heuristic model important for establishing a context for the discussion of memory that reaches across time and shows memory to be an evolved system of structures and functions at the core of all human activity, but nevertheless interconnected with structures from the human phylogenetic past. Human memory appears to depend on several brain systems working in concert across many levels of neuronal organization, rather than on a single brain center (Dobzhansky 1964; Luria 1973; Damasio 1999; Kandel, Schwartz, and Jessell 2000).

Although memory has been a topic of inquiry for centuries, there is still no overarching, comprehensive, well specified, and integrative framework that can account for the many important but disparate, piecemeal findings related to memory in dementia of the Alzheimer type. Unlike work on the higher cortical function of thought, where Piaget's (1952) hierarchic, developmental stage theory had utility for years as an overarching, well-specified framework, or language, where the hierarchic semiotic system can serve as a comprehensive, encompassing paradigm (Bloomfield 1933; Yngve 1986; Emery 1986, 1996, 1999, 2000a), the study of memory is lacking a paradigmatic conceptualization that can account for memory in DAT, or any other population, in a systematic, hierarchic, diachronic, encompassing, integrative, or adequately specified way. Light and Burke (1993, p. 244), for example, stated, "In the study of memory there is general agreement that memory is not a unitary system, but there is no consensus on the nature of its subsystems."

Method

To identify published studies on memory in dementia of the Alzheimer type, an exhaustive computerized literature search spanning the past forty years was performed. The use of Medline, PsychLIT, PsychINFO, and Dartmouth Biomedical INFO/ED computerized databases resulted in 1035 references that were examined. A methodological difficulty encountered was that the nosologic entity or construct of DAT has changed over time (see chaps. 3 and 6) (Reisberg et al. 1997), so work from different time periods involved variations in composition of patient samples. The term *Alzheimer disease* was used originally and continued to be used through the mid-1960s to describe a progressive dementia in persons with symptom onset before 65 years of age. Since the 1960s, primarily because of histopathologic observations that senile plaques and neurofibrillary tangles are found in brains of persons with both early-onset and late-onset symptomatology, these disorders came to be regarded as a single, homogeneous disease entity (Blennow, Wallin, and Gottfries 1994; Paul Janssen Medical Institute 1997). However, most recently, because neurochemical deficits, neuropathologic changes, and neuropsychological symptoms may be more severe, or more accurately, have an accelerated disease course in early-onset as compared to late-onset DAT, some investigators are questioning the scientific basis for combining these disorders, and have come to regard DAT as a heterogeneous syndrome with subtypes (see chaps. 6, 14, and 19) (Emery and Breslau 1987; Emery 1988, 1996; Blennow, Wallin, and Gottfries 1994; Emery and Oxman 1997; Paul Janssen Medical Institute 1997; Londos et al. 1999; Emery, Gillie, and Smith 2000). Because of these definitional changes across time, reviewing studies of memory in DAT involved methodologic problems such as that of phenomenal identity, whereby different patient populations are labeled with an identical term and identical populations are labeled with different terms, as well as other uncontrolled variation across samples compared.

The computerized literature search found that multiple overlapping sets of constructs were used to describe memory in dementia of the Alzheimer type. Memory frameworks or distinctions prominent in the literature on memory in DAT included *short-term memory* versus *long-term memory; primary memory, secondary memory*, and *tertiary memory; episodic memory* versus *semantic memory;*

autobiographical memory versus *generic memory;* and *procedural memory* versus *declarative memory.* These memory frameworks will now be reviewed and evaluated as they relate to the goal of understanding the nature and pattern of memory deficits in DAT.

Short-term Memory versus Long-term Memory Framework

Of memory frameworks in use, *short-term memory* versus *long-term memory* is a basic useful distinction that captures a fundamental reality about the nature of memory: some information is retained only briefly, whereas other information is retained indefinitely. Support for the validity of this distinction comes from well-replicated data that demonstrate that the following basic features of short-term memory differ from those of long-term memory: (1) in short-term memory only a small amount of material is processed or retained at any one time (Morris 1996; Neath 1998; Howe 2000); and (2) material in short-term memory is lost very rapidly unless processed continuously (Hebb 1945; Neath 1998; Howe 2000).

Pioneering in the explanation of differences between short-term memory and long-term memory, Hebb (1945) suggested that short-term memory involved a temporary activation of neural circuits that declines very rapidly, whereas long-term memory involved longer-lasting traces that occur with lasting changes in actual memory structures. Work on short-term and long-term memory has advanced since Hebb proposed this explanation (e.g., Baddeley 1992; Morris 1996; Saykin et al. 1999b; Escobar and Bermudez-Rattoni 2000; Howe 2000; Laming 2000); nevertheless, the basic concepts of temporary and weak activation of neural circuits in short-term memory and long-lasting synaptic changes as part of the neural plasticity of long-term memory appear still to hold, although the terminology for these concepts, as well as the concepts themselves, have undergone development (Hochner and Kandel 1986; Squire 1987; Black and Greenough 1998; Gluck and Myers 1998; Kesner 1998; Damasio 1999; Escobar and Bermudez-Rattoni 2000; Howe 2000). Multiple systems and processes underlie the formation of memories, including neurochemical processes, such as potassium activation of metabolic processes in the glycogenolysis and glycolysis of specific kinds of cells (Laming 2000), and neuroelectrical processes, such as long-term potentiation associated with long-lasting changes in synaptic strength (Escobar and Bermudez-Rattoni 2000). Degree of strength and other variations in such variables appear to underlie some of the essential differences between short-term memory and long-term memory.

Other terms used synonymously with short-term memory are *short-term store*, *immediate memory*, and *primary memory* (Kaszniak, Poon, and Riege 1986; Neath 1998). Although the term *working memory* is also often used interchangeably with short-term memory (e.g., Kesner 1998), the concept of working memory includes, additionally, specified components of executive processing and language (phonological components) (Baddeley 1992; Morris 1996).

Terms used synonymously with long-term memory include *long-term store* and *secondary memory* (Neath 1998). However, there are a number of different kinds or subtypes of long-term memory, as will be described throughout this chapter, but this fact generally is not apparent in studies using the framework of short-term versus long-term memory per se.

Short-term Memory versus Long-term Memory in Dementia of the Alzheimer Type

Investigations of short-term memory in dementia of the Alzheimer type compared to normal controls generally have found (1) greater reduction in memory span or short-term memory capacity in dementia of the Alzheimer type (Morris 1986; Seifert 2000); (2) greater rate at which material is lost from short-term memory in dementia of the Alzheimer type (Corkin 1982; Seifert 2000); (3) greater encoding deficits in short-term memory in dementia of the Alzheimer type (Kesner 1998; Greene, Prepscius, and Levy 2000); and (4) greater decrement on short-term memory tasks under the condition of divided attention in dementia of the Alzheimer type (Morris 1986, 1996). Investigations comparing short-term memory with long-term memory in DAT have generally suggested that the decrement of long-term memory, especially of the new learning and delayed new learning types, is even greater than that of short-term memory (Moss et al. 1986; Emery 1988, 1992, 1993, 1999; Graham et al. 2000).

A main problem with the short-term versus long-term memory framework lies in its generality. There is nothing in the terminology itself, or in the way the framework is usually used in DAT and other research, that lets you know there are at least two kinds or stages in short-term memory and several kinds of long-term memory. For example, as often used in DAT research, the term *short-term memory* incorporates without distinguishing, and thus confounds, *sensory memory*. However, sensory memory constitutes a first and separate phase or stage in memory formation (Broadbent 1984; Cowan 1997; Neath 1998). Further, there are a number of kinds of long-term memory, but this is usually not adequately reflected in studies of memory that use the term *long-term memory* per se. These studies of long-term memory in DAT consistently find significant decrement; but these findings are of global decrement in the long-term memory of persons with DAT and tend not to be sufficiently specific regarding the nature, type, pattern, or comparatives of long-term memory (Emery 1985, 1988, 1999).

The categories of short-term memory and long-term memory have not been sufficiently theoretically specified as to subcategories of each. The categories of short-term memory and long-term memory constitute fundamental dimensions of memory that should be used to represent an overarching, superordinate categorical level with well-defined subordinate subcategories. This has not happened partly because consensus does not exist as to subcategories (Light and Burke 1993). Another reason that a hierarchical organization of the theory and data on memory has not occurred is because, overall, basic principles of hierarchic classification (Piaget 1952) and nosologic hierarchy (see chaps. 10 and 14) (Emery, Gillie, and Smith 1996) have failed to penetrate the literature on memory adequately.

Primary, Secondary, and Tertiary Memory Framework

Primary memory is a term used interchangeably with short-term memory, short-term store, immediate memory, and sometimes working memory (Kaszniak, Poon, and Riege 1986; Cowan 1997; Neath 1998), with some nuances. As such, the descriptions and analyses of short-term memory in the preceding section of this chapter apply also to primary memory.

Even though William James is generally given credit for coining the term *primary memory*, it appears the term was used first by Sigmund Exner (James 1890, p. 600). James conceived of primary memory as the temporary memory that occurs with the initial encounter of a stimulus or information, and attributed to primary memory the two stages of (1) sensory afterimage that automatically preserves vividness of an experience for a short time, and (2) a more abstract or cognitive, as opposed to sensory, mental impression that captures and encodes some components of experience when internally or externally reinforced soon enough (James 1890, p. 645).

Overall, most later models of primary memory combined this early version of a short-term store with computer metaphors to develop an *information-processing* approach (Kaszniak, Poon, and Riege 1986; Neath 1998; Emery 1999, 2000b). However, the fundamental characteristics of limited capacity, short duration, and temporary processing remain core components of recent information-processing variations of primary memory. Primary memory is thought to lose information by rapid fading or displacement as new incoming information displaces other information.

Secondary memory refers to the long-term, more permanent processing and storage of newly acquired information (Schmidt 1978; Neath 1998; Emery 1999, 2000b). Prototypic models dividing memory into primary and secondary memory posit that (1) primary and secondary memory involve separate memory systems; (2) primary memory has limited capacity, whereas secondary memory has no known capacity limits; and (3) secondary memory receives the adequately rehearsed or reinforced information transferred from primary memory (Schmidt 1978; Kaszniak, Poon, and Reige 1986).

Tertiary memory is another kind or stage of long-term memory, which pertains to material previously learned that is highly overlearned, well-known material of both a personal nature (e.g., name, date of birth, mother's birth name) and a nonpersonal, general nature (e.g., alphabet, months of year) (Kaszniak, Poon, and Riege 1986; Emery 1988, 1992, 1999, 2000b).

Tertiary memory is sometimes referred to as *remote memory*, which I would suggest only gives us part of the picture and, therefore, represents an incomplete characterization. The highly overlearned material of tertiary memory can be personal from the remote past (e.g., birth date) or personal from recent times (e.g., present age); the highly overlearned material of tertiary memory can also be nonpersonal from the remote past (e.g., alphabet, days of week) or nonpersonal from recent times (e.g., president) (Emery 1992).

The memory framework of primary, secondary, and tertiary memory improves on the more global short-term versus long-term framework, as it is usually used, because long-term memory is subdivided into two stages or subtypes. A problem with this framework is that there appear to be even more than two subtypes of long-term memory, as will be discussed in later sections of this chapter, where a new model of memory will be introduced.

A paradox of temporal order exists in relation to short-term and long-term memory (Broadbent 1984; Cowan 1997), which, therefore, applies also to primary memory and the two forms of long-term memory, secondary and tertiary memory. To be more specific, it appears that old information is accessed from long-term memory to form a context for and create a short-term memory representation; however, the newly formed memory can be saved in long-term memory (secondary, tertiary) only after it is constructed in short-term (primary) memory (Cowan 1997).

Primary Memory in Dementia of the Alzheimer Type

In dementia of the Alzheimer type research, the construct of primary memory is most often operationalized using tasks of digit span forward, word span, block span, or immediate verbal free recall in which number of words recalled constitutes the task. There have been numerous investigations of primary memory in DAT using these indicators. The well-replicated and robust findings are that (1) primary memory in DAT is significantly impaired, and (2) the degree of impairment of primary memory is positively correlated with the degree of impairment in behavioral indices (e.g., ADL) and cerebral dysfunction (e.g., EEG, fMRI) (Corkin 1982, 1998; Emery 1982, 1985, 1992, 1999; Kesner 1998; Greene, Prepscius, and Levy 2000; Seifert 2000). (Also, see discussions of DAT short-term memory deficits in a previous section of this chapter.)

Secondary Memory in Dementia of the Alzheimer Type

The investigation of secondary memory in dementia of the Alzheimer type often uses as an indicator the tasks of verbal or nonverbal paired associate learning, verbal shopping lists, story recall, delayed story recall, and the task of learning progressively longer lists above word span. As part of the investigation of secondary memory processing in DAT, the variables of encoding, storage, and retrieval have been systematically manipulated. The numerous investigations of secondary memory in DAT have resulted in well-replicated findings. Persons with DAT, for example, are significantly impaired in learning, recognition, recall, percentage retention, encoding semantic and organizational features, and overall memory efficiency (Corkin 1982, 1998; Emery 1982, 1985, 1988, 1992, 1999, 2000b; Saykin et al. 1999a, b, 2000). Additional findings include that scores for primary and secondary memory are correlated for persons with DAT but not for normal elderly persons (Wilson and Kaszniak 1986). In the same vein, there is a significantly greater correlation between deficit in secondary memory and language deficit in DAT than in normal aging (Emery 1999). A study by Emery (1999) concluded that the positive correlation between memory and language increases with an increase in population organicity. Put another way, the less severe the organic decrement of a population, the fewer the positive correlations between memory and language; thus, severity of organic decrement is an intervening variable in the positive relation between memory and language (Emery 1999).

The Hippocampus and Associated Medial Temporal Lobe Structures as Substrates of Secondary Memory in Dementia of the Alzheimer Type

The hippocampus has been implicated in the process of new learning and memory at least since the discovery that bilateral removal of medial temporal lobes results in profound memory loss (Smith and Milner 1981). The well-known patient H.M., who underwent this surgery, never recovered his ability for new learning and never again navigated normally in new environments (Barnes 1998). Although H.M. was significantly more impaired than patients with hippocampal damage restricted to the right temporal lobe (Smith and Milner 1981), patients with one-sided hippocampal damage, nevertheless, evidence significant learning and memory deficits (Damasio 1994, 1999; Van Hoesen, Solodkin, and Hyman 1995; Barnes 1998; Saykin et al. 2000). Recent studies have implicated variables of damage and volume in hippocampal and associated medial temporal lobe structures in DAT memory deficits (Van Hoesen, Solodkin, and Hyman 1995; Saykin et al. 2000). More specifically, fMRI studies have found hippocampal damage to be an underlying substrate in the significant deterioration of secondary memory in persons with DAT (Saykin et al. 1999, 2000). An investigation by Saykin and colleagues (2000) of DAT fMRI hemodynamic responses to a secondary memory task (one-hour delayed memory for words) showed significant absence of prefrontal activity when compared to normal controls. In contrast, persons with DAT showed greater medial temporal lobe activity than did controls. Covariance analysis relating total hippocampal volume to activation indicated that the extent of prefrontal activity was positively correlated with hippocampal volume. Also, DAT performance was related to the ability to activate remaining medial temporal lobe tissue (Saykin et al. 2000).

Underlying brain substrates in dementia of the Alzheimer type memory processing will be discussed further in the final part of the chapter.

Tertiary Memory in Dementia of the Alzheimer Type

Tertiary memory is the form of long-term memory that pertains to often rehearsed, highly overlearned material of both a personal nature (e.g., place of birth, schools attended) and a nonpersonal nature (e.g., days of week), and is often operationalized by tasks of personal information, general information, and more specific tasks, such as recognition of landmarks and of well-known faces or voices, and other overlearned personal or cultural information. Even though clinical observations of patients with DAT sometimes suggest that tertiary memory might be spared because the patient seems to remember things from the past, systematic investigations of tertiary memory in DAT have found that this form of memory is significantly impaired (Kaszniak, Poon, and Riege 1986; Emery 1988, 1992, 1999).

In sum, research results suggest that primary, secondary, and tertiary memory all evidence significant decrement in dementia of the Alzheimer type. However, although there are numerous studies showing that all three of these types of memory are impaired in DAT, there is relatively little data comparing the memory deficits of memory processing in each of these categories with one another. Put another way, what is the degree of deterioration in each of these memory categories, and how do they compare with one another on the parameter of impairment? Addressing this question, a series of studies found that, in terms of percentages or correct answers, persons with DAT showed greatest preservation on a measure of primary memory (Digit Span Forward), followed by tertiary memory, with secondary memory most deteriorated (Emery 1988, 1992, 1993, 1999). And in terms of other comparisons, the greatest discriminant function between DAT and normal aging, as well as between DAT and major depression/unipolar, occurred with measures of tertiary memory (Emery 1992). It is the person with DAT who is unsure how many days there are in a week (Emery 1985, 1988, 1989).

The comparative deficits of differing memory categories in dementia of the Alzheimer type will be described further in the final part of this chapter.

Episodic Memory versus Semantic Memory Framework

Possibly the most influential and most often used memory framework during the past three decades has been that of *episodic memory* versus *semantic memory*. In his seminal exposition of episodic and semantic memory, Tulving (1972) credited Quillian (1966) for first using the term *semantic memory* and credited Reiff and Scheerer (1959) for their work on "remembrances and memoria," which are clear forerunners of episodic and semantic memory. In turn, "remembrances and memoria" originated in Aristotle's essay *De Memoria et Reminiscentia*.

Definition and Construct Validity of Episodic Memory

Episodic and semantic memory are defined as two information-processing systems that differ from one another in terms of what kind of information is stored or "autobiographical versus cognitive reference" (Tulving 1972; Schacter and Tulving 1994). By definition, "episodic memory receives and stores information about temporally dated episodes or events, and temporal-spatial relations among these events" (Tulving 1972, p. 385). These temporally dated episodes or events are always stored in terms of autobiographical reference. The definition of episodic memory requires that an event, episode, or fact be recorded as part of the individual's own past or personal history. Additionally, it was proposed that "the episodic memory system does not include the capabilities of inferential reasoning or generalization" (Tulving 1972, p. 390). This latter criterion I would disagree with; in fact, the generalization of personal, episodic memories constitutes the core of many mental disorders (e.g., phobias, post-traumatic stress disorder) (American Psychiatric Association 1994).

Tulving provides the following examples of episodic memory (Tulving 1972, p. 387): (1) I met a retired sea captain who knew more jokes than any other person I have met; (2) I know the word paired with DAX in this list was FRIGID. Tulving, in delineating the definition of episodic memory, stated, "consider now a typical memory experiment in which a subject is asked to study and remember a list of familiar words or pairs of words; this is an episodic memory task" (1972, p. 390). Thereafter, this particular memory task became and has continued to be the prototypic example and major indicator for episodic memory (Neath 1998; Howe 2000), including for most research on episodic memory in DAT. I will suggest as part of the discussion that follows that this particular memory task violates Tulving's own definitional requirement that all episodic memory be autobiographical.

Construct validity involves the process of refining understanding of the meaning of a concept and the procedures by which a concept is operationally defined (see chap. 2) (Nunnally 1978). Let us open to question whether the study and remembering of lists and pairs of words or nonsense syllables is really a valid measure of personal, autobiographic experience and memory. The pairing of DAX with FRIGID is the essence of the impersonal or nonpersonal. Individuals might recall that they were tested by someone at a certain location on a specific day as part of their episodic memories, but is it valid to expect that the actual pairs of words or nonsense syllables (e.g., DAX was paired with FRIGID) will also become encoded as part of their personal, autobiographic memory system? Perhaps a reevaluation of the validity of this operational definition for autobiographical memory is in order.

Episodic Memory in Dementia of the Alzheimer Type

It is generally accepted that investigations of what is termed episodic memory in dementia of the Alzheimer type find significant decrement and that this particular form of memory failure constitutes a cardinal symptom of dementia of the Alzheimer type (e.g., Backman and Herlitz 1996). Furthermore, decrement in what is referred to as episodic memory is seen very early in the pathogenesis of DAT (Small et al. 1994; Backman and Herlitz 1996; Saykin et al. 1999b, 2000; Celsis 2000), and is regarded as a preclinical marker for future development of DAT (Almkvist and Winblad 1999). Overall, investigators of episodic memory in DAT define the construct, as do Backman and Herlitz (1996, p. 89), as "the ability to encode, store, and retrieve temporally and spatially bound information." The majority of studies of episodic memory in DAT operationalize this construct by testing for recognition or recall of new learning and delayed new learning of nonpersonal material (i.e., word lists, pairs of words, nonsense syllables). As has been stated previously in this chapter, the validity of using an indicator that is the essence of the nonpersonal to measure personal, autobiographical memory is controvertible. Although a person may remember that someone tested him or her at a particular time (temporally bound) in a particular place (spatially bound), is it valid to expect that the actual test materials (nonpersonal words and nonsense syllables) would in reality also become encoded and stored as autobiographical memory? Accordingly, it is debatable whether there should be continued use of a memory construct that involves a constant error or disconnect between theoretical definition and operational definition, thereby compromising construct validity of research designs, data, and interpretations based on this construct (see chap. 2) (Nunnally 1978).

Nevertheless, the following findings relating to the specific form of memory measured in these studies of so-called episodic memory in dementia of the Alzheimer type are well replicated and appear to be robust and reliable: (1) in dementia of the Alzheimer type the capacity for recognition or recall of new learning and delayed new learning of nonpersonal material, such as word lists, pairs of words, and so forth, is profoundly impaired; and (2) this profound impairment in the capacity for recognition or recall of new learning and delayed new learning of nonpersonal material, such as word lists, occurs early in disease course and constitutes a preclinical marker for dementia of the Alzheimer type (Small et al. 1994; Almkvist and Winblad 1999).

To conclude this discussion of episodic memory in dementia of the Alzheimer type, it is suggested that because of inherent contradictions between theoretical definition and usual operational definition, we no longer use this term. Instead, because the data are clear, consistent, and robust that new learning and delayed new learning are significantly impaired early in the disease course, we can validly call a spade a spade. At least for the time being, we can refer to these data by their operational definition rather than the higher-order construct.

It is suggested in this chapter that "episodic" memory, as measured by learning of word lists and so forth, is actually a *measure of the process of new learning.* Further, it is suggested that episodic memory as an indicator of new learning in process contrasts with semantic memory as a *measure of information already learned in the past,* and thus, already known.

Definition and Construct Validity of Semantic Memory

Semantic memory refers to a culturally shared knowledge base that provides a context of meaning for discrete bits of information and experience. In contrast to episodic memory, semantic memory was originally defined and continues to be defined as "the memory necessary for the use of language; it is the mental thesaurus, organized knowledge a person possesses about words and other verbal symbols, their meaning and referents, about relations among them, and about rules, formulas, and algorithms for the manipulation of these symbols, concepts, and relations" (Tulving 1972, p. 386). A problem with this definition that I have never seen addressed is that it borrows heavily, without seeming awareness it does so, from the definition of semantics as a linguistic rank in the semiotic theory of signs, which predates it (Bloomfield 1933; Emery 1985, 1999, 2000a; Yngve 11986). Phonology, morphology, syntax, semantics, and pragmatics are the ranks of the semiotic system of signs. Semantics, as one of these ranks, refers to the analysis, interpretation, organization, and integration of meaning in the context of language and its rules (Bloomfield 1933; Emery 1985, 1999, 2000a; Yngve 1986; Huck and Ojeda 1987). If the core of the definition of semantic memory is going to depend on the linguistic rank of semantics, then the reason for this and the relation between the two should be discussed or at least mentioned. The relation between semantic memory and semantics as a linguistic rank is nowhere mentioned, with an exception (Emery 1992, 1999).

In the original description of semantic memory, it was conceptualized that the "semantic system may be quite independent of the episodic system" (Tulving 1972, p. 386), although in later work the independence of the two systems was questioned and reworked theoretically to some extent (Tulving 1983, 1985; Tulving et al. 1994). What has not been addressed, however, is an inherent logical lapse between the definitions of semantic and episodic memory. The core defining characteristic of the organized knowledge of the semantic system is that it is nonpersonal, nonautobiographic, and nonepisodic compared to the autobiographic, spatially bound, temporally bound attributes constituting episodic memory. But the organized knowledge of the semantic system, however ultimately impersonal, was of necessity at some time (temporally bound) and in some place (spatially bound) learned by the person having the semantic memory. Therefore, is it not logically required, by the very way episodic memory has been defined, to conclude that a semantic memory was in the first instance episodic, even if individuals no longer remember when and where they first learned the material that later became part of their semantic memory system. This then is another problem with the construct of semantic memory that requires some resolution.

Operational definitions or research tasks used as indicators of semantic memory include the generation of exemplars for category fluency, generation of definitions for spoken words, confrontation object naming, and answering general knowledge based questions, such as "What is the freezing point of water?" (Greene and Hodges 1996).

This chapter proposes that a core problem with the episodic-semantic model is that it is a static model lacking the dimension of time—a diachronic dimension, which I would suggest, is at the crux of some of the inherent contradictions of this framework. If episodic memory, as measured by word lists and the like, is a measure of new learning in process, and semantic memory is a measure of knowledge or information already learned in the past and thus already known, then episodic and semantic memory can be viewed as *two different points on a continuum of time in the learning process.* This explanation—this introduction of the variable of time into the framework—can resolve a number of issues. For example, the argument introduced earlier, that the material of semantic memory, no matter how ultimately impersonal, had to be at some time and in some place learned by the person, thus making semantic material in the first instance episodic, is now comprehensible.

There are *actually three variables rather than just two* that crosscut episodic and semantic memory: new learning in process, old learning or information already known, and autobiography. These variables will be detailed later in the context of the introduction of a reconceptualization of memory.

The memory framework of *autobiographical memory* versus *generic memory* is sometimes used synonymously or interchangeably with episodic memory versus semantic memory (Neath 1998). This framework of autobiographical memory and generic memory appears to have greater construct validity than the framework of episodic and semantic memory, partly because (1) the terminology captures the essence of each memory system more directly, (2) the variable of autobiography is not confounded with nonpersonal new learning, and (3) the terminology does not confound the basic definition of memory with concepts from the domain of linguistics. However, the framework of autobiographical-generic memory is not fully synonymous with the episodic-semantic framework because, in fact, it deals with a different set of the three relevant variables. Whereas the autobiographical-generic memory framework captures primarily the variables of autobiographical memory and culturally shared old learning, the episodic-semantic memory framework primarily measures new learning and culturally shared old learning. Accordingly, generic memory and semantic memory appear to be synonymous, whereas autobiographical memory and episodic memory are not fully coextensive.

Semantic Memory in Dementia of the Alzheimer Type

The process of new learning, which is indicated by the construct of episodic memory, shows some deterioration in normal aging (Johansson et al. 1999; Karpel, Hoyer, and Toglia 2001) and profound deterioration in dementia of the Alzheimer type (Backman and Herlitz 1996; Celsis 2000). But what about semantic memory in DAT? Do persons with DAT evidence reliable decrement in semantic memory also? Put another way, how much of their long-standing total stock of culturally shared knowledge do persons with DAT lose because of a failure of memory? The total cultural database is vast and includes multitudinous domains. How does a researcher or clinician evaluate how much and which knowledge is lost due to the dementing process of Alzheimer syndrome?

The original definition of semantic memory emphasized the linguistic domain of preexisting knowledge (Tulving 1972, 1983; Backman and Herlitz 1996; Neath 1998). Accordingly, many studies of semantic memory in DAT have used language tasks, such as category fluency, confrontation object naming, and definition of spoken words (Greene and Hodges 1996). It is of interest that all of these tasks are also prominent in instruments for language assessment per se, such as the Boston Diagnostic Aphasia Examination (Goodglass and Kaplan 1972), Western Aphasia Battery (Kertesz 1982), and Boston Naming Test (Kaplan, Goodglass, and Weintraub 1983). Thus, it can be noted here that evaluating semantic memory through language assessment instruments involves a confound between memory and language processing. Some other studies of semantic memory tap into domains other than language, such as arithmetic and other calculation (e.g., Emery 1985, 1988, 1993). However, methodologic issues notwithstanding, the results of all these types of tasks show reliable and significant impairment of semantic memory in DAT (e.g., Saykin et al. 1999a; Johnson et al. 2000). Further, impairment in semantic memory was found in up to half of clinically referred patients early in the disease course of DAT (Grossman et al. 1996).

To be more specific, there is overall agreement among investigators that naming impairment is prominent in dementia of the Alzheimer type (e.g., Greene and Hodges 1996; Collette et al. 1999). Kertesz (1994) pointed out that the most common finding related to integrity of language knowledge in DAT "is an impoverishment of vocabulary and difficulty finding words" (p. 125). Also, studies show that low-frequency words are generated with more difficulty than words in common use (Huff 1993). However, data suggest that confrontation naming improves when persons with DAT are permitted to handle test objects (Hart 1988), thus implicating a moderating influence of sensory cues in the deficit of language knowledge. Further, there is a direct correlation between ability to name in DAT and low task demand and low task complexity, such as exists when the correct answer is a high-frequency term, cliché, stereotype, or overlearned expression (Emery 1985, 1993, 1999, 2000a).

There is additional evidence for the correlation between task complexity and dementia of the Alzheimer type impairment on semantic tasks. A number of studies have found that category fluency or generative naming is substantially more impaired, and also impaired earlier, than confrontation naming in DAT (Bayles and Kaszniak 1987; Emery and Breslau 1988, 1989; Greene and Hodges 1996; Emery 1996, 1999). This finding, while robust, has been puzzling. Why does the person with DAT show more decrement when asked to name as many category constituents as possible (e.g., grocery items, animals, clothing) than when asked to name an object or fill in a missing word in a commonplace sentence? An investigation that addressed this question found that generative naming is inherently more complex and creates greater task demand on both memory and language because it involves meta-naming, meta-memory, and components of executive function (Emery and Breslau 1988; Emery 2000a).

Compared to the many studies of various kinds of naming, there don't appear to be any studies of syntax per se in the body of literature on semantic memory in dementia of the Alzheimer type, despite the definition that "semantic memory is the memory necessary for the use of language; about rules . . . for the manipulation of these symbols" (Tulving 1972, p. 386). Syntax refers to rules of language use (Huck and Ojeda 1987). Nonetheless, there do exist some data on syntactic knowledge in DAT that are part of research on language in DAT (e.g., Emery 1985, 1988, 1996, 1999; Kempler 1991; Kemper et al. 1993; DeVreese et al. 1996), as opposed to research on semantic memory per se.

In perhaps the first empirical study of syntactic knowledge in dementia of the Alzheimer type, it was found that persons with dementia of the Alzheimer type had trouble understanding sentences when the meaning of those sentences depended on complex syntax without extrasyntactic cues (Emery 1982, 1985). Data from this investigation showed a positive correlation between DAT syntactic knowledge, lesser complexity, and early acquisition of a syntactic form in the developmental sequence of language. Consistent with this, another investigation of syntactic knowledge found persons with mild DAT to be significantly more impaired in syntactic knowledge than demographically equivalent normal elderly persons (DeVreese et al. 1996). Furthermore, this study found that both diffuse and focal damage to the right hemisphere can disrupt syntax, and that both hemispheres are impacted by the neurodegenerative process of DAT, even early in disease course. It was concluded that language knowledge is a higher cortical function with bilateral representation; more specifically, syntactic knowledge is dependent on the integrity of both hemispheres and becomes impaired early in the DAT disease course (DeVreese et al. 1996). Finally, Grossman and colleagues (1995) concluded that although early descriptions of language in persons with DAT emphasized the fluency of speech (e.g., Irigaray 1967), the preservation of grammatical (syntactic) knowledge cannot be inferred from fluent speech; rather, fluent speech does not prevent persons with DAT from having significant grammatical (syntactic) deficits.

In contrast to the investigations described above, all of which found syntactic knowledge to be seriously impaired in dementia of the Alzheimer type, several other researchers have suggested that dementia of the Alzheimer type syntactic knowledge is less impaired (Bayles and Kaszniak 1987; Kempler 1991; Kemper et al. 1993; Rochon, Waters, and Caplan 1994). Importantly, the actual data from all the investigations of syntactic knowledge cited are more similar than not. At the crux of disagreement is how to interpret the variable of preservation/deterioration of syntactic knowledge. To focus on the core issue with an analogy, if once you were able to walk, skip, and run normally but now you are no longer able to skip or run, although you can still walk to all appearances normally, albeit for only a few blocks, should we conclude that your mobility is still preserved?

In summary, semantic memory undergoes significant deterioration as part of the dementing process of dementia of the Alzheimer type, and this deterioration of preexisting cultural knowledge is observed early in the disease course (Grossman et al. 1996; Saykin et al. 1999a). Although there has been longstanding debate on whether this deterioration of semantic memory represents impaired access to intact knowledge stores or breakdown of semantic networks, recent research favors the deterioration of stored representations as an explanation (Greene and Hodges 1996; Saykin et al. 1999a; Johnson et al. 2000).

To conclude this discussion of the episodic-semantic memory framework, there has been analysis of some unresolved problems related to construct validity. However, despite the validity issues of the higher-order constructs of episodic and semantic memory, the underlying variables of new learning, old learning or preexisting knowledge, and autobiography appear to be valid lower-level constructs that are fundamental dimensions of memory. These dimensions as applied to DAT memory research have yielded robust and consistent data pertaining to decrements of memory in Alzheimer dementia.

Declarative Memory versus Procedural Memory Framework

In the early 1980s, Mishkin and colleagues proposed two retention systems that store information in fundamentally different ways: a corticolimbic "memory" system and a corticostriatal "habit" system that are, respectively, analogous to declarative and procedural memory (Mishkin et al. 1982; Zola-Morgan, Squire, and Mishkin 1982; Mishkin, Malamut, and Bachevalier 1984). The authors concluded that the corticolimbic system involves neural substrates in the medial temporal and diencephalic regions and that the corticostriatal system is subserved by the striatum or basal ganglia; retention of the corticolimbic system is lost in amnesia and retention of the corticostriatal system is relatively spared in amnesia (for review, see Mishkin, Malamut, and Bachevalier 1984).

Similarly, Squire and associates also described two memory systems, which they termed *declarative memory* and *nondeclarative memory*, each characterized by specific operations (Squire 1983). In this conceptualization, the declarative memory system is said to be based on explicit information that is consciously accessible and involves specific facts or data; it includes both episodic and semantic memory as two qualitatively different expressions of the overarching declarative memory system (Squire 1983; Kesner 1998; Howe 2000). In contrast, nondeclarative memory is purportedly based on implicit information and is said to be not consciously accessible; it includes unaware representations of simple (motor) classical conditioning and nonassociative learning (Squire 1983; Parkin 1997; Howe 2000). It was proposed that declarative memory was mediated by the hippocampus and interconnected neural regions, such as the parahippocampal gyrus, entorhinal cortex, and perirhinal cortex (Squire 1983). More recently, Squire (1995) suggested that habits and skills of nondeclarative memory are subserved by the striatum, whereas the simple classical conditioning of emotion in the nondeclarative memory system is subserved by the amygdala. Support for the declarative-nondeclarative memory distinction comes from research with human amnestic patients, including the well-known H.M. (Damasio 1994; Kesner 1998).

In the same vein, the *declarative memory* versus *procedural memory* framework was proposed by Cohen and Eichenbaum (1993) and represents an extension of the declarative versus nondeclarative memory model. Declarative memory in this framework is again subserved by the hippocampus and associated neural networks. It is characterized by conscious processing of information and has the capability for relational representation and representational flexibility in novel situations (Cohen and Eichenbaum 1993). In contrast, procedural memory is characterized as relatively independent of the hippocampus; it is inflexible in novel situations. Neural networks that subserve sensory and motor processing of information during learning are at the core of procedural memory (Cohen and Eichenbaum 1993; Kesner 1998).

Procedural memory is involved in the "how to" rather than the "what" of knowledge, for example, how to ride a bicycle or touch type (Schacter and Tulving 1994; Neath 1998; Howe 2000). Schacter and Tulving (1994) proposed that the categories of declarative memory and procedural memory met criteria for fundamentally different memory systems because they are characterized by convergent dissociation; that is, using a variety of materials, populations, techniques, and tasks, there is a convergence on the same conclusion that there exists a multiple dissociation between the two forms of memory. The criterion of convergent dissociation (Schacter and Tulving 1994) is similar in essence to the statistical multitrait, multimethod matrix (Campbell and Fiske 1959). It would appear that procedural memory is, in fact, a form or kind of memory that differs fundamentally from declarative (episodic, semantic) memory. This will be discussed further in following sections of this chapter.

In terms of construct validity, the characterization of procedural or nondeclarative memory as inaccessible to consciousness (e.g., Parkin 1997) seems problematic. For example, bicycle riding and touch typing are often given as exemplars of procedural memory, but, indeed, if one wants to or needs to, one can make conscious what one does in the process of learning or doing these activities and teach them to someone else. Touch typing is taught to students in typing class, and what is taught is accessible to consciousness. However, there is a fundamental difference between these two types of memory that is not adequately apprehended by the conceptualization of consciousness as the mediating variable, which will be discussed in the final part of this chapter.

Declarative Memory versus Procedural Memory in Dementia of the Alzheimer Type

By examining episodic and semantic memory deficits in dementia of the Alzheimer type, we have already demonstrated that the overarching category of declarative memory, of which episodic and semantic memory are two different subtypes (Squire 1983), is significantly impaired by the process of Alzheimer dementia. But what about procedural memory in DAT? Although procedural memory shows some impairment in DAT, usually late in the disease course, it is significantly less impaired in DAT than are the differing forms of declarative memory (see chap. 9) (Massman, Butters, and Delis 1994; Salmon and Fennema-Notestine 1996). To understand the relative and fundamental difference between procedural and declarative memory in DAT, it is useful at this point in the discussion to invoke the concepts of subcortical dementia and cortical dementia (see chap. 9).

The distinctive pattern of cognitive impairment with pathology predominantly in the subcortical nuclei was first described by Albert, Feldman, and Willis (1974) and McHugh and Folstein (1975) and was termed *subcortical dementia.* Diseases associated with subcortical dementia include basal ganglia disorders (e.g., progressive supranuclear palsy, Huntington disease, Parkinson disease), white matter diseases (e.g., multiple sclerosis, acquired immunodeficiency syndrome), white matter cerebrovascular syndromes (e.g., Binswanger disease, lacunar state), and other disorders, such as spinocerebellar degeneration, thalamic degeneration, and others (see chaps. 9, 12, and 13). Subcortical dementia is contrasted with *cortical dementia*, which has pathology predominating in the temporoparietal-occipital regions, association cortices, and projections in contrast to the subcortical-frontal pathology of subcortical dementia (see chaps. 4, 6, 7, and 9). Dementia of the Alzheimer type is regarded as a prototypical cortical dementia. Cognitive functions significantly more impaired in subcortical dementia than in DAT include procedural memory and articulation (i.e. dysarthria) (see chap. 9) (Kertesz 1994; Libon et al. 1998). In contrast, all forms of declarative memory are more impaired in DAT than in subcortical dementia (see chaps. 6 and 9). Data from MRI research show, for example, that persons with ischemic vascular dementia (subcortical dementia) have greater white matter alterations, but larger hippocampal formations than persons with DAT (cortical dementia), and that the two populations can be dissociated on the basis of differing patterns of impairment on tests of procedural and declarative memory (Libon et al. 1998).

New Synthesis: A Three-Tiered Evolutionary Memory Framework

The Missing Evolutionary Perspective in Memory Frameworks

What follows is a new synthesis and reconceptualization of memory. In no way do I propose that this new synthesis is the summum bonum or end all of memory frameworks. Rather, the reconceptualization is presented as a heuristic model signifying a starting point for a new understanding of how the puzzle pieces of memory fit together. Why do we need a new framework at all when other memory frameworks have provided constructs for thousands of studies over many decades? This rhetorical question has for years been a source of puzzlement and unease for me; how could it be that all the splendid frameworks analyzed throughout earlier sections of this chapter somehow did not fully do the job for which they were intended? Why was it that the memory puzzle still didn't quite fit together and the data on memory impairment in DAT did not show a goodness-of-fit with frameworks available? I have tried in earlier sections of this chapter to discuss the most often used memory frameworks and point to problems of validity that, after all is said and done, interfere with valid and comprehensive understanding of what memory is all about. After years of working with various memory paradigms, it seems clear to me that what is missing from all these frameworks is an evolutionary perspective. The various memory constructs analyzed in foregoing sections are juxtaposed in dichotomous relation to one another uninformed by the dimension of time. They all lack a diachronic dimension, and because of this fact, the memory frameworks described fail to reflect the reality that memory is an *evolved* "organ" of adaptation.

Memory is a phylogenetically evolved structural and functional set of systems working in concert to enable organismic survival. The receipt, storage, and retrieval of information are general properties of neuronal networks serving to adapt behavior to environment (Schmidt 1978; Guyton 2000; Kandel, Schwartz, and Jessell 2000). Phylogenetically speaking, human memory is the result of new brain parts and modified old brain parts working together, having evolved over millions of years of evolution (Darwin 1955 [1859]; Luria 1973; Damasio 1999; Guyton 2000). In consequence, memory traces are not localized to any one brain structure, but are widely distributed throughout the nervous system (Dobzhansky 1964; Nauta and Fiertag 1979; Damasio 1999; Guyton 2000; Kandel, Schwartz, and Jessell 2000). The long, complex phylogenetic background of human memory necessitates the idea that human memory is a multitiered, hierarchically organized tool of adaptation; the three different tiers to be described have origins at different points in evolutionary time. However, memory frameworks currently in use, lacking the dimension of time, fail to reflect the realities and the vicissitudes of phylogenetics.

A Three-Tiered Evolutionary Memory Framework

As stated before, the reconceptualization to be presented is a starting point, and, therefore, is not yet complete. The memory framework to be introduced consists of three tiers or systems of memory, the origins of which represent differing times in evolutionary history: *movement (motor, subcortical) memory*, *emotional memory*, and *higher cortical memory*. In terms of the phyletic scale, the phylogenesis of movement, as well as memory for motor information and programmed motor sequences, preceded phylogenesis of emotion; in turn, the phylogenesis of both movement and emotion preceded phylogenesis of the neocortex and its functions, one of which is neocortical or higher cortical memory (Darwin 1955 [1859], 1955 [1871]; Dobzhansky 1964; Nauta and Fiertag 1979; Guyton 1981, 2000; Udalova and Karas 1996). Thus, there is a hierarchic organization underlying the three forms of memory, which is based on phylogenesis. These three tiers of memory, hierarchic in organization, are not isolated from one another, but rather have interconnections and the capacity to function in concert (Luria 1973; Nauta and Fiertag 1979; Guyton 1981, 2000). The three tiers or systems of movement (motor, subcortical) memory, emotional memory, and higher cortical memory will be introduced and sketched out; most of the focus will be on higher cortical memory, for which six stages will be described.

Movement (Motor, Subcortical) Memory

Of the three tiers of memory to be introduced, movement (motor, subcortical) memory is phylogenetically earliest to have evolved and is thus "lowest" on the phyletic hierarchy or scale (Darwin 1955 [1859], 1955 [1871]; Dobzhansky 1964; Nauta and Fiertag 1979; Guyton 1981, 2000; Udalova and Karas 1996). The two-neuron jellyfish, in which one class of neurons were sensory and the other class were motor neurons that made contact with contractile cells, preceded the three-neuron jellyfish phylogenetically. In the three-neuron jellyfish, as in man, sensory and motor neurons, as a rule, no longer communicate directly; between sensory and motor neurons there developed a barrier of neurons that have interconnections not only with motor neurons, but also with one another (Nauta and Fiertag 1979; Guyton 2000). Thus, motor neurons and concomitant memory for motor information and programmed movement sequences were relatively early evolutionary developments in the genesis of man.

Movement memory can also be termed *motor memory;* however, the term *movement memory* is broader than *motor memory*. Although motor neurons are at the basis of movement, a typical motor neuron forms synapses with enormous numbers of axons put out by neurons in the great intermediate net (Nauta and Fiertag 1979; Guyton 2000); accordingly, movement memory is broader than its essential motor components. Also, in analogue to the concept of subcortical dementia (see chap. 9), the term *subcortical memory* captures essential features of this form of memory, and contrasts well with cortical memory, as analogue to cortical dementia. But a dichotomy of subcortical memory versus cortical memory, although roughly descriptive of core components corresponding to what in this chapter is introduced as movement memory and higher cortical memory, leaves out emotional memory, which does not fit neatly into this dichotomy. Finally, the concept of movement memory encompasses many attributes of *procedural memory*. There was consideration as to whether to retain the term *procedural memory* rather than introduce a new term, an advantage to the former being the term is well established. A decision was made not to reuse the term, however, because of some semantic ambiguities. A close look at the dictionary definition of *procedural* shows the term refers essentially to procedure or proceeding in socioculturally defined contexts. The term does not lend itself as well to description of biological or neural processes, under which are subsumed structures, functions, and motor neuron networks at the core of this type of memory. And further, the most commonly given examples of procedural memory, such as touch typing and bicycle riding, have been defined to be unconscious motor sequences as an integral part of the construct of procedural memory (e.g., Parkin 1997). In reality, as has been stated before in this chapter, the performance of these procedures can be and is sometimes taught, and is thereby ipso facto, conscious. In the same vein, procedural memory is sometimes referred to as *implicit memory* in dichotomous relation to declarative (explicit) memory. However, echoing the logic militating against use of the descriptor unconscious to describe procedural memory, to the extent that cognitive skills or motor skills are sometimes explicitly taught or learned, they are, logically speaking, explicit. Thus, it would appear that the concept of implicit does not always apply to procedural memory as it must for definitional purposes. The same argument holds for the equation between declarative memory and the term *explicit memory*. It is stated that because one can declare or make explicit the material of declarative memory, it is therefore explicit. The problem is that one also can sometimes learn the material of declarative memory (e.g., semantic facts) without knowing one was learning the material, as in priming studies (e.g., Light and Burke 1993; Howe 2000), and not be able to make the material explicit.

What is really at issue here is that movement can be *voluntary* or *involuntary* (Guyton 2000). Accordingly, parameters of voluntary-involuntary have greater validity than do conscious-unconscious or explicit-implicit when applied to movement (procedural) memory. The issue is further obscured by the fact that memory in and of itself is a construct that cannot be observed directly but needs to be inferred or implied from operationally defined measures; this is true for all forms of memory, they are *all* inferred from more tangible indicators.

There have been a number of scholarly discussions of construct validity in which criteria for valid constructs have been delineated (see chap. 2) (Campbell and Fiske 1959; Nunnally 1978). An additional criterion should be added to requirements for construct validity, namely, that parameters of standard logic are met. Several constructs discussed in this chapter have shown logical inconsistency, which in turn confounds and obfuscates understanding of memory.

Some terms that seem to apply to the type of memory involved in the automatized or mechanical performance of movement sequences, going from the voluntary to the involuntary end of a spectrum, are cognitive skills learning, motor skills learning, rote learning, simple associative learning, habituation, simple conditioning, reflexive responses, and so forth until we reach the point of debate as to what counts as memory. As stated in the introductory material of this chapter, although memory is usually defined as a cognitive process, the capacity for memory is not limited to the brain. For example, genetic components of the reproductive process represent a form of patterned memory whereby attributes of the parents are genetically remembered and reproduced in offspring. As a second example, by definition immunization depends on a form of memory intrinsic to the immune system (Lanzavecchia and Sallusto 2000). Finally, as a third example, much behavior in animals is based on "genetic memory" (Udalova and Karas 1996).

To conclude, movement (motor, subcortical) memory refers to the type of memory involved in the patterning of automatic movement sequences that can result from practice, drill, habit formation, rote learning, conditioning, and so on down the line to involuntary patterned, programmed movement sequences that result from numerous structures and functions, to include reflexes, autonomic nervous system control, and genetic programming, among others.

Movement (Motor, Subcortical) Memory in Dementia of the Alzheimer Type

Earlier in the discussion, data and theory were presented suggesting that dementia of the Alzheimer type is a *cortical* dementia in contrast to subcortical dementing illnesses, such as basal ganglia disorders (e.g., Huntington disease, Parkinson disease), white matter diseases (e.g., multiple sclerosis), white matter cerebrovascular syndromes (e.g., Binswanger disease), and others (see chaps. 7, 9, 12, and 13). In consequence, higher cortical memory evidences significantly greater impairment earlier in the DAT disease course than does its subcortical counterpart of memory for motor information. Put another way, forms of memory predominantly subserved by temporoparietal-occipital regions, association cortices, and projections are severely impaired early in DAT; in contrast, movement memory is subserved predominantly by subcortical-frontal or corticostriatal substrates and is impacted relatively less and later in the DAT disease course (see chaps. 6, 7, and 9) (Mishkin et al. 1982; Kertesz 1994; Byrne 1997; Libon et al. 1998).

To be more specific, overall, persons with dementia of the Alzheimer type demonstrate relative ability to acquire and perform motor-based skills (e.g., Perani et al. 1993; Emery, Gillie, and Smith 2000). In investigations of motor-based skills, such as pursuit rotor tasks (Eslinger and Damasio 1986), mirror-reversed visuoperceptual motor tasks (Perani et al. 1993), and weight-judgment tasks (Heindel, Salmon, and Butters 1991), persons with DAT showed significantly greater ability to learn motor-based tasks and improve over trials than did persons with subcortical dementia (e.g., Huntington dementia). It has been concluded that persons with DAT can still acquire and modify motor programs, whereas the compromised corticostriatal system of persons with Huntington disease, for example, results in severe impairment in motor program acquisition and execution (Heindel, Salmon, and Butters 1991; Massman, Butters, and Delis 1994).

Similarly, another series of investigations found that persons with dementia of the Alzheimer type could continue the mechanics of reading aloud, even after they no longer understood the meaning of what they read (Emery 1985, 1988, 1996, 1999). In contrast, the motor dysfunction of dysarthria in stroke patients tended to interfere with the mechanics of reading aloud even when the patients still understood the meaning of the text (Emery, Gillie, and Ramdev 1995, 1996; Emery, Gillie, and Smith 1996, 2000). Dysarthria, stuttering, perseveration, and slowness of speech are consistent features of subcortical syndromes (see chaps. 7 and 9). (See the previous section on procedural memory in DAT for more material.)

Although the memory deficits of dementia of the Alzheimer type have been characterized as cortical in the foregoing discussion, it is important at this point to bring into focus the fact that dementia of the Alzheimer type is a syndrome and not a homogeneous singular disease entity (see chaps. 6, 10, 14, and 19). Alzheimer syndrome represents an overarching superordinate phenotype with a spectrum of subtypes. Among the heterogeneous profiles of Alzheimer syndrome is a subgroup of patients with motor symptoms that include extrapyramidal signs, such as rigidity, tremor, bradykinesia, myoclonus, and seizures, and primitive reflexes such as grasp, snout, glabellar, and palmomental reflexes. Further, some persons with DAT evidence ideomotor apraxia, motor impersistence, motor perseveration, and utilization behavior (see chaps. 6, 7, and 9). Pyramidal signs, such as extensor plantar responses and hyperreflexia, are also found in a subgroup of persons with DAT (see chap. 7). It should be noted here that NINCDS-ADRDA criteria include motor symptoms of myoclonus, increased muscle tone, and seizures, especially late in the disease course, as part of the diagnostic category of "probable AD" (McKhann et al. 1984). One investigation of neurological signs and neuropathological correlates in autopsy-verified DAT found snout reflex in 44.6%, grasp reflex in 33.9%, rigidity in

35.7%, myoclonus in 21.4%, and motor seizures in 10.7% of persons with DAT (see chaps. 3, 7, and 9). Extrapyramidal symptoms in DAT often seem to be associated with the taking of neuroleptic medications; however, extrapyramidal symptoms were found also in 12–28% of persons with DAT with drug-free history (Burns, Jacoby, and Levy 1991).

The existence of movement symptoms in some but not most patients with dementia of the Alzheimer type brings into focus the issue of why many patients seem to retain relative integrity of memory for motor information and patterned motor sequences, whereas a subgroup of patients present with prominent motor symptoms. A question that still remains unanswered is whether the motor program dysfunction of a subgroup of persons with DAT represents a DAT spectrum subtype in which motor symptoms are an integral part of the DAT process or the result of two separate but coexisting and interacting disease entities.

Emotional Memory

Emotional memory is presented here as the second major memory system in the hierarchic organization of memory. Emotional memory has been defined as a category of memory for events arousing emotion (Ikeda et al. 1998; Mori et al. 1999). Emotional memory has also been referred to as *personal memory* (Mori et al. 1999). Further, it is a thesis of this chapter that *autobiographical memory* is a phylogenetically later and higher-order development of the emotional memory system. It will be proposed that in autobiographical memory, the emotional memory system interfaces the neocortical memory stage representing autobiographically based, overlearned personal material (see the following chapter sections on the higher cortical memory system, as well as the previous section on tertiary memory).

Reference to emotional memory is infrequent in the body of work on memory per se, and yet, it will be argued that the complex network of interacting brain regions subserving the structures and functions of memory cannot be understood without the concept of emotional memory. It already has been stated that synapses change according to previous experience, and that accordingly, formation of memories creates synaptic change and can be viewed as a specific form of neural plasticity (Gluck and Myers 1998; Jessell and Sanes 2000).

The relationship between emotional memory and neural plasticity has been better understood in the literature on post-traumatic stress disorder, which can be defined as the pathological replay of emotional memory formed in response to life-threatening or traumatic events (Emery, Emery, and Berry 1993; Post et al. 1998).

The word *emotion* has roots in the Latin word *emotus*, which refers to moving away. So in this section on emotional memory, we are shifting our focus from motion to emotion, from motion to organismic biochemical and electrochemical internal and behavioral motional responses to and away from motion, in the most elemental sense of the word.

Phylogenetically, emotion developed after motion, but before the neocortex (Darwin 1872; Dobzhansky 1964; Stebbins 1977; Nauta and Fiertag 1979; Kandel, Schwartz, and Jessell 2000). Emotion developed as a mechanism or set of mechanisms to aid organismic survival (Darwin 1872; Damasio 1999). Darwin conducted extensive investigations of emotions in large numbers of species in many places, and concluded that human emotion developed phylogenetically from emotion found in lower species (Darwin 1872). The basic structure of emotions can be found in simple organisms, even in unicellular organisms (Damasio 1999). For example, if the gill of a marine snail (*Aplysia californica*) is touched, the gill will recoil instantly and the heart rate of the snail will increase as it releases ink into its environs to aid in hiding itself; this programmed behavioral response is triggered by the emotion of fear or something akin to fear (Kandel et al. 1987). Emotional memory is an evolved mechanism to aid organismic avoidance of things previously proven dangerous to survival and aid organismic approach to things previously proven to favor survival.

Damasio (1999) categorized emotions as being primary emotions (e.g., fear, anger), secondary or social emotions (e.g., guilt, embarrassment), and background or organismic milieu emotions (e.g., calm, tension). Emotions are defined as complicated collections of neural and chemical responses that form patterns and have homeostatic, bioregulatory functions. Damasio (1994, 1999) describes emotions as biologically determined processes that depend on innate brain devices, which were laid down during a long evolutionary history. These brain devices function automatically, and despite great individual variance across persons and cultures, there is some fundamental automaticity, stereotypicity, and bioregularity in emotions. All emotions involve the body for expression (e.g., visceral, vestibular, musculoskeletal, autonomic systems), and affect the mode of operation of brain circuits (e.g., monoamine nuclei, somatosensory cortices, cingulate cortices) (Damasio 1999).

Data from studies of human and animal lesions suggest that substrates underlying emotions involve neural dispositions in a number of brain regions located predominantly in subcortical nuclei of the brain stem, hypothalamus, basal forebrain, and amygdala, but also in the ventromedial prefrontal region (Damasio 1994, 1999; Hyman 1998; Phelps et al. 1998; Canli et al. 1999; Iversen, Kupfermann, and Kandel 2000; Kandel 2000; Kandel, Schwartz, and Jessell 2000). For example, a region known as periaqueductal gray appears to be a major coordinator of emotional responses; periaqueductal gray acts through nuclei or cranial nerves, such as the vagus nerve, and through motor nuclei of the reticular formation (Bandler and Shipley 1994; Damasio 1994, 1999; Kandler, Schwartz, and Jessell 2000). A consistent and reliable finding of both lesion and brain imaging studies is that the amygdala plays a crucial role in emotional memory (Damasio 1994, 1999; Hyman 1998; Phelps et al. 1998; Akirav and Richter-Levin 1999; Canli et al. 1999; Mori et al. 1999; Mory et al. 1999; Iversen, Kupfermann, and Kandel 2000). For example, in an investigation of primate prefrontal cortex, Barbas (2000) found distinct domains with different complexes of neural connections suggesting different functions in cognitive and emotional memory; it was found that orbitofrontal and caudal medial (limbic) prefrontal cortices received robust projections from the amygdala in the processing of emotional memory. Among other functions, the amygdala appears to mediate affect-laden information based on reward-punishment reinforcement schedules (Squire 1995; Kesner 1998). Further, different emotions (e.g., fear, pleasure-related emotions) activate different neural as well as biochemical responses (Canli et al. 1999; Damasio 1999). In fact, the entire field of psychopharmacology is based on the premise of differential neurochemical or synaptic responses in different states of emotional memory. And, in terms of the neural substrates of emotion, sadness, for example, consistently activates the ventromedial prefrontal cortex, hypothalamus, and brain stem, while anger or fear appears to activate neither the prefrontal cortex nor the hypothalamus (Damasio 1999; Kandel, Schwartz, and Jessell 2000). I would posit that anger and fear were phylogenetically earlier-to-evolve, more primitive emotions than the more socialized affect of sadness, and therefore, are represented in earlier-to-evolve and lower organismic regions (for example, brain stem as compared to ventromedial prefrontal cortex).

In a comparison between the much-written-about patient H.M. and an encephalitis patient named David, Damasio (1999) described how H.M. and David were similar in their incapacity to learn new facts, but differed significantly in memory for recall of old or overlearned material of a personal nature, most notably, autobiographical material. The two patients shared one site of damage, the hippocampus, which has been found critical for the learning of new facts (episodic list learning) (Damasio 1994, 1999; Van Hoesen, Solodkin, and Hyman 1995; Barnes 1998; Saykin et al. 1999b, 2000; Kandel, Kupfermann, and Iversen 2000). Unlike H.M., David also had damage in the remainder of the temporal lobe, especially in the inferotemporal and polar regions; H.M. could remember personal history, whereas David had severely impaired autobiographical memory (Damasio 1999). This comparison of patient lesions suggests at least two important points: (1) these data indicate, yet again, the association between hippocampal damage and impairment of new learning, and (2) these data point to a dissociation between new learning (episodic memory) and autobiographical memory. The chapter section on episodic memory discussed the three variables of nonpersonal new learning, nonpersonal old learning or knowledge (semantic memory), and autobiographical memory. It was suggested that the construct of episodic memory (as indicated by learning of nonpersonal word lists, etc.) confounds nonpersonal new learning with autobiographical memory and that the two are not coterminous. The lesion data above point to a dissociation between episodic memory (nonpersonal list learning) and autobiographical memory because they appear to be subserved by different neural substrates.

As part of the three-tiered memory framework being introduced in this chapter, it is proposed that autobiographical memory developed phylogenetically from the emotional memory system and that autobiographical memory is represented in the neural convergence zone of emotional memory and the neocortical memory stage involved in overlearned, personal information, such as is found, for example, on mental status questionnaires (e.g., date of birth, place of birth, mother's birth name, schools attended, and so forth) (see the following sections on higher cortical memory). Autobiographical memory may be thought of or provisionally defined as the recording in memory of the collection of facts, events, patterns of internal and external responses, patterns of thought and behaviors, and other variables that are part of a lifelong ontogenetically emergent bioelectrochemical neural complex and continuity experienced as a self. Phylogenetically, there evolved a number of critical mechanisms between the programmed emotional responses of a unicellular organism (Kandel et al. 1987) and human autobiographical memory; these evolved mechanisms included the development of consciousness (Damasio 1999; Kandel 2000; Saper 2000) and the development of the conscious, reflective self (Mead 1964; Damasio 1994, 1999). In an analysis of lesion data and the multisite network of autobiographical memory, Damasio (1999, p. 221) stated that the key elements of autobiography that need to be reliably recorded in "nearly permanent fashion are those that correspond to our identity . . . those critical elements arise from a continuously reactivated network based on convergence zones which are located in the temporal and the frontal higher-order cortices, as well as in the subcortical nuclei such as those in the amygdala."

Emotional Memory in Dementia of the Alzheimer Type

In one of the very few investigations of emotional memory in dementia of the Alzheimer type, an electrophysiological study was made of free recall and recognition of emotionally pleasant, unpleasant, and neutral photographs in comparison groups of early dementia of the Alzheimer type and normal control subjects (Hamann, Monarch, and Goldstein 2000). The study found that although there were no significant differences between DAT and normal controls in emotional arousal, persons with DAT failed to show the enhanced memory effect that follows emotional arousal in neurologically intact individuals.

In an investigation of actual autobiographical memory, in which the emotional stimulus was the actual experience of the Kobe earthquake by persons with dementia of the Alzheimer type, forty-four (86.3%) of the fifty-one dementia of the Alzheimer type subjects remembered their own terrible experience during the earthquake six to ten weeks after its occurrence (emotional/autobiographical memory), but could not remember any of the objective facts about the earthquake (semantic memory) (Ikeda et al. 1998). This study points to the dissociation between memory of an emotional, autobiographical, or personal kind and memory for objective knowledge based information. Another study of autobiographical memory in thirty-six persons with DAT who had themselves experienced the Kobe earthquake found that, irrespective of generalized brain atrophy and cognitive impairments, emotional (autobiographical) memory was correlated more with normalized amygdalar volume (right and left averaged) than with normalized hippocampal volume (Mori et al. 1999). This study concluded that impairment of emotional, autobiographical memory in DAT is related to amygdalar damage and that the amygdala is heavily involved in emotional (autobiographical) memory (Mori et al. 1999). This investigation provides evidence for the relatedness of autobiographical memory to emotional memory. Also, this investigation provides further evidence for the dissociation between emotional/autobiographical memory, which has strong underpinnings in the amygdala, and types of memory having a dominant underpinning in the hippocampus (e.g., episodic memory).

Further, in a study of emotion processing in visual and auditory domains in persons with dementia of the Alzheimer type, Koff and colleagues (1999) concluded that persons with dementia of the Alzheimer type do not have a primary deficit in processing emotion; rather, the data suggest that difficulties of persons with dementia of the Alzheimer type in perceiving and interpreting emotion are secondary to the cognitive impairments of dementia of the Alzheimer type.

Finally, one of the first empirical investigations of language deterioration in dementia of the Alzheimer type (Emery 1982, 1985) found that even after patients with dementia of the Alzheimer type lost their ability for normative denotation and connotation, language was used as a vehicle for expression of emotionally laden memories, which appeared to remain with patients with dementia of the Alzheimer type long after language ceased its function in normative social discourse.

This and other research (Emery 1985, 1988, 1996, 1999, 2000a) suggested that cognitive decline in dementia of the Alzheimer type is hierarchical in nature and occurs in reverse order of ontogenetic development, with complex, later-developing cognitive forms first to decline. I will term this phenomenon *retroontogenesis.* This same effect of ontogenetic retrogenesis was found and conceptualized by Reisberg (1999) in DAT activities of daily living and cognitive decline. I suggest that there is probable retrogenesis in DAT along dimensions of the phylogenetic hierarchy as well as in ontogenesis. This would explain the foregoing data whereby persons with DAT evidence greater preservation in subcortical motor memory and emotional memory than in neocortical functions, such as higher cortical memory. This can be termed *retrophylogenesis.*

Higher Cortical Memory

The third and final memory system of the three-tiered evolutionary memory framework that is being introduced is *higher cortical memory*. Higher cortical memory is dependent on the neocortex, the latest form of cortex to appear in evolution. This part of the human cerebral cortex has enormous extent and structural complexity, and is estimated to contain at least 70% of all neurons in the central nervous system (Nauta and Fiertag 1979; Kandel, Schwartz, and Jessell 2000). Neocortical structures evolved not simply on top of other cortical structures, but from them and with them (Damasio 1994). Thus, the higher cortical memory stages to be introduced are not totally independent of and isolated from lower brain structures. Connection between brain structure and memory function is not isomorphic; the brain works as an integrated system (Luria 1973; Damasio 1994, 1999; Kandel, Schwartz, and Jessell 2000). Accordingly, higher cortical memory is part of a larger synergistic neurocognitive set of systems, even while it is dependent on the neocortex.

The higher cortical memory tier will integrate fundamental dimensions of different memory frameworks described previously in this chapter, as well as define new parameters for understanding higher cortical memory. My reconceptualization of higher cortical memory will consist of the reconfiguration of well-established, well-investigated memory categories already described in previous sections, along with newly introduced dimensions.

The higher cortical memory system to be described involves three processing levels and six stages. These stages could also be called phases, but the term *stage* will be used in its dictionary definition of "a single step or degree in a process." The three processing levels are short-term memory, *intermediate-term memory*, and long-term memory. Short-term memory and long-term memory are defined in this framework essentially the same as they have been described and defined in previous sections of this chapter, with some nuances. Additionally, an intermediate level of processing is being introduced as part of what is a continuous model, as opposed to a dichotomous model. Short-term memory, intermediate-term memory, and long-term memory are conceptualized as consisting of two stages each, thus resulting in a six-stage model of higher cortical memory, which will be described below. Short-term memory consists of stage 1 memory (sensory) and stage 2 memory (select, recode, encode); intermediate-term memory consists of stage 3 memory (new learning) and stage 4 memory (delayed new learning); and long-term memory consists of stage 5 memory (old learning or knowledge) and stage 6 memory (overlearned material).

Higher Cortical Short-term Memory: Stage 1 Memory (Sensory)

All information used in the formation of memories must enter the human organism through the senses. Thus, the senses provide the raw data as part of a first step or stage in the making of memories. The senses have traditionally been categorized as visual, auditory, chemical (gustatory and olfactory), and tactile senses. More recently, senses have been recategorized to include vestibular senses (position of body in vestibular field) and somatosenses (pain, temperature, itch, proprioception) (Gardner, Martin, and Jessell 2000).

Despite the diversity of senses, all sensory systems communicate four basic kinds of information: modality, location, intensity, and timing. This sameness of function is subserved by similar neuronal organization across sensory systems; the various sensory systems appear to use similar neural codes for these four basic properties of sensory feedback (Gardner and Martin 2000). When a sensory neuron fires, it communicates to the brain that a certain form of energy has been received at a specific location in the sense organ; the details of the action potential communicate to the brain the amount of energy, when it began and stopped, and how quickly the energy changed in intensity (Gardner and Martin 2000). Humans have four classes of sensory receptors, each of which is sensitive to primarily one form of physical energy: chemical, mechanical, thermal, or electromagnetic (Gardner and Martin 2000). As an example of the common ground plan or organization subserving all senses, irrespective of modality, all somatosensory data from the trunk and limbs are communicated by dorsal root ganglion neurons, whereas somatosensory data from cranial structures are transmitted by trigeminal sensory neurons, which are morphologically and functionally homologous to dorsal root ganglion neurons (Gardner, Martin, and Jessell 2000).

Sensory memory is in essence a sensory playback system that permits fleeting sensory information to be *re-presented* long enough that it can be selected for further processing. For example, you hear a loud bang, see a light flash, see something pass by you before there is time to think; sensory memory provides a system to play back sensory stimuli for further processing. Cowan (1997) pointed out that we think about things at a finite pace and sensory memory allows the sensation and experience of things to linger while we think about them. Defining features of sensory memory include processing modality-specific information, as well as discrimination between fine gradations of modality-specific information (e.g., discrimination between two acoustically different sounds of the vowel *e*) (Cowan 1997). The visual playback system has been referred to as *iconic memory* and the auditory playback system as *echoic memory* (Neath 1998).

Cowan (1997) concluded there are two phases of sensory memory with different properties: a brief afterimage and a more processed, perceptually resolved phase of sensory memory, which preserves sensory features, but also involves other processes to recode and categorize sensory information. The duration of these two phases of sensory memory has been the subject of a number of investigations and dispute regarding numbers of hundred milliseconds and seconds (Cowan 1997; Neath 1998).

Although sensory memory, when included in a memory framework at all, is conceptually delimited to the first phase in formation of memories, I wish to point out here that sensory memory also exists as part of some long-term memories, especially autobiographical memories. Preliminary data from a research project on life cycle impact of early life experiences, which is in progress, suggests that recollection of earliest memories involves visual imagery and sometimes other forms of sensory memory (e.g., echoic recollection and so forth) (Emery unpublished data). You can verify this idea with your own experience: when you recollect one of your own earliest memories, do you not have some visual imagery as part of the recollection? Thus, sensory memory would appear to have a function in long-term autobiographical memory, which is a stage 6 memory in the framework being developed in this chapter.

Stage 1 Memory (Sensory) in Dementia of the Alzheimer Type

With the exception of the growing literature on olfaction in dementia of the Alzheimer type, data on sensory memory in dementia of the Alzheimer type are scant.

Visual, or *iconic*, *memory* is often measured by backward masking, whereby a letter or number is presented for very brief duration (10–150 milliseconds), followed by a masking (interfering) stimulus that blocks display. Experimental paradigms such as backward masking are difficult to execute with persons with DAT, partly because of the confound between task performance and failure to understand task demands (Kaszniak, Poon, and Riege 1986). Nevertheless, in one study of iconic memory using backward masking, presenile patients with DAT recalled significantly fewer letters in an array than did normal control subjects (Miller 1996).

By definitional criteria, persons with dementia of the Alzheimer type demonstrate significantly poorer performance on tasks of the Dementia Rating Scale (Mattis 1988), including visual memory subtests, than do normal controls. Further, in comparing patients with DAT and patients with severity-matched vascular dementia on the Dementia Rating Scale, Kertesz (1994) found patients with DAT scored significantly worse than vascular patients on memory subtests, including subtests of visual memory. Similarly, Massman, Butters, and Delis (1994) found that patients with DAT had significantly worse visual retention than did persons with Huntington disease, depressed persons, or normal controls. Also, it has been both clinically observed and empirically demonstrated that persons with DAT evidence impairment for visual memory of faces (Damasio 1999). In the same vein, Schneidman (1952) found persons with DAT had significant impairment in visual memory for pictures compared to persons with Huntington disease or normal controls.

However, data for visual memory in dementia of the Alzheimer type are variable. Salmon and Fennema-Notestine (1996) point out that investigations of perceptual priming in DAT fail to demonstrate significant impairment in comparisons with age-matched controls. Consistent with this, Fleischman et al. (1995) found preservation of perceptually based repetition priming in persons with DAT and concluded that perceptually based priming may be mediated by a putative visual memory mechanism in the right occipital cortex, a brain area not affected as early or severely in DAT as other brain regions.

Part of this variability in research results can be explained by the parameter of relative complexity of task demand in the differing studies; good dementia of the Alzheimer type performance is inversely correlated with task complexity (Emery 1988, 1999, 2000a; Emery and Breslau 1989). Also, DAT performance correlates inversely with severity of illness (Emery 1985, 1999) and severity of illness was not constant across investigations cited.

In sum, it must be kept in mind that one core clinical and defining characteristic of dementia of the Alzheimer type is impairment of visual memory for places; the patient with dementia of the Alzheimer type has a failure in visual memory and gets lost in both new and familiar surroundings (Emery 1985, 1988; American Psychiatric Association 1994).

Turning now to *vestibular senses* and balance, one-third to one-half of healthy older adults over 65 years of age fall each year; in persons with dementia of the Alzheimer type the occurrence of falls and hip fractures is three times higher than in healthy older people (Chong et al. 1999). In an investigation of sensory organization for balance, some specific deficits in vestibular senses were found in DAT but not in Parkinson disease or normal aging (Chong et al. 1999). Although persons with DAT appeared to have vestibular function in the normative range, they had decreased ability to suppress incongruent visual stimuli when trying to maintain balance. It would appear that the increased incidence of falls in DAT is in part a function of the inability to screen incongruent visual input (Chong et al. 1999).

Finally, there are consistent and robust data pertaining to impairment of *olfactory memory* in dementia of the Alzheimer type (Nordin and Murphy 1998; Solomon et al. 1998; Murphy 1999; Devanand et al. 2000). In establishing normative data for olfactory event-related potentials, Murphy and colleagues (2000) found olfactory processing speed decreased at a constant rate over decades for sensory, as well as for cognitive, components in normal aging; decline in amplitude over decades was also found. Nevertheless, decline in olfactory memory is significantly less in normal elderly persons than in persons with DAT (Nordin and Murphy 1998). Also, impairment of olfactory memory discriminates DAT from major depression, as well as from normal aging; olfactory assessment can be an adjunctive screening measure in differential diagnosis of DAT from old age depression (Solomon et al. 1998). It appears that persons with DAT evidence neuropathological changes in areas of brain central to olfactory processing, suggesting the potential diagnostic utility of olfactory function (Solomon et al. 1998; Murphy 1999). Early in the DAT disease course, degeneration occurs in the entorhinal-hippocampal-subicular complex, and neurons of the olfactory epithelium evidence numerous neurofibrillary tangles (Talamo et al. 1989; Devanand et al. 2000). There is evidence not only that impairment of olfactory memory is positively correlated with both age and severity of dementia, but also that impaired olfaction has been observed in first-degree relatives of persons with DAT (Devanand et al. 2000). On the basis of investigation of impaired olfactory memory in persons with mild cognitive deficits, Devanand and associates (2000) concluded that impaired olfactory memory can predict DAT at follow-up. It would appear that dysfunction in olfactory memory can have substantial clinical utility for early differential diagnosis of DAT (Nordin and Murphy 1998; Murphy 1999; Devanand et al. 2000).

Higher Cortical Short-term Memory: Stage 2 Memory (Selection, Recoding, Encoding)

We have said that the higher cortical memory tier of the three-tiered evolutionary framework of movement (motor) memory, emotional memory, and higher cortical memory consists of three processing levels: short-term memory, intermediate-term memory, and long-term memory, each processing level being comprised of two stages. We look now at stage 2 of higher cortical memory.

Stage 2 incorporates some definitional features described earlier in this chapter in discussions of primary memory (Schmidt 1978; Kaszniak, Poon, and Riege 1986), immediate memory (Cowan 1997), and working memory (Baddeley 1992). Stage 2 is defined by fundamental characteristics of limited capacity, short duration, and rapidly lost material. Stage 2 of the higher cortical memory tier is also defined by weaker synaptic potentiation in contrast to the tetanic potentiation and lasting synaptic structural changes that occur in long-term memory as part of neural plasticity (Schmidt 1978; Hochner and Kandel 1986; Gluck and Myers 1998; Escobar and Bermudez-Rattone 2000; Guyton 2000; Kandel 2000). In this regard, stage 2 memory takes on functional as opposed to structural dimensions.

In thinking about stages of memory, an analogy can be made whereby the raw material for memories passes through an assembly line for the formation of memories. The more stages the material passes through, the greater the degree of processing, the greater the synaptic changes, the greater and longer lasting the structural changes, and the longer material potentially can be remembered.

Thus far we have described how raw material from which memories can be formed entered the organism through the senses, passed through two phases of stage 1, and was processed next in stage 2, where sensory material undergoes selection and a more "cognitive" processing and recoding/encoding. Only a very small percentage of sensory stimuli bombarding a person gets selected out for further memory processing (Schmidt 1978; Kandel, Schwartz, and Jessell 2000). Such selection appears to take place in the memory processing continuum of stage 1/phase 2 and stage 2 memory. As material from which memories are formed passes through stage 1 memory into stage 2 memory, sensory information from unimodal areas of the cortex converges in multimodal association areas; sensory pathways dedicated exclusively to visual, auditory, somatic, and similar information converge in multimodal association areas in the prefrontal, parietotemporal, and limbic cortices (Kandel, Kupfermann, and Iversen 2000; Saper, Iversen, and Frackowiak 2000). Neurons in these multimodal areas appear to respond to combinations of signals representing different sensory modalities by constructing internal representations of sensory stimuli concerned with specific aspects of behavior (Saper, Iversen, and Frackowiak 2000). Further, recent research suggests the prefrontal association area is critical in progression of stage 1 sensory material into stage 2, where sensory material undergoes higher cortical "cognitive" processing and recoding; major functions of the prefrontal association areas are to weigh consequences for future actions, plan, and organize actions accordingly (Funchashi, Bruce, and Goldman-Rakic 1989; Kandel, Kupfermann, and Iversen 2000; Saper, Iversen, and Frackowiak 2000). As part of stage 2 memory, to select appropriate behavioral responses to stage 1 sensory signals, the frontal association areas appear to integrate sensory information from both the outside world and the body (Kandel 2000; Kandel, Kupfermann, and Iversen 2000; Saper, Iversen, and Frackowiak 2000). The cortex surrounding the principal sulcus appears to be involved in tasks and behavioral responses that require stage 2 memory functions of selection, interpretation, and cognitive recoding (Saper, Iversen, and Frackowiak 2000). Baddeley (1992) in delineating working memory and Cowan (1997) in discussions of immediate memory posited that only a subset of information can be in a state of heightened activation, whereby memory is integrated with attention and other executive processes. Recent data of cellular recordings from neurons in the prefrontal association area suggest these neurons are concerned with executive functions (see chap. 9) and short-term activated memory (Saper, Iversen, and Frackowiak 2000).

Stage 2 Memory in Dementia of the Alzheimer Type

Discussion related to basic variables of stage 2 memory in dementia of the Alzheimer type can be found in earlier sections of this chapter on short-term memory and primary memory.

In investigations of short-term memory in dementia of the Alzheimer type, stage 2 is typically indicated by measures of digit span forward, block span, word span, or immediate verbal free recall.

In comparisons with normal elderly persons, robust data show persons with dementia of the Alzheimer type evidence significant decrement in stage 2 memory; the degree of decrement is associated with the degree of cerebral dysfunction and impairment in activities of daily living (Corkin 1982, 1998; Emery 1985, 1996, 1999; Greene, Prepscius, and Levy 2000; Siefert 2000). Dementia of the Alzheimer type decrement in stage 2 memory includes greater encoding deficits, greater reduction in memory span, accelerated loss of material, and greater incapacity to perform with divided attention (Corkin 1982; Emery 1985, 1993, 1996; Morris 1986, 1996; Siefert 2000).

Although data evidence significant decrement in stage 2 memory in dementia of the Alzheimer type, the question remains as to how persons with dementia of the Alzheimer type perform stage 2 memory tasks relative to their own performance at other stages of memory. In other words, we know persons with DAT are significantly impaired compared to normal elderly persons on all stage 2 measures of memory, but what is the pattern of DAT deficits relative to themselves? In addressing this question, data indicate persons with DAT do significantly better on stage 2 memory tasks (i.e., digit span forward) than on tasks at subsequent stages (Emery 1988, 1998, 1999). This will be discussed further in following sections.

Higher Cortical Intermediate-term Memory: Stage 3 Memory (New Learning) and Stage 4 Memory (Delayed New Learning)

Generally, throughout the literature on memory, forms of memory not classified as short-term memory are categorized as long-term memory (e.g., Neath 1998). For example, the form of memory termed *secondary memory* (new learning and delayed new learning) and the form of memory termed *tertiary memory* (overlearned material) are both considered long-term memory (e.g., Kaszniak, Poon, and Riege 1986). As part of the reconceptualization of memory presented in this chapter, the term *intermediate-term memory* will be coined. The idea that new learning, such as DAX is paired with FRIGID (Tulving 1972), is categorized as being the same as knowing one's own name or date of birth strikes me as lacking in proportionality. There has already been discussion earlier in this chapter regarding the facts that synapses change according to previous experience and, thus, formation of memories creates synaptic change; therefore, memory can be viewed as a specific form of neural plasticity (Hochner and Kandel 1986; Squire 1987; Black and Greenough 1998; Gluck and Myers 1998; Almkvist 2000). Further, we have said previously that a difference between short-term memory and long-term memory lies in synaptic potentiation or tetanic potentiation; repeated use of a synapse can result in synaptic potentiation. This phenomenon often appears during repeated (tetanic) stimulation of a synapse and is thus called tetanic potentiation (Schmidt 1978; Guyton 1981, 2000). Putting these facts together into a deductive paradigm leads to the conclusion that new learning by definition involves less repetitive action in the organism than old or overlearned learning, and therefore involves less synaptic or tetanic potentiation and less synaptic structural change. Accordingly, the concept of *intermediate-term memory* is being introduced here to conceptually take into account the continuum of repetitive action on synapses and synaptic potentiation and resulting structural changes.

Using the same logic, along with consistent data-driven observations that brand-new learning and delayed new learning are not exactly one and the same (Emery 1985, 1988, 1992, 1993, 1999; Emery, Gillie, and Smith 1996, 2000), we introduce here the higher cortical intermediate-term memory stages of stage 3 memory (new learning) and stage 4 memory (delayed new learning). These will be discussed further in the next section on new learning and delayed new learning in DAT.

Stage 3 Memory and Stage 4 Memory in Dementia of the Alzheimer Type

Data regarding fundamental features of stage 3 memory and stage 4 memory in dementia of the Alzheimer type have been analyzed in earlier sections on secondary memory and episodic memory in dementia of the Alzheimer type. Both the constructs of secondary memory and episodic memory combine new learning and delayed new learning into a single entity, indicated by tasks such as recall of word lists and verbal and nonverbal paired associate learning, and do not distinguish between tasks such as story recall and delayed story recall (see discussions in earlier sections). Nonetheless, despite combining, and therefore in my view confounding, memory at stage 3 and stage 4, investigations using constructs of secondary memory and episodic memory result in consistent and robust findings of significant impairments in DAT in encoding, storage, retrieval, and overall memory efficiency (e.g., Corkin 1982; Wilson and Kaszniak 1986; Saykin et al. 1999a, b, 2000). Data indicate that in DAT, capacity for recognition or recall of new learning and delayed new learning of nonpersonal material, such as word lists and the like, is profoundly impaired; this impairment of encoding new learning and remembering delayed new learning is so significant it constitutes a preclinical marker for DAT (Small et al. 1994; Almkvist and Winblad 1999).

But what, then, is the case for distinguishing between new learning (stage 3) and delayed new learning (stage 4)? We turn now to the few investigations that separated new learning (stage 3) and delayed new learning (stage 4), and demonstrate why, despite solid data described above, there appears to be a need for secondary memory to be divided into several stages.

In the process of investigating significant differences between dementia of the Alzheimer type and depressive dementia, persons with dementia of the Alzheimer type did significantly worse on measures of delayed new learning compared to nondelayed new learning (Emery 1988). For example, the twenty patients with DAT of the study as a group averaged 15% correct answers on a new learning paired associates task, but only 2% correct answers on delayed new learning, resulting in a 0.0001 significant difference. This study found that of eight memory tasks, relative to themselves, DAT performance was worst at stage 4/delayed new learning (2%) and next most impaired at stage 3/new learning

(15%); performance was most preserved at short-term stage 2/digits forward with 57% correct answers (Emery 1988). In another investigation comparing twenty-three patients with DAT with twenty patients with major depression/unipolar and twenty normal elderly persons, research results showed mean performance on story recall (stage 3) and delayed story recall (stage 4) was significantly different for all three groups (Emery 1992). On the statistical measure of mean percentage correct answers for within-sample comparisons (Emery 1988, 1992), the mild DAT subgroup of this study got 12% correct answers on delayed story recall (stage 4) and 26% correct answers on story recall (stage 3), resulting in a 0.0001 significant difference; mild DAT best performance was on digits forward (stage 2) with 75% correct answers (Emery 1992). Finally, in a comparison of three different patient populations, data again evidenced significant difference in DAT performance at stage 3 and stage 4 (Emery 1999). In sum, data from these investigations suggest that information for understanding basic nature and patterns of memory is lost when new learning and delayed new learning are combined without distinction into a single entity.

Higher Cortical Long-term Memory: Stage 5 Memory (Old Learning/Knowledge, Semantic Memory)

This is yet another stage of memory that is subsumed without distinction as part of secondary memory (e.g., Kaszniak, Poon, and Riege 1986), which, for reasons given in previous sections of this chapter, should constitute a separate memory stage. In contrast, the episodic-semantic memory framework has at its core the distinction between old learning/factual knowledge (semantic memory) and new learning (episodic memory) (Tulving 1972; Neath 1998), but fails to integrate these two isolated categories into a broader framework of memory. Hopefully, the heuristic model being developed in this chapter can at least point the way for an integration of these various important components of differing memory frameworks.

Basic features of stage 5 memory have been delineated previously in sections on semantic memory. Stage 5 memory refers to old learning that has become part of a person's culturally shared knowledge base. Stages 3, 4, and 5 reflect increases in synaptic or tetanic potentiation (Schmidt 1978; Guyton 1981, 2000). Something just learned differs from something known for an hour, which in turn differs from something known for years and years; these differences in memory reflect quantitative differences in repeated synaptic use and resulting qualitative structural changes underlying long-term memory, which in turn appear to correspond to degree of consolidation of memories (Schmidt 1978; Guyton 1981, 2000; Hochner and Kandel 1986; Black and Greenough 1998; Gluck and Myers 1998). Stage 5 memory (old learning, knowledge) is marked by a degree of consolidation of memories that does not characterize memory at stage 3 or stage 4.

Hippocampal function is at the core of the evolutionary tier of higher cortical memory and plays a crucial, integrative role in learning and memory at stages 3, 4, and 5 (Alvarez and Squire 1994; McClelland, McNaughton, and O'Reilly 1994; Gluck and Myers 1998). In describing memory consolidation, several models propose that (1) a stimulus enters the neocortex via the sensory system and activates cells in the hippocampus; (2) the hippocampus in turn feeds back to the neocortex, initiates activation patterns, and activates new cell populations that are added to the existing representation or allow connections to form between active cells in the neocortex; (3) the hippocampus represents memories to the neocortex repeatedly, over time, to allow the neocortex to integrate new knowledge without overwriting the old (McClelland, McNaughton, and O'Reilly 1994; Gluck and Myers 1998). There appears to be an inverse relation between memory age and hippocampal independence with concomitant susceptibility to disruption; this inverse relation is known as the Ribot gradient of retrograde amnesia (Ribot 1882; Alvarez and Squire 1994; Gluck and Myers 1998). Accordingly, the probability for memories to be disrupted is greater at stage 3 and stage 4 than at stage 5, where old learning/knowledge has attained greater or increased consolidation with passage of time (i.e., greater memory age).

In sum, material described above would seem to constitute a valid reason to make a separate stage of old learning/knowledge (stage 5) rather than continue to include it with no differentiation as part of the more global category of secondary memory. Further, the extensive theoretical and empirical material presented by Tulving (1972, 1983, 1985; Tulving et al. 1994; Schacter and Tulving 1994) as he makes the case for differentiation of old learning/knowledge (semantic memory) from other memory categories adds cogency to the conclusion of this chapter that old learning/knowledge constitutes a memory category of its own.

Stage 5 Memory in Dementia of the Alzheimer Type

We have seen that dementia of the Alzheimer type involves consistent and profound deficits at stage 3/new learning and stage 4/delayed new learning (Backman and Herlitz 1996; Celsis 2000). But what is the degree of decrement at stage 5? In other words, how much of their long-standing total stock of culturally shared knowledge do persons with DAT lose because of the process of Alzheimer-type dementia?

Numerous studies have been discussed previously in this chapter as they pertain to old learning/knowledge in dementia of the Alzheimer type (see the sections on semantic memory and declarative memory in dementia of the Alzheimer type). For example, stage 5 memory in DAT involves prominent deficits in naming (e.g., Collette et al. 1999), with generative naming significantly more impaired, and impaired earlier in the disease course, than confrontation naming, because of greater task complexity (Bayles and Kaszniak 1987; Emery and Breslau 1988, 1989; Emery 1999, 2000a). Good performance on the part of persons with DAT is positively correlated with low task demand and complexity (Emery 1985, 1993, 1999, 2000a). There are also serious deficits in stage 5 memory in DAT on tasks of complex syntax without extrasyntactic cues (see section on semantic memory/syntactic knowledge in DAT). Data suggest syntactic knowledge is a higher cortical function with bilateral representation; syntactic knowledge is dependent on the integrity of both hemispheres and becomes impaired early in the DAT disease course (DeVreese et al. 1996).

The process of Alzheimer dementing appears to involve progressive dissociation between mechanistic speech sound without reference to sound (phonology) and meaning (semantic knowledge) such that the person with dementia of the Alzheimer type increasingly uses words and speech separated from or divested of normative denotation and connotation (Emery 1985, 1993, 2000a). Vygotsky (1962) made the original observation that meaning and sound represent two separate lines of development until around age 2, after which the two developmental lines intersect and become merged. The material presented in this chapter suggests DAT is a disease process in which the two merged lines of meaning and sound once again are separated. Once it is realized that DAT involves a process of dissociation of culturally shared knowledge/meaning from sound, various symptoms fall into place; the vague, stereotyped, imprecise use of language with circumlocutory phrases that are part of diagnostic criteria (American Psychiatric Association 1994) can be better understood by both physician and family. The language tasks persons with DAT do best all require a minimal integration of culturally shared knowledge/meaning with sound (e.g., repetition, clichés, rote speech, stereotypes, overlearned phrases, preprogrammed chunks, etc.) (Emery 1982, 1985, 1988, 1993, 2000a; Kempler 1991).

Consistent with this, stage 5 memory in dementia of the Alzheimer type also involves decrement in idea density, with deficits in idea density already in evidence early in life (Snowdon 2001). Finally, stage 5 in DAT evidences significant deficits in calculation (Emery 1985, 1988, 1993).

There has been extensive reference to the fact that higher cortical memory stage 3, stage 4, and stage 5 are heavily subserved by the hippocampus and associated neural networks for processes of encoding, consolidation, and retrieval (see previous sections for discussion). Neural science data suggest that old learning and knowledge of stage 5 memory are stored in a distributed fashion; there does not appear to be a general semantic memory store (e.g., Kandel, Kuperfermann, and Iversen 2000). Rather, each time knowledge is recalled, it appears the recall is built up from distinct bits of information, each of which is stored in a specialized (dedicated) memory store (e.g., Kandel, Kuperfermann, and Iversen 2000). In consequence, a diffuse progressive disorder such as DAT would result in increasing fragmentation of knowledge.

Higher Cortical Long-term Memory: Stage 6 Memory (Overlearned Knowledge)

We discuss now the final stage of the higher cortical memory tier of the three-tiered overarching memory framework. Stage 6 refers to often rehearsed, highly overlearned factual material of both a nonpersonal nature (e.g., days of week, alphabet) and a personal nature (e.g., name, place of birth, birth date); stage 6 factual knowledge comprises the major content of mental status questionnaires (e.g., Folstein, Folstein, and McHugh 1975). Stage 6 incorporates the construct of tertiary memory (Schmidt 1978; Kaszniak, Poon, and Riege 1986; Emery 1988, 1992, 1999, 2000b). The material of tertiary memory (stage 6) has sometimes been referred to as remote memory, but this gives us only part of the picture. Stage 6 overlearned knowledge can be nonpersonal from the remote past (e.g., numbers, months of year) or nonpersonal from the present (e.g., president); and highly overlearned knowledge can be personal from the remote past (e.g., schools attended, mother's birth name) or personal from recent times (e.g., present age) (Emery 1992).

We discussed in the previous section how the process of consolidation involves repetitive synaptic action, synaptic potentiation, and tetanic/post-tetanic potentiation; memory age is positively correlated with consolidation and negatively correlated with susceptibility for hippocampal disruption (Schmidt 1978; Alvarez and Squire 1994; McClelland, McNaughton, and O'Reilly 1994; Gluck and Myers 1998). The hippocampus and associated networks are critical for encoding of new learning and repetitive synaptic action of consolidation as new learning becomes old learning (that is, material goes from stage 3 to stage 5). But neural science data suggest that over time, with great increases in consolidation, sensory input is able to activate memory cells directly, without the hippocampus playing a central role (Alvarez and Squire 1994; McClelland, McNaughton, and O'Reilly 1994; Gluck and Myers 1998). Putting these data together into a deductive paradigm leads to the conclusion that stage 6 memories are the most consolidated, the least dependent on the hippocampus, and therefore, the least vulnerable to disruption when compared to higher cortical memory at stage 3 (new learning), stage 4 (delayed new learning), and stage 5 (old learning/knowledge).

In the discussion of emotional memory in a previous section of this chapter, I postulated that autobiographical memory developed phylogenetically from the evolutionary tier of emotional memory, and that autobiographical memory is represented in the neural convergence zone of emotional memory and neocortical memory stage 6. Autobiographical memory is defined as the recording in memory of the collection of facts, events, experiences, patterns of internal and external responses, patterns of cognition, conation, affect, and behavior that are part of the lifelong ontogenetically emergent bioelectrochemical complex and continuity experienced as a self. Lesion data suggest the critical variables of autobiography that need to be recorded in memory with near permanency are those related to identity; these critical elements of identity arise from a continuously reactivated network based on convergence zones that are located in the temporal and frontal higher-order cortices, as well as in the subcortical nuclei such as those in the amygdala (Damasio 1994). A consistent finding is that the amygdala plays a crucial role in emotional memory (Damasio 1994, 1999; Hyman 1998; Phelps et al. 1998; Akirav and Richter-Levin 1999; Canli et al. 1999; Mori et al. 1999; Mory et al. 1999; Iversen, Kupfermann, and Kandel 2000). Accordingly, autobiographical memory as an evolutionary development of emotional memory, in its intersection with neocortical stage 6, would be subserved at a convergence zone of the amygdala and the hippocampus and associated neural networks. The overlearned personal factual knowledge of the hippocampally subserved neocortical memory tier stage 6 (name, birth date, place of birth) intersects or converges with the amygdalar subserved emotional memory developmental line of autobiographical memory. I suggest that it is at this convergence zone that lifelong emotional memory converges with overlearned factual personal knowledge to form autobiography. Further, as I stated previously, preliminary data from a life themes study I am conducting indicate that autobiographical memory may undergo dual-coding (Paivio 1986), such that memorable autobiographical events are stored in both visual code (pictures) and verbal code (words).

Finally, trauma psychology (Emery, Emery, and Berry 1993) teaches us that a trauma need happen only once to be remembered (Terr 1983; American Psychiatric Association 1994), and does not appear to require for consolidation the repeated synaptic stimulation and tetanic potentiation across time that neocortical memories require (Schmidt 1978; Gluck and Myers 1998). Diagrammatically, it is as if one severe trauma in the emotional memory tier will go straight to the equivalent of neocortical stage 6 factual knowledge, which in contrast appears to have gone through six stages to attain the degree of processing, consolidation, and memorability of one trauma. Finally, as discussed in earlier sections, it does not appear that learning word lists, a common indicator for episodic memory, is valid representation of emotional/autobiographical memory, but rather represents the new learning of neocortical stage 3 memory (see the sections on episodic memory and neocortical memory stage 3).

Stage 6 Memory in Dementia of the Alzheimer Type

Stage 6 overlearned factual knowledge constitutes a solid core in mental status examinations and dementia screening instruments (e.g., Folstein, Folstein, and McHugh 1975). Thus, as part of the structure and standardization of dementia scaling, persons with DAT do significantly worse than demographically equivalent normal subjects on stage 6 overlearned material.

But how do persons with dementia of the Alzheimer type do on overlearned, highly rehearsed personal and nonpersonal factual material compared to their performance on other memory stages? What is the pattern of memory deficits in DAT? Addressing this question and using the measure of mean percentage correct answers for within-sample comparisons, an investigation found that patients with DAT got 29% correct answers on stage 6 overlearned factual knowledge (e.g., information, orientation, mental control); this compared with 2% correct answers on delayed new learning (stage 4), 15% correct answers on new learning (stage 3), and 57% correct answers on short-term memory/digits forward (stage 2) (Emery 1988, 1998, 1999). Thus, the DAT pattern of memory deficits is such that patients with DAT did neither their best nor their worst on stage 6 overlearned knowledge. This was in sharp contrast to the pattern of deficits evidenced by normal elderly persons and persons with major depression/unipolar, who did best on stage 6 overlearned factual material with 98%

and 81% correct answers, respectively (Emery 1999). Finally, in the difficult task of differential diagnosis between depressive dementia (see chaps. 14–17) and DAT, stage 6 overlearned factual material was the single most discriminating or best differential diagnostic tool; whereas the two populations had very similar memory patterns, they did differ significantly on overlearned knowledge; the person with DAT cannot tell you how many days there are in a week or months in a year (Emery 1988, 1998, 1999).

Summary

This chapter has provided theoretical, empirical, and clinical discussion about memory. It has been suggested that the key problem with memory frameworks currently in use is that they lack an evolutionary dimension and, in consequence, fail to reflect the phylogenetic reality that memory is an evolved organ of adaptation. The point of view developed in this chapter is that memory is a phylogenetically evolved structural and functional set of systems working in concert to enable organismic survival. As part of this chapter, a three-tiered evolutionary memory framework was introduced, consisting of three phylogenetically based tiers of motor (movement) memory, emotional memory, and higher cortical (neocortical) memory. The new memory framework reconceptualizes memory constructs currently in use, along with introducing new parameters. New terms introduced include *retrophylogenesis* and *retroontogenesis*. Theory and data are presented suggesting the disease process of DAT involves retrophylogenesis: memory structures last to evolve in phylogenesis appear to deteriorate first. Whereas the term *retrophylogenesis* has as its context species evolutionary history across millennia, *retroontogenesis* has as its context life-span ontogenetic development. Within the neocortical tier of the three-tiered evolutionary framework, the term *retroontogenesis* suggests hierarchic deterioration of neocortical memory in DAT because there is evidence for a negative relation between sequence in ontogenetic development and sequence of deterioration (Emery 1982, 1985, 1992, 1996, 1998, 1999, 2000a,b; Reisberg 1988, 1999; Reisberg, Auer et al. 1996; Reisberg, Franssen et al. 2001). This new framework involves theory construction heavily buttressed by deductive and inductive paradigms in addition to empirical and clinical data on memory in DAT, which are at the core of the framework. This synthesis is presented as a heuristic model with the hope that it will break through old paradigms, generate new perspectives on memory, and stimulate new constructs and hypotheses for empirical work.

Clinical Conclusions

The material in this chapter enables new clinical understandings of dementia of the Alzheimer type disease progression across time. The material developed adds both phylogenetic and ontogenetic dimensions to clinical understanding and enables increased prediction about what to expect in clinical aspects of DAT deterioration. The clinician will come to understand that the process of Alzheimer dementing involves both *retrophylogenesis* and *retroontogenesis*. For example, data are presented that demonstrate that even while the person with DAT can no longer remember the facts of an emotional event, the emotions remain; this is an example of retrophylogenesis whereby neocortical memory is lost but emotional memory remains. Relative to themselves and to other populations, the memory deficit of DAT appears greatest on tasks of neocortical memory, as compared to subcortical memory tasks or tasks of emotional remembrance. Both clinicians and family members will be aided in understanding the person with DAT as they come to realize that DAT is a disease process akin to desocialization involving retrophylogenesis and retroontogenesis. In illustration, language is a system of rule-governed or socialized behavior. The progressive incapacity of the person with DAT to code and decode within normative range is akin to desocialization (Emery 1985, 2000a). The material of the chapter shows DAT to be a disease process that destroys progressively capacity for participation in rule-governed or socialized behavior. Further, data are presented that suggest DAT is a disease process in which the two lines of sound and meaning/knowledge, which became merged at around age 2 (Vygotsky 1962), are becoming progressively separated, such that sound is made without it being integrated with normative meaning. It is clinically useful to understand that DAT involves progressive separation of meaning from sound because various symptoms of DAT can then be better understood: the vague, stereotyped, imprecise use of language with circumlocutory phrases now has a context. It can be clinically helpful to know that language tasks persons with DAT do best all require the most minimal integration of thought or meaning with sound, such as repetition, rote speech, clichés, overlearned phrases, and so forth. In sum, it is clinically useful to gain the perspective of this chapter that

DAT involves fundamental dedifferentiation in the context of the evolved memory capacities of humans.

REFERENCES

Akirav, I., and G. Richter-Levin. 1999. Biphasic modulation of hippocampal plasticity by behavioral stress and basolateral amygdala stimulation in the rat. *Journal of Neuroscience* 19:10530–35.

Albert, M.L., R.G. Feldman, and A.L. Willis. 1974. The "subcortical dementia" of progressive supranuclear palsy. *Journal of Neurology, Neurosurgery and Psychiatry* 37: 121–30.

Almkvist, O. 2000. Functional brain imaging as a looking-glass into the degraded brain: Reviewing evidence from Alzheimer disease in relation to normal aging. *Acta Psychologica* 105:255–77.

Almkvist, O., and B. Winblad. 1999. Early diagnosis of Alzheimer dementia based on clinical and biological factors. *European Archives of Psychiatry and Clinical Neuroscience* 249:3–9.

Alvarez, P., and L. Squire. 1994. Memory consolidation and the medial temporal lobe: A simple network model. *Annals of the New York Academy of Sciences* 91:7041–45.

American Psychiatric Association. 1994. *Diagnostic and Statistical Manual of Mental Disorders.* 4th ed. Washington, D.C.: American Psychiatric Association.

Backman, L., and A. Herlitz. 1996. Knowledge and memory in Alzheimer-type dementia: A relationship that exists. In *The Cognitive Neuropsychology of Alzheimer-type Dementia*, edited by R.G. Morris. Oxford: Oxford University Press, pp. 89–105.

Baddeley, A.D. 1992. Working memory. *Science* 255:556–69.

Bandler, R., and M.T. Shipley. 1994. Columnar organization in the midbrain periaqueductal gray: Modules for emotional expression? *Trends in Neuroscience* 17:379–89.

Barbas, H. 2000. Connections underlying the synthesis of cognition, memory, and emotion in primate prefrontal cortices. *Brain Research Bulletin* 52:319–30.

Barnes, C.A. 1998. Memory changes during normal aging: Neurobiological correlates. In *Neurobiology of Learning and Memory*, edited by J. Martinez and R. Kesner. San Diego: Academic Press, pp. 247–87.

Bayles, K.A., and A.W. Kaszniak. 1987. *Communication and Cognition in Normal Aging and Dementia.* Boston: College Hill Press.

Black, J.E., and W.T. Greenough. 1998. Developmental approaches to the memory process. In *Neurobiology of Learning and Memory*, edited by J. Martinez and R. Kesner. San Diego: Academic Press, pp. 55–88.

Blennow, K., A. Wallin, and C.G. Gottfries. 1994. Clinical subgroups of Alzheimer disease. In *Dementia: Presentations, Differential Diagnosis, and Nosology*, edited by V.O.B. Emery and T.E. Oxman. Baltimore: Johns Hopkins University Press, pp. 95–107.

Bloomfield, L. 1933. *Language.* New York: Henry Holt.

Broadbent, D.E. 1984. The Maltese Cross: A new simplistic model for memory. *Behavioral and Brain Sciences* 7:55–94.

Burns, A., R. Jacoby, and R. Levy. 1991. Neurological signs in Alzheimer's disease. *Age and Aging* 20:45–51.

Byrne, E.J. 1997. Overview of differential diagnosis. *International Psychogeriatrics* 9:39–50.

Campbell, D.T., and D.W. Fiske. 1959. Convergent and discriminant validation by the multitrait-multimethod matrix. *Psychological Bulletin* 56:81–105.

Canli, T., Z. Zhao, J.E. Desmond, et al. 1999. fMRI identifies a network of structures correlated with retention of positive and negative emotional memory. *Psychobiology* 27:441–52.

Celsis, P. 2000. Age-related cognitive decline, mild cognitive impairment, or preclinical Alzheimer's disease? *Annals of Medicine* 32:6–14.

Chong, R.K., F.B. Horak, J. Frank, et al. 1999. Sensory organization for balance: Specific deficits in Alzheimer's but not in Parkinson's disease. *Journal of Gerontology* 54A: 122–28.

Cohen, N.J., and H. Eichenbaum. 1993. *Memory, Amnesia, and the Hippocampal System.* Cambridge, Mass.: MIT Press.

Collette, F., M. VanderLinden, S. Bechet, et al. 1999. Phonological loop and central executive functioning in Alzheimer's disease. *Neuropsychologia* 37:905–18.

Corkin, S. 1982. Some relationships between global amnesias and the memory impairments in Alzheimer's disease. In *Alzheimer's Disease: A Report of Progress in Research,* edited by S. Corkin, K.L. Davis, J.H. Growdon, et al. New York: Raven Press, pp. 149–64.

Corkin, S. 1998. Functional MRI for studying episodic memory in aging and Alzheimer's disease. *Geriatrics* 53:13–15.

Cowan, N. 1997. *Attention and Memory: An Integrated Framework.* New York: Oxford University Press.

Damasio, A.R. 1994. *Descartes' Error.* New York: Avon Books.

Damasio, A.R. 1999. *The Feeling of What Happens: Body and Emotion in the Making of Consciousness.* New York: Harcourt, Brace, and Company.

Darwin, C. 1955 [1859]. *The Origin of Species.* New York: Modern Library.

Darwin, C. 1955 [1871]. *The Descent of Man.* New York: Modern Library.

Darwin, C. 1872. *The Expression of the Emotions in Man and Animals.* London: Murray.

Devanand, D., K. Michaels-Marston, X. Liu, et al. 2000. Olfactory deficits in patients with mild cognitive impairment predict Alzheimer's disease at follow up. *American Journal of Psychiatry* 157:1399–1405.

DeVreese, L.P., M. Neri, G. Salvioli, et al. 1996. Bihemispheric language disorders in early-stage dementia of the Alzheimer type. *International Psychogeriatrics* 8:63–81.

Dobzhansky, T. 1964. *Heredity and the Nature of Man.* New York: Harcourt, Brace, and World.

Emery, P.E., V.O.B. Emery, and N. Berry. 1993. Trauma psychology: A psychoanalytic model and approach. *Journal of Social Behavior and Personality* 8:29–48.

Emery, V.O.B. 1982. *Linguistic Patterning in the Second Half of the Life Cycle.* Doctoral dissertation, University of Chicago.

Emery, V.O.B. 1985. Language and aging. *Experimental Aging Research* 11:3–62.

Emery, V.O.B. 1986. Linguistic decrement in normal aging. *Language and Communication* 6:47–62.

Emery, V.O.B. 1988. *Pseudodementia: A Theoretical and Empirical Discussion.* Cleveland: Case Western Reserve University School of Medicine.

Emery, V.O.B. 1992. Interaction of language and memory in major depression and senile dementia of Alzheimer's type. In *Memory Functioning in Dementia*, edited by L. Backman. Amsterdam: Elsevier, pp. 175–204.

Emery, V.O.B. 1993. Language and memory processing in senile dementia Alzheimer's type. In *Language, Memory, and Aging*, edited by L. Light and D. Burke. New York: Cambridge University Press, pp. 221–43.

Emery, V.O.B. 1996. Language functioning. In *The Cognitive Neuropsychology of Alzheimer-type Dementia*, edited by R.G. Morris. Oxford: Oxford University Press, pp. 166–93.

Emery, V.O.B. 1998. A stage model of memory decline in dementia of the Alzheimer type. *Neurobiology of Aging* 19:137.

Emery, V.O.B. 1999. On the relationship between memory and language in the dementia spectrum of depression, Alzheimer syndrome, and normal aging. In *Language and Communication in Old Age: Multidisciplinary Perspectives*, edited by H. Hamilton. New York: Garland Publishing, pp. 25–62.

Emery, V.O.B. 2000a. Language impairment in dementia of the Alzheimer type: A hierarchical decline? *International Journal of Psychiatry in Medicine* 30:145–64.

Emery, V.O.B. 2000b. Phases of memory decline in dementia of the Alzheimer type (DAT). *The Gerontologist* 40:217–18.

Emery, V.O.B., and L.D. Breslau. 1987. The acceleration process in Alzheimer's disease: Thought dissolution in Alzheimer's disease early onset and senile dementia Alzheimer's type. *American Journal of Alzheimer's Care* 2:24–32.

Emery, V.O.B., and L.D. Breslau. 1988. The problem of naming in SDAT: A relative deficit. *Experimental Aging Research* 14:181–93.

Emery, V.O.B., and L.D. Breslau. 1989. Language deficits in depression: Comparisons with SDAT and normal aging. *Journal of Gerontology* 44:85–92.

Emery, V.O.B., and T.E. Oxman. 1997. Depressive dementia: A 'transitional dementia'? *Clinical Neuroscience* 4:23–30.

Emery, V.O.B., E.X. Gillie, and P.T. Ramdev. 1995. Noninfarct vascular dementia. In *Treating Alzheimer's and Other Dementias*, edited by M. Bergener and S. Finkel. New York: Springer, pp. 184–203.

Emery, V.O.B., E.X. Gillie, and P.T. Ramdev. 1996. Noninfarct vascular dementia: A new subtype of dementing disorder. *Journal of Clinical Geropsychology* 2:197–213.

Emery, V.O.B., E.X. Gillie, and J.A. Smith. 1996. Reclassification of the vascular dementias: Comparisons of infarct and noninfarct vascular dementias. *International Psychogeriatrics* 8:33–61.

Emery, V.O.B., E.X. Gillie, and J.A. Smith. 2000. Interface between vascular dementia and Alzheimer syndrome: Nosologic redefinition. *Annals of the New York Academy of Sciences* 903:229–38.

Escobar, M.L., and F. Bermudez-Rattoni. 2000. Long-term potentiation in the insular cortex enhances conditioned taste aversion retention. *Brain Research* 852:208–12.

Eslinger, P.J., and A.R. Damasio. 1986. Preserved motor learning in Alzheimer's disease: Implications for anatomy and behavior. *Journal of Neuroscience* 6:3006–9.

Fleischman, D.A., J. Gabrieli, S. Reminger, et al. 1995. Conceptual priming in perceptual identification for patients with Alzheimer's disease and a patient with right occipital lobectomy. *Neuropsychology* 9:187–97.

Folstein, M.F., S. Folstein, and P.R. McHugh. 1975. "Mini-Mental State": A practical method for grading the mental state of patients for the clinician. *Journal of Psychiatry Research* 12:189–98.

Funchashi, S., C.J. Bruce, and P.S. Goldman-Rakic. 1989. Mnemonic coding of visual space in the monkey's dorsolateral prefrontal cortex. *Journal of Neurophysiology* 61: 331–49.

Gardner, E.P., and J.H. Martin. 2000. Coding of sensory information. In *Principles of Neural Science*, edited by E.R. Kandel, J. Schwartz, and T.M. Jessell. New York: McGraw-Hill, pp. 411–29.

Gardner, E.P., J.H. Martin, and T.M. Jessell. 2000. The bodily senses. In *Principles of Neural Science*, edited by E.R. Kandel, J. Schwartz, and T.M. Jessell. New York: McGraw-Hill, pp. 430–50.

Gluck, M.A., and Myers, C.E. 1998. Psychobiological models of hippocampal function in learning and memory. In *Neurobiology of Learning and Memory*, edited by J. Martinez and R. Kesner. San Diego: Academic Press, pp. 417–48.

Goodglass, H., and E. Kaplan. 1972. *The Assessment of Aphasia and Related Disorders*. Philadelphia: Lea and Febinger.

Graham, K.S., J. Simons, K. Pratt, et al. 2000. Insights from semantic dementia on the relationship between episodic and semantic memory. *Neuropsychologia* 38:313–24.

Greene, A.J., C. Prepscius, and W. Levy. 2000. Primacy versus recency in a quantitative model: Activity is the critical distinction. *Learning and Memory* 7:48–57.

Greene, J.D.W., and J.R. Hodges. 1996. Semantic processing. In *The Cognitive Neuropsychology of Alzheimer-type Dementia*, edited by R.G. Morris. Oxford: Oxford University Press, pp. 128–48.

Grossman, M., J. Mickanin, K. Onishi, et al. 1995. An aspect of sentence processing in Alzheimer's disease: Quantifier-noun disagreement. *Neurology* 45:85–91.

Grossman, M., M. D'Esposito, E. Hughes, et al. 1996. Language comprehension difficulty in Alzheimer's disease, vascular dementia, and fronto-temporal degeneration. *Neurology* 47:183–89.

Guyton, A.C. 1981. *Basic Human Physiology*. Philadelphia: W.B. Saunders.

Guyton, A.C. 2000. *Medical Physiology*. New York: Mosby.

Hamann, S.B., E.S. Monarch, and F. Goldstein. 2000. Memory enhancement for emotional stimuli is impaired in early Alzheimer's disease. *Neuropsychology* 14:82–92.

Hart, S. 1988. Language and dementia: A review. *Psychological Medicine* 18:99–112.

Hebb, D.O. 1945. Man's frontal lobes: A critical review. *Archives of Neurology and Pathology* 54:11–24.

Heindel, W., D. Salmon, and N. Butters. 1991. The biasing of weight judgements in Alzheimer's and Huntington's disease: A priming or programming phenomenon? *Journal of Clinical and Experimental Neuropsychology* 13:189–203.

Hochner, B., and E.R. Kandel. 1986. Action potential duration and the modulation of transmitter release from the sensory neurons of Aplasia in presynaptic facilitation and behavioral sensitization. *Proceedings of the National Academy of Sciences USA* 83: 8410–14.

Howe, M.L. 2000. *The Fate of Early Memories*. Washington, D.C.: American Psychological Association.

Huck, G., and A. Ojeda. 1987. *Syntax and Semantics*. San Diego: Academic Press.

Huff, J. 1993. The disorder of naming in Alzheimer's disease. In *Language, Memory and Aging*, edited by L. Light and D. Burke. New York: Cambridge University Press, pp. 209–21.

Hyman, S.E. 1998. A new image of fear and emotion. *Nature* 393:417–18.

Ikeda, M., E. Mori, N. Hirono, et al. 1998. Amnestic people with Alzheimer's disease who remembered the Kobe earthquake. *British Journal of Psychiatry* 172:425–28.

Irigaray, L. 1967. Approach psycholinguistique du langage des dements. *Neuropsychologia* 5:25–52.

Iversen, S., I. Kupfermann, and E.R. Kandel. 2000. Emotional states and feelings. In *Principles of Neural Science*, edited by E.R. Kandel, J. Schwartz, and T.M. Jessell. New York: McGraw-Hill, pp. 982–97.

James, W. 1890. *The Principles of Psychology*. New York: Henry Holt and Company.

Jessell, T.M., and J.R. Sanes. 2000. The generation and survival of nerve cells. In *Principles of Neural Science*, edited by E.R. Kandel, J. Schwartz, and T.M. Jessell. New York: McGraw-Hill, pp. 1041–62.

Johansson, B., K. Whitfield, N. Pedersen, et al. 1999. Origins of individual differences in episodic memory in the oldest-old: A population based study of identical and same-sex fraternal twins aged 80 and older. *Journal of Gerontology* 54B:P173–79.

Johnson, S.C., A.J. Saykin, L.C. Baxter, et al. 2000. The relationship between fMRI activation and cerebral atrophy: Comparison of normal aging and Alzheimer disease. *NeuroImage* 11:179–87.

Kandel, E.R. 2000. From nerve cells to cognition: The internal cellular representation required for perception and action. In *Principles of Neural Science*, edited by E.R. Kandel, J. Schwartz, and T.M. Jessell. New York: McGraw-Hill, pp. 381–403.

Kandel, E.R., I. Kupfermann, and S. Iversen. 2000. Learning and memory. In *Principles of Neural Science*, edited by E.R. Kandel, J. Schwartz, and T.M. Jessell. New York: McGraw-Hill, pp. 1227–45.

Kandel, E.R., J. Schwartz, and T.M. Jessell (Eds.). 2000. *Principles of Neural Science*. New York: McGraw-Hill.

Kandel, E.R., S. Schacher, V. Castellucci, et al. 1987. The long and short of memory in Aplysia: A molecular perspective. In *Fidia Research Foundation Neuroscience Award Lectures*. Padova: Liviana Press.

Kaplan, E., H. Goodglass, and S. Weintraub. 1983. *The Boston Naming Test*. Philadelphia: Lea and Febiger.

Karpel, M., W.J. Hoyer, and M. Toglia. 2001. Accuracy and qualities of real and suggested memories: Nonspecific age differences. *Journal of Gerontology* 56B:P103–10.

Kaszniak, A., L. Poon, and W. Riege. 1986. Assessing memory deficits: An information processing approach. In *Handbook for Clinical Memory Assessment of Older Adults*, edited by L. Poon. Washington, D.C.: American Psychological Association, pp. 168–89.

Kemper, S., E. LaBarge, R. Farraro, et al. 1993. On the preservation of syntax in Alzheimer's disease. *Archives of Neurology* 50:81–86.

Kempler, D. 1991. Language changes in dementia of the Alzheimer type. In *Dementia and Communication*, edited by R. Lubinski. Philadelphia: B.C. Decker, pp. 98–114.

Kertesz, A. 1982. *The Western Aphasia Battery*. New York: Grune and Stratton.

Kertesz, A. 1994. Language deterioration in dementia. In *Dementia: Presentations, Dif-*

ferential Diagnosis, and Nosology, edited by V.O.B. Emery and T.E. Oxman. Baltimore: Johns Hopkins University Press, pp. 108–22.

Kesner, R.P. 1998. Neurobiological views of memory. In *Neurobiology of Learning and Memory*, edited by J. Martinez and R.P. Kesner. San Diego: Academic Press, pp. 361–416.

Koff, E., D. Zaitchik, J. Montepare, et al. 1999. Emotion processing in the visual and auditory domains by patients with Alzheimer's disease. *Journal of the International Neuropsychological Society* 5:32–40.

Laming, P.R. 2000. Potassium signaling in the brain: Its role in behavior. *Neurochemistry International* 36:271–90.

Lanzavecchia, A., and F. Sallusto. 2000. From synapses to immunological memory: The role of sustained T cell stimulation. *Current Opinion in Immunology* 12:92–98.

Libon, D., B. Bogdanoff, B. Cloud, et al. 1998. Declarative and procedural learning, quantitative measures of the hippocampus, and subcortical white alterations in Alzheimer's disease and ischemia vascular dementia. *Journal of Clinical and Experimental Neuropsychology* 20:30–41.

Light, L., and D. Burke. 1993. Patterns of language and memory in old age. In *Language, Memory, and Aging*, edited by L. Light and D. Burke. New York: Cambridge University Press, pp. 244–71.

Londos, E., U. Passant, A. Brun, et al. 1999. Clinical Lewy body dementia—Alzheimer's disease with vascular components? *International Psychogeriatrics* 11:185–86.

Luria, A. 1973. *The Working Brain.* New York: Basic Books.

MacLean, P.D. 2001. *The Triune Brain in Evolution.* New York: Plenum Press.

Massman, P.J., N. Butters, and D. Delis. 1994. Some comparisons of verbal deficits in Alzheimer dementia, Huntington disease, and depression. In *Dementia: Presentations, Differential Diagnosis, and Nosology*, edited by V.O.B. Emery and T.E. Oxman. Baltimore: Johns Hopkins University Press, pp. 232–48.

Mattis, S. 1988. *Dementia Rating Scale Professional Manual.* Odessa, Fla.: Psychological Assessment Resources.

McClelland, J., B. McNaughton, and R. O'Reilly. 1994. *Why We Have Complementary Learning Systems in the Hippocampus and Neocortex.* Pittsburgh: Carnegie Mellon University.

McHugh, P.R., and M. Folstein. 1975. Psychiatric syndromes of Huntington's chorea: A clinical and phenomenologic study. In *Psychiatric Aspects of Neurologic Disease*, edited by D. F. Benson and D. Blumer. New York: Grune and Stratton, pp. 267–86.

McKhann, G., D. Drachman, M. Folstein, et al. 1984. Clinical diagnosis of Alzheimer's disease. *Neurology* 34:939–44.

Mead, G.H. 1964. *On Social Psychology.* Chicago: University of Chicago Press.

Miller, E. 1996. The assessment of dementia. In *The Cognitive Neuropsychology of Alzheimer-type Dementia*, edited by R. G. Morris. Oxford: Oxford University Press, pp. 291–309.

Mishkin, M., B. Malamut, and J. Bachevalier. 1984. Memories and habits: Two neural systems. In *Neurobiology of Learning and Memory*, edited by G. Lynch, J. McGaugh, and N. Weinberger. New York: Guilford Press, pp. 65–77.

Mishkin, M., B. Siegler, R. Saunders, et al. 1982. An animal model of global amnesia. *Alzheimer's Disease: A Report in Progress* 19:235–47.

Mori, E., M. Ikeda, N. Hirono, et al. 1999. Amygdalar volume and emotional memory in Alzheimer's disease. *American Journal of Psychiatry* 156:216–22.

Morris, R.G. 1986. Short-term forgetting in senile dementia of the Alzheimer's type. *Cognitive Neuropsychology* 3:77–97.

Morris, R.G. 1996. Attentional and executive dysfunction. In *The Cognitive Neuropsychology of Alzheimer-type Dementia*, edited by R.G. Morris. Oxford: Oxford University Press, pp. 49–70.

Mory, S., B. Berdel, H. Jagalska-Majewska, et al. 1999. The basolateral amygdaloid complex: Its development, morphology, and functions. *Folia Morphologica* 58:29–46.

Moss, M.B., M.S. Albert, N. Butters, et al. 1986. Differential patterns of memory loss among patients with Alzheimer's disease, Huntington's disease, and alcoholic Korsakoff's syndrome. *Archives of Neurology* 43:239–46.

Murphy, C. 1999. Loss of olfactory function in dementing disease. *Physiology and Behavior* 66:177–82.

Murphy, C., C. Morgan, M. Geisler, et al. 2000. Olfactory event-related potentials and aging: Normative data. *International Journal of Psychophysiology* 36:133–45.

Nauta, W., and M. Feirtag. 1979. The organization of the brain. In *The Brain*, edited by Scientific American. San Francisco: W.H. Freeman, pp. 40–53.

Neath, I. 1998. *Human Memory: An Introduction to Research, Data, and Theory*. Pacific Grove, Calif.: Brooks/Cole Publishing.

Nordin, S., and C. Murphy. 1998. Odor memory in normal aging and Alzheimer's disease. *Annals of the New York Academy of Sciences* 855:686–93.

Nunnally, J. 1978. *Psychometric Theory*. New York: McGraw-Hill.

Paivio, A. 1986. *Mental Representation: A Dual-Coding Approach*. Oxford: Oxford University Press.

Parkin, A. 1997. *Memory and Amnesia*. Oxford: Basil Blackwell.

Paul Janssen Medical Institute. 1997. *Postgraduate Dementia Course: Heterogeneity of Alzheimer's Disease*. Amsterdam: Reed Elsevier.

Perani, D., S. Bressi, S. Cappa, et al. 1993. Evidence of multiple memory systems in the human brain. *Brain* 116:903–19.

Phelps, E., K. LaBar, A. Anderson, et al. 1998. Specifying the contributions of the human amygdala to emotional memory: A case study. *Neurocase: Case Studies in Neuropsychology, Neuropsychiatry, and Behavioral Neurology* 4:527–40.

Piaget, J. 1952. *The Origins of Intelligence in Children*. New York: International Universities Press.

Post, R., S. Weiss, H. Li, et al. 1998. Neural plasticity and emotional memory. *Development and Psychopathology* 10:829–55.

Quillian, M.R. 1966. *Semantic Memory*. Doctoral dissertation, Carnegie Institute of Technology, Pittsburgh, Pa.

Reiff, R., and M. Scheerer. 1959. *Memory and Hypnotic Age Regression*. New York: International Universities Press.

Reisberg, B. 1988. Functional Assessment Staging (FAST). *Psychopharmacology Bulletin* 24:653–59.

Reisberg, B., S.R. Auer, I. Monteiro, et al. 1996. Behavioral disturbances of dementia: An overview of phenomenology and methodologic concerns. *International Psychogeriatrics* 8:169–82.

Reisberg, B. 1999. Towards a science of Alzheimer's disease management: A model based upon current knowledge of retrogenesis. *International Psychogeriatrics* 11:9–10.
Reisberg, B., A. Burns, H. Brodaty, et al. 1997. Diagnosis of Alzheimer's disease. *International Psychogeriatrics* 9:11–38.
Reisberg, B., E.H. Franssen, L. Souren, et al. 2001. Overview of severe dementia. *International Psychogeriatrics* 13 (Supp.2):S 78.
Ribot, T. 1882. *The Diseases of Memory.* New York: Appleton.
Rochon, E., G. Waters, and D. Caplan. 1994. Sentence comprehension in patients with Alzheimer's disease. *Brain and Language* 46:329–49.
Salmon, D., and C. Fennema-Notestine. 1996. Implicit memory. In *The Cognitive Neuropsychology of Alzheimer-type Dementia,* edited by R.G. Morris. Oxford: Oxford University Press, pp. 105–27.
Saper, C. 2000. Brain stem, reflexive behavior, and the cranial nerves. In *Principles of Neural Science,* edited by E.R. Kandel, J. Schwartz, and T.M. Jessell. New York: McGraw-Hill, pp. 873–908.
Saper, C., S. Iversen, and R. Frackowiak, 2000. Integration of sensory and motor function: The association areas of the cerebral cortex and the cognitive capabilities of the brain. In *Principles of Neural Science,* edited by E.R. Kandel, J. Schwartz, and T.M. Jessell. New York: McGraw-Hill, pp. 349–80.
Saykin, A., L. Flashman, S. Frutiger, et al. 1999a. Neuroanatomic substrates of semantic memory impairment in Alzheimer's disease: Patterns of functional MRI activation. *Journal of the International Neuropsychological Society* 5:377–92.
Saykin, A., S. Johnson, L. Flashman, et al. 1999b. Functional differentiation of medial temporal and frontal regions involved in processing novel and familiar words: An fMRI study. *Brain* 122:1963–71.
Saykin, A., L. Flashman, S. Johnson, et al. 2000. Frontal and hippocampal memory circuitry in early Alzheimer's disease: Relation of structural and function MRI changes. *NeuroImage* 11 (Suppl. 5):S123.
Schacter, D., and E. Tulving. 1994. *Memory Systems 1994.* Cambridge, Mass.: MIT Press.
Schmidt, R.F. 1978. Synaptic transmission. In *Fundamentals of Neurophysiology,* edited by R.F. Schmidt. New York: Springer-Verlag, pp. 72–105.
Schneidman, E. 1952. *Make a Picture Story Test.* New York: The Psychological Corporation.
Siefert, L. 2000. Customized art activities for individuals with Alzheimer-type dementia. *Activities, Adaptation, and Aging* 24:65–74.
Small, G., A. Okonek, M. Mandelkern, et al. 1994. Age-associated memory loss: Initial neuropsychological and cerebral metabolic findings of longitudinal study. *International Psychogeriatrics* 6:23–44.
Smith, M., and B. Milner. 1981. The role of the right hippocampus in the recall of spatial location. *Neuropsychologia* 19:781–93.
Snowdon, D. 2001. *Aging with Grace.* New York: Bantam Books.
Solomon, G., W. Petrie, J. Hart, et al. 1998. Olfactory dysfunction discriminates Alzheimer's dementia from major depression. *Journal of Neuropsychiatry and Clinical Neurosciences* 10:64–67.
Squire, L. 1983. The hippocampus and the neuropsychology of memory. In *Neurobiology of the Hippocampus,* edited by W. Seifert. New York: Academic Press.

Squire, L. 1987. *Memory and Brain.* New York: Oxford University Press.

Squire, L. 1995. Biological foundations of accuracy and inaccuracy in memory. In *Memory Distortion*, edited by D. Schacter. Cambridge, Mass.: Harvard University Press, pp. 197–255.

Stebbins, G.L. 1977. *Process of Organic Evolution.* Englewood Cliffs, N.J.: Prentice-Hall.

Talamo, B., R. Rudel, K. Kosik, et al. 1989. Pathological changes in olfactory neurons in patients with Alzheimer's disease. *Nature* 337:736–39.

Terr, L. 1983. Chowchilla revisited: The effects of psychic trauma four years after a schoolbus kidnapping. *American Journal of Psychiatry* 140:1543–50.

Tulving, E. 1972. Episodic and semantic memory. In *Organization of Memory*, edited by E. Tulving and W. Donaldson. New York: Academic Press, pp. 381–403.

Tulving, E. 1983. *Elements of Episodic Memory.* Oxford: Clarendon Press.

Tulving, E. 1985. How many memory systems are there? *American Psychologist* 40:385–98.

Tulving, E., H. Markowitsch, S. Kapur, et al. 1994. Novelty encoding networks in the human brain: Positron emission tomography data. *NeuroReport* 5:2525–28.

Udalova, G., and A. Karas. 1996. Learning, memory, and motivation in ants. In *Russian Contributions to Invertebrate Behavior*, edited by C. Abramson, Z. Shuranova, and Y. Burmistrov. Westport, Conn.: Praeger, pp. 145–75.

Van Hoesen, G., A Solodkin, and B. Hyman. 1995. Neuroanatomy of Alzheimer's disease: Hierarchical vulnerability and neural system compromise. *Neurobiology of Aging* 16:278–80.

Vygotsky, L. 1962. *Thought and Language.* Cambridge, Mass.: MIT Press.

Wilson, R., and A. Kaszniak, 1986. Longitudinal changes: Progressive idiopathic dementia. In *Clinical Memory Assessment of Older Adults*, edited by L. Poon. Washington, D.C.: American Psychological Association, pp. 285–93.

Yngve, V. 1986. *Linguistics as a Science.* Bloomington: Indiana University Press.

Zola-Morgan, S., L. Squire, and M. Mishkin. 1982. The neuroanatomy of amnesia: Amygdala-hippocampus versus temporal stem. *Science* 218:1337–39.

Part III / Vascular Dementias and Subcortical Dementias

CHAPTER NINE

Cortical and Frontosubcortical Dementias

Differential Diagnosis

Frédéric Assal, M.D., and Jeffrey L. Cummings, M.D.

This chapter will review cognitive and behavioral characteristics of frontosubcortical dementias (FSCD) and compare them to the features of cortical dementias, mainly Alzheimer disease (AD). The main etiologies of FSCD and relevant associated neurologic features are summarized, with special emphasis for clinicians. Finally, the pathophysiology of FSCD is discussed, focusing on the connections of the basal ganglia and the frontal lobes.

Albert, Feldman, and Willis (1974) were the first to emphasize the distinctive pattern of mental impairment (including forgetfulness, slowing of thought processes, emotional or personality changes, and impaired ability to manipulate acquired knowledge) characterized as "subcortical dementia" (SCD) and characteristic of progressive supranuclear palsy (PSP). Since the pathology of PSP is mainly subcortical, this pattern of mental impairment was called SCD, in contrast to dementias such as AD, in which primarily cortical pathological changes produce aphasias, apraxias, agnosias, and amnesia. Other authors had pointed out some aspects of the syndrome previously. In 1912, Wilson described the "narrowing of mental horizons" in hepatolenticular degeneration. Ten years later, Naville (1922) brought up the concept of bradyphrenia, referring to slowness of thought processes. Finally, in 1932, von Stockert introduced the term *subcortical dementia.* A year after Albert and colleagues described SCD, McHugh and Folstein (1975) attributed the intellectual decline of Huntington disease (HD) to SCD. Emphasizing the subcortical distribution of the pathology of HD, they postulated that the degeneration of subcortical nuclei in HD and other subcortical diseases such as Parkinson disease (PD) was responsible for the cognitive and mood disturbances commonly observed in these conditions.

These first descriptions of subcortical dementia suggested that behavioral symptoms (mood disturbances, personality changes) and specific cognitive changes (bradyphrenia, poor verbal fluency, retrieval deficit type of memory disturbance, and impaired executive function) distinguished subcortical and cortical dementias. These features of SCD have since been described in various neurologic disorders associated clinically with dementias. However, patients with intellectual compromise secondary to subcortical pathology may not meet criteria for a dementing syndrome as required by the *Diagnostic and Statistical Manual of Mental Disorders*, 4th edition (American Psychiatric Association 1994). These patients may, however, fit with the definition proffered by Cummings, Benson, and LoVerm (1980), which defines dementia as an acquired persistent disturbance in neuropsychological function involving at least three of the following spheres of mental activity: language, memory, visuospatial function, executive function, personality, and emotion. Because in SCD these deficits are not always sufficient to warrant a diagnosis of dementia, many authors refer to "subcortical syndromes." These distinctions are important because some data presented here derive from patients without dementia.

With the recognition of atrophy in the nucleus basalis as a pathological hallmark in Alzheimer disease and of cortical pathology in many subcortical disorders, objections have arisen concerning the validity of the concept of subcortical dementia (Whitehouse 1986). Recent pathological data reported significant changes in some brainstem nuclei in AD compared to normals (Parvizi, Van Hoesen, and Damasio 2001). Issues regarding methodology also have challenged the validity of SCD (Mayeux and Stern 1987; Rosen 1987). Distinguishing subcortical and cortical dementias has proven to be clinically useful because these profiles aid in identification of diseases that reflect cortical or subcortical dysfunction, even when the pathological changes are not so discrete.

Since the first edition of this book, various entities with overlapping features of cortical and subcortical dementias have been identified. Dementia with Lewy bodies (DLB), frontotemporal dementias (FTDs), and corticobasal ganglionic degeneration (CBGD) involve cortical and subcortical structures, and their contribution to understanding dementia is currently under study. Nevertheless, when these "new" diseases were compared to AD or PSP using qualitative and quantitative measures, various authors showed that cortical versus subcortical neuropsychological profiles increased the level of clinical diagnostic accuracy (Pillon et al. 1994, 1995a, b; Litvan, Cummings, and Mega 1998; Lopez et al. 1999).

Because of the connections of subcortical structures with the frontal lobes and similarities in neuropsychological testing in subcortical and frontal pathologies (Rodgers et al. 1998; Dimitrov et al. 1999), we will use the term *frontosubcortical dementias* (FSCD).

Cognitive Features

Attention and Concentration

Classically, attentional processes are impaired in delirium but not in either Alzheimer disease or frontosubcortical dementias, at least in early stages. Nevertheless, certain deficits of complex attention, such as divided attention and aspects of selective attention, manifest early on in AD (Perry and Hodges 1999). Likewise, aspects of attention also are compromised in FSCD. Sustained attention tested with digit span or other tests is generally preserved in patients with PD (Huber et al. 1986; Pillon et al. 1986) but may be impaired in patients with PSP (Pillon et al. 1986), HD (Salmon et al. 1989; Pillon et al. 1991), and multiple sclerosis (MS) (Rao et al. 1991). Selective or focused attention is spared in PD, although patients were slower in their response time (Lee et al. 1999). Other authors showed that maintenance of attention was defective in PD (Wright et al. 1990). These results provide evidence for the heterogeneity of attentional dysfunction among FSCD, but may also be the consequence of methodological and conceptual problems. The term *attention* denotes not a single function, but rather a complex set of related functions dependent on several separate subsystems. Since attentional processes and concentration are subserved by the frontal lobes and linked to executive functions and working memory, these differences could also be explained by differences in severity of frontal lobe lesions.

Language and Speech

Language is generally intact in patients with frontosubcortical dementias, whereas aphasia is a consistent feature of the cortical dementias such as AD (Pillon et al. 1991). Dysarthria is frequent in all FCSD. In a comparison of AD and PD subjects with similar severity of dementia, Cummings and colleagues (1988) found patients with PD to have impaired speech mechanics (including loudness, pitch, articulation, rate, and intelligibility) as well as impaired writing mechanics and diminished grammatical complexity (shorter phrase length, fewer dependent clauses), while other linguistic abilities were intact. Patients with AD exhibited fluent but impoverished spontaneous output with a severe anomia. Repetitive speech phenomena, resembling palilalia and stuttering, also have been described in FCSD, in particular in PD (Benke et al. 2000). Relatively preserved language abilities have been demonstrated in PSP (Albert, Feldman, and Willis 1974) and in MS (Rao et al. 1991). Comprehension deficits frequently occur in longitudinal follow-up of HD (Bachoud-Levi et al. 2001). When compared to AD patients with a similar severity of dementia, however, patients with FSCD generally have a milder naming deficit and lack paraphasic errors (Huber, Shuttleworth, and Freidenberg 1989). Patients with frontotemporal dementia may exhibit all the classic symptoms of FSCD plus an aphasic syndrome, a unique combination of deficits.

Visuospatial Functions

Impaired visuospatial abilities are characteristic of Alzheimer disease. Similar deficits have been found in patients with MS (Rao et al. 1991) and in patients with PD with dementia, even when tasks minimize motor demands. In some studies, patients with PD performed even worse on visuospatial skills than patients with AD (Stern et al. 1993). In other studies, PD caused more impairment than AD on Raven's matrices; but in contrast, patients with PD performed better on Block Design than did the group with AD (Huber, Shuttleworth, and Friedenberg 1989). In a recent study comparing AD, vascular dementia (VaD), PD, and normal controls, the drawing of a modified Rey-Osterrieth Complex Figure was superior for normal controls compared to all dementias (Freeman et al. 2000). Patients with AD outperformed both VaD and PD groups, and there were few differences between VaD and PD. The drawings of VaD and PD were very fragmented and contained numerous perseverations and omissions. In neuropathologically proven dementia with Lewy bodies, pentagon copying is more impaired than in neuropathologically proven AD, which may reflect a synergistic effect of cortical and subcortical impairments on visuospatial and visuoconstructive functions (Ala et al. 2001).

Memory

In general, memory deficits in frontosubcortical dementias are not as severe as those in Alzheimer disease (Huber et al. 1986; Pillon et al. 1986; Salmon et al. 1989), but recent studies of patients with frontosubcortical dementias have demonstrated abnormalities in some memory processes. The characteristic pattern of FCSD is different from that of AD.

Working memory is a form of short-term memory or immediate recall linked with executive functions and frontal lobes: its characterization derives from modern cognitive neuroscience (D'Esposito et al. 1995). A simple way to test verbal working memory at the bedside is to have the patient memorize and immediately recall in ascending order a series of seven digits. This task has been shown to be severely affected in patients with PD (Hoppe et al. 2000) and subcortical vascular disease (Reed et al. 2000).

In Parkinson disease, Huntington disease, and progressive supranuclear palsy, the diminished ability to learn and remember new information, which is part of episodic memory, is characterized by a prominent retrieval deficit, as evident from relatively preserved recognition, poor free recall, benefit from cueing, and a lack of intrusions (Pillon et al. 1994; Knoke, Taylor, and Saint-Cyr 1998). Severely impaired recall with only mildly impaired recognition also has been documented in MS (Caine et al. 1986). In AD, both recall and recognition are impaired, reflecting the inability of patients to store new information.

On memory tasks involving interference following information presentation, patients with progressive supranuclear palsy are impaired on both recall and recognition; when interference is minimized, recognition processes are better preserved than recall (Litvan et al. 1989). This increased sensitivity to interference is postulated to be secondary to impaired temporal sequencing and inability to maintain a strategic search of stored information due to frontal systems impairment.

Remote memory is less affected in Parkinson disease than in Alzheimer disease (Huber, Shuttleworth, and Paulsen 1986). Furthermore, in FSCD, the retrograde amnesia is not characterized by a temporal gradient like in AD, where there is a relative preservation of memories of more distant than recent events.

Semantic memory alludes to the memory of facts and general knowledge. It is disrupted in AD, in the temporal variant of FTD (or semantic dementia), and in DLB (Perry and Hodges 2000; Lambon Ralph et al. 2001). Usually not observed in FSCD, semantic memory impairments in HD were attributed to a retrieval deficit (van der Hurk and Hodges 1995).

Procedural memory refers to the memory of skill acquisition. Although challenged by some authors (Bondi and Kaszniak 1991), most have confirmed that patients with PD (Saint-Cyr, Taylor, and Lang 1988; Koenig, Thomas-Anterion, and Laurent 1999) or with ischemic VaD (Libon et al. 1998) exhibit impairment in various tests of procedural memory, in contrast to the preservation of procedural memory observed in amnestic patients, normal controls, and those with early AD. These results confirm animal data and emphasize the role of the prefrontal cortex in procedural memory.

In summary, memory performance in patients with frontosubcortical dementias appears to have a distinct clinical profile, as summarized in table 9.1. These clinical differences highlight the anatomical basis of the different subcomponents of memory and contrast with the type of memory impairment observed in AD.

Executive Functions

Executive function refers to the ability to plan or program new information, to use and manipulate it effectively, to shift mental sets, and to inhibit incorrect responses or resist the environment, and is also concerned with drive, motivation, and will. Executive deficits are especially notable on tasks requiring self-initiated

Table 9.1. Memory impairment in frontosubcortical dementia and Alzheimer disease

Memory Feature	Frontosubcortical Dementias	Alzheimer Disease
Overall severity	Less impaired	More impaired
Working memory	Impaired	Impaired late
Recall	Impaired	Impaired
Recognition	Intact	Impaired
Response to verbal clue	Good	Poor
Intrusions	Absent	Present
Remote memory	Less impaired (without temporal gradient)	Impaired (with temporal gradient early in the clinical course)
Procedural memory	Impaired	Intact

Table 9.2. Comparison of nonmemory cognitive impairments, behavioral symptoms, and motor anomalies in frontosubcortical dementias and Alzheimer disease

Feature	Frontosubcortical dementias	Alzheimer Disease
Cognitive symptoms		
Attention	Normal (slow) or impaired (sustained attention)	Normal or impaired (divided attention and selective attention)
Speed of cognitive processing	Slow	Normal
Language	Most often preserved	Impaired
Speech	Dysarthric	Normal
Visuospatial skills	Impaired (poor planning, preservation errors)	More impaired
Executive functions		
Set planning and shifting	Severely impaired	Impaired late
Verbal fluency	Severely impaired (esp. letter fluency)	Impaired (esp. category fluency)
Delayed alternation	Intact	Impaired
Delayed response	Impaired	Impaired
Behavioral symptoms		
Psychosis	Variably present	Common
Mood disturbances	Common	Less common
Others	Irritability, apathy, obsessive-compulsive behaviors, anxiety	Anxiety
Motor anomalies		
Movement disorder	Present early (chorea, tremor, bradykinesia, dystonia	Absent or late myoclonus
Posture and gait	Abnormal early	Normal until late

or internally guided planning and execution of information-processing strategies. Executive functions are linked to the frontal lobes and frontosubcortical circuits as shown by lesion (Stuss and Benson 1984) and functional neuroimaging studies (Konishi et al. 1998). As noted earlier, patients with frontal and subcortical lesions present similar cognitive deficits (Rodgers et al. 1998; Dimitrov et al. 1999).

Recently, evidence has begun to emerge that executive deficits are present early in Alzheimer disease (Perry and Hodges 1999) and are more prominent in the so-called frontal variant of Alzheimer disease (Johnson et al. 1999). Nevertheless, these deficits are much less severe than in FSCD (tab. 9.2). When compared to patients with AD, performances of patients with PSP (Pillon et al. 1986; Grafman et al. 1990; Lange et al. 1995; Watkins et al. 2000), lacunar state (Wolfe et al. 1990), or MS (Rao et al. 1991; Arnett et al. 1997) were significantly worse on the Wisconsin Card Sorting Test or the Tower of London, which measure planning and set-shifting ability.

Performance on verbal fluency tasks was shown to be significantly more impaired in progressive supranuclear palsy, Parkinson disease, Huntington disease, and vascular dementia than Alzheimer disease (Pillon et al. 1986; Huber, Shuttleworth, and Freidenberg 1989; Lafosse et al. 1997). Impaired verbal fluency also is reported in preclinical HD (Lawrence et al. 1998). Other studies confirmed that letter (or phonemic or lexical) fluency was significantly decreased in FCSD (PSP, HD) and not in AD, but category (or semantic) fluency was significantly impaired in both FCSD and AD (Rosser and Hodges 1994). Therefore, it was argued that the deficits of category fluency in AD were secondary to breakdown of semantic knowledge, reflecting temporal lobe involvement. Deficits in both letter and category fluency reflect initiation and retrieval problems, which are common to both tasks, secondary to disruption of frontostriatal circuits. More recent studies have shown that both letter and category fluency scores of PD with dementia, HD, and MS were poor, but, in contrast to previous research, patients with AD also had decreased letter fluency scores and patients with PD without dementia had normal scores (Tröster et al. 1998).

Bradyphrenia

Bradyphrenia is a clinical sign characterized by slowing of cognitive processes or psychomotor retardation. Poor motivation, initiation, verbal fluency, or working memory and diminished attentional processes were described in FSCD earlier in this chapter. They all contribute to bradyphrenia, which is common in FSCD.

Behavioral Features

Since the original description of behavioral disturbances in patients with Huntington disease (McHugh and Folstein 1975), many studies confirmed that these were common in frontosubcortical dementias. In addition to classic phenomenological data, the Neuropsychiatric Inventory (NPI), a tool with established validity and reliability, has been used to assess and quantify the most common behavioral disturbances in AD and FSCD (Cummings et al. 1994).

Depression is frequent in frontosubcortical dementias such as multiple sclerosis (Diaz-Olavarrieta et al. 1999), Parkinson disease (Cummings and Mastermann 1999), or Huntington disease (Cummings 1995). In a retrospective clinicopathologic study, depression was more common in PD and DLB than AD (Klatka, Louis, and Schiffer 1996). When PD and AD patients with similar levels of severity were compared to normal controls, the patients with PD had significantly more severe depressive symptoms than the two other groups (Huber, Shuttleworth, and Freidenberg 1989). The severity of depression in PD was unrelated to the degree of motor impairment, suggesting that depression was not simply a reaction to physical disability (Huber et al. 1986). The relationship between depression and executive deficits and their anatomical basis remain controversial. In PD, the severity of depression was unrelated to degree of cognitive impairment (Huber, Shuttleworth, and Freidenberg 1989). In PSP, depression was found to be common but did not correlate with cognitive impairment and in particular was unrelated to executive deficits (Esmonde et al. 1996). Depression is more prevalent in VaD than in AD (Cummings et al. 1987; Newman 1999). Moreover, higher depression scores were associated with frontal white matter changes (Barber et al. 1999).

Episodes of secondary mania occur in frontosubcortical dementias such as Huntington disease, multiple sclerosis, and acquired immune deficiency syndrome dementia (Mendez 2000). They are less frequent than episodes of depression. In AD, elevated mood is rare (Burns, Jacoby, and Levy 1990; Lyketsos, Corazzini, and Steele1995).

Patients with Huntington disease exhibited significantly more anxiety than patients with progressive supranuclear palsy (Litvan et al. 1998). Anxiety is frequent in both AD and VaD, whereas it is unrelated to the severity of the cognitive disorder (Aharon-Peretz, Kliot, and Tomer 2000).

Irritability has been described in Huntington disease (McHugh and Folstein 1975) and is significantly more present than in patients with progressive supranuclear palsy (Litvan et al. 1998).

Apathy, defined as reduced motivation and involvement, is more prominent in progressive supranuclear palsy than in Huntington disease (Litvan et al. 1998) or PD (Aarsland et al. 2001a, b). Apathy is more marked than depression in AD and is associated with significantly more severe frontal lobe-related deficits

(Kuzis et al. 1999). Apathy, as assessed by the NPI, has been related to deficits in right cingulate on single-photon emission computed tomography (SPECT) (Benoit et al. 1999). These data confirm the involvement of frontosubcortical circuits in this symptom.

Obsessive-compulsive symptoms have not been described in Alzheimer disease; they are not rare in patients with Huntington disease (Cummings 1995). In a sample of patients with PD but not dementia or depression, obsessive-compulsive symptoms were significantly more frequent than in normal controls and were correlated with severity and duration of illness (Alegret et al. 2001). Obsessive-compulsive symptoms are common in FTD. These results support the involvement of the basal ganglia and frontal lobes in obsessive-compulsive symptomatology.

Delusions are common in some frontosubcortical dementias as well as Alzheimer disease. The nature and prevalence of delusions do not distinguish AD and VaD (Cummings et al. 1987). They tend to be uncomplicated, loosely held, persecutory beliefs involving fears of theft and infidelity. Delusions and hallucinations were significantly more common in DLB than PD with dementia and also in PD with dementia compared to PD without dementia (Aarsland et al. 2001a, b). These findings may support the hypothesis that delusions and hallucinations are associated with subcortical and superimposed cortical pathologies.

Diseases Associated with Frontosubcortical Dementias

Table 9.3 lists a variety of diseases that have in common the syndrome of frontosubcortical dementias. The main disorders and their contribution to our understanding of the pathophysiology of FSCD are discussed below.

Basal Ganglia Disorders

Progressive supranuclear palsy was first described as a distinctive clinical syndrome in 1964 by Steele, Richardson, and Olszewski. They reported eight patients with a progressive neurologic illness characterized by supranuclear ophthalmoplegia, axial dystonia, pseudobulbar palsy, bradykinesia, postural instability, dysarthria, and dementia. Although PSP is a prototype of FSCD, early dementia is rare (Litvan et al. 1996). Pathology consists of cerebral atrophy with pallor of the substantia nigra and shrinkage of the internal globus pallidus. Histologically, there exists substantial neuronal loss and gliosis with abundant

Table 9.3. Diseases associated with frontosubcortical dementias

Degenerative	Nondegenerative
Parkinson disease	Vascular dementias
Progressive supranuclear palsy	Binswanger disease
Huntington disease	Lacunar state
Multiple system atrophy	CADASIL
Wilson disease	Infectious dementias
Neuroacanthocytosis	AIDS dementia complex
Fahr disease	Whipple disease
Hallervorden-Spatz disease	Neurosyphillis
Spinocerebellar ataxias	Creutzfeldt-Jakob disease
Frontotemporal dementia	Demyelinating dementias
Amyotrophic lateral sclerosis	Multiple sclerosis
Progressive subcortical gliosis	Inherited leukoencephalopathies
	Miscellaneous
	Normal pressure hydrocephalus
	Sarcoidosis
	Behcet disease

neurofibrillary tangles and neuropil threads. The tangles and threads are localized primarily to subcortical regions and are composed of hyperphosphorylated tau (Daniel, de Bruin, and Lees 1995). Recently, a clinicopathologic analysis of nine patients with PSP showed greater frontal lobe atrophy compared to controls, which correlated with increasing neurofibrillary tangle densities and with clinical dementia (Cordato et al. 2000). These findings concur with neuroimaging data showing reduced frontal perfusion or metabolism in PSP and impaired executive functions (Blin et al. 1990; Johnson et al. 1992).

Huntington disease is a progressive, autosomal dominant neurodegenerative disorder with 100% penetrance characterized by chorea and cognitive and behavioral changes (Cummings 1995). Traditionally it is accepted that these signs and symptoms are usually present at the onset of the disease, although one may precede the other by a matter of years. A large survey including 1238 individuals with symptomatic HD revealed that involuntary movements were the earliest reported symptom, then respectively mental and emotional symptoms. As the disease progressed, behavioral and cognitive symptoms were manifested (Kirkwood et al. 2001). Huntington disease is caused by an increased number of CAG trinucleotide repeats affecting the IT15 gene at chromosome 4p16.3 (Huntington's Disease Collaborative Research Group 1993). Normal alleles contain 34 or fewer CAG repeats, whereas repeats of 37 to 150 or more occur in affected individuals. A negative correlation has been observed between the number of repeats and the age of onset of disease. There is currently no effective treatment.

Reported prevalence of dementia in Parkinson disease ranges around 40%, with important variations, depending on the ascertainment methods (Cummings et al. 1988). The risk for developing dementia in patients with PD relative to controls, according to DSM-III (American Psychiatric Association 1987) criteria, after adjusting for age, sex, and education, was 5.9 (95% CI, 3.9 to 9.1) in a recent prospective study (Aarlsand et al. 2001a). It is generally accepted that the pattern of dementia corresponds to a FSCD, as opposed to AD (Huber et al. 1986; Pillon et al. 1986), although it is likely that there are several dementia syndromes in PD (Cummings et al. 1988). These different clinical syndromes reflect different pathologies. Coexistent findings of AD (neuritic plaques, neurofibrillary tangles, granulovacuolar degeneration) with characteristic findings of PD (loss of pigmented neurons in the pars compacta of the substantia nigra, Lewy bodies in the substantia nigra, various subcortical nuclei and cerebral cortex) have been reported (Boller et al. 1980). More recently, cortical Lewy bodies, detected by alpha-synuclein immunostaining, were better correlated with cognitive impairment in patients with PD than AD histological findings (Hurtig et al. 2000; Mattila et al. 2000). The spectrum of DLB includes several histological variants (pure Lewy body and AD variants), and their link with PD and AD is still debated. Thus, the contributions of cortical Lewy bodies, AD-type pathology, and the PD pathology to the dementia of PD is uncertain. In clinical practice, it is important to be aware that some patients with PD and dementia may meet the criteria of DLB, since symptomatic treatments are available.

Multiple system atrophy (MSA) is another neurodegenerative disease with alpha-synuclein positive glial cytoplasmic inclusions. Multiple system atrophy includes Shy-drager syndrome and striatonigral and olivopontocerebellar degenerations. They manifest parkinsonian features, which respond poorly to treatment, and may exhibit cerebellar signs or dysautonomia. Patients show significant deficits in executive functions similar to PD but less severe than in PSP (Pillon et al. 1995a, b). In a clinicopathological survey, patients with MSA lacked criteria for dementia and, when compared to PD, did not develop levodopa-induced confusion (Wenning et al. 2000).

Wilson disease (WD), or hepatolenticular degeneration, is an inherited disorder of copper metabolism caused by mutations of the gene ATP7B on chromosome 13q14. Wilson disease is characterized, clinically, by liver, ocular (Kayser-Fleischer ring), and neurological signs. The latter include extrapyramidal features due to putaminal changes and mild FSCD with personality and mood disturbances (Wilson 1912; Medalia, Isaace-Glaberman, and Scheinberg 1988; Lauterbach et al. 1998).

Hepatic cirrhosis may also be associated with putaminal involvement due to probable manganese deposition (Butterworth 2000). These changes may explain the parkinsonism and the subclinical hepatic encephalopathy which exhibits a subcortical pattern (McCrea et al. 1996).

Fahr disease, or idiopathic basal ganglia calcification (IBGC), is a familial progressive disorder variably associated with extrapyramidal signs and frontosubcortical dementias with psychosis and mood disturbance (Lauterbach et al. 1998). A locus on chromosome 14q has been identified in a family with dominantly inherited IBCG (Geschwind, Loginov, and Stern 1999).

Vascular Diseases

Vascular dementia (VaD) is a heterogeneous group of disorders associated with vascular risk factors or ischemic or hemorrhagic brain injury. Vascular dementia may have features of FSCD, cortical dementia, or both, depending on the distribution of infarctions. Compared to AD, there is no consensus gold standard for pathological diagnosis of VaD. Uniform premortem criteria requiring neuroimaging have been developed only recently by a committee of experts from the National Institute of Neurological Disease and Stroke and the Association Internationale pour la Recherche et l'Enseignement en Neurosciences (NINCDS-AIREN) (Roman et al. 1993). Even with the recommendations of the NINCDS-AIREN consensus panel, a study found that dementia could not be attributed to the effects of cerebrovascular disease alone in any patients coming to autopsy (Nolan et al. 1998). Another clinicopathologic study using the same criteria found a low sensitivity and high specificity for the diagnosis of probable VaD, but the pathologic definition of VaD arbitrarily excluded cases with vascular lesions confined to subcortical structures (Gold et al. 1997). Although VaD accounted for 15.8% of cases of dementia in a recent population study (Lobo et al. 2000), the frequency of pure VaD is controversial compared to mixed AD-cerebrovascular disease. Frontosubcortical dementias occur in at least three forms of VaD: lacunar state, Binswanger disease, and cerebral autosomal dominant arteriopathy with subcortical infarcts and leukoencephalopathy (CADASIL).

In lacunar state (LS), the number of lacunes, the extent of periventricular lucency, and the severity of ventricular enlargement were associated with cognitive deficits dependent on frontal-executive function (Corbett, Bennet, and Kos 1994). Moreover, in a prospective study, frontal lobe hypometabolism on functional neuroimaging predicted cognitive decline in patients with LS (Reed et al. 2001).

Binswanger disease (BD) is a gradually progressive frontosubcortical dementia (McPherson and Cummings 1996) caused by ischemic injury to the deep periventricular white matter of the cerebral hemispheres. Binswanger disease also is characterized by pseudobulbar palsy, small-stepped gait, and urinary urgency.

Migraine, recurrent ischemic episodes leading to gait disturbances, urinary urgency, pseudobulbar palsy, and psychiatric disturbances in patients without risk factors for vascular dementia are the most common presentations of cerebral autosomal dominant arteriopathy with subcortical infarcts and leukoencephalopathy (Dichgans et al. 1998). The disorder is autosomal dominant and is due to severe alterations of vascular smooth-muscle cells secondary to mutations of the Notch 3 gene on chromosome 19q12 (Bousser and Tournier-Lasserve 2001).

Demyelinating and Infectious Diseases

Multiple sclerosis is the most common demyelinating disorder of the central nervous system. Its etiology is still unknown. The clinical course of MS has three forms: relapsing-remitting, acute progressive, and chronic progressive. The most common pattern in those with late-onset MS is a chronic, slowly progressive course. Cognitive dysfunction occurs in more than 40% of patients with MS and shows a pattern suggestive of FSCD (Caine et al. 1986; Rao et al. 1991). It is generally accepted that the cognitive deficits are correlated with the lesion burden in the frontal lobe (Rovaris and Filippi 2000). It is still not known if the immunomodulatory treatments will be able to delay or diminish the occurrence of dementia.

Acquired immune deficiency syndrome dementia complex (ADC), or human immunodeficiency virus dementia, affected 15–20% of all patients with acquired immune deficiency (Power and Johnson 1995), but incidence rates for acquired immune deficiency syndrome dementia complex decreased in the past few years probably following the introduction of highly active antiretroviral therapy (HAART) in 1996 (Sacktor et al. 2001). Acquired immune deficiency syndrome dementia complex occurs most often at moderate and advanced degrees of immunodeficiency. However, with the advent of HAART, ADC may occur at higher CD4 cell counts than previously (Sacktor et al. 2001). The progressive FSCD and accompanying motor dysfunction are hypothesized to reflect injury induced by HIV-1 viral proteins and the subsequent release of chemokines, cytokines, and toxins (Brew 1999). These changes are predominant in the frontal lobe and also affect the basal ganglia.

Creutzfeldt-Jakob disease (CJD) is the most common human transmissible subacute spongiform encephalopathy or prion disease (Weihl and Roos 1999). It is mostly sporadic but can occur in families, with an autosomal dominant pattern of inheritance. Creutzfeldt-Jakob disease results in a rapidly progressive dementia with myoclonic jerks, ataxia, and frequent initial symptoms such as anorexia, insomnia, mood changes, and malaise. The dementia has both cortical and subcortical features and often begins with predominant frontosubcortical features. It rapidly evolves into a mute and akinetic state.

Pathophysiology

The common attribute linking the diverse etiologies of frontosubcortical dementias is the location of structural or functional changes in subcortical nuclei, frontal cortical regions projecting to these nuclei, or the connecting white matter tracts. Injuries to different components within these circuits lead to similar clinical deficits, thus explaining the similarity of frontal lobe and frontosubcortical syndromes (Rodgers et al. 1998; Dimitrov et al. 1999).

Based on animal data, five different basal ganglia-thalamocortical circuits were proposed (Alexander, DeLong, and Strick 1986; Alexander, Crutcher, and DeLong 1990). The authors suggested that they were "segregated and parallel circuits," and each one of those circuits subserved different aspects of movement or complex behavior (motor, associative, and limbic). For each circuit, striatal output reaches the basal ganglia output nuclei (the substantia nigra pars reticulata and the internal segment of the globus pallidus) via a "direct pathway" and an "indirect pathway"; the latter traverses the external segment of the globus pallidus and the subthalamic nucleus. Later studies showed that the number of circuits could be expanded (Middleton and Strick 2000) and that, besides the segregated or closed circuits, open connections involving the circuits or interconnections of different functional circuits existed (Joel 1997).

The dorsolateral prefrontal circuit originates in the convexity of the frontal lobes and projects primarily to the dorsolateral head of the caudate nucleus, which projects to the globus pallidus and substantia nigra. The latter project to the medial dorsal thalamic nucleus, that in turn projects to the dorsolateral prefrontal cortex. Damage to this circuit produces most of the classic executive deficits associated with FSCD.

The orbitofrontal circuit originates in the inferolateral prefrontal cortex and projects to the ventromedial caudate nucleus, which in turn projects to the globus pallidus and substantia nigra. The latter project to the ventral anterior and medial dorsal thalamic nuclei that connect with the orbitofrontal cortex. The orbitofrontal cortex is further subdivided both anatomically and functionally into a lateral and a medial region, the medial region being considered as an integrator of visceral drives, probably through amygdalar connections (Mega, Cummings, and Salloway 1997). Lesions involving this circuit are characterized by changes in emotional and social behaviors with irritability and elevated mood. Because of its connections with the dorsolateral prefrontal cortex, this circuit also is involved in executive functions such as the Wisconsin Card Sorting Test (Stuss et al. 2000).

The anterior cingulate circuit begins in the anterior cingulate gyrus and projects to the ventral striatum (nucleus accumbens and ventromedial portions of the caudate and putamen). This circuit is involved in motivation as well as speech and word generation and suppression of standard responses in novel circumstances (Stroop, antisaccade tests). Lesions of the anterior cingulate cortex may produce apathy or akinetic mutism.

The motor circuit originates from neurons in the supplementary motor area, premotor cortex, and somatosensory cortex. Motor initiation abnormalities (akinesia) are associated with lesions in the supplementary motor area; parkinsonism and dystonia are observed with putaminal dysfunction and choreiform movements with caudate and subthalamic nucleus damage.

The oculomotor circuit originates in the frontal eye field and prefrontal and posterior parietal cortices. Lesions in this circuit produce supranuclear gaze palsy as seen in PSP.

Involvement of these circuits results in the deficits characteristic of frontosubcortical dementias. As an example, lesions in the caudate nuclei would predict all cognitive, behavioral, oculomotor, and motor anomalies encountered in Huntington disease: frontosubcortical dementias, conduct and mood disturbances, gaze anomalies, and choreiform movements.

Research Conclusions and Future Directions

The cognitive and behavioral studies of dementia with subcortical involvement share common features called frontosubcortical dementias. These cognitive, behavioral, and motor features are predicted from a model of segregated and parallel basal ganglia-thalamocortical circuits. Functional neuroimaging data exploring various FSCD, such as lacunar state (Reed et al. 2001) or PSP (Blin et al. 1990; Johnson et al. 1992), confirmed hypotheses regarding FSCD derived from animal data. Electrophysiological recordings during stereotaxic surgery of patients with PD supported the functional segregation of the motor and cognitive circuits in the human globus pallidus (Lombardi et al. 2000). These circuits may subserve various psychiatric diseases sharing features of FSCD (for a review, see Krystal et al. 2001). For example, subtle structural or neurochemical anomalies of the orbitofrontal and dorsolateral prefrontal cortex may explain executive deficits, psychiatric features, and motor akinesia encountered in major depression. Future research directions include investigation of these possible explanations.

Clinical Conclusions

Ample cognitive and behavioral evidence exists for differentiating Alzheimer disease from frontosubcortical dementias, although there may be some clinical and pathologic overlaps. Frontosubcortical dementias are characterized by relative absence of aphasia, apraxia, agnosia, and amnesia, in contrast to AD. Because we still do not have sensitive and specific biological markers for most dementias, this clinical distinction is important for many reasons, especially at the onset of the symptoms. First, recognizing FSCD may lead to diagnostic tests and genetic counseling for HD or CADASIL. Second, the distinction may lead to specific treatment such as levodopa for PD, or more important, to preventive measures such as better blood pressure control in patients with lacunar state. Third, AD is frequent and one may be tempted to prescribe acetylcholinesterase inhibitors to any dementia, but these drugs have not been proven to benefit FSCD and have negative side effects. More basic research and clinicopathologic correlations are needed in order to improve diagnostic criteria and quality of care.

ACKNOWLEDGMENTS

This project was supported by an National Institute on Aging Alzheimer disease grant (AG16570), an Alzheimer's Disease Research Center of California grant, the Sidell-Kagen Foundation (JLC), and a scholarship from the University Hospital, Geneva, Switzerland (FA).

REFERENCES

Aarsland, D., I. Litvan, and J.P. Larsen. 2001. Neuropsychiatric symptoms of patients with progressive supranuclear palsy and Parkinson's disease. *Journal of Neuropsychiatry and Clinical Neurosciences* 13:42–49.

Aarlsand, D., K. Andersen, J.P. Larsen, et al. 2001a. Risk of dementia in Parkinson's disease: A community-based, prospective study. *Neurology* 56:730–36.

Aarsland, D., C. Ballard, J.P. Larsen, et al. 2001b. A comparative study of psychiatric symptoms in dementia with Lewy bodies and Parkinson's disease with and without dementia. *International Journal of Geriatric Psychiatry* 16:528–36.

Aharon-Peretz, J., D. Kliot, and R. Tomer. 2000. Behavioral differences between white matter lacunar dementia and Alzheimer's disease: A comparison on the Neuropsychiatric Inventory. *Dementia and Geriatric Cognitive Disorders* 11:294–98.

Ala, T.A., L.F. Hughes, G.A. Kyrouac, et al. 2001. Pentagon copying is more impaired in dementia with Lewy bodies than in Alzheimer's disease. *Journal of Neurology, Neurosurgery, and Psychiatry* 70:483–88.

Albert, M.L., R.G. Feldman, and A.L. Willis. 1974. The "subcortical dementia" of progressive supranuclear palsy. *Journal of Neurology, Neurosurgery, and Psychiatry* 37: 121–30.

Alegret, M., C. Junque, F. Vallderiola, et al. 2001. Obsessive-compulsive symptoms in Parkinson's disease. *Journal of Neurology, Neurosurgery, and Psychiatry* 70:394–96.

Alexander, G.E., M.D. Crutcher, and M.R. DeLong. 1990. Basal ganglia-thalamocortical circuits: Parallel substrates for motor, oculomotor, "prefrontal," and "limbic" functions. *Progress in Brain Research* 85:119–46.

Alexander, G.E., M.R. DeLong, and P.L. Strick. 1986. Parallel organization of functionally segregated circuits linking basal ganglia and cortex. *Annual Review of Neuroscience* 9:357–81.

American Psychiatric Association. 1987. *Diagnostic and Statistical Manual of Mental Disorders.* 3rd revised ed. Washington, D.C.: American Psychiatric Association.

American Psychiatric Association. 1994. *Diagnostic and Statistical Manual of Mental Disorders.* 4th ed. Washington, D.C.: American Psychiatric Association.

Arnett, P.A., S.M. Rao, J. Grafman, et al. 1997. Executive functions in multiple sclerosis: An analysis of temporal ordering, semantic encoding, and planning abilities. *Neuropsychology* 11:535–44.

Bachoud-Levi, A.-C., P. Maison, P. Bartolomeo, et al. 2001. Retest effects and cognitive decline in longitudinal follow-up of patients with early HD. *Neurology* 56:1052–58.

Barber, R., P. Scheltens, A. Gholkar, et al. 1999. White matter lesions on magnetic resonance imaging in dementia with Lewy bodies, Alzheimer's disease, vascular dementia, and normal aging. *Journal of Neurology, Neurosurgery, and Psychiatry* 67:66–72.

Benke, T., C. Hohenstein, W. Poewe, et al. 2000. Repetitive speech phenomena in Parkinson's disease. *Journal of Neurology, Neurosurgery, and Psychiatry* 69:319–24.

Benoit, M., I. Dygai, O. Migneco, et al. 1999. Behavioral and psychological symptoms in Alzheimer's disease: Relation between apathy and regional cerebral perfusion. *Dementia and Geriatric Cognitive Disorders* 10:511–17.

Blin, J., J.C. Baron, B. Dubois, et al. 1990. Positron emission tomography study in progressive supranuclear palsy: Brain hypometabolic pattern and clinico-metabolic correlations. *Archives of Neurology* 47:747–52.

Boller, F., R. Mizutani, U. Roessmann, et al. 1980. Parkinson's disease, dementia, and Alzheimer's disease: Clinicopathologic correlations. *Annals of Neurology* 7:329–35.

Bondi, M.W., and A.W. Kaszniak. 1991. Implicit and explicit memory in Alzheimer's disease and Parkinson's disease. *Journal of Clinical and Experimental Neuropsychology* 13:339–58.

Bousser, M.G., and E. Tournier-Lasserve. 2001. Cerebral autosomal dominant arteriopathy with subcortical infarcts and leukoencephalopathy: From stroke to vessel wall physiology. *Journal of Neurology, Neurosurgery, and Psychiatry* 70:285–87.

Brew, B.J. 1999. AIDS dementia complex. *Neurologic Clinics* 17:861–81.

Burns, A., R. Jacoby, and R. Levy. 1990. Psychiatric phenomena in Alzheimer's disease. III: Disorders of mood. *British Journal of Psychiatry* 157:92–94.

Butterworth, R.F. 2000. Complications of cirrhosis III. Hepatic encephalopathy. *Journal of Hepatology* 32 (Suppl. 1):S171–80.

Caine, E.D., K.A. Bamford, R.B. Schiffer, et al. 1986. A controlled neuropsychological comparison of Huntington's disease and multiple sclerosis. *Archives of Neurology* 43: 249–54.

Corbett, A.J., H. Bennet, and S. Kos. 1994. Cognitive dysfunction following subcortical infarction. *Archives of Neurology* 51:999–1007.

Cordato, N.J., G.M. Halliday, A.J. Harding, et al. 2000. Regional brain atrophy in progressive supranuclear palsy and Lewy body diseases. *Annals of Neurology* 47:718–28.

Cummings, J.L. 1995. Behavioral and psychiatric symptoms associated with Huntington's disease. *Advances in Neurology* 65:179–86.

Cummings, J.L., and D.L. Mastermann. 1999. Depression in patients with Parkinson's disease. *International Journal of Geriatric Psychiatry* 14:711–18.

Cummings, J.L., D.F. Benson, and S.J. LoVerme. 1980. Reversible dementia. *Journal of the American Medical Association* 243:2434–39.

Cummings, J.L., B. Miller, M.A. Hill, et al. 1987. Neuropsychiatric aspects of multi-infarct dementia and dementia of the Alzheimer's type. *Archives of Neurology* 44: 389–93.

Cummings, J.L., A. Darklins, M. Mendez, et al. 1988. Alzheimer's disease and Parkinson's disease: Comparison of speech and language alterations. *Neurology* 38:680–84.

Cummings, J.L., M. Mega, K. Gray, et al. 1994. The Neuropsychiatric Inventory: Comprehensive assessment of psychopathology in dementia. *Neurology* 44:2308–14.

Daniel, S.E., V.M. de Bruin, and A.J. Lees. 1995. The clinical and pathological spectrum of Steele-Richardson-Olszewski syndrome progressive supranuclear palsy: A reappraisal. *Brain* 118:759–70.

D'Esposito, M., J.A. Detre, D.C. Alsop, et al. 1995. The neural basis of the central executive system of working memory. *Nature* 378:279–81.

Diaz-Olavarrieta, C., J.L. Cummings, J. Velazquez, et al. 1999. Neuropsychiatric manifestations of multiple sclerosis. *Journal of Neuropsychiatry and Clinical Neurosciences* 11: 51–57.

Dichgans, M., M. Mayer, I. Uttner, et al. 1998. The phenotypic spectrum of CADASIL: Clinical findings in 102 cases. *Annals of Neurology* 44:731–39.

Dimitrov, M., J. Grafman, A.H. Soares, et al. 1999. Concept formation and concept shifting in frontal lesion and Parkinson's disease patients assessed with the California Card Sorting Test. *Neuropsychology* 13:135–43.

Esmonde, T., E. Giles, M. Gibson, et al. 1996. Neuropsychological performances, disease severity, and depression in progressive supranuclear palsy. *Journal of Neurology* 243:638–43.

Freeman, R.Q., T. Giovannetti, M. Lamar, et al. 2000. Visuoconstructional problems in dementia: Contributions of executive systems functions. *Neuropsychology* 14:415–26.

Geschwind, D.H., M. Loginov, and J.M. Stern. 1999. Identification of a locus on chromosome 14q for idiopathic basal ganglia calcification Fahr disease. *American Journal of Human Genetics* 65:764–72.

Gold, G., P. Giannakopoulos, C. Montes-Paixao Jr., et al. 1997. Sensitivity and specificity of newly proposed clinical criteria for possible vascular dementia. *Neurology* 49:690–94.

Grafman, J., I. Litvan, C. Gomez, et al. 1990. Frontal lobe function in progressive supranuclear palsy. *Archives of Neurology* 47:553–58.

Hoppe, C.D., U.D. Muller, K.D. Werheid, et al. 2000. Digit Ordering Test: Clinical, psychometric, and experimental evaluation of a verbal working memory test. *Clinical Neuropsychology* 14:38–55.

Huber, S.J., E.C. Shuttleworth, and D.L. Freidenberg. 1989. Neuropsychological differences between the dementias of Alzheimer's and Parkinson's disease. *Archives of Neurology* 46:1287–91.

Huber, S.J., E.C. Shuttleworth, and G.W. Paulson. 1986. Dementia in Parkinson's disease. *Archives of Neurology* 43:987–90.

Huber, S.J., E.C. Shuttleworth, G.W. Paulson, et al. 1986. Cortical vs. subcortical dementia. Neuropsychological differences. *Archives of Neurology* 43:392–94.

Huntington's Disease Collaborative Research Group. 1993. A novel gene containing a trinucleotide repeat that is expanded and unstable on Huntington's disease chromosomes. *Cell* 72:971–83.

Hurtig, H.I., J.Q. Trojanowski, J. Galvin, et al. 2000. Alpha-synuclein cortical Lewy bodies correlate with dementia in Parkinson's disease. *Neurology* 54:1916–21.

Joel, D. 1997. The connections of the primate subthalamic nucleus: Indirect pathways and the open-interconnected scheme of basal ganglia-thalamocortical circuitry. *Brain Research Review* 23:62–78.

Johnson, J.K., E. Head, R. Kim, et al. 1999. Clinical and pathological evidence for a frontal variant of Alzheimer's disease. *Archives of Neurology* 56:1233–39.

Johnson, K.A., R.A. Sperling, B.L. Holman, et al. 1992. Cerebral perfusion in progressive supranuclear palsy. *Journal of Nuclear Medicine* 33:704–9.

Kirkwood, S.C., J.L. Su, P.M. Conneally, et al. 2001. Progression of symptoms in the early and middle stages of Huntington disease. *Archives of Neurology* 58:273–78.

Klatka, L.A., E.D. Louis, and R.B. Schiffer. 1996. Psychiatric features in diffuse Lewy body disease: A clinicopathologic study using Alzheimer's disease and Parkinson's disease comparison groups. *Neurology* 47:1148–52.

Knoke, D., A.E. Taylor, and J.A. Saint-Cyr. 1998. The differential effects of cueing on recall in Parkinson's disease and normal subjects. *Brain and Cognition* 38:261–74.

Koenig, O., C. Thomas-Anterion, and B. Laurent. 1999. Procedural learning in Parkinson's disease: Intact and impaired components. *Neuropsychologia* 37:1103–9.

Konishi, S., K. Nakajima, I. Uchida, et al. 1998. Transient activation of inferior prefrontal cortex during cognitive set shifting. *Nature Neuroscience* 1:80–84.

Krystal, J.H., D.C. D'Souza, G. Sanacora, et al. 2001. Advances in the pathophysiology and treatment of psychiatric disorders: Implication for internal medicine. *Medical Clinics of North America* 85:559–77.

Kuzis, G., L. Sabe, C. Tiberti, et al. 1999. Neuropsychological correlates of apathy and depression in patients with dementia. *Neurology* 52:1403–7.

Lafosse, J.M., B.R. Reed, D. Mungas, et al. 1997. Fluency and memory differences between ischemic vascular dementia and Alzheimer's disease. *Neuropsychology* 11: 514–22.

Lambon Ralph, M.A., J. Powell, D. Howard, et al. 2001. Semantic memory is impaired in both dementia with Lewy bodies and dementia of Alzheimer's type: A comparative neuropsychological study and literature review. *Journal of Neurology, Neurosurgery, and Psychiatry* 70:149–56.

Lange, K.W., B.J. Sahakian, N.P. Quinn, et al. 1995. Comparison of executive and visuospatial memory function in Huntington's disease and dementia of Alzheimer type matched for degree of dementia. *Journal of Neurology, Neurosurgery, and Psychiatry* 58: 598–606.

Lauterbach, E.C., J.L. Cummings, J. Duffy, et al. 1998. Neuropsychiatric correlates and treatment of lenticulostriatal diseases: A review of the literature and overview of research opportunities in Huntington's, Wilson's, and Fahr's disease. *Journal of Neuropsychiatry and Clinical Neurosciences* 10:249–66.

Lawrence, A.D., J.R. Hodges, A.E. Rosser, et al. 1998. Evidence for specific cognitive deficits in preclinical Huntington's disease. *Brain* 121:1329–41.

Lee, S.S., K. Wild, C. Hollnagel, et al. 1999. Selective visual attention in patients with frontal lobe lesions or Parkinson's disease. *Neuropsychologia* 37:595–604.

Libon, D.J., B. Bogdanoff, B.S. Cloud, et al. 1998. Declarative and procedural learning, quantitative measures of the hippocampus and subcortical white alterations in Alzheimer's disease and ischaemic vascular dementia. *Journal of Clinical and Experimental Neuropsychology* 20:30–41.

Litvan, I., J.L. Cummings, and M. Mega. 1998. Neuropsychiatric features of corticobasal degeneration. *Journal of Neurology, Neurosurgery, and Psychiatry* 65:717–21.

Litvan, I., J. Grafman, C. Gomez, et al. 1989. Memory impairment in patients with progressive supranuclear palsy. *Archives of Neurology* 46:765–67.

Litvan, I., Y. Agid, J. Jankovic, et al. 1996. Accuracy of clinical criteria for the diagnosis of progressive supranuclear palsy Steele-Richardson-Olszewski syndrome. *Neurology* 46:922–30.

Litvan, I., J.S. Paulsen, M.S. Mega, et al. 1998. Neuropsychiatric assessment of patients with hyperkinetic and hypokinetic movement disorders. *Archives of Neurology* 55: 1313–19.

Lobo, A., L. J. Launer, L. Fratiglioni, et al. 2000. Prevalence of dementia and major subtypes in Europe: A collaborative study of population-based cohorts. Neurologic Disease in the Elderly Research Group. *Neurology* 54 (Suppl. 5):S4–9.

Lombardi, W.J., R.E. Gross, L.L. Trepanier, et al. 2000. Relationship of lesion location to cognitive outcome following microelectrode-guided pallidotomy for Parkinson's disease: Support for the existence of cognitive circuits in the human pallidum. *Brain* 123:746–58.

Lopez, O.L., I. Litvan, K.E. Catt, et al. 1999. Accuracy of four clinical diagnostic criteria for the diagnosis of neurodegenerative dementias. *Neurology* 53:1292–99.

Lyketsos, C.G., K. Corazzini, and C. Steele. 1995. Mania in Alzheimer's disease. *Journal of Neuropsychiatry and Clinical Neurosciences* 7:350–52.

Mattila, P.M., J.O. Rinne, H. Helenius, et al. 2000. Alpha-synuclein-immunoreactive cortical Lewy bodies are associated with cognitive impairment in Parkinson's disease. *Acta Neuropathologica* 100:285–90.

Mayeux, R., and Y. Stern. 1987. Subcortical dementia. *Archives of Neurology* 34:642–46.

McCrea, M., J. Cordoba, G. Vessey, et al. 1996. Neuropsychological characterization and detection of subclinical hepatic encephalopathy. *Archives of Neurology* 53:758–63.

McHugh, P.R., and M.F. Folstein. 1975. Psychiatric syndromes of Huntington's chorea: A clinical and phenomenologic study. In *Psychiatric Aspects of Neurologic Disease*, edited by D. F. Benson and D. Blumer. New-York: Grune and Stratton, pp. 267–86.

McPherson, S.E., and J.L. Cummings. 1996. Neuropsychological aspects of vascular dementia. *Brain and Cognition* 31:269–82.

Medalia, A., K. Isaacs-Glaberman, and I.H. Scheinberg. 1988. Neuropsychological impairment in Wilson's disease. *Archives of Neurology* 45:502–4.

Mega, M.S., J.L. Cummings, S. Salloway, et al. 1997. The limbic system: An anatomic, phylogenetic, and clinical perspective. *Journal of Neuropsychiatry and Clinical Neuroscience* 6:315–30.

Mendez, M.F. 2000. Mania in neurologic disorders. *Current Psychiatry Reports* 2:440–45.

Middleton, F.A., and P.L. Strick. 2000. Basal ganglia output and cognition: Evidence from anatomical, behavioral, and clinical studies. *Brain and Cognition* 42:183–200.

Naville, F. 1922. Etude sur les complications et les séquelles mentales de l'encéphalite épidemique: La bradyphrénie. *L'Encéphale* 17:369–75, 423–36.

Newman, S.C. 1999. The prevalence of depression in Alzheimer's disease and vascular dementia in a population sample. *Journal of Affective Disorders* 52:169–76.

Nolan, K.A., M.M. Lino, A.W. Seligmann, et al. 1998. Absence of vascular dementia in an autopsy series from a dementia clinic. *Journal of the American Geriatric Society* 46: 597–604.

Parvizi, J., G.W. Van Hoesen, and A. Damasio. 2001. The selective vulnerability of brainstem nuclei to Alzheimer's disease. *Annals of Neurology* 49:53–66.

Perry, R.J., and J.R. Hodges. 1999. Attention and executive deficits in Alzheimer's disease. A critical review. *Brain* 122:383–404.

Perry, R.J., and J.R. Hodges. 2000. Differentiating frontal and temporal variant frontotemporal dementia from Alzheimer's disease. *Neurology* 54:2277–84.
Pillon, B., B. Dubois, F. Lhermitte, et al. 1986. Heterogeneity of cognitive impairment in progressive supranuclear palsy, Parkinson's disease, and Alzheimer's disease. *Neurology* 36:1179–85.
Pillon, B., B. Dubois, A. Ploska, et al. 1991. Severity and specificity of cognitive impairment in Alzheimer's, Huntington's, and Parkinson's, and progressive supranuclear palsy. *Neurology* 41:634–43.
Pillon, B., B. Deweer, A. Michon, et al. 1994. Are explicit memory disorders of progressive supranuclear palsy related to damage to striatofrontal circuits? Comparison with Alzheimer's, Parkinson's, and Huntington's diseases. *Neurology* 44:1264–70.
Pillon, B., J. Blin, M. Vidailhet, et al. 1995a The neuropsychological pattern of corticobasal degeneration: Comparison with progressive supranuclear palsy and Alzheimer's disease. *Neurology* 45:1477–83.
Pillon, B., N. Gouider-Khouja, B. Deweer, et al. 1995b. Neuropsychological pattern of striatonigral degeneration: Comparison with Parkinson's disease and progressive supranuclear palsy. *Journal of Neurology, Neurosurgery, and Psychiatry* 58:174–79.
Power, C., and R.T. Johnson. 1995. HIV-1 associated dementia: Clinical features and pathogenesis. *Canadian Journal of Neurological Sciences* 22:92–100.
Rao, S.M., G.J. Leo, L. Bernardin, et al. 1991. Cognitive dysfunction in multiple sclerosis. I. Frequency, patterns, and prediction. *Neurology* 41:685–91.
Reed, B.R., J.L. Eberling, D. Mungas, et al. 2000. Memory failure has different mechanisms in subcortical stroke and Alzheimer's disease. *Annals of Neurology* 48:275–84.
Reed, B.R., J.L. Eberling, D. Mungas, et al. 2001. Frontal lobe hypometabolism predicts cognitive decline in patients with lacunar infarcts. *Archives of Neurology* 58:493–97.
Rodgers, R.D., B.J. Sahakian, J.R. Hodges, et al. 1998. Dissociating executive mechanisms of task control following frontal lobe damage and Parkinson's disease. *Brain* 121:815–42.
Roman, G.C., T.K. Tatemichi, T. Erkinjuntti, et al. 1993. Vascular dementia: Diagnostic criteria for research studies. *Neurology* 43:250–60.
Rosen, T.J. 1987. Cortical vs. subcortical dementia: Neuropsychological similarities. *Archives of Neurology* 44:131.
Rosser, A., and J.R. Hodges. 1994. Initial letter and semantic category fluency in Alzheimer's disease, Huntington's disease, and progressive supranuclear palsy. *Journal of Neurology, Neurosurgery, and Psychiatry* 57:1389–94.
Rovaris, M., and M. Filippi. 2000. MRI correlates of cognitive dysfunction in multiple sclerosis. *Journal of Virology* 6 (Suppl. 2):S172–75.
Sacktor, N., R.H. Lyles, R. Skolasky, et al. 2001. HIV-associated neurologic disease incidence changes: Multicenter AIDS cohort study, 1990–1998. *Neurology* 56:257–60.
Saint-Cyr, J.A., A.E. Taylor, and A.E. Lang. 1988. Procedural learning and neostriatal dysfunction in man. *Brain* 111:941–59.
Salmon, D.P., P.F. Kwo-on-Yuen, W.C. Heindel, et al. 1989. Differentiation of Alzheimer's disease and Huntington's disease with Dementia Rating Scale. *Archives of Neurology* 46:1204–8.
Steele, J.C., J.C. Richardson, and J. Olszewski. 1964. Progressive supranuclear palsy. A heterogeneous degeneration involving the brainstem, basal ganglia, and cerebellum

with vertical gaze, and pseudobulbar palsy, nuchal dystonia, and dementia. *Archives of Neurology* 10:333–58.

Stern, Y., M. Richards, M. Sano, et al. 1993. Comparison of cognitive changes in patients with Alzheimer's and Parkinson's disease. *Archives of Neurology* 50:1040–45.

Stuss, D.T., and D.F. Benson. 1984. Neuropsychological studies of the frontal lobe. *Psychological Bulletin* 95:3–28.

Stuss, D.T., B. Levine, M.P. Alexander, et al. 2000. Wisconsin card sorting test performance in patients with focal frontal and posterior brain damage: Effects of lesion location and test structure on separable cognitive process. *Neuropsychologia* 38:388–402.

Tröster, A.I., J.A. Fields, J.A. Testa, et al. 1998. Cortical and subcortical influences on clustering and switching in the performance of verbal fluency tasks. *Neuropsychologia* 36:295–304.

van der Hurk, P.R., and J.R. Hodges. 1995. Episodic and semantic memory in Alzheimer's disease and progressive supranuclear palsy: A comparative study. *Journal of Clinical and Experimental Neuropsychology* 17:459–71.

von Stockert, F.G. 1932. Subcorticale Demenz. *Archives of Psychiatry* 97:77–100.

Watkins, L.H.A., R.D. Rogers, A.D. Lawrence, et al. 2000. Impaired planning but intact decision making in early Huntington's disease: Implication for specific fronto-striatal pathology. *Neuropsychologia* 38:1112–25.

Weihl, C.C., and R.P. Roos. 1999. Creutzfeldt-Jakob disease, new variant Creutzfeldt-Jakob disease and bovine spongiform encephalopathy. *Neurologic Clinics* 17:835–59.

Wenning, G.K., Y. Ben-Shlomo, A. Hughes, et al. 2000. What clinical features are most useful to distinguish definite multiple system atrophy from Parkinson's disease? *Journal of Neurology, Neurosurgery, and Psychiatry* 68:434–40.

Whitehouse, P.J. 1986. The concept of subcortical dementia: Another look. *Annals of Neurology* 19:1–6.

Wilson, S.A.K. 1912. Progressive lenticular degeneration. *Brain* 34:296–508.

Wolfe, N., R. Linn, V.L. Babikian, et al. 1990. Frontal systems impairment following multiple lacunar infarcts. *Archives of Neurology* 47:129–32.

Wright, M.J., R.J. Burns, G.M. Geffen, et al. 1990. Covert orientation of visual attention in Parkinson's disease: An impairment in the maintenance of attention. *Neuropsychologia* 28:151–59.

CHAPTER TEN

Noninfarct Vascular Dementia

The Spectrum of Vascular Dementia and Alzheimer Syndrome

V. Olga B. Emery, Ph.D., Edward X. Gillie, M.D., and Joseph A. Smith, M.D.

In this chapter the nosologic construct of vascular dementia (VaD) is redefined and broadened to include what we term *noninfarct vascular dementia:* vascular dementia caused by underlying vascular factors other than cerebral infarction (Emery, Gillie, and Ramdev 1995; Emery, Gillie, and Smith 1996, 2000). The results of our investigations of cognitive impairment in a broad spectrum of vascular disorders are summarized and analyzed in this chapter. The findings indicate that cerebral infarction is not the only path to the phenotypic presentation of VaD. Data are presented that indicate vascular disease without cerebral infarction results in a continuum of cognitive impairment, with one end of this continuum represented by the concept of noninfarct VaD. Definition, nomology, and nosology are critical methodologic components in the understanding of mechanisms underlying VaD. It is crucial that VaD be conceptualized as an overarching superordinate nosologic category with subtypes. Not all subtypes of VaD involve cerebral infarction.

Vascular dementia is reported to be the second most common dementing illness in North America and Europe (Lobo et al. 2000; Gauthier and Ferris 2001). A recent study of 5092 community residents of a Utah county, who were

65 years of age or older, found that 329 had dementia (0.065). Of these elderly persons with dementia, 65% had Alzheimer syndrome and 19% had VaD (Lyketsos et al. 2000). A recent European population-based study of dementia prevalence found that VaD accounted for about 16% of dementia cases (Lobo et al. 2000). In Japan, China, and Korea, it is reported that VaD was the most prevalent dementing illness until the 1990s, after which Alzheimer syndrome increasingly became greater in prevalence, with VaD now second most common (Suh and Shah 2001) (see chap. 11). For India, data are contradictory: some studies show Alzheimer syndrome and other studies show VaD with highest prevalence (Suh and Shah 2001).

Despite this documented high frequency and concomitant medical and sociocultural impact of vascular dementia, the clinical and pathophysiologic characterizations remain controversial (Aguero-Torres and Winblad 2000; Erkinjuntti et al. 2000; Feldman and Kertesz 2001; Gauther and Ferris 2001). How VaD is defined is a core dimension in the understanding of clinicopathophysiologic features of the syndrome. Further, valid differential diagnosis and rationally based treatment of the class of dementing conditions linked to different cerebrovascular disorders are, in part, a function of the validity and reliability of constructs and classification of VaD. Definitions and conceptualizations are determinants of operationalizations and circumscribe interpretation of empiric and clinical findings. It is a requisite for progress in medical science that constructs (concepts and their operationalization) faithfully reflect empirical reality (that is, that they have validity and reliability) (Campbell and Stanley 1969; Tanur et al. 1985). This chapter is concerned with the validity of the construct of VaD.

Changes in Concepts

An analysis of the nosologic history of vascular dementia during the twentieth century uncovers a constant error of misidentification of the overarching category of vascular dementia, first with one and then with some other of its subtypes. Overall, the classification history of VaD indicates a failure to place the construct of VaD in a superordinate hierarchical position, with a number of subtypes comprising the broader category. The results of our investigations of a broad spectrum of vascular disorders indicate that the term *vascular dementia* should not be regarded as coextensive nor be used interchangeably with any of its subtypes.

To be more specific, in analyzing the evolution of the construct of vascular dementia during the twentieth century, one sees that during the mid-1900s the term *vascular dementia* was equated with arteriosclerotic psychosis or cerebral arteriosclerosis (Mayer-Gross, Slater, and Roth 1960; Slater and Roth 1969). Reflecting the prevailing descriptions of VaD, the first edition of the *Diagnostic and Statistical Manual of Mental Disorders* (DSM-I) (American Psychiatric Association 1952), in its section on organic brain syndromes, incorporated VaD in the nosologic category "chronic brain syndrome associated with cerebral arteriosclerosis." The second edition of this manual (DSM-II) (American Psychiatric Association 1968) retained this concept, but changed the terminology related to VaD to "psychosis with cerebral arteriosclerosis." The disorder was described as "a chronic disorder attributed to cerebral arteriosclerosis that may be impossible to differentiate from senile dementia and presenile dementia, which may coexist with it" (p. 28). The DSM-II also included a second nosologic category of VaD called "psychosis with other cerebrovascular disturbance," which included such "circulatory disturbances as cerebral thrombosis, cerebral embolism, arterial hypertension, cardiorenal disease, and cardiac disease" (p. 28).

A fundamental reconceptualization of vascular dementia occurred when Fisher (1968) and Hachinski, Lassen, and Marshall (1974) proposed that vascular dementia was caused by multiple cerebral infarcts. Hachinkski, Lassen, and Marshall (1974) coined the term *multi-infarct dementia* (MID), and thereafter, for the past three decades, there has been an equation between VaD and MID (Roman 1987; Roman et al. 1993; Erkinjuntti 1997). Inhering in this shift in terminology was a major nosologic problem; rather than being conceptualized as one specific subtype of the overarching category of VaD, the concept of MID was used as a replacement for all of previously described kinds of VaD, and further, was regarded as coterminous with the entirety of the category of VaD (Emery, Gillie, and Ramdev 1994, 1996; Emery, Gillie, and Smith 2000). It is the perspective of this chapter that the construct validity of VaD would have been better served had MID been conceptualized as an additional distinct subtype of VaD rather than as a substitute for all previous subtypes. Our data point to the idea that MID is only one subtype of VaD, although possibly the most prevalent one, and that VaD is broader than any one subtype.

As the two terms *vascular dementia* and *multiinfarct dementia* became virtually synonymous, this delimitation of vascular dementia as multiinfarct dementia became reflected in formal classification. The DSM-III and DSM-III-R specifically, and DSM-IV more generally and with less closure, have equated VaD with MID (American Psychiatric Association 1980, 1987, 1994), thus defining VaD more narrowly than either DSM-I or DSM-II. In contrast, ICD-10 placed VaD in a superordinate position with a number of subtypes comprising the broader category (World Health Organization 1992). Conflictually, however, in its actual research criteria, the ICD-10 requires cerebral infarction for the diagnosis of VaD (World Health Organization 1993), thus contradicting what potentially would and should have been a broader, hierarchic classification of the vascular dementias. Finally, in the DSM-IV-TR (American Psychiatric Association 2000), for the first time in thirty years, one does find that diagnostic criteria for VaD are no longer delimited by the infarct concept. This represents a significant step forward.

Our ongoing investigations of the vascular dementias arose from frustration in attempting to diagnose patients with long-standing histories of vascular disorders who were cognitively impaired but who met neither criteria for vascular dementia (patients without cerebral infarction), nor criteria for probable Alzheimer disease (patients with higher ischemia scores than criteria permit or gait or seizure disorder early in illness) (Hachinski 1983; McKhann et al. 1984; Wade and Hachinski 1987; Reisberg et al. 1997; American Psychiatric Association 2000). The nosologic criterial equation between VaD and cerebral infarction during the past three decades has resulted in a standard practice by both researchers and clinicians whereby patients with long-standing histories of serious vascular disease, who lack actual cerebral infarction, are placed (or, in our view, forced) into the diagnostic category of dementia of the Alzheimer type (DAT), where they might not belong. Possible ramifications of this standard practice include years of contaminated Alzheimer research samples, inflated incidence and prevalence figures for DAT, and lack of appropriate medical treatment for patients carrying the misdiagnosis of Alzheimer dementia.

Although there have been neuropsychologic studies comparing vascular dementia with other dementing disorders (e.g., Bowen et al. 1990; Kontiola et al. 1990; Mahler and Cummings 1991; Pohjasvaara et al. 2000; Feldman and Kertesz 2001) (see chaps. 9 and 12), with few exceptions (Erkinjuntti 1987; Emery, Gillie, and Ramdev 1994, 1995, 1996; Emery, Gillie, and Smith 1996, 2000), there have been virtually no studies comparing cognitive deficits across different types of vascular dementia. This lack of investigation within the population of VaD is the result of the equation of the entirety of VaD with one subtype. Put another way, if the belief exists that there is only one type of VaD, then the idea of comparisons between several types is inhibited by prevailing nosologic thinking; you don't investigate something you think doesn't exist. Accordingly, the research to be described represents a major paradigm shift.

The research to be reported tests the following null hypotheses/hypotheses: (1) the cognitive impairment of patients with cerebral infarct and noninfarct vascular disorder is not/is significantly greater than and outside the range of normal aging, as indicated by performance on mental status and other cognitive measures, and (2) there are/are not significant differences between patients with cerebral infarction and those with cerebral noninfarct vascular disorders on measures of mental status and other cognitive functions. When these hypotheses are plugged into a deductive paradigm, the data will provide information on the relation between the broader construct of VaD and its subtypes. If the cerebral infarct and noninfarct vascular groups do not differ significantly from one another, then VaD cannot be validly equated with just one of these groups while excluding the other subgroup from the possibility of being classified as VaD.

Method

Participants

This report involves a total of 117 elderly participants: 81 patients with vascular disorders and 36 normal controls. The 81 patients with vascular disorders formed two vascular samples: cerebral infarction ($n = 43$) and cerebral noninfarction ($n = 38$). The cerebral infarct, noninfarct, and normal elderly samples had mean ages of 71.9, 77.1, and 70.2 years, respectively. Mean education of infarct, noninfarct, and normal elderly samples was 11.3, 11.8, and 11.9 years, in turn. Variables of race, native birth, native language, and occupation were also comparable across the three samples.

The vascular samples were composed of eighty-one consecutive patients with vascular disorders meeting sample criteria. Patients were recruited through the Geriatric Service of the Manchester Veterans Affairs Medical Center (VAMC). Overall, the patients represent a stable population of New Hampshire residents who have been treated by the same physicians for several decades and for whom complete records dating back many years were available. Excluded from vascular samples were patients with major head trauma, substance abuse, and suspected dementing disorder other than VaD. The eighty-one vascular patients were being evaluated at the VAMC Geriatric Evaluation Unit for medical problems of a noncognitive nature related to vascular disorders; for example, hypertension, hypotension, high cholesterol, bradycardia, abnormal electrocardiogram (ECG), peripheral vascular disease, coronary disease, cardiomegaly, atrial fibrillation, calcified carotid, ventricular hypertrophy, aneurysm, vasculitis. Screening procedures included medical examination, medical history, and physical, neurologic, psychiatric, and psychosocial assessments. All vascular patients had laboratory tests, chest radiography, ECG, and computed tomographic (CT) scanning of the brain; some patients also underwent magnetic resonance imaging (MRI). CT scans were performed without contrast enhancement with 10-mm continuous slices using Phillips Tomo Scan 60. All scans were reexamined for this research by the same neuroradiologist without knowledge of clinical diagnosis. Morphologic changes analyzed included (1) focal/localized changes suggesting cerebral infarction; (2) white matter changes/white matter low attenuation (Valentine, Moseley, and Kendall 1980; Brun and Englund 1986; Wallin et al. 1989; Diaz et al. 1991; Parnetti 1999; Rockwood et al. 1999; Seno et al. 2000; Auer et al. 2001); and (3) absence or presence of cerebral atrophy. Gray matter and white matter changes were noted. White matter changes were rated mild if less than one-fourth of total white matter area were involved, moderate if less than one-half of total white matter were involved, and severe if more than one-half of total white matter showed changes.

Further, all patients were evaluated for vascular variables of myocardial infarction, heart block, ischemic heart disease, and lipid levels. Also, patients were evaluated for additional vascular risk factors, such as diabetes mellitus and other chronic problems, such as chronic obstructive pulmonary disease. Hypertension was defined as long-term systolic blood pressure over 160 mmHg or long-term diastolic blood pressure over 90 mmHg. Arteriosclerosis was defined as a broad category denoting arterial or vascular sclerosis consisting of several subtypes, including atherosclerosis, Monckeberg, and arteriolosclerosis (Stedman 1990). Atherosclerosis was graded using the World Federation of Neurology Code (National Institute of Neurological and Communicative Disorders and Stroke 1975).

Patients were selected for infarct and noninfarct samples on the basis of brain scan/imaging evidence for cerebral infarction (gray matter or white matter) and on the basis of clinical history. Patients in the infarct sample had to have both clinical and brain imaging evidence of cerebral infarction. The following disorders were included in the category of cerebral infarction: (a) transient ischemic attack, (b) reversible ischemic neurological deficit, and (c) prolonged neurolog-

Table 10.1. Vascular factors in vascular patients with and without cerebral infarction

	Vascular Group	
Vascular Factor	With Cerebral Infarction (n = 43) (in %)	Without Cerebral Infarction (n = 38) (in %)
Cerebral infarction—gray matter	100	0
White matter infarction	28	0
Myocardial infarction	33	55
Heart block	28	24
Cardiomegaly	21	24
Ischemic heart disease	58	79
Arteriosclerosis	77	84
Abnormal electrocardiogram	72	84
Abnormal blood pressure	86	97
Hypertension*	86	79
Hypotension	0	18
Diabetes mellitus	37	42
Peripheral vascular disease	40	53
Chronic obstructive pulmonary disease	47	47

*Hypertension (160 mmHg+/90 mmHg+).

ical deficit or completed stroke (National Institute of Neurological and Communicative Disorders and Stroke 1975).

Of the 43 research participants with cerebral infarction, 16 patients had had a single stroke in gray matter area of the brain and 27 patients had had multiple infarctions in gray matter of the brain. Twelve (28%) of these 43 patients with gray matter infarction additionally had white matter infarction (tab. 10.1).

Inclusion in the cerebral noninfarct sample required that patients have had a long-standing history (minimum of five years) of vascular disorders and that there existed neither clinical nor brain imaging evidence of cerebral infarction of either gray matter or white matter. Of these patients without cerebral infarction, 97% had abnormal blood pressure, 84% had an abnormal ECG, 84% had arteriosclerosis, 79% had ischemic heart disease, 55% had myocardial infarction, 53% had peripheral vascular disease, 47% had chronic obstructive pulmonary disease, and 42% had diabetes mellitus (tab. 10.1). Other conditions of these patients with cerebral noninfarct vascular disorders included vascular collagen disease, aortic aneurysm, atrial fibrillation, left ventricular hypertrophy, cardiomegaly, bradycardia, carotid stenosis, pacemaker complications, hypercholesterolemia, heart murmur, progressive angina, and calcified iliac heart vessels. Although none of the thirty-eight patients comprising the vascular noninfarct sample had cerebral infarction of gray matter or white matter, eight evidenced white matter changes (white matter low attenuation or white matter lucencies) (Brun and Englund 1986; Diaz et al. 1991; Seno et al. 2000; Auer et al. 2001). However, the white matter changes of these eight patients did not reach the point of being actual infarcts per se as evidenced on brain imaging (CT or MRI). It should be noted that the same brain imaging equipment and neuroradiologists did detect actual white matter infarction in twelve patients in the cerebral infarct sample. Finally, all of the subjects comprising the cerebral noninfarct sample had Hachinski Ischemia Scale scores of 7 or higher, thereby being excluded for probable Alzheimer disease (Hachinski 1983; McKhann et al. 1984; Reisberg et al. 1997).

Normal elderly persons were recruited from the community at large. Requirements for participation in the normal elderly sample included noncompromised major organ systems, vital signs within normal range, lack of chronic illness, and self-sufficiency in activities of daily living. No normal elderly participant had either a history of or current vascular disorder.

Mental Status Measures

Two instruments for assessment of mental status and organic deterioration were administered: Mini-Mental State Examination (MMSE) (Folstein, Folstein, and McHugh 1975) and Dementia Rating Scale (DRS) (Mattis 1988).

The Mini-Mental State Examination is a thirty-item brief screening instrument evaluating awareness of time and place, registration, new learning, delayed new learning, construction, attention, writing, and ability to hold in mind and reverse digits (e.g., serial sevens) or letters (e.g., spelling of "world" backward). Also the MMSE includes a brief assessment of oral language dimensions of repetition, naming, and sequential commands. The MMSE has a suggested cut point of 23 out of the 30-point total to indicate the boundary between normal aging and dementia (Folstein, Folstein, and McHugh 1975). The MMSE scores of 16 to 23 correspond to the Global Deterioration Scale, stage 4, indicating moderate cognitive decline and a late confusional clinical phase (Reisberg et al. 1985). The scores in this range cannot be construed to be those of normal aging (Reisberg et al. 1986) (see chap. 1).

Also administered was the Dementia Rating Scale, which was designed to assess cognitive status in persons with known dementing disorder (Mattis 1988). The DRS has a 144-point total and consists of 36 different tasks divided into 5 subscales: (1) attention (37 points), (2) initiation/perseveration (37 points), (3) memory (25 points), (4) conceptualization (39 points), and (5) construction (6 points). Although some constructs constituting the subscales might need work to establish construct validity (e.g., initiation/perseveration), the DRS is a very useful measure of cognitive status when tasks are operationally defined. The DRS has high split-half reliability, content validity, and concurrent validity (Rosen, Mohs, and Davis 1986). It also has high test-retest reliability (Niederehe and Oxman 1994) (see chap. 2). The DRS has a cutoff score of 123 of the 144-point total to indicate the border between normal aging and dementia (Mattis 1988).

Other Cognitive Measures

Oral Language Measures

Oral language processing was measured by six subtests from the Western Aphasia Battery (WAB) (Kertesz 1982) and by the Boston Naming Test (BNT) (Kaplan, Goodglass, and Weintraub 1983). Oral language variables assessed were repetition, naming, auditory verbal comprehension, and grammatical-syntactic processing (Kertesz 1982, 1994; Emery 1985, 1986, 1988, 1993, 1996, 1999, 2000; Huck and Ojeda 1987; Emery and Breslau 1988, 1989; Emery, Gillie, and Ramdev 1995, 1996; Emery, Gillie, and Smith 1996).

The Western Aphasia Battery Repetition test requires the participant to repeat fourteen items. The three WAB tests for naming impairment are sentence completion, responsive speech, and word fluency. Naming is also assessed by the Boston Naming Test, which is a confrontation naming test consisting of fifteen black-and-white pictures that must be named; three levels of word frequency are represented with five pictures per level (Kaplan, Goodglass, and Weintraub 1983). Auditory verbal comprehension was assessed through WAB Yes/No Questions and WAB Sequential Commands. WAB Sequential Commands also provides an assessment for processing of grammatical-syntactic forms.

Because oral language is sensitive to focal lesions (Kertesz, 1982, 1994; Emery 1985, 1996, 1999; Bayles and Kaszniak 1987; Kertesz, Bayles, and Kirshner 1991; Pohjasvaara et al. 2000) (see chap. 7), measures of oral language were included to determine if there would be significant differences and predictor measures among cerebral infarct, noninfarct, and normal elderly persons.

Reading Comprehension Measures

The Western Aphasia Battery Reading Comprehension of Sentences and Paragraphs test was administered. The test has eight items to be answered, and correct answers depend on reading comprehension: for example, "Shovels and saws are common tools; they have parts made of (farmer, forest, metal, cutting)." The test has a 40-point total.

Statistical Measures

To determine significance of difference in means, a one-way ANOVA was used to compare samples, followed by two general linear model post hoc tests: (a) the T test (lowest significant difference), which controls for type I comparison-wise error rate, and (b) Tukey's Studentized Range Test (highest significant difference), which controls for type I experiment-wise error (Statistical Analysis Systems Institute 1982). Additionally, a difference of means test using Student's t distribution, the model for either equal or unequal variances, was used to obtain more specific information, such as exact alpha values (Blalock 1972). Two-tailed tests were used to interpret statistical significance.

This chapter describes the combined or meta-analytic results from smaller, independent studies of our ongoing investigations of cognitive deficits in vascular dementia reported elsewhere (Emery, Gillie, and Ramdev 1994, 1995; Emery, Gillie, and Smith 1996, 1999).

All subjects gave informed consent. For patients with vascular disorders, consent was obtained from family or legal guardians as well.

Results

Results are organized to address the research null hypotheses/hypotheses: (1) the cognitive impairment of patients with cerebral infarct and noninfarct vascular disorders is not/is significantly greater than and outside the range of normal aging; and (2) there are/are not significant differences between patients with cerebral infarction and those with noninfarct vascular disorder on measures of mental status and other cognitive measures.

Comparisons between Vascular and Normal Elderly Samples

Mental Status Measures

On the Mini-Mental State Examination, comparisons between the 43 patients with cerebral infarcts and 36 normal elderly persons were significant at the 0.0001 level. Similarly, comparisons between the 38 vascular patients with no cerebral infarction and the 36 normal elderly persons on the MMSE were also significant at the 0.0001 level (tabs. 10.2 and 10.3).

Turning next to the Dementia Rating Scale, comparisons between patients with cerebral infarction and normal elderly persons were all significant at the 0.0001 level, as were comparisons between noninfarct vascular patients and normal elderly persons (tabs. 10.2 and 10.3). Further, all comparisons between patients with cerebral infarction and normal elderly persons, as well as noninfarct patients and normal elderly persons, on DRS subscale factors of memory, attention, conceptualization, initiation, and construction were significant at the 0.0001 level.

Thus, the data indicate that a broad spectrum of vascular disorders, which crosscut the parameter of cerebral infarction-noninfarction, result in significantly impaired mental status when contrasted with the deficits of normal aging.

Language Measures

Both the infarct and the noninfarct samples were significantly impaired at the 0.0001 level when contrasted with normal elderly persons on the Boston Naming Test (tabs. 10.2 and 10.3).

Analysis of the seven subtests of the Western Aphasia Battery revealed that both vascular samples had deficits at the 0.0001 level when compared with normal elderly persons on the WAB Word Fluency test, which comprises a metanaming task (Emery and Breslau 1988) assessing capability for generative naming (e.g., "name as many foods as you can"). Patients with cerebral infarction also were impaired at the 0.0001 level when compared to normal elderly persons on sequential commands and reading comprehension tasks, whereas patients with noninfarct vascular disorders when contrasted with normals were impaired on sequential commands and reading comprehension at the 0.0004 and 0.004 levels (tab. 10.3). Comparisons between both vascular samples and normal elderly persons on repetition and auditory comprehension were also statistically significant (tab. 10.3). Of the eight language assessments made, only two were not statistically significant (tab. 10.3). There were no significant differences between either the infarct or noninfarct patients in relation to normal elderly persons on oral language tasks of responsive speech and sentence completion, which are the simplest of language tasks involving overlearned language sequences (e.g., "roses are red, violets are what?") (Emery, 1988, 1992, 2000) (see chap. 8).

In sum, these data indicate that, irrespective of cerebral infarction, a broad

Table 10.2. Comparisons of means by sample on measures of mental status and language processing

	Infarct (1) (n = 43)		Noninfarct (2) (n = 38)		Normal (3) (n = 36)		
	M	SD	M	SD	M	SD	Group Comparisons*
Mini-Mental State Examination (30)	22.38	4.14	21.95	5.33	29.37	1.39	1,2<3**
Dementia Rating Scale (144)	112.39	25.54	115.36	22.12	141.75	3.92	1,2<3**
Boston Naming Test (15)	12.46	2.39	12.41	2.08	14.97	0.12	1,2<3**
WAB Repetition (100)	87.67	11.86	89.12	11.44	95.92	7.56	1,2<3**
WAB Sentence Completion (10)	9.68	1.12	9.79	0.63	9.90	0.47	
WAB Responsive Speech (100)	9.84	0.62	9.89	0.44	10.00	0.00	
WAB Word Fluency (20)	9.69	5.50	10.01	5.71	17.71	3.68	1,2<3**
WAB Yes/No Questions (60)	59.70	0.8	59.35	1.89	60.00	0.00	
WAB Sequential Commands (80)	66.24	19.87	65.46	22.62	79.55	1.88	1,2<3**
WAB Reading Comprehension (40)	30.39	11.14	34.08	7.48	38.17	3.72	1,2<3**

Source: Emery, Gillie, and Smith 2000.

*Results of t-test comparisons. Degrees of freedom for the respective comparisons are: 79 (1 versus 2), 77 (1 versus 3), and 72 (2 versus 3). Differences are significant at $p \leq 0.005$.

**Notation means groups 1 and 2 did significantly less well on those tests than did group 3.

Table 10.3. Difference of means on measures of mental status and language processing

	Infarct versus Noninfarct		Infarct versus Normal		Noninfarct versus Normal	
Measure	t-value	*P*	t-value	*P*	t-value	*P*
Mini-Mental State Examination (30)	0.41	0.68	−9.68	0.0001	−8.09	0.0001
Dementia Rating Scale (144)	−0.56	0.58	−6.82	0.0001	−7.05	0.0001
Boston Naming Test (15)	0.10	0.92	−6.29	0.0001	−7.37	0.0001
WAB Repetition (100)	−0.56	0.58	−3.60	0.0006	−3.00	0.004
WAB Sentence Completion (10)	−0.54	0.59	−1.10	0.28	−0.85	0.40
WAB Responsive Speech (100)	−0.41	0.68	−1.55	0.13	−1.50	0.14
WAB Word Fluency (20)	−0.26	0.80	−7.50	0.0001	−6.85	0.0001
WAB Yes/No Questions (60)	1.09	0.28	−2.09	0.04	−2.06	0.04
WAB Sequential Commands (80)	0.17	0.87	−4.00	0.0001	−3.72	0.0004
WAB Reading Comprehension (40)	−1.73	0.09	−4.00	0.0001	−2.95	0.004

Source: Emery, Gillie, and Smith 2000.

spectrum of vascular disorders have significant disadvantage in relation to demographically comparable normal elderly persons on assessments of mental status, oral language, reading comprehension, and other cognitive parameters.

Comparisons between Cerebral Infarct and Noninfarct Vascular Patients

Mental Status Measures

Statistical analyses resulted in no significant differences in means between vascular patients with cerebral infarction and vascular patients with no cerebral infarction on the Mini-Mental State Examination (tabs. 10.2 and 10.3).

On overall scores on the Dementia Rating Scale, there were no significant differences between vascular patients with and without cerebral infarction (tabs. 10.2 and 10.3). Further, in looking at comparisons between patients with and without cerebral infarction on DRS subscale factors of attention, initiation, conceptualization, and memory, there were again no significant differences; however; the DRS subscale factor of construction approached significance, with cerebral infarct patients doing less well than their cerebral noninfarct counterparts. The post hoc procedure that corrected for type I comparison-wise error resulted in a significant difference between infarct and noninfarct patients on the DRS subscale of construction (tab. 10.4). This is consistent with a previous finding where there was a significant difference between cerebral infarct and noninfarct patients on the related parameter of apraxia, with infarcted patients showing greater apractic decrement (Emery, Gillie, and Smith 1996).

Language Measures

On the seven measures of oral language, there were no statistical differences between cerebral infarct and noninfarct patients; oral language means of the two vascular groups were comparable (tabs. 10.2 and 10.3). However, on the WAB Reading Comprehension of Sentences/Paragraphs, although there was no significant difference between means of infarct and noninfarct patients, there was a trend toward significance (tab. 10.3).

Discussion

Vascular Disorders and Normal Aging

In comparisons between vascular patients comprising a broad spectrum of vascular disorders and demographically comparable normal elderly persons, the

Table 10.4. General linear model procedure post hoc comparisons of cerebral noninfarct vascular patients with cerebral infarct patients

Measure	T Tests (LSD) Comparison Error Control	Turkey's Studentized Range (HSD) Experimentwise Error Control
Mental status measure		
Mini-Mental State Examination	ns	ns
Dementia Rating Scale	ns	ns
Dementia Rating Scale/Attention	ns	ns
Dementia Rating Scale/Initiation	ns	ns
Dementia Rating Scale/Conceptualization	ns	ns
Dementia Rating Scale/Memory	ns	ns
Dementia Rating Scale/Construction	***	ns
Language measure		
WAB Repetition	ns	ns
WAB Sentence Completion	ns	ns
WAB Responsive Speech	ns	ns
Word Fluency	ns	ns
WAB Yes/No Questions	ns	ns
WAB Sequential Commands	ns	ns
Reading Comprehension	***	ns

***$p \leq 0.05$; ns = not significant.

patients with vascular disorders performed significantly worse on all measures of mental status, as well as on all measures of language assessment except two. Thus, in addressing the first research question of how patients with a spectrum of vascular disorders compare with normal controls, we conclude that vascular disorders involve decrements in higher cortical processing that are reliably greater and outside the range of normal aging. This is not to say, however, that all patients with vascular disorders have VaD. Elsewhere the relevance of the continuum concept for medical diagnostics has been pointed out (Emery 1988, 1999; Emery, Gillie, and Smith 1996; Emery and Oxman 1997) (see chap. 19). The cognitive impairments of vascular disorders can be conceptualized as a continuum, with minimal cognitive impairment on one end and VaD on the other end. If one adds a diachronic dimension, then the possibility of progression from the mild to the severe end of this cognitive impairment continuum comes into focus. Longitudinal data will be required to better elucidate the relationship between different vascular disorders and the progression of cognitive impairment over time.

Cerebral Infarct and Cerebral Noninfarct Vascular Disorders

Turning now to the second research question pertaining to comparisons between the patients with cerebral infarction (e.g., completed gray matter stroke, reversible ischemic neurologic deficit, transient ischemic attack, white matter infarction) and patients with no cerebral infarction of any kind, the data indicate there are no significant differences between these two groups of vascular patients on any of the mental status, language, or other cognitive measures, except for the significant difference on assessment of construction.

How can one explain the overall similarity in cognitive deficits between patients with cerebral infarction and vascular patients with no cerebral infarction? This question requires further work and also a new perspective on VaD. We have introduced the concept of noninfarct vascular dementia: vascular dementia caused by underlying vascular factors other than cerebral infarction. The introduction of noninfarct VaD as a nosologic entity presents a changed paradigm from which to work. However, some directions follow from the data presented. The data suggest that the distinction of focal versus diffuse or generalized cerebral dysfunction has less explanatory significance for understanding cognitive impairment in vascular disorders than do some shared factors of vascular abnormality.

Vascular abnormalities crosscutting both the cerebral infarct and noninfarct groups include hypertension, abnormal ECG, arteriosclerosis, ischemic heart disease, peripheral vascular disease, chronic obstructive pulmonary disease, and other pathogenic vascular factors (tab. 10.1). The pathogenetic mechanisms underlying these disorders that crosscut both infarct and noninfarct vascular samples have yet to be defined. Although VaD has by convention been associated with focality, focal lesions are in reality not purely localized. Focal lesions, such as stroke, may precipitate a diffuse encephalopathy or dementia in the aging brain (see chap. 7). The distinction between focal and generalized or diffuse disease is in reality not clear-cut. Focal lesions may disrupt functions of other areas of the brain through a number of mechanisms, including edema, disruption of cortical connections, and diaschisis (i.e., reduced metabolic activity of distant but synaptically connected areas of the brain) (Luria 1980; Wallin et al. 1990) (see chap. 7). Furthermore, MID, the definitional and nosologic prototype of focal vascular disorder is, in reality, a multifocal (i.e., multiple infarction equals multiple focality) disorder (Emery, Gillie, and Ramdev 1994; Emery, Gillie, and Smith 1996). Where does one draw the line between multifocality and diffuse or generalized disease? These issues are at the core of questions relevant to the lack of significant differences in cognitive decrement between infarct and noninfarct vascular patients.

During the 1950s and 1960s, it was believed that the cognitive deficits of vascular disorders were caused by arteriosclerosis (Mayer-Gross, Slater, and Roth 1960; Slater and Roth 1969). This line of explanation was abandoned when VaD became equated with MID (Hachinski et al. 1974; American Psychiatric Association 1980, 1987, 1994; Roman et al. 1993; World Health Organization 1993). We submit it was an error to completely throw out the arteriosclerotic explanation in favor of the concept of MID. We propose that multiple infarction be considered only one proximal cause of VaD, while the arteriosclerotic process be considered a major vascular variable in the distal causality of what appears to be a substantial percentage of cases of VaD. By crosscutting both infarct and noninfarct groups, arteriosclerosis is implicated in the causal chain of vascular events related to cognitive decline in both vascular populations. This same reasoning should be applied to abnormalities of blood pressure (tab. 10.1). Our data, as well as the data of others (see chap. 11), indicate that hypertension and hypotension are distal determinants in the vascular chain of events leading to many cases of cognitive impairment in vascular patients. Thus, vascular factors such as arteriosclerosis and hypertension/hypotension can be viewed as "causal" in many instances of VaD.

At this point in our discussion, we would like to introduce the concept of *preinfarct state*. We think that the conceptualization of a preinfarct state will assist in the definition of noninfarct dementia. Whereas all white matter changes are not infarcts per se, it is possible that white matter changes that are not actually infarcts constitute and define a preinfarct state. Thus, it is useful to conceptualize white matter changes as part of a spectrum, going from the preinfarct state on one end of the spectrum to a single infarct to multiple infarction at the other end of the spectrum of white matter changes. Throughout the literature, one finds the interchangeable use of the terms *changes*, *lesions*, and *infarcts*. Such global equation works against construct validity and adds to the confusion surrounding VaD. All changes are not necessarily either lesions or infarcts, and all lesions are not infarcts. The spectrum concept has utility because it saves us from forcing all white matter changes into the infarct category when in fact the data do not support the coterminous definition or equation of all white matter changes with infarction; the two are not categorically identical.

Similarly, gray matter changes can be thought of in the context of a continuum or spectrum. Our data indicate that arteriosclerosis, for example, crosscuts patient groups both with and without cerebral infarcts. Thus, arteriosclerotic changes may constitute a preinfarct condition at one point in the continuum of such changes. As a rule, infarcts do not come out of nowhere. The vascular pathogenic processes that lead up to multiple infarction constitute continua, and the idea of a preinfarct state should have utility for clinicians as well as researchers. We have had the experience of being part of the diagnostic teams where a vascular diagnosis is totally discounted in the absence of actual infarction when, in fact, the diagnosis of vascular cognitive impairment would have been accurate.

What are the pathophysiologic mechanisms underlying the preinfarct state that cause cognitive decline? The data do not support a one-to-one linear relation between the infarct continuum and cognitive deterioration continuum. It appears there are intervening mechanisms, mediating variables, or other causes of cognitive decline besides infarction. The two vascular groups of our study constitute opposing sides of the infarct spectrum, yet the cognitive performance of the two groups is statistically similar. Thus, we conclude that vascular or brain mechanisms as yet unidentified exist in the explication of VaD.

To summarize, although the concept of a preinfarct state adds to the explanatory power of the infarct spectrum in its function of cognitive decline, a careful analysis of data from our investigation indicates that vascular dementia represents a broader category than what can be accounted for with the infarct concept, even when that concept is extended to include a preinfarct state. The data suggest that a wide variety of vascular disorders result in cognitive deterioration and that the underlying pathogenetic mechanisms have yet to be delineated. Therefore, it follows that VaD is not a homogeneous, single disease entity, and VaD is not coextensive with MID. In sum, VaD is an end point (the final common pathway) for a spectrum of vascular disorders. Vascular dementia can be understood best as a phenotype (Emery 1988). Vascular dementia is a final end-point presentation.

How, then, should the nosology or classification of vascular dementia be structured? Vascular dementia should continue to be, as it is now, subsumed under the superordinate classification of dementia (World Health Organization 1992, 1993; American Psychiatric Association 1994, 2000). As such, VaD is on the same hierarchic level as Alzheimer dementia, Pick dementia, HIV dementia, and others. In turn, the category of VaD must have codes for subtypes, such as

MID, Binswanger disease, and others not yet typologically delineated. On the basis of the data presented as part of this chapter, we urge that a subtype category or code be added for noninfarct VaD. The category of noninfarct vascular dementia should also have codes for its own subtypes, such as arteriosclerotic dementia, when there is no evidence of infarction but clear evidence of both arteriosclerosis and dementia, as was the case with a preponderant number of noninfarct patients in our study. Finally, the category of noninfarct dementia would also have a formal nosologic provision (subcategory code) for severe cognitive impairment associated with such disorders as collagen vascular disease.

The Spectrum of Vascular Dementia and Alzheimer Syndrome

Of essence in the spectrum of vascular dementia and Alzheimer syndrome is the ambiguous transition between these two syndromes, which parallels the ambiguous transition between multifocality and diffuse or generalized disease. Our previous discussion of arteriosclerosis in the distal causality of VaD is of interest here. Atherosclerosis, a subtype of the broader category of arteriosclerosis (Stedman 1990), is basically an inflammatory disease, which can lead to ischemia of the brain, heart, or extremities (Ross 1999). The underlying mechanisms of atherosclerosis are fundamentally no different than those in other inflammatory syndromes (Ross 1993a, 1993b, 1999; Lukacs and Ward 1996; Johnson 1997; Tormey et al. 1997). Thus, inflammation is a core process in substantial numbers of cases of VaD, the exact percentage as yet not clear. One causal sequence in the vascular chain of events involving inflammation and subsequent VaD is as follows. Atherosclerosis, a process by which fatty deposits form plaques on interior walls of blood vessels, results in increased heart pumping but decreased efficiency with concomitant decreases in nutrients and oxygen to the brain; in consequence, first, nerve cells die, and then brain tissue becomes inflamed. This initiates what is called an inflammatory cascade (see chap. 5), whereby cells release toxic chemicals, killing more brain cells and further damaging blood vessels (Ross 1993a, 1993b, 1999; Snowdon 2001).

We are interested at this point in the chapter in the common function of inflammation at the interface of vascular dementia and Alzheimer syndrome. Recent research has brought into focus the key role of inflammation in Alzheimer syndrome (see chap. 5). The underlying process of inflammation is in its essence the same irrespective of syndrome. Accordingly, one finds great similarity between VaD and Alzheimer syndrome in descriptions of how the inflammatory process contributes to brain disintegrity. In Alzheimer syndrome, postmortem studies have shown a state of chronic inflammation in affected regions of Alzheimer brain tissue (McGeer et al. 1989; Akiyama and McGeer 1990; McGeer, Schulzer, and McGeer 1996; McGeer and McGeer 2000, in press). Immunohistological investigations have indicated that many inflammatory markers newly appear or are upregulated in affected regions of Alzheimer brain (see chap. 5). Recent data suggest that inflammation is killing neurons as part of Alzheimer syndrome (Rogers et al. 1988; McGeer and McGeer 2000, in press). The complement system, as part of the innate immune system, appears to be playing a major role in Alzheimer syndrome through the mechanism of autotoxicity. Autotoxicity refers to self-attack by the innate immune system, as distinguished from autoimmunity, which refers to self-attack by the phylogenetically later to evolve adaptive immune system (McGeer and McGeer 2000, in press) (see chap. 5). Activated complement cascade, activated microglia, and other factors inhering in the inflammatory process appear to play a major role in converting DAT into a malignant inflammatory condition (McGeer and McGeer 2000). More than twenty epidemiological studies have indicated that taking nonsteroidal anti-inflammatory drugs greatly reduces incidence of DAT; it is suggested that nonsteroidal anti-inflammatory treatment may inhibit neuronal death (Rogers et al. 1988; McGeer, Shulzer, and McGeer 1996; Rogers 1997; McGeer and McGeer 2000; Veld et al. 2000). In sum, although the initial causes of pathology in VaD and DAT may be said to be different (i.e., plaque deposition in vessel walls in VaD and amyloid deposition in cerebral vascular walls, tangles, and plaques in DAT), a secondary process involving inflammation is common to both. Thus, we conclude that the role of inflammation is key to understanding the existence and nature of the spectrum of VaD and DAT.

Further evidence for common factors in the spectrum of vascular dementia and dementia of the Alzheimer type comes from recent research on the role of blood vessels in producing pathological changes in Alzheimer brain tissue (Miyakawa et al. 2000). It is well known that deposition of amyloid-β protein is a cardinal feature of DAT (see chap. 4). But only recently are mechanisms of amyloid-β production starting to be understood (see chap. 4). Recent data indicate that microvessels in Alzheimer brain are highly involved in deposition of amyloid-β protein found in Alzheimer brain tissue (Miyakawa et al. 2000). This research underscores the conceptualization of this chapter that VaD and DAT represent a spectrum with pathophysiologic processes common to both.

Other recent research, which relates to the data described above, focuses on the fact that cerebral capillary ultrastructure is significantly more damaged in patients with dementia of the Alzheimer type than in normal age-matched controls (Farkas et al. 2000). Based on these data, it has been suggested that decreased blood supply and cerebrovascular alterations contribute to DAT as they do to VaD (Farkas et al. 2000).

Converging with the studies described in the foregoing, a recent investigation of cerebrovascular pathology in Alzheimer syndrome found a high percentage of Alzheimer patients evidenced chronic ischemic white matter leukoaraiosis (Brown et al. 2000). The investigation found that the periventricular veins in a large number of Alzheimer patients were significantly occluded by multiple layers of collagen in vessel walls, and that such collagen deposition is especially excessive in leukoaraiosis lesions. The investigation also found severe loss of oligodendrocytes in leukoaraiosis lesions due to extensive apoptosis in Alzheimer patients (Brown et al. 2000).

Finally, another study found aberrant nitric oxide synthase-3 expression in cerebrovascular degeneration and vascular-mediated injury in dementia of the Alzheimer type (De La Monte et al. 2000). Nitric oxide is an important signaling molecule that is generated through catalytic activity of nitric oxide synthase: in the brain, nitric oxide mediates neuronal survival, synaptic plasticity, vascular smooth muscle relaxation, and endothelial cell permeability (De La Torre 1994; Pasquier and Leys 1997; De La Monte et al. 2000). Significant abnormalities were found in nitric oxide synthase-3 expression in DAT, which in turn contributed to diminished capacity to remove respiratory waste products and toxins from extracellular space due to reduced capillary permeability and cerebral hypoperfusion due to impaired vasodilation responses (De La Monte et al. 2000).

The foregoing demonstrates there is now evidence for common factors of pathophysiology in vascular dementia and dementia of the Alzheimer type. The common function of vascular factors in both VaD and DAT makes it clear that one should no longer view these two syndromes as separate, discrete homogeneous disease entities. Rather, VaD and DAT appear to represent two phenotypic presentations of the overarching class of dementia with numerous underlying vascular pathogenetic mechanisms in common.

Clinical Conclusions

One goal of this chapter has been to free the clinician from having to diagnostically "force" patients with long-standing histories of vascular problems into the Alzheimer category because of the lack of frank cerebral infarct. Rationally based treatment depends on integrity of diagnosis, and the placement of long-standing vascular patients into the Alzheimer category has often resulted in lack of treatment for vascular components of dementing disorder. We have argued that infarcts don't come out of nowhere and that preceding cerebral infarction is a *preinfarct state.* These vascular patients in a preinfarct condition are often nosologically forced into the Alzheimer category, where treatment for their vascular disorders is not in focus.

Vascular dementia has the characteristics of a syndrome and appears to be caused by a number of vascular disorders with several underlying mechanisms. Thus, to equate VaD with any single subtype is invalid. Accordingly, the classification of VaD should not be delimited by the infarct concept. There should be nosologic provision for the classification of *noninfarct vascular dementia:* vascular dementia caused by underlying vascular factors other than cerebral infarction (Emery, Gillie, and Randev 1995; Emery, Gillie, and Smith 1996, 2000). Vascular dementia is a broad, overarching category comprised of a number of subtypes. Our investigations suggest that one form of the subtype of noninfarct VaD is *alzheimerized VaD* (Emery, Gillie, and Smith 1996) at the interface of VaD and Alzheimer syndrome.

It has been a thesis of this chapter that vascular dementia and Alzheimer syndrome comprise a spectrum. Vascular factors involved in pathogenetic mechanisms of both VaD and Alzheimer syndrome have been discussed, including the roles of activated complement cascade and activated microglia as part of inflammation of brain tissue; deposition of amyloid-β protein by microvessels; and damaged cerebral capillary ultrastructure in both syndromes. Knowledge that inflammation crosscuts both VaD and Alzheimer syndrome is useful for its clinical application. For example, knowledge that nonsteroidal anti-inflammatory drugs greatly reduce incidence of disease at the Alzheimer end of the vascular-Alzheimer spectrum (McGeer, Shulzer, and McGeer 1996; McGeer and McGeer 2000) is useful for rationally based treatment of DAT. And, the use of aspirin in treatment of vascular disorders is well known. The conceptualization of VaD and Alzheimer syndrome as a spectrum is clinically useful because it brings into focus vascular factors in Alzheimer syndrome that are at least somewhat amenable to treatment but which have historically been left untreated. A spectrum perspective on VaD and Alzheimer syndrome results in a concomitant wider treatment spectrum; the possibilities for rationally based treatment of patients defined in the context of a vascular-Alzheimer spectrum are by definition immediately broader, more efficacious, and more hopeful than the treatment of these same patients defined dichotomously in the context of Alzheimer disease alone.

This chapter has focused on the ambiguous transition underlying the distinction of focal versus diffuse or generalized cerebral dysfunction. We have pointed to nosologic, empiric, and clinical problems that come into existence in and around this ambiguous transition, but it has also been suggested that this very ambiguous transition opens up possibilities for improved diagnostics and clinical treatments when bridged by a spectrum approach to these dementias.

REFERENCES

Aguero-Torres, H., and B. Winblad. 2000. Alzheimer's disease and vascular dementia: Some points of confluence. *Annals of the New York Academy of Sciences* 903:547–52.

Akiyama, H., and P.L. McGeer. 1990. Brain microglia constitutively express b2 integrins. *Journal of Neuroimmunology* 30:81–93.

American Psychiatric Association. 1952. *Diagnostic and Statistical Manual of Mental Disorders*. Washington, D.C.: American Psychiatric Association.

American Psychiatric Association. 1968. *Diagnostic and Statistical Manual of Mental Disorders*. 2nd ed. Washington, D.C.: American Psychiatric Association.

American Psychiatric Association. 1980. *Diagnostic and Statistical Manual of Mental Disorders*. 3rd ed. Washington, D.C.: American Psychiatric Association.

American Psychiatric Association. 1987. *Diagnostic and Statistical Manual of Mental Disorders*. 3rd ed., revised. Washington, D.C.: American Psychiatric Association.

American Psychiatric Association. 1994. *Diagnostic and Statistical Manual of Mental Disorders*. 4th ed. Washington, D.C.: American Psychiatric Association.

American Psychiatric Association. 2000. *Diagnostic and Statistical Manual of Mental Disorders*. 4th ed., text revision. Washington, D.C.: American Psychiatric Association.

Auer, D., B. Putz, C. Gossl, et al. 2001. Differential lesion patterns in Cadasil and sporadic subcortical arteriosclerotic encephalopathy: MR imaging study with statistical parametric group comparison. *Radiology* 218:443–51.

Bayles, K., and A. Kasnziak. 1987. *Communication and Cognition in Normal Aging and Dementia*. Boston: College Hill Press.

Blalock, H. 1972. *Social Statistics*. New York: McGraw-Hill.

Bowen, B., W. Barker, D. Loewenstein, et al. 1990. MR signal abnormalities in memory disorder and dementia. *American Journal of Neuroradiology* 11:283–90.

Brown, W., D. Moody, C. Thore, et al. 2000. Cerebrovascular pathology in Alzheimer's disease and leukoaraiosis. *Annals of the New York Academy of Sciences* 903:39–45.

Brun, A., and E. Englund. 1986. A white matter disorder in dementia of the Alzheimer type: A pathoanatomical study. *Annals of Neurology* 19:253–62.

Campbell, D., and J. Stanley. 1969. *Experimental and Quasi-Experimental Designs for Research*. Chicago: Rand McNally.

De La Monte, S., Y. Sohn, D. Etienne, et al. 2000. Role of aberrant nitric oxide synthase-3 expression in cerebrovascular degeneration and vascular mediated injury in Alzheimer's disease. *Annals of the New York Academy of Sciences* 903:61–71.

De La Torre, J. 1994. Impaired brain microcirculation may trigger Alzheimer's disease. *Neuroscience Biobehavior Review* 18:397–401.

Diaz R., V. Hachinski, H. Merskey, et al. 1991. Leukoaraiosis and cognitive impairment in Alzheimer's disease. In *Alzheimer's Disease: Basic Mechanisms, Diagnosis, and Therapeutic Strategies*, edited by K. Iqbal, D. McLachlan, B. Winblad, et al. New York: John Wiley, pp. 9–11.

Emery, V.O.B. 1985. Language and aging. *Experimental Aging Research Monograph* Series 11 (1).

Emery, V.O.B. 1986. Linguistic decrement in normal aging. *Language and Communication* 6:47–62.

Emery, V.O.B. 1988. *Pseudodementia: A Theoretical and Empirical Discussion.* Cleveland: Case Western Reserve University School of Medicine.

Emery, V.O.B. 1992. Interaction of language and memory in major depression and senile dementia of Alzheimer's type. In *Memory Functioning in Dementia*, edited by L. Backman. Amsterdam: Elsevier, pp. 175–204.

Emery, V.O.B. 1993. Language and memory processing in senile dementia Alzheimer's type. In *Language, Memory and Aging*, edited by L. Light and D. Burke. New York: Cambridge University Press, pp. 221–43.

Emery, V.O.B. 1996. Language functioning. In *The Cognitive Neuropsychology of Alzheimer-type Dementia*, edited by R. Morris. Oxford: Oxford University Press, pp. 166–93.

Emery, V.O.B. 1999. On the relationship between memory and language in the dementia spectrum of depression, Alzheimer syndrome, and normal aging. In *Language and Communication in Old Age: Multidisciplinary Perspectives*, edited by H. Hamilton. New York: Garland Publishing, pp. 25–62.

Emery, V.O.B. 2000. Language impairment in dementia of the Alzheimer type: A hierarchical decline? *International Journal of Psychiatry in Medicine* 30:145–64.

Emery, V.O.B., and L. Breslau. 1988. The problem of naming in SDAT: A relative deficit. *Experimental Aging Research* 14:181–93.

Emery, V.O.B., and L. Breslau. 1989. Language deficits in depression: Comparisons with SDAT and normal aging. *Journal of Gerontology* 44:85–92.

Emery, V.O.B., and E.X. Gillie. 1999. The interface between vascular dementia and Alzheimer syndrome. *Alzheimers Report* 2:22–23.

Emery, V.O.B., E.X. Gille, and P. Ramdev. 1994. Vascular dementia redefined. In *Dementia: Presentations, Differential Diagnosis, and Nosology*, edited by V.O.B. Emery and T.E. Oxman. Baltimore: Johns Hopkins University Press, pp. 162–94.

Emery, V.O.B., E.X. Gille, and P. Ramdev. 1995. Noninfarct vascular dementia. In *Treating Alzheimer's and Other Dementias*, edited by M. Bergener and S. Finkel. New York: Springer, pp. 184–203.

Emery, V.O.B., E.X. Gille, and P. Ramdev. 1996. Noninfarct vascular dementia: A new subtype of dementing disorder. *Journal of Clinical Geropsychology* 2:197–213.

Emery, V.O.B., E.X. Gille, and J. Smith. 1996. Reclassification of the vascular dementias: Comparisons of infarct and noninfarct vascular dementias. *International Psychogeriatrics* 8:33–61.

Emery, V.O.B., E.X. Gille, and J. Smith. 2000. Interface between vascular dementia and

Alzheimer syndrome: Nosologic redefinition. *Annals of the New York Academy of Sciences* 903:229–38.

Emery, V.O.B., and T.E. Oxman. 1997. Depressive dementia: A 'transitional dementia'? *Clinical Neuroscience* 4:23–30.

Erkinjuntti, T. 1987. Types of multi-infarct dementia. *Acta Neurologica Scandinavica* 75:391–99.

Erkinjuntti, T. 1997. Vascular dementia: Challenge of clinical diagnosis. *International Psychogeriatrics* 9:51–58.

Erkinjuntti, T., D. Inzitari, L. Pantoni, et al. 2000. Research criteria for subcortical vascular dementia in clinical trials. *Journal of Neural Transmission* 59:23–30.

Farkas, E., G. DeJong, E. Apro, et al. 2000. Similar ultrastructural breakdown of cerebrocortical capillaries in Alzheimer's disease, Parkinson's disease, and experimental hypertension. *Annals of the New York Academy of Sciences* 903:72–82.

Feldman, H., and A. Kertesz. 2001. Diagnosis, classification, and natural history of degenerative dementias. *Canadian Journal of Neurological Sciences* 28:17–27.

Fisher, C.M. 1968. Dementia in cerebrovascular disease. In *Cerebral Vascular Disease*, edited by J. Toole, R. Sickert, and J. Whisnant. New York: Grune and Stratton, pp. 232–36.

Folstein, M., S. Folstein, and P.R. McHugh. 1975. "Mini-Mental State": A practical method for grading the mental state of patients for the clinician. *Journal of Psychiatry Research* 12:189–98.

Gauthier, S., and S. Ferris. 2001. Outcome measures for probable vascular dementia and Alzheimer's disease with cerebrovascular disease. *International Journal of Clinical Practice* 120:29–39.

Hachinski, V.C. 1983. Multi-infarct dementia. *Neurologic Clinics* 1:27–36.

Hachinski, V.C., N. Lassen, and J. Marshall. 1974. Multi-infarct dementia: A cause of mental deterioration in the elderly. *Lancet* ii:207–10.

Hachinski, V.C., L. Iliff, M. Phil, et al. 1975. Cerebral blood flow in dementia. *Archives of Neurology* 32:632–37.

Huck, G., and A. Ojeda. 1987. *Syntax and Semantics*. San Diego: Academic Press.

Johnson, R.J. 1997. What mediates progressive glomerulosclerosis? The glomerular endothelium comes of age. *American Journal of Pathology* 151:1179–81.

Kaplan, E., H. Goodglass, and S. Weintraub. 1983. *Boston Naming Test*. Philadelphia: Lea and Febiger.

Kertesz, A. 1982. *Western Aphasia Battery*. New York: Grune and Stratton.

Kertesz, A. 1994. Language deterioration in dementia. In *Dementia: Presentations, Differential Diagnosis, and Nosology*, edited by V.O.B. Emery and T.E. Oxman. Baltimore: Johns Hopkins University Press, pp. 123–38.

Kertesz, A., K. Bayles, and H. Kirshner. 1991. Language in dementia. *Journal of Clinical and Experimental Neuropsychology* 13:79–81.

Kontiola, P., R. Laaksonen, R. Sulkava, et al. 1990. Pattern of language impairment is different in Alzheimer's disease and multi-infarct dementia. *Brain and Language* 38:364–83.

Lobo, A., L. Launer, L. Fratiglioni, et al. 2000. Prevalence of dementia and major subtypes in Europe: A collaborative study of population-based cohorts. *Neurology* 54 (Suppl. 5):S4–9.

Lukacs, N.W., and P. Ward. 1996. Inflammatory mediators, cytokines, and adhesion molecules in pulmonary inflammation and injury. *Advance in Immunology* 62:257–304.

Luria, A. 1980. *Higher Cortical Functions in Man.* New York: Basic Books.

Lyketsos, C., M. Steinberg, J. Tschanz, et al. 2000. Mental and behavioral disturbances in dementia: Findings from the Cache County Study on Memory in Aging. *American Journal of Psychiatry* 157:708–14.

Mahler, M.E., and J.L. Cummings. 1991. The behavioral neurology of multi-infact dementia. *Alzheimer Disease and Related Disorders* 5:122–30.

Mattis, S. 1988. *Dementia Rating Scale Professional Manual.* Odessa, Fla.: Psychological Assessment Resources.

Mayer-Gross, W., E. Slater, and M. Roth. 1960. *Clinical Psychiatry.* 2nd ed. London: Bailliere, Tindall, and Cassell.

McGeer, P.L., H. Akiyama, S. Itagaki, et al. 1989. Immune system response in Alzheimer's disease. *Canadian Journal of Neurological Science* 16:516–27.

McGeer, P.L., and E.G. McGeer. 2000. Autotoxicity and Alzheimer disease. *Archives of Neurology* 57:789–90.

McGeer, P.L., and E.G. McGeer. In press. Polymorphisms in inflammatory genes enhance the risk of Alzheimer disease. *Archives of Neurology.*

McGeer, P.L., M. Schulzer, and E.G. McGeer. 1996. Arthritis and antiinflammatory agents as possible protective factors for Alzheimer's disease: A review of 17 epidemiological studies. *Neurology* 47:425–32.

McKhann, G., D. Drachman, M. Folstein, et al. 1984. Clinical diagnosis of Alzheimer's disease. *Neurology* 34:939–44.

Miyakawa, T., T. Kimura, S. Hirata, et al. 2000. Role of blood vessels in producing pathological changes in the brain with Alzheimer's disease. *Annals of the New York Academy of Sciences* 903:46–54.

National Institute of Neurological and Communicative Disorders and Stroke. 1975. A classification and outline of cerebrovascular disease II. *Stroke* 6:564–616.

Niederehe, G., and T.E. Oxman. 1994. The dementias: Construct and nosologic validity. In *Dementia: Presentations, Differential Diagnosis, and Nosology,* edited by V.O.B. Emery and T.E. Oxman. Baltimore: Johns Hopkins University Press, pp. 19–46.

Nunnally, J.C. 1967. *Psychometric Theory.* New York: McGraw-Hill.

Parnetti, L. 1999. Pathophysiology of vascular dementia and white matter changes. *Revue Neurologique* 155:754–58.

Pasquier, F., and D. Leys. 1997. Why are stroke patients prone to develop dementia? *Journal of Neurology* 244:135–42.

Pohjasvaara, T., R. Mantyla, R. Ylikoski, et al. 2000. Comparison of different clinical criteria for the diagnosis of vascular dementia. *Stroke* 31:2952–57.

Reisberg, B., S. Ferris, M. deLeon, et al. 1985. Age-associated cognitive decline and Alzheimer's disease: Implications for assessment and treatment. In *Thresholds in Aging,* edited by M. Bergener, J. Ermini, and H. Stahelin. London: Academic Press, pp. 255–92.

Reisberg, B., S. Ferris, J. Borenstein, et al. 1986. Assessment of presenting symptoms. In *Handbook for Clinical Memory Assessment of Older Adults,* edited by L. Poon. Washington, D.C.: American Psychological Association, pp. 108–38.

Reisberg, B., A. Burns, H. Brodaty, et al. 1997. Diagnosis of Alzheimer's disease. *International Psychogeriatrics* 9:11–38.

Rockwood, K., K. Howard, C. MacKnight, et al. 1999. Spectrum of disease in vascular cognitive impairment. *Neuroepidemiology* 18:248–54.

Rogers, J. 1997. Anti-inflammatory approaches to the treatment of Alzheimer's disease. In *Postgraduate Dementia Course: Heterogeneity of Alzheimer's Disease*, edited by Excerpta Medica Medical Communications. Amsterdam: Excerpta Medica, pp. 32–33.

Rogers, J., J. Luber-Narod, S.D. Styren, et al. 1988. Expression of immune-system associated antigens by cells of the human central nervous system: Relationship to the pathology of Alzheimer's disease. *Neurobiology of Aging* 9:339–49.

Roman, G.C. 1987. Senile dementia of the Binswanger type: A vascular form of dementia in the elderly. *Journal of the American Medical Association* 258:1782–88.

Roman, G.C., T. Tatemichi, T. Erkinjuntti, et al. 1993. Vascular dementia: Diagnostic criteria for research studies. Report of the NINDS-AIREN International Workshop. *Neurology* 43:250–60.

Rosen, W., R. Mohs, and K. Davis. 1986. Longitudinal changes: Cognitive, behavioral, and affective patterns in Alzheimer's disease. In *Clinical Memory Assessment of Older Adults*, edited by L. Poon. Washington, D.C.: American Psychological Association, pp. 294–301.

Ross, R. 1993a. Atherosclerosis: A defense mechanism gone awry. *American Journal of Pathology* 143:987–1002.

Ross, R. 1993b. The pathogenesis of atherosclerosis. *Nature* 362:801–9.

Ross, R. 1999. Mechanisms of disease: Atherosclerosis: an inflammatory disease. *New England Journal of Medicine* 340:115–26.

Seno, H., H. Ishino, T. Inagaki, et al. 2000. Comparison between multiple lacunar infarcted patients with and without dementia in nursing homes in Shimane Prefecture, Japan. *Dementia and Geriatric Cognitive Disorders* 11:161–65.

Slater, E., and M. Roth. 1969. *Clinical Psychiatry*. 3rd ed. London: Bailliere, Tindall, and Cassell.

Snowdon, D. 2001. *Aging with Grace*. New York: Bantam Books.

Statistical Analysis Systems Institute. 1982. *Statistical Analysis System: User's Guide*. Cary, N.C.: Statistical Analysis Systems Institute.

Stedman, T.L. 1990. *Stedman's Medical Dictionary*. Baltimore: Williams & Wilkins.

Suh, G., and A. Shah. 2001. A review of the epidemiological transition in dementia: Cross-national comparisons of the indices related to Alzheimer's disease and vascular dementia. *Acta Psychiatrica Scandinavica* 104:4–11.

Tanur, J., F. Mosteller, W. Kruskal, et al. 1985. *Statistics: A Guide to the Unknown*. Monterey, Calif.: Wadsworth and Brooks/Cole.

Tormey, V., J. Faul, C. Leonard, et al. 1997. T-cell cytokines may control the balance of functionally distinct macrophage populations. *Immunology* 90:463–69.

Valentine, A., I. Moseley, and B. Kendall. 1980. White matter abnormality in cerebral atrophy: Clinicoradiological correlations. *Journal of Neurology, Neurosurgery, and Psychiatry* 43:139–42.

Veld, B.A.I., A. Ruitenberg, L. Launer, et al. 2000. Duration of non-steroidal anti-inflammatory drug use and risk of Alzheimer's disease: The Rotterdam Study. *Neurobiology of Aging* 21 (Suppl. 3):S204.

Wade, J., and V.C. Hachinski. 1987. Multi-infarct dementia. In *Dementia*, edited by B. Pitt. London: Churchill Livingstone, pp. 209–28.

Wallin, A., K. Blennow, and C.G. Gottfries. 1990. Subcortical symptoms predominate in vascular dementia. *International Journal of Geriatric Psychiatry* 5:1–9.

Wallin, A., K. Blennow, C. Uhlemann, et al. 1989. White matter low attenuation on computed tomography in Alzheimer's disease and vascular dementia: Diagnosis and pathogenetic aspects. *Acta Neurologica Scandinavica* 80:518–23.

World Health Organization. 1992. *The ICD-10 Classification of Mental and Behavioral Disorders: Clinical Descriptions and Diagnostic Guidelines.* Geneva: World Health Organization.

World Health Organization. 1993. *The ICD-10 Classification of Mental and Behavioral Disorders: Diagnostic Criteria for Research.* Geneva: World Health Organization.

CHAPTER ELEVEN

The Relationship of Hypertension to Vascular Dementia

Shotai Kobayashi, M.D., Ph.D., FAJSIM, FACP, FRCP

Vascular dementia (VaD) may arise as a sequel to any form of cerebrovascular disease, but it is more likely to occur in the context of recurring bilateral events (e.g., cardiac embolism) or as the result of widespread small vessel disease (e.g., hypertensive arteriopathy).

The most common form of vascular dementia appears to be multilacunar dementia. Meyer and associates (1988) reported the incidence of multilacunar dementia was 43%, followed by multiple bilateral cerebral embolization (30%) and abnormal perfusion due to severe extracranial and intracranial occlusive disease (26%) in 173 patients with VaD. Dementia due to severe, diffuse white matter lesions caused by arteriosclerosis of medullary arteries (subcortical arteriosclerotic encephalopathy, or Binswanger type) is also an important, associated form of VaD (Goto, Ishii, and Fukasawa 1981; Babikian and Ropper 1987). Moreover, multilacunar infarction is usually part of Binswanger disease. Vascular dementia of Binswanger type may represent the end-stage pathology of lacunar state (Pantoni, Rossi, and Garcia 1995). Therefore, a significant number of so-called multilacunar cases of dementia may overlap with VaD of Binswanger type.

It is well known that lacunar infarction is closely related to hypertensive small artery disease. Fisher (1969) described hypertensive vasculopathy, which produces almost the same type of hypertensive hemorrhage as found in 90% of lacunar infarctions. In one magnetic resonance imaging (MRI) study, 88% of the patients with hypertensive hemorrhage had silent lacunar infarction (Okada et al. 1997). Although some authors have suggested that hypertension is not a specific risk factor for lacunar infarction (Lodder et al. 1990), it is generally agreed that hypertension is a major risk factor for multilacunar type of VaD. Clinical and pathological studies of VaD have provided evidence that hypertension is a main risk factor (Clair and Whalley 1983; Meyer et al. 1988; Furuta et al. 1991).

However, the multilacunar state alone does not often cause dementia. Diffuse subcortical white matter lesions have been reported to be significantly associated with both multilacunar dementia and with Binswanger disease (BD). A study by Goto, Ishii, and Fukasawa (1981) found that most cases of severe VaD are associated with diffuse white matter lesions (diffuse demyelination with multiple lacunar state). Goto, Ishii, and Fukasawa concluded that subcortical arteriosclerotic encephalopathy was a common pathology found in VaD. Tomonaga and associates (1980) emphasized that progressive subcortical vascular encephalopathy, which is similar to subcortical arteriosclerotic encephalopathy, is common in elderly persons; progressive subcortical vascular encephalopathy was found in 3.8% of 1000 serial autopsied brains of elderly patients from Tokyo Metropolitan Geriatric Hospital.

Binswanger original cases showed prominent white matter lesions, especially in the occipital lobe (Babikian and Ropper 1987). However, Furuta and colleagues (1991) reported hypertensive arteriosclerotic changes of medullary arteries existed more often in frontal subcortical white matter. Based on an examination of 500 autopsied patients with cerebrovascular diseases, Kameyama (1973) reported that 60% of elderly vascular patients with prefrontal white matter lesions had dementia, whereas 27% without such lesions had dementia. Thus, a strong association between VaD and diffuse prefrontal white matter lesions (association area) appears to exist. These data are compatible with the finding that most patients with progressive subcortical vascular encephalopathy or multiple infarction show evidence of frontal dementia and reduction of frontal lobe cerebral blood flow as measured by positron emission tomography (PET) (Yao et al. 1990).

Although vascular dementia is the second major cause of dementing illness in elderly people, the prevalence of vascular dementia is lower than that of dementia of the Alzheimer type (DAT) in Europe and in the United States. In contrast, Japanese epidemiological and clinicopathological studies have shown that VaD is the most common cause of dementia in Japanese elderly patients (VaD: DAT = 3:2) (Karasawa 1989). The prevalence rate of dementia among Hisayama residents age 65 or older was estimated at 6.7%. Among fifty cases of dementia in which brain morphology was examined, the frequency of VaD was 56%; this rate was 2.2 times higher than that for DAT (Ueda et al. 1992). The cause of this difference is not known, but it may be related to the higher incidence of small cerebral vessel disease in Japanese who are living in Japan than for those living elsewhere, which was a finding of the Hawaii–Japan study (Reed et al. 1994).

Leukoaraiosis (a term used to describe white matter changes seen on computed tomography [CT] or MRI) (Hachinski, Potter, and Mersky 1987) is observed frequently in the elderly population without any neurological symptoms. However, whether leukoaraiosis is related to mental functions remains controversial (Hunt et al. 1989; Junque et al. 1990). Nevertheless, leukoaraiosis is clearly related to cerebrovascular disease, hypertension, and age (Inzitari et al. 1987). Overall, the data suggest that leukoaraiosis is far more severe in persons with VaD than in normal elderly people. Thus, the severe form of leukoaraiosis may be associated with decline of mental functions.

In the presence of leukoaraiosis, regional cerebral blood flow as measured by Xenon-computed tomography demonstrates a 50% decrease in normal white matter both in clinically asymptomatic elderly people and in patients with vascular dementia (Kawamura et al. 1991). This finding suggests that leukoaraiosis may be a consequence of either low perfusion or incomplete white matter infarction.

Fazekas and colleagues (1988) emphasized that extracranial vascular disease was more highly associated with white matter lesions than was hypertension in normal subjects. Herholz et al. (1990), however, found no correlation between severity of extracranial carotid artery disease and white matter lesions.

Clinicopathological studies have shown that small, silent white matter lesions, especially nonconfluent patchy lesions recognized on T2 weighted images of magnetic resonance imaging, rarely correspond to lacunar infarction in asymptomatic elderly people. These lesions are considered to be related to age and hypertension (e.g., Awad et al. 1986). Diffuse, confluent white matter lesions, however, have been attributed to diffuse white matter demyelination secondary to a lacunar state (Révész et al. 1989). Hypertension has been the most significant risk factor for confluent white matter lesions as well as for lacunar infarction.

Blood Pressure and Vascular Dementia

Binswanger disease is characterized pathologically by severe white matter changes with multiple lacunes due to advanced arteriosclerosis in medullary arteries that irrigate deep white matter (Babikian and Ropper 1987). The pathogenesis of this disease appears to be related to persistent hypertension. A review of data relating to Binswanger disease (Babikian and Ropper 1987) showed that most reported cases (thirty-nine of forty-one) had severe hypertension; only one patient with Binswanger disease had normal blood pressure.

Prototypical Binswanger disease seems to be relatively rare, but it has been suggested that the disease has clinicopathological features similar to multiinfarct dementia (Goto, Ishii, and Fukasawa 1981). Goto, Ishii, and Fukasawa (1981) investigated clinicopathological correlates of severe cases of VaD associated with diffuse white matter lesions, and concluded that subcortical arteriosclerotic encephalopathy may occur in most cases of multilacunar dementia.

To determine the pathophysiological mechanisms associated with white matter lesions, Furuta et al. (1991) examined sclerotic changes of the medullary arteries (small arteries and arterioles) in 110 non-neuropsychiatric patients, 20 patients with subcortical arteriosclerotic encephalopathy and Binswanger disease, and 20 patients with dementia of the Alzheimer type. Furuta et al. found that arteriosclerotic changes increased with age, but were significantly more prominent in patients with subcortical arteriosclerotic encephalopathy and Binswanger disease than in control subjects or in patients with DAT. Arteriosclerotic rate correlated significantly with severity of diffuse ischemic white matter changes, as well as with blood pressure.

A clinical study of blood pressure in 27 patients with multiinfarct dementia, 46 patients with dementia of the Alzheimer type, and 16 patients with mixed-type dementia found that no patients with multiinfarct dementia alone had a systolic blood pressure below 140 mmHg, whereas 26 patients from the other groups had a systolic pressure below 140 mmHg (Clair and Whalley 1983). This cutoff point for blood pressure is lower than the World Health Organization criteria for hypertension. However, an epidemiological study by Ueda et al. (1988) showed that the prevalence of stroke is higher for patients with borderline hypertension, as well as for definitive hypertensives. The average annual incidence of cerebral infarction is 9.2 in subjects with diastolic hypertension, 4.1 in those with borderline hypertension, and 1.9 in normotensive subjects (Ueda et al. 1988). These data suggest that even mild hypertension might be a significant risk factor for multiinfarct dementia. The Honolulu–Asia aging study showed that the risk for dementia was 4.8 (confidence interval: 2.0–11.0) in those with systolic blood pressure 160 mmHg and higher compared to those with systolic blood pressure of 110 to 139 mmHg during midlife. This study suggests elevated levels of blood pressure in middle age can increase the risk for late-age dementia in persons never treated with antihypertensive medication (Launer et al. 2000). These data suggest that hypertension might be the most important risk factor for VaD.

Blood Pressure and Leukoaraiosis in Cerebral Infarction

Bougouslavsky, Regli, and Uske (1987) reported that in a large sample of 1000 consecutive ischemic stroke patients confirmed by computed tomography, leukoencephalopathy was observed with greater frequency following deep infarcts (8%) than cortical infarcts (0.8%). Eighty-four percent of these ischemic stroke patients had mental impairment; hypertension was the most significant risk factor for leukoencephalopathy. Kozachuk and associates (1990) found no difference in severity of leukoaraiosis between normotensive elderly control patients and patients with DAT without risk factors for stroke. However, systolic blood pressure correlated with severity of leukoaraiosis only in elderly control subjects. This investigation suggests that blood pressure is significantly associated with leukoaraiosis even in normotensive elderly people.

We investigated the relationships between white matter changes, brain atrophy, mental function, blood pressure, and cerebral blood flow in a group of patients with cerebral infarction, then compared them to patients with dementia of the Alzheimer type (Kobayashi, Okada, and Yamashita 1991). The study consisted of 34 patients with multiple lacunar cerebral infarction with an age range of 52 to 84 years. Twenty patients did not have dementia (mean age, 70 years), and 14 patients had dementia (mean age, 71 years). The Alzheimer sample consisted of 13 patients (age range, 53–84 years; mean age, 71 years). White matter changes were evaluated on absolute T1-weighted images and T2-weighted images using 0.15T magnetic resonance imaging. Brain areas exceeding 400 milliseconds of T1 value were defined as white matter lesions (Fukuda et al. 1990). The maximum distance of the brain area from the ventricle (white matter lesion index, WMLI) was measured in frontal, central, and posterior regions on CT scan. Brain atrophy index (percentage of brain parenchymal area divided by intracranial area) was also calculated by digitizer. The regional cerebral blood flow was measured by 133Xe inhalation method. Mental function was evaluated using Hasegawa Dementia Rating Scale for Japanese aged people (full scale score, 32.5) (Hasegawa 1983). This scale consists of items similar to the MMSE, except for figure copying.

Patients with dementia and multilacunar cerebral infarction showed a significantly greater total white matter lesion index than did patients with multilacunar cerebral infarction but no dementia and patients with dementia of the Alzheimer type ($p < 0.001$). Scores in the study by Hasegawa (1983) significantly correlated with bilateral frontal (right, $r = -0.7$; left, $r = -0.79$) and total WMLI ($r = -0.66$, $p < 0.001$) only in patients with multilacunar cerebral infarction (fig. 11.1).

Mean regional cerebral blood flow correlated inversely with total white matter lesion index in patients with multilacunar cerebral infarction ($r = -0.496$, $p < 0.02$) but not in patients with dementia of the Alzheimer type ($r = -0.1$). There was a strong correlation ($r = 0.79$, $p < 0.001$) between age and WMLI in DAT but not in patients with multilacunar cerebral infarction. Brain atrophy index correlated with WMLI in the both groups. Mean arterial blood pressure (both systolic and diastolic) during several months preceding MRI significantly correlated with WMLI only in patients with multilacunar cerebral infarction ($r = 0.65$, $p < 0.005$) (fig. 11.1B).

Other risk factors for stroke, such as diabetes mellitus, hyperlipidemia, smoking, ischemic change of electrocardiogram, and so on did not significantly correlate with white matter lesion index. These results indicate that cerebral white matter changes may contribute to the cause of dementia in multiple lacunar cerebral infarction, and persistent hypertension may be the most important risk factor. This study also suggests that the pathophysiological mechanism leading to white matter changes may be different in multiple lacunar cerebral infarct dementia and Alzheimer disease.

Brun and Englund (1986) studied the relationship between blood pressure and white matter changes in autopsied patients with Alzheimer disease. Their results showed that white matter changes in Alzheimer disease related both to hyaline vascular stenosis without hypertensive vasculopathy and to cardiovascular disorders associated with hypotension.

Variation of blood pressure is also thought to play an important role in white matter lesions. Cerebral circulation is maintained by the cerebral vascular au-

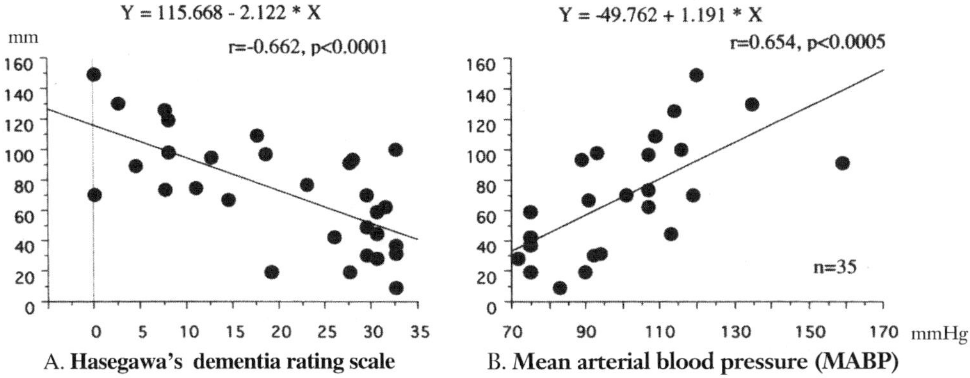

Figure 11.1. A: Severity of white matter lesion (WMLI) negatively correlated with mental function (Hasegawa's dementia rating scale) in the patients with multilacunar infarction. *B*: Severity of WMLI positively correlated with mean arterial blood pressure in the patients with multilacunar infarction.

toregulatory system in normal subjects, but both the lower and upper limits of autoregulation are shifted to the higher levels in patients with hypertension as compared with normotensive persons (Strandgaard 1978).

Based on a study of 13 of 28 pathologically proven cases of vascular dementia, Brun and Englund (1986) suggested that white matter disorder was related to hypertensive arteriopathy and long-standing or episodic hypotension associated with cardiovascular disorders. MaQuinn and O'Leary (1987) found that 10 of 11 patients (4 with dementia) with white matter lucencies on CT scan had disordered blood pressure regulation with hypertension, labile systolic blood pressure, or orthostatic hypotension. Tohgi, Chiba, and Kimura (1991) reported that hypertension, short-term variations in blood pressure, and sustained nighttime elevation of blood pressure were important for the pathogenesis of both Binswanger-type and lacunar-type dementia. These conclusions were based on data from 24-hour recordings of blood pressure in 35 patients with Binswanger-type dementia and 43 patients with lacunar-type dementia. We examined cerebral blood flow autoregulation during the tilt-up loading using infra-red spectroscopy attached frontal head in the patients with VaD of Binswanger type. Mild but significant impairment of autoregulation was observed in these patients compared to those with lacunar infarction without leukoaraioasis (Shirasawa et al. 2000). These research results suggest blood pressure disregulation based on hypertension may be one of the critical factors in the etiology of VaD.

Although hypertension is the most common risk factor for vascular dementia, especially for Binswanger type, some patients have no history of hypertension. Vinters (1987) suggested that amyloid angiopathy was frequently found in Binswanger-type dementia. Tomonaga, Chiba, and Kimura (1981) demonstrated a high frequency of amyloid angiopathy in the brains of elderly patients. It is well known that most patients with DAT have amyloid deposition in cerebral vascular walls. This amyloid is β-protein (Glenner and Wong 1984), and this type of amyloid angiopathy rarely causes cerebrovascular disorders. On the other hand, hereditary amyloid angiopathy with cystatin C deposition has been found to be associated with recurrent cerebral hemorrhage (Grubb et al. 1984). We reported a dementia case with multiple hemorrhage caused by cystatin C amyloid angiopathy (Fujihara et al. 1989). We also experienced a sporadic case of VaD of Binswanger type with cystatin C amyloid angiopathy (Shimode et al. 1996). The cystatin C amyloid is thought to be more harmful to cerebral arteries than β-amyloid protein. This type of amyloid angiopathy might cause not only vascular stenosis but also impairment of cerebrovascular autoregulation. Amyloid angiopathy must be recognized as one cause of VaD, especially in normotensive elderly patients. Recently, hereditary VaD with leukoencephalopathy similar to Binswanger type was recognized as cerebral autosomal dominant arteriopathy with subcortical infarcts and leukoencephalopathy (CADASIL) due to Notch 3 gene mutation (Joutel et al. 2000).

Hypertension and Silent Lacunar Lesions: Leukoaraiosis in Normal Adults

Lechner et al. (1988) reported that the frequency of white matter lesions on magnetic resonance imaging significantly increased based on the number of risk factors for stroke in neurologically normal subjects. Patients with a single risk factor had a 32% frequency of white matter lesions, and patients with two factors had a 92% frequency. Patients with three or more risk factors had a 100% frequency of white matter lesions. The prevalence of hypertension was 9%, 69.2%, and 100%, respectively.

We studied the incidence of silent subcortical brain infarction and leukoaraiosis by magnetic resonance imaging and its relation to risk factors in 1522 neurologically normal adults (mean age, 57 years) who received health checkups of the brain (Kobayashi, Okada, and Yamashita 1991; Kobayashi et al. 1997; Kobayashi 2001). Incidence of possible silent subcortical brain infarction was 15.6% and that of leukoaraiosis was 7% in all subjects, but these incidences

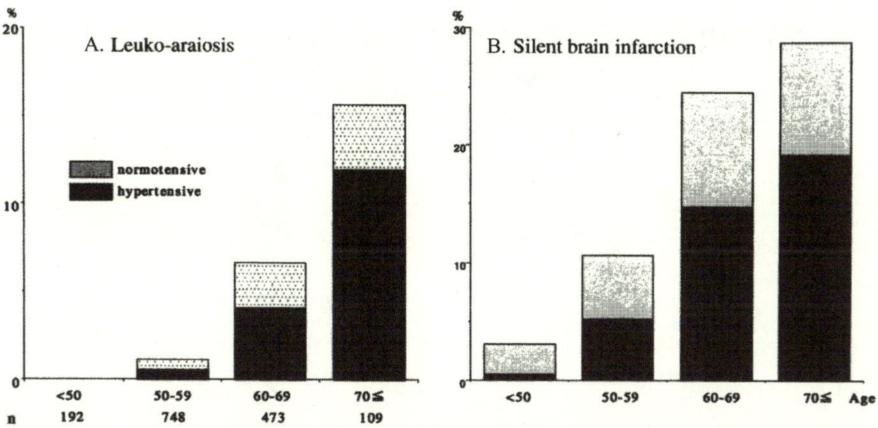

Figure 11.2. Incidence of leukoaraiosis (*A*) and silent subcortical infarction (SSBI; *B*) in the neurologically normal subjects who received our brain health check-up. Both incidences increased with aging. There is significantly higher incidence of hypertension in the subjects with leukoaraiosis or SSBI than in those without.

were significantly increased with aging. And hypertension was the most important risk factor for silent ischemic lesions (fig. 11.2).

We are continuing the health check-ups of the brain, and have been conducting a prospective study since 1988, now using magnetic resonance imaging. Annual incidence of stroke was 2.8% in the subjects with silent subcortical brain infarction. It was significantly higher than in subjects without silent subcortical brain infarction. Our results showed that leukoaraiosis and silent subcortical brain infarction were highly significant risk factors for symptomatic stroke (OR:10.6, CI: 5.0–22.3 and 8.8, 4.8–16.4, respectively). Hypertension was the most significant risk factor for silent subcortical brain infarction (OR: 4.1, CI: 3.1–5.5). But for leukoaraiosis, aging was the strongest risk factor, and hypertension was the second one (OR: 10.5, CI: 4.9–22.3 and 4.8, 2.7–8.4). The subjects with silent subcortical brain infarction complicated hypertension showed significantly higher incidence of stroke than those without hypertension (fig. 11.3).

These results suggest that the essential mechanism of these two phenomena involved a common basic pathological process caused by small artery disease, but leukoaraiosis represents more complex features, including the aging process.

Our longitudinal investigation of risk factors for impaired mental function in normal elderly persons showed that subjects who had worsened magnetic reso-

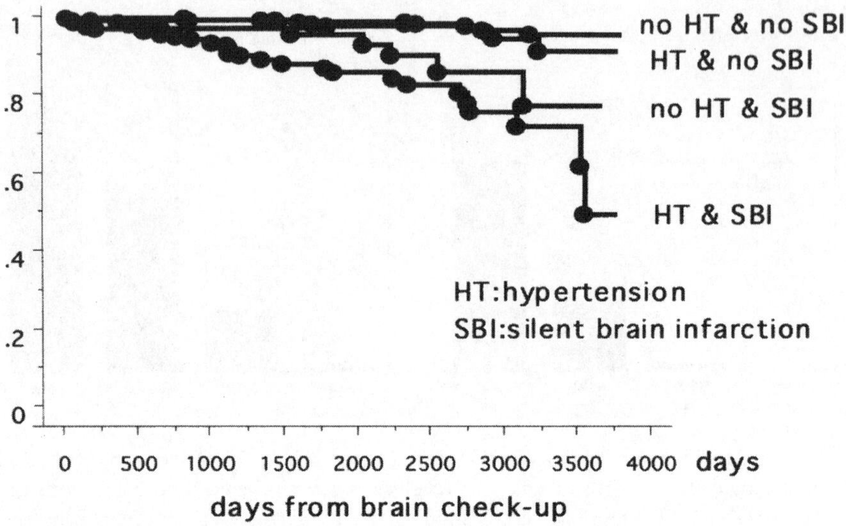

Figure 11.3. The incidence of stroke onset in the normal subjects who received our brain health check-up. Kaplan-Meier life table analysis revealed significantly higher incidence of stroke in the hypertensive subjects with SSBI than in those without.

nance imaging findings after six-year follow-up had declined mental function and their systolic blood pressure was elevated significantly (Yamaguchi et al. 1996). These results suggest that hypertension is one of the most important risk factors for mental decline caused by small artery disease, especially in elderly persons.

Effect of Antihypertensive Therapy in Vascular Dementia

Large controlled epidemiological studies have demonstrated that the incidence of stroke is significantly reduced by antihypertensive therapy (Hypertension Detection and Follow-up Program Cooperative Group 1982). Experimental studies of the spontaneous hypertensive stroke-prone rat also have demonstrated that antihypertensive therapy improved cerebral blood flow and prevented stroke (Yamori et al. 1976). However, Meissner, Whisnant, and Garraway(1988) reported that recurrence of stroke was only slightly higher in the nontreated control group than in the treated control group. Neither blood pressure before stroke nor management of hypertension had any apparent effect on stroke recurrence rates throughout the follow-up. Stroke recurrence, however, may increase the risk for VaD. Nevertheless, Hisayama's cohort study revealed that hypertensive cerebral hemorrhage and lacunar infarctions were significantly decreased during the past twenty years in Japan (Ueda et al. 1988). Longitudinal epidemiological studies also have shown a tendency for VaD to decrease over the past fifteen to twenty-five years (Schoenberg 1988). However, few controlled studies have prospectively determined whether antihypertensive therapy has a significant effect in preventing the development of VaD. Meyer et al. (1986) reported that optimal control of blood pressure in the range of 135 to 150 mmHg significantly improved the cognition and clinical course in seventeen hypertensive patients with VaD during a three-year follow-up study. They also showed excessive reduction of systolic blood pressure (to 128 mmHg) worsened dementia in these patients with hypertension.

Randomized controlled study of nimodipine for vascular dementia ($n = 259$) revealed that only the subcortical vascular dementia group ($n = 92$) improved after six-month treatment by subgroup analysis (Pantoni, Rossi, and Inzitari 2000).

In patients included in the dementia substudy of SYST-EUR, a beneficial effect of antihypertensive therapy on the risk of cognitive decline and of dementia of the Alzheimer type has been shown (Leys and Pasquier 1999). These results could be explained by the following hypothesis. Many cases of dementia occurring in stroke patients are probably the consequence of the cumulative effect of cerebrovascular lesions, Alzheimer pathology, and white matter changes. Even when these changes do not lead to dementia by themselves, their cumulative effect may reach the threshold of lesions required to produce dementia (Pasquier and Leys 1997). Therefore, antihypertensive drugs could prevent the overt dementia in borderline patients with Alzheimer pathology by reducing the vascular risk factor.

Recently, a large international randomized controlled study (PROGRESS) for prevention of stroke recurrence in minor stroke patients by antihypertensive drug (perindpril; ACE inhibitor) was completed, and results showed a significant beneficial effect on the risk of cognitive decline evaluated by Mini-Mental Status Examination in the recurrent stroke cases (OR: 0.55, CI: 0.39–0.79). These large trials gave us some hope of being able to prevent VaD. Although management of vascular risk factors is most important to prevent VaD, we should not forget that disuse deterioration of brain function is common in poststroke patients with apathy (Okada et al. 1997). It is necessary not only to develop preventive drugs for vascular risk factors but also to treat apathy.

Clinical Conclusions

Multilacunar dementia and subcortical arteriosclerotic encephalopathy are strongly associated with hypertension. Subcortical arteriosclerotic encephalopathy or Binswanger-type dementia is not uncommon in elderly patients with VaD. Therefore, white matter lesions may play a significant role in the etiology of dementia in patients with multiple cerebral infarctions. We confirmed that hypertension is significantly correlated with severity of white matter lesions in multilacunar infarction, and also that severity of white matter lesions is significantly correlated with decrements in mental function. Furthermore, we have shown that the severity of white matter lesions is closely related to hypertension, even in neurologically normal adults.

Treatment studies have shown that systematic management of hypertension significantly reduces the incidence of stroke. Therefore, proper treatment of hypertension before or after symptomatic stroke without dementia could prevent the development of VaD. Our large controlled prospective study to determine whether optimum control of hypertension can reduce VaD has revealed that ACE inhibitor can reduce VaD after recurrence of stroke.

REFERENCES

Awad, I.A., P.C. Johanson, R.F. Spetzler, et al. 1986. Incidental subcortical lesions identified on magnetic resonance imaging in the elderly. II. Postmortem pathological correlations. *Stroke* 17:1090–97.

Babikian, V., and A.H. Ropper. 1987. Binswanger disease: A review. *Stroke* 18:2–12.

Bougousslavsky, J., F. Regli, and A. Uske. 1987. Leukoencephalopathy in patients with ischemic stroke. *Stroke* 18:896–99.

Brun, A., and E. Englund. 1986. A white-matter disorder in dementia of the Alzheimer type: A pathoanatomical study. *Annals of Neurology* 19:253–62.

Clair, D.St., and L.J. Whalley. 1983. Hypertension, multi-infarct dementia and Alzheimer's disease. *British Journal of Psychiatry* 143:274–76.

Fazekas, F., K. Niederkorn, R. Schmidt, et al. 1988. White-matter signal abnormalities in normal individuals: Correlation with carotid ultrasonography, cerebral blood flow measurements, and cerebrovascular risk factors. *Stroke* 19:1285–88.

Fisher, C.M. 1969. The arterial lesions underlying lacunes. *Acta Neuropathologica* (Berlin) 12:1–15.

Fujihara, S., K. Shimode, M. Nakamura, et al. 1989. Cerebral amyloid angiopathy with the deposition of cystatine C (gamma-trace) and β-protein. Vol. 317, Progress in clinical and biological research. In *Alzheimer's Disease and Related Disorders*, edited by K. Iqbal, H.M. Wisniewski, and B. Winblad. New York: Alan R. Liss.

Fukuda, H., S. Kobayashi, K. Okada, et al. 1990. Frontal white-matter lesions and dementia in lacunar infarction. *Stroke* 21:1143–49.

Furuta, A., N. Ishii, Y. Nishihara, et al. 1991. Medullary arteries in aging and dementia. *Stroke* 22:442–46.

Glenner, G.G., and C.W. Wong. 1984. Initial report of purification of a novel cerebrovascular amyloid protein. *Biochemistry and Biophysiology Research Communication* 120:885–90.

Goto, K., N. Ishii, and H. Fukasawa. 1981. Diffuse white-matter disease in the geriatric population. *Radiology* 141:687–95.

Grubb, A., O. Jensson, G. Gudmundsson, et al. 1984. Abnormal metabolism of gamma-trace alkaline microprotein: The basic defect in hereditary cerebral hemorrhage with amyloidosis. *New England Journal of Medicine* 311:1547–49.

Hachinski, V.C., P. Potter, and H. Merskey. 1987. Leukoaraiosis. *Archives of Neurology* 44:21–23.

Hasegawa, K. 1983. The clinical assessment of dementia in the aged: A dementia screening scale for psychogeriatric patients. In *Aging in the Eighties and Beyond*, edited by M. Bergener. New York: Springer.

Herholz, K., W. Heindel, A. Rackl, et al. 1990. Regional cerebral blood flow in patients with leukoaraiosis and atherosclerotic carotid artery disease. *Archives of Neurology* 47:392–96.

Hunt, A.L., W.W. Orrison, R.A. Yeo, et al. 1989. Clinical significance of MRI white-matter lesions in the elderly. *Neurology* 39:1470–74.

Hypertension Detection and Follow-up Program Cooperative Group. 1982. Five-year findings of the hypertension detection and follow-up program: III. Reduction in stroke incidence among persons with high blood pressure. *Journal of the American Medical Association* 247:633–88.

Inzitari, D., F. Diaz, A. Fox, et al. 1987. Vascular risk factors and leukoaraiosis. *Archives of Neurology* 44:42–47.

Joutel, A., F. Andreux, S. Gaulis, et al. 2000. The ectodomain of the Notch 3 receptor accumulates within the cerebrovasculature of CADASIL patients. *Journal of Clinical Investigation* 105 (5):597–605.

Junque, C., J. Pujol, P. Vendrell, et al. 1990. Leukoaraiosis on magnetic resonance imaging and speed of mental processing. *Archives of Neurology* 47:151–56.

Kameyama, M. 1973. Prefrontal cerebrovascular lesions and dementia. *Psychiatry and Medicine Japan* 15:357–66.

Karasawa, A. 1989. Epidemiology of vascular dementia. *Journal of Senile Dementia* (Japan) 3:37–44.

Kawamura, J., J.S. Meyer, Y. Terayama, et al. 1991. Leukoaraiosis and lCBF reduction among patients with vascular dementia. *Journal of Cerebral Blood Flow Metabolism* 11 (Suppl. 2):S800.

Kobayashi, S. 2001. Clinical significance of silent brain infarction. *Advances in Neurological Sciences* (Japan) 45:450–60.

Kobayashi, S., K. Okada, and K. Yamashita. 1991. Incidence of silent lacunar lesion in normal adults and its relationship to cerebral blood flow and risk factors. *Stroke* 22: 564–71.

Kobayashi, S., K. Okada, H. Koide, et al. 1997. Subcortical silent brain infarction as a risk factor for clinical stroke. *Stroke* 28:1932–39.

Kozachuk, W.E., C. DeCarli, M.B. Schapiro, et al. 1990. White-matter hyperintensities in dementia of Alzheimer's type and in healthy subjects without cerebrovascular risk factors. *Archives of Neurology* 47:1306–10.

Launer, L.J., G.W. Ross, H. Petrovitch, et al. 2000. Midlife blood pressure and dementia: The Honolulu-Asia aging study. *Neurobiology of Aging* 21:49–55.

Lechner, H., R. Schmidt, G. Bertha, et al. 1988. Nuclear magnetic resonance image white-matter lesions and risk factors for stroke in normal individuals. *Stroke* 19: 263–65.

Leys, D., and E. Pasquier. 1999. Prevention of dementia: Syst-Eur trial. *Lancet* 353: 236–37.

Lodder, J., J.M. Bamford, P.A.G. Sandercock, et al. 1990. Are hypertension or cardiac embolism likely causes of lacunar infarction? *Stroke* 21:375–81.

MaQuinn, B.A., and D.H. O'Leary. 1987. White-matter lucencies on computed tomography, subacute arteriosclerotic encephalopathy (Binswanger disease), and blood pressure. *Stroke* 18:900–905.

Meissner, I., J.P. Whisnant, and W.M. Garraway. 1988. Hypertension management and stroke recurrence in a community. *Stroke* 19:459–63.

Meyer, J.S., B.W. Judd, T. Tawaklna, et al. 1986. Improved cognition after control of risk factors for multi-infarct dementia. *Journal of the American Medical Association* 256: 2203–9.

Meyer, J. S., K. McClintic, P. Sims, et al. 1988. Etiology, prevention, and treatment of vascular and multi-infarct dementia. In *Vascular and Multi-Infarct Dementia*, edited by J.S. Meyer, H. Lechner, J. Marshall, et al. New York: Futura Publishing, pp. 129–47.

Mirsen, T., and V. Hachinski. 1988. Epidemiology and classification of vascular and multi-infarct dementia. In *Vascular and Multi-Infarct Dementia*, edited by J.S. Meyer, H. Lechner, J. Marshall, et al. New York: Futura Publishing, pp. 61–76.

Okada, K., S. Kobayashi, S. Yamagata, et al. 1997. Post-stroke apathy and regional cerebral blood flow. *Stroke* 28:2437–41.

Omae, T., and K. Ueda. 1988. Editorial review. Hypertension and cerebrovascular disease—the Japanese experience. *Journal of Hypertension* 6:343–49.

Pantoni, L., R. Rossi, and J.H. Garcia. 1995. The significance of cerebral white-matter abnormalities 100 years after Binswanger report: A review. *Stroke* 26:1293–1301.

Pantoni, L., R. Rossi, and D. Inzitari. 2001. Efficacy and safety of nimodipine in subcortical vascular dementia: A subgroup analysis of the Scandinavian Multi-Infarct Dementia Trial. *Journal of Neurological Science* 175:124–34.

Pasquier, E., and D. Leys. 1997. Why are stroke patients prone to develop dementia? *Journal of Neurology* 244:135–42.

Reed, D., D. Jacobs, T. Hayashi., et al. 1994. A comparison of lesions in small intracerebral arteries among Japanese men in Hawaii and Japan. *Stroke* 25:60–65.

Révész, T., C.P. Hawkins, E.P.G.H. du Boulay, et al. 1989. Pathological findings correlated with magnetic resonance imaging in subcortical arteriosclerotic encephalopathy (Binswanger disease). *Journal of Neurology, Neurosurgery, and Psychiatry* 52:1337–44.

Schoenberg, B.S. 1988. Epidemiology of vascular and multi-infarct dementia. In *Vascular and Multi-Infarct Dementia,* edited by J.S. Meyer, H. Lechner, J. Marshall, et al. New York: Futura Publishing, pp. 47–59.

Shimode, K., S. Fujihara, M. Nakamura, et al. 1991. Diagnosis of cerebral amyloid angiopathy by enzyme-linked immunosorbent assay of cystatic C in cerebrospinal fluid. *Stroke* 22:860–66.

Shirasawa., A., N. Sjyama, S. Kobayaski, et al. 2000. Cerebrovascular autoregulation and silent cerebrovascular lesions. *Journal of Stroke and Cerebrovascular Disease* 9 (Suppl.): S277–78.

Strandgaard, S. 1978. Autoregulation of cerebral circulation in hypertension. *Acta Neurologica Scandinavica* 57 (Suppl. 66):S1–82.

Tohgi, H., K. Chiba, and M. Kimura. 1991. Twenty-four-hour variation of blood pressure in vascular dementia of the Binswanger type. *Stroke* 22:603–8.

Tomonaga, M. 1981. Cerebral amyloid angiopathy in the elderly. *Journal of the American Geriatrics Society* 29:151–57.

Tomonaga, M., H. Yamanouchi, H. Tohgi, et al. 1980. A clinicopathological study on the progressive subcortical vascular encephalopathy (Binswanger type) observed in the elderly persons. *Japanese Journal of Stroke* 2:49–54.

Ueda, K., T. Omae, Y. Hasuo, et al. 1988. Prognosis and outcome of elderly hypertensive in a Japanese community: Results from a long-term prospective study. *Journal of Hypertension* 6:991–97.

Ueda, K., H. Kawano, Y. Hasuo, et al. 1992. Prevalence and etiology of dementia in a Japanese community. *Stroke* 23:798–803.

Vinters, H.V. 1987. Cerebral amyloid angiopathy: A critical review. *Stroke* 18:311–24.

Yamaguchi, S., S. Kobayashi, K. Okada, et al. 1996. Cognitive decline associated with worsening of white-matter lesions: A six-year follow-up study. *Journal of Stroke and Cerebral Vascular Disease* 6 (Suppl. 1):S106–9.

Yamori, Y., R. Horie, M. Sato, et al. 1976. Regional cerebral blood flow in stroke-prone SHR. A preliminary report. *Japanese Heart Journal* 17:378–80.

Yao, H., S. Sadoshima, Y. Kuwabara, et al. 1990. Cerebral blood flow and oxygen metabolism in patients with vascular dementia of the Binswanger type. *Stroke* 21:1694–99.

CHAPTER TWELVE

Vascular Dementias and Alzheimer Disease

Differential Diagnosis

Tuula Pirttilä, M.D., Ph.D.,
Timo Erkinjuntti, M.D., Ph.D.,
and Vladimir Hachinski, M.D.,
FRCP(C), MSC, DSC, DMHC

Vascular dementia (VaD) is a common cause of dementia, second only to Alzheimer disease (AD) and accounting for 10–50% of all dementia cases, depending on the age of the patient (Rocca et al. 1991; Fratiglioni et al. 2000; Lobo et al. 2000; Rockwood et al. 2000a). The primary cause of VaD is cerebrovascular disease (CVD) with ischemic brain injury (Erkinjuntti 1999). However, the multiplicity of vascular causes, associated risk factors, and clinical manifestations of dementia related to CVD make VaD a complex area of research (Wallin and Blennow 1993; Erkinjuntti 1999; Pohjasvaara et al. 2000). Even though a number of sets of diagnostic criteria have been produced for epidemiological studies of VaD, opinions are divided over the definition of subtypes, how wide the definition should be, and which patients should be excluded from a diagnosis of VaD.

Further debate centers on difficulties in distinguishing dementia due to Alzheimer disease from that arising from cerebrovascular disease, as there are large overlaps in clinical signs and symptoms. Both result in cognitive, functional, and behavioral impairment. There are also similarities in pathophysiological mechanisms (e.g. white matter lesions, delayed neuronal death, and apoptosis) (Pantonini and Garcia 1997; Snowdon et al. 1997; Pantoni et al. 1999; Skoog,

Kalaria, and Breteler 1999), associated risk factors (e.g., age, education, arterial hypertension) (Leibson et al. 1997; Skoog 1997; Notkola et al. 1998; Skoog, Kalaria, and Breteler, 1999; Breteler 2000; Kivipelto et al. 2001), and neurochemical deficits (e.g., cholinergic dysfunction) (Wallin, Blennow, and Gottfries 1989; Gottfries et al. 1994; Tohgi et al. 1996).

Even more relevant is the fact that Alzheimer disease and vascular dementia coexist in a large proportion of patients (Gearing et al. 1995; Kalaria and Ballard 1999; Rockwood et al. 1999b). Alzheimer disease with CVD (sometimes referred to as mixed dementia) could present clinically either as AD with evidence of cerebrovascular lesions in brain imaging, or with features of both AD and VaD (Rockwood et al. 1999a). Based on the findings from the Nun Study, it has been suggested that CVD may play an important role in determining the presence and severity of clinical symptoms of AD (Snowdon et al. 1997). Either way, the prevalence of AD with CVD has previously been underestimated, and may be more than 30% (Kalaria and Ballard 1999).

Aside from Alzheimer disease, the large number of different vascular etiologies and accessory risk factors in vascular dementia introduce a high degree of heterogeneity in clinical subtypes of vascular dementia (tab. 12.1). Varied progression paths are seen, including abrupt onset and stepwise progression in some patients, while in others insidious onset with a uniformly progressive course may be observed (Chui and Gonthier 1999; Desmond et al. 1999; Erkinjuntti 1999). This heterogeneity gives rise to difficulties in clinical and neuropathological diagnosis, and the classification and monitoring of VaD. Neuroimaging findings showing vascular lesions and the associated brain pathology, combined with epidemiological evidence from surveys of clinical deficits, are vital in establishing classifications of VaD subtypes. Findings from such studies have so far succeeded in identifying the most common types of cerebrovascular lesions associated with the onset of dementia. These include multiple cortico-subcortical infarcts, strategically located single infarcts, and small vessel disease with lacunar infarcts and ischemic white matter disease. The clinical deficits frequently associated with these subtypes have also been elucidated (Hachinski, Lassen, and Marshall 1974; Bowler, Steenhuis, and Hachinski 1999; Erkinjuntti 1999). Vascular dementia can now be seen a group of syndromes rather than a single disease. Indeed, recent debate has raised the possibility of using the umbrella term, *vascular cognitive impairment* (*VCI*), which can encompass all patients with dementia associated with CVD, and may or may not include AD with CVD (Bowler, Steenhuis, and Hachinski 1999; Rockwood et al. 2000b).

Table 12.1. Subtypes of vascular dementia

Cortical vascular dementia, or multiinfarct dementia
Subcortical vascular dementia, or small vessel dementia
Strategic infarct dementia
Hypoperfusion dementia
Hemorrhagic dementia
Hereditary vascular dementia, including CADASIL
Other vascular dementia
Alzheimer disease with cerebrovascular disease (mixed dementia)

Greater understanding of any disease leads to better chances of successful treatment, and vascular dementia is no exception. A number of drugs have been studied for the symptomatic treatment of VaD, but have shown largely negative results. It is thought this has been largely due to small study numbers, short treatment periods, different study end points, and, in particular, variations in diagnostic criteria and the inconsistent inclusion of different patient populations (Görtelmeyer and Erbler 1992; Pantoni et al. 1996a; Rother et al. 1998; Erkinjuntti 1999).

Critical elements of the concept and diagnosis of vascular dementia include the identification of vascular changes and subsequent brain pathology, and description of the characteristics of cognitive dementia syndrome (type, extent, and combination of impairments in different cognitive domains). Accessory clinical deficits, such as focal neurological symptoms, also form an important part of the overall clinical picture in VaD. This chapter will focus on the pathology and clinical diagnosis of the most common VaD subtypes. It will also address similarities and differences with AD relating to differential diagnoses in VaD.

Main Subtypes of Vascular Dementia

Cortical Vascular Dementia or Multiinfarct Dementia

This subtype relates to large vessel disease, cardiac embolic events, and hypoperfusion (tab. 12.2). Typical neuroimaging presentations of multiinfarct dementia (MID) show predominantly cortical and corticosubcortical arterial territorial and distal field (watershed) infarcts (Erkinjuntti et al. 1988; Erkinjuntti 1999). This group shows heterogeneity in regards to etiology, vascular mechanisms, changes in the brain, as well as clinical manifestations (Erkinjuntti 1987a; Rockwood et al. 1999a).

Strategic Infarct Vascular Dementia and Dementia after Stroke

Strategic infarct vascular dementia is characterized by small, focal ischemic lesions involving specific sites that are critical for higher cortical functions. Specific cortical areas affected often include the hippocampal formation, angular gyrus, and gyrus cinguli. Subcortical areas affected include the thalamus, fornix, basal forebrain, caudate nucleus, globus pallidus, and the genu or anterior limb of the internal capsule (Tatemichi 1990; Erkinjuntti and Hachinski 1993). This group shows even more heterogeneity, especially in regard to lesion site and clinical manifestations.

Subcortical Vascular Dementia or Small Vessel Dementia

Subcortical vascular dementia incorporates two entities, both of which involve small vessel disease. The lacunar state and Binswanger disease both involve lacunar infarcts, focal and diffuse ischemic white matter lesions (WMLs), and incomplete ischemic brain injury (Erkinjuntti et al. 2000; Roman 2000; Chui 2001). In particular, ischemic lesions affect elements of the prefrontal subcortical circuit, including the prefrontal cortex, caudate nucleus, pallidum, thalamus, and thalamocortical circuit (genu or anterior limb of the internal capsule, anterior semiovale, and anterior corona radiata) (Cummings 1993). The clinical presentation of subcortical VaD is more homogeneous than that of two other main entities, cortical VaD or strategic infarct.

Table 12.2. Pathogenesis of vascular dementia syndromes

Vascular Mechanism	Change in the Brain
Cortical or multiinfarct vascular dementia	
Large vessel disease	Arterial territorial infarct
Cardiac embolic events	Distal field (watershed) infarct
Hypoperfusion	
Strategic infarct dementia	
Large vessel disease	Arterial territorial infarct
Cardiac embolic events	Distal field (watershed) infarct
Small vessel disease	Lacunar infarct
Hypoperfusion	Focal and diffuse white matter lesions
Subcortical vascular dementia	
Small vessel disease	Lacunar infarct
Hypoperfusion	Focal and diffuse white matter lesions
Incomplete ischemic injury	

Alzheimer Disease with Cerebrovascular Disease, or "Mixed Dementia"

Given the possible significance of Alzheimer disease with cerebrovascular disease, biological markers for this subtype are undeniably needed. However, there are currently no specific markers to diagnose this entity. Potentially useful neuroimaging signs for detection of AD include early and significant medial temporal lobe atrophy on MRI or bilateral parietal hypoperfusion on single-positron emission tomography (SPECT) analysis (Scheltens et al. 1992; Erkinjuntti et al. 1993; Laakso et al. 1996; Jack et al. 1997; Jagust et al. 2001).

Pathology

So far, no large and systematic study has been carried out to evaluate the pathological aspects of subtypes of vascular dementia. Knowledge is extrapolated mainly from selected case series and from studies that have assessed the pathological-radiological correlates in patients with a clinical-radiological picture consistent with that of different VaD subtypes. Pathological subtypes of VaD are given in table 12.2.

Large cortical lesions by definition exclude the diagnosis of subcortical vascular dementia. However, cortical gliosis or granular atrophy of the cortex, related to incomplete ischemic injury in areas of selective vulnerability, may coexist with damage of subcortical structures (Garcia and Brown 1992). Characteristic lesions that are consistently recognized in subcortical VaD include white matter lesions (WMLs) and lacunar infarcts. The pathogenesis of lacunar infarcts is considered a quite well established issue (Fisher 1982; Donnan and Yasaka 1998), despite discordant opinions (Millikan and Futrell 1990). Conversely, the pathogenesis of white matter changes is less well established. A number of clinical observations and instrumental and experimental data suggest that vascular, and more specifically ischemic, mechanisms are responsible for these alterations (Erkinjuntti 1987a; Pantoni et al. 1996b; Pantoni and Garcia 1997; Chui 2001). The small vessel pathology that results in white matter pathology is related to aging, arterial hypertension, and diabetes mellitus (Alex et al. 1962; Furuta 1991; Ostrow and Miller 1993). These changes may lead to stenosis or occlusion of the vessels with consequent sudden or more chronic ischemia of the parenchyma (Chui 2001). The effect of ischemia can be either acute, severe, and localized, leading to small areas of veritable necrosis (lacunar infarction), or chronic, less severe, and diffuse, with histological alterations consistent with the definition of incomplete infarct (Garcia et al. 1996; Pantoni and Garcia 1997).

Experimental data show that white matter components are extremely vulnerable to ischemia and can be damaged in the absence of neuronal injury (Pantoni et al. 1996; Petito et al. 1998). White matter lesions can be diffuse or focal, but often the two types coexist. The changes are mainly found in the deep hemispheric white matter (centrum semiovale, watershed areas), but in most cases of ischemic subcortical VaD alterations of the white matter are also evident in the periventicular regions. The diffuse changes of white matter are characterized by myelin pallor sparing the U fibers with or without astrogliosis (Janota et al. 1989; Révész et al. 1989; Chimowitz et al. 1992; Fazekas et al. 1993; Pantoni et al. 1996b). The white matter rarefaction corresponds to spongiosis (vacuolization of white matter), état criblé (widening of perivascular spaces), loss of myelinated axons, and decreased number of oligodendrocytes without clear aspects of necrosis (Awad et al. 1986; Janota et al. 1989; Révész et al. 1989; Muñoz et al. 1993; Erkinjuntti et al. 1996). In these areas, alterations of the small penetrating vessels including thickening of the wall, replacement of the smooth muscle cells by fibrohyaline-lipidic material, and lumen narrowing are almost invariably found (Marshall et al. 1988; Révész et al. 1989; Leifer, Buonanno, and Richardson 1990; Fazekas et al. 1991; van Swieten et al. 1991; Pantoni et al. 1996b).

The focal, nonconfluent, small (< 15 mm) alterations of white matter are mainly regarded as lacunar infarcts. Lacunar infarcts are areas of coagulative necrosis and are mostly found in the chronic stage of ischemic subcortical VaD (Fisher 1982). They correspond to cavitated lesions seated in the regions of the small penetrating vessels including the deep thalamoperforating and long medullary arteries and in caudate, globus pallidus, thalamus, internal capsule, corona radiata, frontal white matter (Braffman et al. 1988; Muñoz et al. 1993; Olsson, Brun, and Englund 1996; Pantoni et al. 1996b). Besides acquired vascular risk factors and conditions, other genetically determined factors could play an important role in the development of subcortical ischemic VaD, and at least one form of subcortical VaD exists with a clearly determined genetic origin. Cerebral autosomal dominant arteriopathy with subcortical infarcts and leukoencephalopathy (CADASIL) is clinically characterized by recurrent strokes and progressive neurological deterioration occurring in middle-aged subjects and eventually resulting in pseudobulbar palsy and dementia (Baudrimont et al. 1993; Chabriat et al. 1995). From the radiological point of view, CADASIL patients present with diffuse cerebral white matter alterations associated with small focal lesions of the lacunar type (Skehan, Hutchinson, and MacErlaine 1995). Histological studies have shown a degeneration of small vessel smooth muscle cells with deposition of granular osmiophilic material in the vessel wall (Ruchoux and Maurage 1997).

Clinical Diagnosis

The main steps in the clinical examination of a patient include at least four objectives: (1) staging the severity of the disorder (e.g., diagnosis of mild cognitive impairment or dementia), (2) identifying the vascular cause for the cognitive syndrome, (3) evaluation of the specific etiology of the cerebrovascular disease (e.g., causes and risk factors), and (4) examination of secondary factors that may worsen the patient's cognitive function (tab. 12.3). Cornerstones in the diagnosis of VaD are evidence of brain ischemia related to the evolution of the dementia syndrome and brain-imaging evidence of vascular lesions in the brain. The pattern of cognitive impairment associated with VaD is highly variable and depends on the size and location of vascular brain injury. Vascular dementia is a spectrum with primarily cortical involvement at the one end and primarily white matter change at the other that may neuropathologically be characterized by a combination of changes related to atherothrombotic strokes, lacunar strokes, ischemic white matter changes, and hemodynamic changes. Due to the heterogeneity of clinical features of VaD, many other conditions may resemble VaD (tab. 12.4).

Careful clinical interview and examination is the core element in the clinical diagnostic work-up. The main emphasis of this chapter is on the diagnosis of vascular cause of cognitive decline and differential diagnosis in respect to AD. The concept of dementia and clinical assessment of cognitive decline and dementia are covered in other chapters in the book. The key elements of the diagnosis of VaD are (1) recognition of the clinical features of the subtype of VaD, (2) demonstration of significant cerebrovascular disorder by neuroimaging, and (3) laboratory examination of causes and risk factors for CVD.

Current Clinical Criteria for Vascular Dementia

The criteria chosen to diagnose vascular dementia influence greatly recognition of vascular dementia, as well as estimates of its incidence and prevalence. Prevalence of VaD varies several-fold in magnitude depending on the criteria

Table 12.3. Diagnostic work-up in a patient with suspected vascular dementia

Assessment of severity of cognitive decline
Cognitive functions
Functioning in daily living
Confirmation of vascular etiology
Clinical history of risk factors and symptomatic cerebrovascular disease
Neurological examination
Neuroimaging
Etiology of cerebrovascular disease
Blood pressure, heart rate
ECG, chest X-ray
Auscultation of carotid vessels
Laboratory
Blood sugar, cholesterol and lipid levels, fibrinogen, Blood coagulation studies, genetic tests (Notch3 mutations), etc.
Orthostatic test
Twenty-four-hour blood pressure monitoring
Holter monitoring
Echocardiography
Ultrasound examination of cervical vessels
Cerebral angiography
Arterial and leptomeningeal biopsies
Exclusion of factors worsening the patient's condition

Table 12.4. Differential diagnosis of vascular dementia

Alzheimer disease
Alzheimer disease and cerebrovascular disease (mixed dementia)
Normal pressure hydrocephalus
White matter lesions and dementia
Frontal lobe tumor
Intracranial mass
Lewy body dementia
Frontotemporal dementia
Parkinson disease and dementia
Progressive supranuclear palsy
Multisystem atrophy

selected (Wetterling, Kanitz, and Borigis 1996; Pohjasvaara et al. 1997; Chui et al. 2000). The Hachinski Ischemic Score (HIS) was originally developed as a clinical tool to aid in the differentiation between MID and AD (Hachinski et al. 1975). The original scale consists of thirteen items considered typical of MID.

Each scale item is assigned a numeric value, with a double weighting applied to clinical features thought to correlate well with ischemic changes found in neuropathological studies. Since the introduction of the HIS, many other criteria have been developed to improve the diagnosis of VaD. The main features of the most commonly used clinical criteria are summarized in table 12.5.

The DSM-IV definition for vascular dementia requires focal neurological signs and symptoms or laboratory evidence of focal neurologic damage clinically judged to be etiologically related to the disturbance (American Psychiatric Association 1994). The course is specified by sudden cognitive and functional losses. The DSM-IV criteria do not require brain imaging. The DSM-IV definition is reasonably broad, but lacks detailed clinical and radiological guidelines.

The ICD-10 criteria (World Health Organization 1993) require unequal, "patchy" distribution of cognitive deficits (with some functions affected and others relative spared), focal neurological signs as evidence of brain damage, and significant cerebrovascular disease judged to be etiologically related to the dementia. The criteria do not require brain imaging. The main shortcomings include lack of detailed guidelines (e.g., unequal cognitive deficits and neuroimaging), lack of etiological cues, and heterogeneity (Wetterling, Kanitz, and Borgis 1994).

The ADDTC criteria are exclusive for ischemic vascular dementia (IVD) (Chui et al. 1992). They require evidence of two or more ischemic strokes by history, neurologic signs or neuroimaging studies (CT or T1-weighted MRI), or in case of a single stroke a clearly documented temporal relationship (not specified in detail). Neuroradiological evidence of at least one infarct outside the cerebellum is compulsory. Ischemic white matter lesions on computed tomography (CT) or magnetic resonance imaging (MRI) do not qualify as brain-imaging evidence of probable IVD, but may support a diagnosis of possible IVD. The criteria include a list of features supporting the diagnosis, as well as a list of features casting doubt on a diagnosis of probable IVD.

NINDS-AIREN criteria for the diagnosis of vascular dementia produced by the National Institute of Neurological Disorders and Stroke and the Association Internationale pour la Recherche et l'Enseignement en Neurosciences International Workshop (Roman et al. 1993) have been neuropathologically validated (Gold et al. 1997). Currently, they are the most specific and widely used for research purposes in VaD. The NINDS-AIREN research criteria for VaD include definitions for the dementia syndrome, CVD, and their relationship. Cerebrovascular disease is defined by the presence of focal neurological signs

Table 12.5 Comparison of clinical criteria for vascular dementia

	DSM-IV	ICD-10	ADDTC Probable IVD	NINDS-AIREN Probable AD
Ischemic stroke	+	+	+	+
Hemorrhage	+	+	−	+
Stepwise deterioration	−	−	−	(+)1
"Patchy" distribution of cognitive deficits	−	+	−	−
Focal neurological signs	+	+	−	+
Focal neurological symptoms	+	−	−	−
Two or more strokes	−	−	+ or one if there is a temporal relation	−
Evidence of significant cerebrovascular disease	+	+	+(2)	+
Etiological relation to the disturbance	+	+	−	+
Temporal relationship between stroke and dementia	−	−	+ in cases where there is a single stroke	(+)1
Structural neuroimaging	−	−	One infarct outside cerebellum	Multiple large vessel strokes or multiple lacunes or extensive WMLs or single strategically placed lesion
List of supporting and nonsupporting features	−	−	+	+
Different levels of certainty	−	−	+	+

1 = either onset of dementia within three months after a recognized stroke or abrupt deterioration in cognitive functions; or fluctuating, stepwise progression of cognitive deficits.

2 = evidence of two or more ischemic strokes by history, neurological signs, or neuroimaging studies, or occurrence of a single stroke with a clearly documented relationship to the onset of dementia.

and detailed brain imaging with evidence of ischemic changes in the brain. A relationship between dementia and CVD is inferred from the onset of dementia within three months following a recognized stroke, or abrupt deterioration in cognitive functions, or fluctuating, stepwise progression of cognitive deficits. The criteria include a list of features consistent with the diagnosis, as well as a list of features that make the diagnosis uncertain or unlikely. Also, different levels of certainty of the clinical diagnosis (probable, possible, definite) are included. By attaching these criteria, antemortem accuracy of the diagnosis of probable VaD rises to nearly 90%. However, many cases with VaD may go undetected using these criteria.

All currently used clinical criteria are "consensus criteria" derived from expert opinion based on prevailing knowledge and pathogenetic hypotheses of dementia causation; they are neither derived from prospective community-based studies, nor based on detailed cohort studies of the natural history of cognitive decline in subjects with cerebrovascular disease or vascular risk factors (Chui et al. 1992; Roman et al. 1993; Erkinjuntti 1994; Rockwood et al. 1994). All criteria are based on the ischemic infarct concept, with the NINDS-AIREN criteria also including hemorrhages. All are designed to have high specificity at the expense of lower sensitivity. Recent retrospective meta-analysis of the application of the HIS in the sample of pathologically verified dementias showed a good differentiation between AD and MID. The standard cutoffs discriminated accurately between AD and MID with a sensitivity of 89% and a specificity of 89% (Moroney et al. 1997). However, identification of mixed dementia remained problematic. Another retrospective study compared three criteria, the HIS, the ADDTC, and the NINDS-AIREN, in a hospital cohort of 113 autopsied elderly persons (Gold et al. 1997). The sensitivities were 63% for the ADDTC, 58% for the NINDS-AIREN, and 43% for the HIS, and the corresponding specificities were 64%, 80%, and 88%, respectively. Prospective longitudinal clinicopathological studies are needed to validate the criteria and to improve diagnostic accuracy for the mixed dementia (Rockwood et al. 1994).

The Clinical Course of Vascular Dementia

Clinical symptoms and signs and the natural history of vascular dementias vary greatly due to the heterogeneity in the pathogenesis of vascular dementia (Rockwood et al. 1999a). Vascular dementia has traditionally been thought to be characterized by a relative abrupt onset (days to weeks), a stepwise deterioration (some recovery after worsening), and fluctuating course (e.g., difference between days) of cognitive functions (Erkinjuntti 1987a). This is seen in patients with multiple lesions affecting cortical and cortical-subcortical brain structures. In patients with subcortical VaD, however, the onset of cognitive symptoms may be relatively insidious and the course slowly progressive (Erkinjuntti 1987a; Roman 1987; Fischer et al. 1990). The mean duration of VaD is around five years (Hébert and Brayne 1995), and patients' survival is shorter than that of the general population of patients with AD (Skoog et al. 1993; Mölsä, Marttila, and Rinne 1995). Detailed studies on the natural history of subcortical VaD are lacking, and little is known or can be predicted about the rate and pattern of cognitive decline and prognosis in subcortical VaD.

The current clinical criteria for vascular dementia implicitly recognize the heterogeneity of lesions capable of causing vascular dementia; however, none of these clinical criteria provide guidelines for subtypes of vascular dementia. The NINDS-AIREN criteria mention the following subtypes: cortical vascular dementia, subcortical vascular dementia, Binswanger disease, and thalamic dementia (Roman et al. 1993). For practical purposes, recognition of two major subtypes of VaD, cortical and subcortical VaD, and their typical clinical symptoms and signs helps the clinician detect most patients with VaD.

Clinical Features of the Subtypes of Vascular Dementia

Cortical Vascular Dementia, or Multiinfarct Dementia

The cognitive syndrome in cortical vascular dementia, or multiinfarct dementia, is primarily determined by localization of the vascular lesions. Memory impairment may be mild with early cognitive impairment (Erkinjuntti 1987a). Heteromodal cortical symptoms (e.g., aphasia, apraxia, agnosia, visuospatial or constructional difficulty) can be seen in various combinations (Mahler and Cummings 1991). In the majority of patients, some decline in executive functions is observed. The course of the syndrome in patients with cortical VaD is characterized by abrupt onset (within days or weeks), stepwise deterioration, and fluctuating course (e.g., difference between days). However, long plateaus in cognitive performance with slow progression can feature in patients taking steps to control vascular risk factors or medication to prevent recurrent stroke.

Accessory clinical symptoms can include focal neurological symptoms. Examples of neurological symptoms include "field cut," lower facial weakness, upper motor neuron signs, and gait impairment that presents either hemiplegic or apractic-atactic disability (Erkinjuntti 1987a).

Strategic Infarct Dementia

Acute-onset cognitive impairments can feature in strategic infarct vascular dementia (e.g., in thalamic dementia). Severe memory impairment is often apparent, and fluctuating consciousness and confusion is observed in many patients. Other cognitive deficits include apathy, lack of spontaneity, perseveration, and mild dysphasia. Depending on the strategic location of infarcts in this subtype, the time course of disease progression and specific profile of clinical features can vary considerably.

Subcortical Vascular Dementia

The term *subcortical dementia* defines the mental changes that are related to prefrontal lobe dysfunction. Patients with subcortical VaD represent a more homogeneous subgroup than patients with other VaD subtypes (Erkinjuntti et al. 2000; tab.12.6). The cognitive syndrome of subcortical VaD is characterized by (1) dysexecutive syndrome, including slowed information processing; (2) memory deficit that may be mild; and (3) behavioral and psychological symptoms. The majority of the patients (60%) show a slow, less abrupt onset, and 80% show both slow progression with or without acute deficits (Babikian and Ropper 1987; Roman 2000).

Dysexecutive syndrome is the core feature of subcortical vascular dementia, characterized by mental slowing and impairment of goal formulation, initiation, planning, organizing, sequencing, executing, set-sifting, set-maintenance, and abstracting (Cummings 1994; Desmond et al. 1999). However, perseveration is also seen and some memory deficit is apparent, although less severe than in, for example, AD (Lamar et al. 1997; Desmond et al. 1999). The memory deficit in subcortical VaD is different from memory disorder seen in AD (Tierney et al. 2001). The patients show less episodic memory dysfunction and more executive dysfunction at an equal overall level of severity. Memory disturbances are characterized by impaired recall and retrieval, relatively intact recognition, less severe forgetting, and benefits from cues (Desmond et al. 1999; Tierney et al. 2001). This pattern is consistent with organizational and retrieval impairment

Table 12.6. Etiology, brain changes, and clinical syndrome of subcortical vascular dementia

- Etiology
  - Primary vascular mechanisms and risk factors
    - Small vessel disease
    - Age, arterial hypertension
  - Secondary vascular mechanisms and risk factors
    - Hemodynamic changes of systemic vascular, cardiac, and carotid origin
    - Arterial hypotension, hypoxic-ischemic events, blood pressure fluctuations, hyperlipidemia, low education
- Brain change
  - Ischemic white matter lesions (WMLs)
    - Extending periventricular and deep WMLs affecting especially the genu or anterior limb, the internal capsule, anterior corona radiata, and anterior centrum semiovale
  - Lacunar infarcts
    - In the caudate, globus pallidus, thalamus, internal capsule, corona radiata, frontal white matter
- Clinical syndrome
  - Cognitive syndrome
    - Dysexecutive syndrome: impairment in goal formulation, initiation, planning, organizing, sequencing, executing, set-sifting and -maintenance, abstracting
    - Memory deficit (may be mild): impairment recall, relative intact recognition, less severe forgetting, benefit from cues
  - Behavioral and psychological symptoms
    - Depression, personality change, emotional incontinence, psychomotor retardation

(frontal functions) as opposed to storage (temporal lobe) difficulties (Ishii, Nishihara, and Imamura 1986). Recent studies have shown that memory deficit in VaD correlates with prefrontal lobe metabolism, whereas in AD memory correlates with hippocampal and temporal lobe metabolism (Reed et al. 2000). Behavioral and psychological symptoms include in particular depression, personality change, emotional lability, and incontinence, as well as inertia, emotional bluntness, and psychomotor retardation (Babikian and Ropper 1987; Mahler and Cummings 1991; Sultzer et al. 1993; Cummings 1994).

Episodic and often subtle focal neurological signs are also seen in subcortical vascular dementia. These include imbalance, altered urinary frequency and incontinence, mild upper motor neuron signs (drift, reflex asymmetry, incoordination), gait disturbance, imbalance and falls, dysarthria, and dysphagia (Roman 1987; Wallin, Blennow, and Gottfries 1991; Roman et al. 1993). Some extrapyramidal symptoms, such as rigidity and hypokinesia, are also often evident.

Neuroimaging

Diagnosis of vascular dementia requires evidence of significant cerebrovascular lesions detected in neuroimaging. A strategy for addressing the large amount of heterogeneity seen in VaD is to describe possible subtypes of VaD that can be associated with different forms of vascular lesions. Changes in the brain associated with CVD are evaluated clinically by CT or MRI scans. By definition, cortical VaD or MID is characterized by multiple cortical infarcts, whereas the radiological hallmarks of subcortical VaD include extending diffuse periventricular and deep ischemic focal WMLs and lacunar infarcts.

The characteristic white matter lesions are detected especially in the genu or anterior limb of the internal capsule, the anterior corona radiata, and centrum semiovale and lacunar infarcts in the caudate nucleus, globus pallidus, thalamus, internal capsule, corona radiata, and frontal white matter (Pohjasvaara et al. 2000). Both WMLs and lacunar infarcts can be detected by CT and MRI, but the two methods have different sensitivity and, possibly, different specificity. Magnetic resonance imaging has higher sensitivity than CT in detecting WMLs, but some of the MRI-detected WMLs are thought to represent normal radiological findings without pathological significance. Particularly small lesions in the periventricular white matter can be found in all age groups, and we suggest not to consider them as characteristic alterations of subcortical VaD (Mäntylä et al. 1999). White matter lesions detected by CT are commonly believed to be more indicative of disease than those detected by MRI.

Clinically significant white matter lesions are seen as bilateral, symmetric areas of hypodensity on computed tomography scans or hyperintensity on T2-weighted magnetic resonance images, located in the periventricular or deep subcortical white matter. They can be distinguished from territorial infarcts because they do not have well-defined margins, are not wedge-shaped, do not involve the cortex, and are not associated with enlargement of ipsilateral sulci or ventricle; moreover, they do not follow specific vascular territory (Inzitari et al. 1987). White matter lesions detected by CT and MRI are not completely superimposable as to number, site, and extension (Brant-Zaeadski et al. 1983; Bradley et al. 1984; Erkinjuntti 1987a; Johnson et al. 1987).

Moreover, many different rating scales exist for white matter lesions (Mäntylä et al. 1997; Scheltens et al. 1998). Most of them are based on the visual evaluation of the WMLs and are subjected to high interrater variability. The simplest scales, especially those based on CT, classify WMLs into periventricular, anterior or posterior, and deep subcortical. Deep subcortical lesions are usually distinguished as focal or diffuse. Almost all the MRI visual rating scales for WMLs are more detailed. Periventricular lesions may be classified as follows: (a) hyperintensities surrounding the tip of the frontal or occipital horns of the lateral ventricles (also called caps); (b) tiny or more extensive hyperintensities along the lateral wall of the cella media of the lateral ventricles (thin lining and smooth halo); these lesions may differently extend from the periventricular areas toward the deeper white matter regions; (c) deep or centrum semiovale lesions, which are usually distinguished as focal, more or less confluent, or diffuse. It has been shown that different scales attribute different significance to the same radiological picture.

Rating of white matter lesions can be based on systematic identification of basic types of white matter lesions as described below. White matter lesions can be rated in distinct white matter areas, including periventricular, deep or centrum semiovale, watershed, and subcortical areas (Mäntylä et al. 1997). On MRI, periventricular WMLs (termed hyperintensities) are in contact with the ventricular wall; deep hyperintensities are separated from the ventricular system by a strip of normal-looking white matter and are located outside watershed areas. The subcortical region is considered to represent an area less than 5 mm beneath the cortex.

Periventricular hyperintensities around the frontal and occipital horns are classified based on size and shape into small caps, large caps, and extending caps. Periventricular hyperintensities along the bodies of lateral ventricles are classified based on thickness and shape into thin lining, smooth halo, and irregular halo. Lacunar infarcts are seen as more or less cavitated lesions according to different stages of evolution, round or oval in shape, with a diameter less than 15 mm, although this limit appears reasonable but arbitrary. Hyperintensities in other white matter areas are classified based on size (greatest diameter) and shape into small focal, large focal, focal confluent, diffusely confluent, and extensive white matter changes.

Clinical Examination of Causes and Risk Factors of Cerebrovascular Disorder

Examination of a patient with vascular dementia should always include the assessment of the causes and risk factors of cerebrovascular disorder (Skoog 1998). History of smoking, cardiac diseases, hypertension, diabetes, and other possible risk factors for cerebrovascular diseases should be taken. The basic evaluation of the cardiovascular system includes careful auscultation of heart and carotid vessels, measurement of heart rate and blood pressure, chest radiography, and electrocardiography. Further tests that may be needed in individual patients are the orthostatic test, twenty-four-hour blood pressure monitoring, Holter monitoring, and two-dimensional echocardiography with additional radioisotope studies. Sonography of cervical vessels may also be useful in selected cases. In some cases cerebral angiography, arterial biopsy, or even brain and leptomeningeal vessel biopsy may be needed, particularly in patients with suspected angiitis of brain vessels. Laboratory examination of risk factors for CVD includes measurements of blood sugar, cholesterol and lipid levels, fibrinogen, and blood coagulation tests in selected cases. Genetic tests such as detection of Notch3 gene mutations are needed if CADASIL is suspected.

The Relationship between Alzheimer Disease and Vascular Dementia

The presence of vascular risk factors per se does not offer diagnostic clues for the etiology of dementia. Recent studies have suggested that many risk factors for vascular diseases such as hypertension, diabetes, and high cholesterol may increase the risk of AD as well (Leibson et al. 1997; Notkola et al. 1998; Skoog, Kalaria, and Breteler 1999; Breteler 2000; Kivipelto et al. 2001). However, the neuropathological confirmation of AD is lacking in all studies. Therefore, it is not clear if cognitive impairment associated with vascular risk factors is due to a direct effect on the development of AD or whether it is mediated through vascular changes that will lower the threshold for the manifestation of cognitive decline. Moreover, comorbidity of AD and VaD is common, particularly in the very old (Kalaria and Ballard 1999; Snowdon et al. 1997).

There is substantial overlap between the pattern of cognitive impairment in vascular dementia and Alzheimer disease, although some differences have been identified (tab. 12.7). However, precise distinctions of cognitive impairment at specific levels of cognition in the two illnesses are still uncertain. The nature, extent, and progression of deterioration in functional abilities have been observed to differ in VaD compared with AD (Groves et al. 2000). Analysis of data from the Canadian Study of Health and Aging showed that capabilities for motoric functions such as walking and getting into bed were different between AD and VaD, as opposed to nonmotoric functions (e.g., handling of money, groom-

Table 12.7. Differential diagnosis between vascular dementia and Alzheimer disease

Vascular Dementia	Alzheimer Disease
Early Cognitive Syndrome	
Dysexecucutive syndrome	Impaired episodic memory
Impaired planning, sequencing, speed of processing, memory; ineffective learning, less forgetting, preserved recognition, good response cues, perseveration	Ineffective learning, increased forgetting, impaired recognition, poor response to cues, intrusion errors
Cortical symptoms (s) (variable)	Anomia (mild), aphasia, apraxia, agnosia, visuospatial impairment (mild), constructive difficulty
Early Clinical Features	
Mild upper motor neuron signs (motor deficit, decreased coordination, brisk tendon reflexes, urine frequency, dysarthria, mood changes, depression)	Absence of focal neurological signs Dysthymia, mild depression, Babinski's sign, gait disorder, imbalance
Onset	
Variable: relatively abrupt, insidious	Insidious
Clinical Course	
Variable: fluctuating, stepwise progressive, stable	Progressive May have plateaus

ing, using the telephone, traveling and taking medicine), where no difference is seen (Gauthier et al. 1999). Impairments in attention and visual perception are thought to be greater in early AD than in VaD, which has been seen to produce differential effects on capabilities in complex activities (e.g., driving) in the two illnesses (Fitten et al. 1995).

Psychiatric comorbidity is a common feature of vascular dementia. Behavioral (neuropsychiatric) disorders that are often reported in patients with vascular disorder include depression, behavioral retardation, psychomotor slowing, anxiety, and apathy. Among these psychiatric comorbidities, most comparative studies have shown that depression occurs more frequently in VaD than in AD (Groves et al. 2000). The severity of behavioral symptoms generally increases with cognitive decline in both AD and VaD. However, mood and personality changes can be more severe in VaD (Hargrave et al. 2000), and may occur earlier in the course of disease progression (Chui and Gonthier 1999).

The NINDS-AIREN criteria for the diagnosis of vascular dementia have attempted to take some of the differences between Alzheimer disease and vascular dementia into account. Probable VaD is characterized in NINDS-AIREN criteria by abrupt onset, or fluctuating and stepwise course with clinical signs of CVD and relevant CVD on brain imaging. In addition, it is specified that functional disability be distinguished as arising from cognitive deficit and not due to physical disability related to brain pathology. In contrast, AD is characterized by NINCDS-ADRDA criteria (McKhann et al. 1984) by insidious onset and progressive course, without clinical signs of CVD or brain changes due to CVD on neuroimaging. It is now becoming more clear that a continuum of pathologies may exist, where "pure" AD and VaD represent only the two extremes. Recent studies have suggested that mixed dementia (i.e., AD with coexistent significant CVD) may be the most common cause of dementia in the very old population (Rockwood et al. 2000b). Because these patients often show extensive WMLs and infarct(s) on brain imaging, the clinical diagnosis is difficult in the absence of defined biological markers for AD. This may in the past have been a leading factor in the previous underestimation of this patient subgroup. Studies showing the frequency and possible causes of dementia after stroke have helped to define the link between dementia and CVD. Findings from studies in Japan and the United States and from the Helsinki Aging Memory Study have estimated the frequency of dementia after stroke at around 25% (Pohjasvaara et al. 1987; Suzuki et al. 1987; Tatemichi et al. 1992). In the U.S. study, stroke was confirmed as the underlying cause of dementia in over 50% of cases, and of these, approximately 36% were thought to be due to the cumulative effects of stroke and AD (Tatemichi et al. 1992).

The presence of cerebrovascular disease may play an important role in determining the presence and severity of the clinical symptoms of Alzheimer disease. The incidence rate of AD after stroke is doubled, suggesting that stroke may induce an earlier expression of AD (Kokmen et al. 1996). Moreover, according to Henon et al. (2001) stroke patients with mild AD developed overt dementia syndrome during the first months after stroke whereas pure VaD may also develop after more prolonged poststroke interval. The Nun Study, as well as other studies, have shown that individuals meeting neuropathological criteria for AD with additional evidence of CVD (e.g., lacunar infarcts) showed poorer cognitive performance and more prevalent dementia than those with AD and no evidence of brain infarcts (Snowdon et al. 1997; Heyman et al. 1998). These studies clearly demonstrate that many different pathologies can contribute to the clinical symptoms of dementia in one single patient.

The identification of coexistent pathologies in patients in practice is of great

Table 12.8. Clinical clues to the diagnosis of a vascular component with otherwise typical presentation of Alzheimer disease

Disease course
Abrupt onset*
Stepwise deterioration*
Fluctuating course*
Prolonged periods of plateau
Other clinical features
Patchy cognitive deficits
History of stroke*
Focal neurological signs and symptoms*
Early onset of a gait disorder
Early onset of a seizure
Early onset of urinary incontinence

Source: Adapted from Rockwood and MacKnight 2000.
*Items derived from the Hachinski Ischaemia Scale.

importance, particularly from therapeutic aspects. In a study conducted by the Consortium for the Investigation of Vascular Impairment of Cognition (CIVIC), typical AD presentations with one or more features pointing to "vascular aspects," derived from the Hachinski Ischemia Scale score, were used successfully to diagnose "mixed dementia" in combination with neuroimaging of ischemic lesions (Rockwood et al. 2000b). Vascular risk factors and focal neurological signs and symptoms were present more often in AD with CVD than in "pure" AD. Other visible clinical clues for a diagnosis of AD with CVD were gained from analyses of disease course characteristics, and presentations of patchy cognitive deficits, early onset of seizures, or gait disorder (tab. 12.8).

Vascular Cognitive Impairment

It is becoming clear that there is a need to diagnose cognitive impairment arising from vascular origins early on, rather than waiting until patients develop symptoms of frank dementia (Hachinski 1992). This is a major problem that arises from the continued assessment of VaD patients from the perspective of Alzheimer-type criteria such as the ICD-10 and DSM-IV, which accentuate memory loss and a linear, irreversible progression of cognitive decline that are not typical features of cognitive impairment in VaD.

Debate over the current classification of dementia types has led to proposals for a new definition of cognitive impairment applying to vascular dementia, termed *vascular cognitive impairment* (VCI) (Rockwood 1997; Bowler, Steenhuis, and Hachinski 1999; Rockwood et al. 1999b, 2000b). Dementia is traditionally diagnosed from the perspective of AD-related criteria that emphasize early episodic memory impairment, a more global cognitive syndrome, and major impairment in day-to-day activities. However, delay in treatment of the patients with significant cognitive decline of vascular origin may have an adverse effect on the outcome. The concept of VCI would be aimed at identifying at-risk patients early, before onset of frank dementia. In doing so, the treatment could offer the potential for prevention of disease progression. The natural course of patients with vascular cognitive impairment is largely unknown. One recent study reported that 52% of 149 patients with VCI died during a five-year follow-up period, and 46% of the patients developed dementia (Wentzel et al. 2001). These results suggest that prognosis of VCI is poor and further emphasize the need for early detection and active treatment of VCI.

Vascular cognitive impairment may encompass a wider range of patients and may in fact be more prevalent than Alzheimer disease. The term *VCI* would incorporate currently recognized subtypes of VaD, including cortical VaD (MID), subcortical (small vessel) VaD, and strategic infarct dementia. The more recently recognized (and previously underestimated) mixed dementia, in which patients have AD coincident with CVD and in which cerebrovascular lesions are thought to play an important role in determining the presence and severity of AD, may also be included under VCI. Such patients have previously been excluded from clinical trials with symptomatic treatments due to regulatory guidelines, although recent evidence suggests that these patients respond to treatment as well as patients with "pure" AD.

Discussion

Vascular dementia can be thought of as an umbrella term comprising a number of heterogeneous syndromes, including cortical (multiinfarct) dementia, strategic infarct dementia, and subcortical (small vessel) dementia. Vascular dementia relates to different vascular mechanisms and changes in the brain, and has a number of different causes and clinical manifestations. Cognitive impairment in VaD has complex interactions with vascular etiologies (CVD and risk factors), changes in the brain (infarcts, WMLs, atrophy), and host factors (age, education). As a result, functional decline, behavioral symptoms, and neurological deficits also vary.

The substantial overlap in clinically observed deficits between Alzheimer disease and vascular dementia, coupled with the variability of symptom progression and the wide range of vascular etiologies and risk factors involved in vascular dementia, can be problematic to diagnosis and clinical study. Debate surrounding optimal methods for differential diagnosis has led to calls for a reconceptualization of previous, narrower definitions of VaD, such as the suggested definition of VCI, which could also include AD with CVD (or mixed dementia). However, further epidemiological, clinical, and neuroimaging data must be collected in order to produce set criteria for VCI. It would be preferable if raw data collected in different studies were available to other researchers for analyses of different scales or elaboration of the results.

An alternative to this approach would be the analysis of more homogeneous vascular dementia subgroups, such as patients with ischemic subcortical disease and dementia (Chui 2000; Erkinjuntti et al. 2000). It is thought that such approaches may be more useful in identifying therapeutic benefits, and thus bring better opportunities for prevention of decline and symptomatic treatment in dementia related to CVD, as seen in VaD.

The verification of brain lesions by neuroimaging analysis and study of their relation to cognitive changes are critical to the concept, diagnosis, and targeted study of vascular dementia. The types of brain changes seen to correlate with a possible diagnosis of VaD include a combination of varied infarct features (sites, number, and volume), the extent and type of white matter lesions, the degree and sites of atrophy, as well as host factors (Pohjasvaara et al. 2000). The extent to which brain pathology due to cerebrovascular lesions causes, compounds, or coexists with cognitive impairment is also important in determining both the presence and subtype of dementia. It can influence the selection of patients in clinical trials. Further research experience on the pathological, mechanistic, and clinical features of VaD/VCI should offer more hope of defining expectations for the future pharmacotherapy of dementia related to CVD (Erkinjuntti 1999).

Clinical Conclusions

Vascular dementia is a common cause of dementia, second only to Alzheimer disease. Alzheimer disease and VaD also coexist in a large proportion of patients. Vascular dementia is best viewed as a spectrum. Varied patterns of cognitive impairment and disease course are seen, including abrupt onset and stepwise progression in some patients, insidious onset with a uniform, progressive course in others.

The cornerstones of the diagnosis of vascular dementia are evidence of brain ischemia related to the evolution of the dementia syndrome and brain-imaging evidence of vascular lesions in the brain. The main steps in the clinical examination of a patient include: (1) staging the severity of the disorder (e.g., diagnosis of mild cognitive impairment or dementia); (2) identifying the vascular cause for the cognitive syndrome; (3) examination for the specific etiology of the CVD (e.g., auscultation of heart and carotid vessels, measurement of heart rate and blood pressure, chest radiography, electrocardiography); and (4) examination of secondary factors that may worsen the patient's cognitive function (e.g., history of smoking, cardiac disease, hypertension, diabetes; laboratory examination of blood sugar, cholesterol, and lipid levels).

Cortical vascular dementia, or multiinfarct dementia, is a subtype that relates to large vessel disease, cardiac embolic events, and hypoperfusion. The cognitive syndrome in cortical VaD or MID is primarily determined by localization of the vascular lesions. The course of the syndrome in patients with cortical VaD is characterized by abrupt onset (within days or weeks), stepwise deterioration, and a fluctuating course.

Strategic infarct vascular dementia is characterized by small, focal ischemic lesions involving specific sites that are critical for higher cortical functions. Like cortical VaD, strategic infarct shows heterogeneity in regards to etiology, vascular mechanisms, changes in the brain, as well as clinical manifestations. Acute severe memory impairment and fluctuating consciousness and confusion are observed in many.

Subcortical vascular dementia incorporates two entities, both of which involve small vessel disease. The lacunar state and Binswanger disease both involve lacunar infarcts, focal and diffuse ischemic white matter lesions (WMLs), and incomplete ischemic brain injury. Subcortical VaD is more homogeneous than the other two types. White matter lesions detected by CT are commonly believed to be more indicative of disease than those detected by MRI. The cognitive pattern is characterized by less episodic memory dysfunction and more executive dysfunction, including slowed information processing and behavioral symptoms. A slow, less abrupt onset and a slow progression with subtle focal neurological signs are seen.

Mixed dementia with Alzheimer disease and vascular dementia is more difficult to diagnose. Potentially useful neuroimaging signs for detection of AD include early and significant medial temporal lobe atrophy on MRI or bilateral parietal hypoperfusion on SPECT analysis.

REFERENCES

Alex, M., E.K. Baron, S. Goldenberg, et al. 1962. An autopsy study of cerebrovascular accident in diabetes mellitus. *Circulation* 25:663–73.

American Psychiatric Association. 1994. *Diagnostic and Statistical Manual of Mental Disorders*. 4th ed. Washington, D.C.: American Psychiatric Association.

Awad, I.A., P.C. Johnson, R.F. Spetzler, et al. 1986. Incidental subcortical lesions identified on magnetic resonance imaging in the elderly. II. Postmortem pathological correlations. *Stroke* 17:1090–97.

Babikian, V., and A.H. Ropper. 1987. Binswanger's disease: A review. *Stroke* 18:2–12.

Baudrimont, M., F. Dubas, A. Joutel, et al. 1993. Autosomal dominant leukoencephalopathy and subcortical ischemic stroke: A clinicopathological study. *Stroke* 24: 122–25.

Bowler, J.V., R. Steenhuis, and V. Hachinski. 1999. Conceptual background to vascular cognitive impairment. *Alzheimer Disease and Associated Disorders* 13 (Suppl. 3):S30–37.

Bradley, W.G., Jr., V. Waluch, R.A. Yadley, et al. 1984. Comparison of CT and MR in 400 patients with suspected disease of the brain and cervical spinal cord. *Radiology* 152:695–702.

Braffman, B.H., R.A. Zimmerman, J.Q. Trojanowski, et al. 1988. Brain MR. Pathologic correlation with gross and histopathology. 1. Lacunar infarction and Virchow-Robin spaces. *American Journal of Neuroradiology* 9:621–28.

Brant-Zawadzki, M., P.L. Davis, L.E. Crooks, et al. 1983. NMR demonstration of cerebral abnormalities: Comparison with CT. *American Journal of Roentgenology* 140: 847–54.

Breteler, M.M. 2000. Vascular risk factors for Alzheimer's disease: An epidemiologic perspective. *Neurobiology of Aging* 21:153–60.

Chabriat, H., K. Vahedi, M.T. Iba-Zizen, et al. 1995. Clinical spectrum of CADASIL: A study of seven families. *Lancet* 346:934–39.

Chimowitz, M.I., M.L. Estes, A.J. Furlan, et al. 1992. Further observations on the pathology of subcortical lesions identified on magnetic resonance imaging. *Archives of Neurology* 49:747–52.

Chui, H.C. 2001. Vascular dementia, a new beginning: Shifting focus from clinical phenotype to ischemic brain injury. *Neurology Clinics* 18:951–77.

Chui, H.C., and R. Gonthier. 1999. Natural history of Vascular Dementia. *Alzheimer Disease and Associated Disorders* 13 (Suppl. 3):S124–30.

Chui, H.C., J.I. Victoroff, D. Margolin, et al. 1992. Criteria for the diagnosis of ischemic Vascular Dementia proposed by the State of California Alzheimer's disease Diagnostic and Treatment Centers. *Neurology* 42:473–80.

Chui, H C., W. Mack, J.E. Jackson, et al. 2000. Clinical criteria for the diagnosis of vascular dementia. *Archives of Neurology* 57:191–96.

Cummings, J.L. 1993. Fronto-subcortical circuits and human behavior. *Archives of Neurology* 50:873–80.

Cummings, J.L. 1994. Vascular subcortical dementias: Clinical aspects. *Dementia* 5: 177–80.

Desmond, D.W., T. Erkinjuntti, M. Sano, et al. 1999. The cognitive syndrome of Vascular Dementia: Implications for clinical trials. *Alzheimer Disease and Associated Disorders* 13 (Suppl 3):S21–29.

Donnan, G.A., and M. Yasaka. 1998. Lacunes and lacunar syndromes. In *Cerebrovascular Disease: Pathophysiology, Diagnosis, and Management*, edited by M.D. Ginsberg and J. Bogousslavsky. Malden, Mass.: Blackwell Science, pp. 1090–1102.

Erkinjuntti, T. 1987a. Types of multi-infarct dementia. *Acta Neurologica Scandinavica* 75: 391–99.

Erkinjuntti, T. 1987b. Differential diagnosis between Alzheimer's disease and vascular dementia: Evaluation of common clinical methods. *Acta Neurologica Scandinavica* 76: 433–42.

Erkinjuntti, T. 1994. Clinical criteria for Vascular Dementia: The NINDS-AIREN criteria. *Dementia* 5:189–92.

Erkinjuntti, T. 1999. Cerebrovascular dementia. Pathophysiology, diagnosis and treatment. *CNS Drugs* 12:35–48.

Erkinjuntti T., and V.C. Hachinski. 1993. Rethinking vascular dementia. *Cerebrovascular Diseases* 3:3–23.

Erkinjuntti, T., M. Haltia, J. Palo, et al. 1988. Accuracy of the clinical diagnosis of Vascular Dementia: A prospective clinical and post-mortem neuropathological study. *Journal of Neurology Neurosurgery and Psychiatry* 51:1037–44.

Erkinjuntti, T., D.H. Lee, F. Gao, et al. 1993. Temporal lobe atrophy on magnetic resonance imaging in the diagnosis of early Alzheimer's disease. *Archives of Neurology* 50: 305–10.

Erkinjuntti, T., O. Benavente, M. Eliasziw, et al. 1996. Diffuse vacuolization (spongiosis) and arteriolosclerosis in the frontal white matter occurs in vascular dementia. *Archives of Neurology* 53:325–32.

Erkinjuntti, T., D. Inzitari, L. Pantoni, et al. 2000. Research criteria for subcortical vascular dementia in clinical trials. *Journal of Neural Transmission* 59 (Suppl. 11):S23–30.

Fazekas, F., R. Kleinert, H. Offenbacher, et al. 1991. The morphologic correlate of incidental punctate white matter hyperintensities on MR images. *American Journal of Neuroradiology* 12:915–21.

Fazekas, F., R. Kleinert, H. Offenbacher, et al. 1993. Pathologic correlates of incidental MRI white matter signal hyperintensities. *Neurology* 43:1683–89.

Fischer, P., G. Gatterer, A. Marterer, et al. 1990. Course characteristics in the differentiation of dementia of the Alzheimer type and multi-infarct dementia. *Acta Psychiatrica Scandanavica* 81:551–53.

Fisher, C.M. 1982. Lacunar strokes and infarcts: A review. *Neurology* 32:871–76.

Fitten, L.J., K.M. Perryman, C.J. Wilkinson, et al. 1995. Alzheimer and vascular dementias and driving. *Journal of the American Medical Association* 273:1360–65.

Fratiglioni, L., L.J. Launer, K. Andersen, et al. 2000. Incidence of dementia and major subtypes in Europe: A collaborative study of population-based cohorts. *Neurology* 54 (Suppl 5):S10–15.

Furuta, A., N. Ishii, Y. Nishihara, et al. 1991. Medullary arteries in aging and dementia. *Stroke* 22:442–46.

Garcia, J.H., and G.G. Brown. 1992. Vascular dementia: Neuropathologic alterations and metabolic brain changes. *Journal of Neurological Science* 109:121–31.

Garcia, J.H., N.A. Lassen, C. Weiller, et al. 1996. Ischemic stroke and incomplete infarction. *Stroke* 27:761–65.

Gauthier, S., K. Rockwood, I. Gelinas, L. Sykes, S. Teunisse, J.M. Orgogozo, T. Erkinjuntti, H. Erzigkeit, M. Gleeson, B. Kittner, M. Pontecorvo, H. Feldman, and P. Whitehouse. 1999. Outcome measures for the study of activities of daily living in vascular dementia. *Alzheimer Disease and Associated Disorders* 13 (Suppl. 3): S143–47.

Gearing, M., S.S. Mirra, J.C. Hedreen, et al. 1995. The Consortium to Establish a Registry for Alzheimer's disease (CERAD) part X: Neuropathology confirmation of the clinical diagnosis of Alzheimer's disease. *Neurology* 45:461–66.

Gold, G., P. Giannakopoulos, C. Montes-Paixao Jr., et al. 1997. Sensitivity and specificity of newly proposed clinical criteria for possible Vascular Dementia. *Neurology* 49:690–94.

Görtelmeyer, R., and H. Erbler. 1992. Memantine in treatment of mild to moderate dementia syndrome. *Drug Research* 42:904–12.

Gottfries, C.G., K. Blennow, I. Karlsson, et al. 1994. The neurochemistry of vascular dementia. *Dementia* 5:163–67.

Groves, W.C., J. Brandt, M. Steinberg, et al. 2000. Vascular dementia and Alzheimer's disease: Is there a difference?: A comparison of symptoms by disease duration. *Journal of Neuropsychiatry and Clinical Neurosciences* 12:305–15.

Hachinski, V. 1992. Preventable senility: A call for action against the Vascular Dementias. *Journal of the American Geriatrics Society* 340:645–48.

Hachinski, V.C., N.A. Lassen, and J. Marshall. 1974. Multi-infarct dementia. A cause of mental deterioration in the elderly. *Lancet* 2 (7874):207–10.

Hachinski, V.C., L.D. Iliff, E. Zilhka, et al. 1975. Cerebral blood flow in dementia. *Archives of Neurology* 32:632–37.

Hargrave, R., L.C. Geck, B. Reed, et al. 2000. Affective behavioural disturbances in Alzheimer's disease and ischaemic vascular disease. *Journal of Neurology, Neurosurgery, and Psychiatry* 68:41–46.

Hébert, R., and C. Brayne. 1995. Epidemiology of Vascular Dementia. *Neuroepidemiology* 14:240–57.

Henon, H., I. Durie, D. Guerouaou, et al. 2001. Poststroke dementia: Incidence and relationship to prestroke cognitive decline. *Neurology* 57:1216–22.

Heyman, A., G.G. Fillenbaum, K.A. Welsh-Bohmer, et al. 1998. Cerebral infarcts in patients with autopsy-proven Alzheimer's disease. CERAD, part XVIII. *Neurology* 51: 159–62.

Inzitari, D., F. Diaz, A. Fox, et al. 1987. Vascular risk factors and leuko-araiosis. *Archives of Neurology* 44:42–47.

Ishii, N., Y. Nishihara, and T. Imamura. 1986. Why do frontal lobe symptoms predominate in vascular dementia with lacunes? *Neurology* 36:340–45.

Jack, C.R. Jr., R.C. Petersen, Y.C. Xu, et al. 1997. Medial temporal atrophy on MRI in normal aging and very mild Alzheimer's disease. *Neurology* 49:786–94.

Jagust, W., R. Thisted, M.D. Devous Sr., et al. 2001. SPECT perfusion imaging in the diagnosis of Alzheimer's disease: A clinical-pathologic study. *Neurology* 56:950–56.

Janota, J., T.R Mirsen, V.C. Hachinski, et al. 1989. Neuropathological correlates of leuko-araiosis. *Archives of Neurology* 46:1124–28.

Johnson, K.A., K.R. Davis, F.S. Buonanno, et al. 1987. Comparison of magnetic resonance and roentgen ray computed tomography in dementia. *Archives of Neurology* 44: 1075–80.

Kalaria, R.N., and C. Ballard. 1999. Overlap between pathology of Alzheimer disease and Vascular Dementia. *Alzheimer Disease and Associated Disorders* 13 (Suppl. 3): S115–23.

Kivipelto, M., E.L. Helkala, M. Laakso, et al. 2001. Midlife vascular risk factors and late-life Alzheimer's disease: A longitudinal, population-based study. *British Medical Journal* 322:1447–51.

Kokmen, E., J.P. Whisnant, W.N. O'Fallon, et al. 1996. Dementia after ischemic stroke: A population-based study in Rochester, Minnesota (1960–1984). *Neurology* 46:154–59.

Laakso, M.P., K. Partanen, P. Riekkinen, et al. 1996. Hippocampal volumes in Alzheimer's disease, Parkinson's disease, and in vascular dementia: A MRI study. *Neurology* 46:678–81.

Lamar, M., K. Podell, T.G. Carew, et al. 1997. Perseverative behaviour in Alzheimer's disease and subcortical ischaemic vascular dementia. *Neuropsychology* 11:523–34.

Leibson, C. L., W.A. Rocca, V.A. Hanson, et al. 1997. Risk of dementia among persons with diabetes mellitus: A population-based cohort study. *American Journal of Epidemiology* 145:301–8.

Leifer, D., F.S. Buonanno, and E.P. Richardson Jr. 1990. Clinicopathologic correlations of cranial magnetic resonance imaging of periventricular white matter. *Neurology* 40: 911–18.

Lobo, A., L.J. Launer, L. Fratiglioni, et al. 2000. Prevalence of dementia and major subtypes in Europe: A collaborative study of population-based cohorts. *Neurology* 54 (Suppl. 5):S4–9.

Mahler, M.E., and J.L. Cummings. 1991. The behavioural neurology of multi-infarct dementia. *Alzheimer Disease and Associated Disorders* 5:122–30.

Mäntylä, R., T. Erkinjuntti, O. Salonen, et al. 1997. Variable agreement between visual rating scales for white matter hyperintensities on MRI: Comparison of 13 rating scales in a poststroke cohort. *Stroke* 28:1614–23.

Mäntylä, R., H.J. Aronen, O. Salonen, et al. 1999. The prevalence and distribution of white-matter changes on different MRI pulse sequences in a post-stroke cohort. *Neuroradiology* 41:657–65.

Marshall, V.G., W.G. Bradley Jr., C.E. Marshall, et al. 1988. Deep white matter infarction: Correlation of MR imaging and histopathologic findings. *Radiology* 167:517–22.

McKhann, G., D. Drachman, M. Folstein, et al. 1984. Clinical diagnosis of Alzheimer's disease: Report of the NINCDS-ADRDA Work Group under the auspices of Department of Health and Human Services Task Force on Alzheimer's disease. *Neurology* 34:939–44.

Millikan, C., and N. Futrell. 1990. The fallacy of the lacune hypothesis. *Stroke* 21: 1251–57.

Mölsä, P.K., R.J. Marttila, and U.K. Rinne. 1995. Long-term survival and predictors of mortality in Alzheimer's disease and multi-infarct dementia. *Acta Neurologica Scandinavica* 91:159–64.

Moroney, J.T., E. Bagiella, D.W. Desmond, et al. 1997. Meta-analysis of the Hachinski Ischemic Score in pathologically verified dementias. *Neurology* 49:1096–1105.

Muñoz, D.G., S.M. Hastak, B. Harper, et al. 1993. Pathologic correlates of increased signals of the centrum ovale on magnetic resonance imaging. *Archives of Neurology* 50: 492–97.

Notkola, I.L., R. Sulkava, J. Pekkanen, et al. 1998. Serum total cholesterol, apolipoprotein E ε4 allele, and Alzheimer's disease. *Neuroepidemiology* 17:14–20.
Olsson, Y., A. Brun, and E. Englund. 1996. Fundamental pathological lesions in vascular dementia. *Acta Neurologica Scandinavica* 168 (Suppl.):S31–38.
Ostrow, P.T., and L.L. Miller. 1993. Pathology of small artery disease. *Advances in Neurology* 62:93–123.
Pantoni, L., and J.H. Garcia. 1997. Pathogenesis of leukoaraiosis: A review [review] [114 refs]. *Stroke* 28:652–59.
Pantoni, L., M. Carosi, S. Amigoni, et al. 1996a. A preliminary open trial with nimodipine in patients with cognitive impairment and leukoaraiosis. *Clinical Neuropharmacology* 19:497–506.
Pantoni, L., J.H. Garcia, and J.A. Gutierrez. 1996b. Cerebral white matter is highly vulnerable to ischemia. *Stroke* 27:1641–46.
Pantoni, L., D. Leys, F. Fazekas, et al. 1999. Role of white matter lesions in cognitive impairment of vascular origin. *Alzheimer Disease and Associated Disorders* 13 (Suppl. 3): S49–54.
Petito, C.K., J.-P. Olarte, B. Roberts, et al. 1998. Selective glial vulnerability following transient global ischemia in rat brain. *Journal of Neuropathology and Experimental Neurology* 3:231–38.
Pohjasvaara, T., T. Erkinjuntti, R. Vataja, et al. 1997. Dementia three months after stroke. Baseline frequency and effect of different definitions of dementia in the Helsinki Stroke Aging Memory Study (SAM) cohort. *Stroke* 28:785–92.
Pohjasvaara, T., R. Mantyla, O. Salonen, et al. 2000. How complex interactions of ischemic brain infarcts, white matter lesions, and atrophy relate to poststroke dementia. *Archives of Neurology* 57 (9):1295–1300.
Reed, B.R., J.L. Eberling, D. Mungas, et al. 2000. Memory failure has different mechanisms in subcortical stroke and Alzheimer's disease. *Annals of Neurology* 48:275–84.
Révész, T., C.P. Hawkins, E.P.G.H. du Boulay, et al 1989. Pathological findings correlated with magnetic resonance imaging in subcortical arteriosclerotic encephalopathy (Binswanger's disease). *Journal of Neurology, Neurosurgery, and Psychiatry* 52:1337–44.
Rocca, W.A., A. Hofman, C. Brayne, et al. 1991. The prevalence of Vascular Dementia in Europe: Facts and fragments from 1980–1990 studies. The EURODEM-Prevalence Research Group. *Annals of Neurology* 30:817–24.
Rockwood, K. 1997. Lessons from mixed dementia. *International Psychogeriatrics* 9:245–50
Rockwood, K., and C. MacKnight. 2000. *Understanding Dementia: A Primer of Diagnosis and Management.* Halifax: Pottersfield.
Rockwood, K., I. Parhad, V. Hachinski, et al. 1994. Diagnosis of Vascular Dementia: Consortium of Canadian Centres for Clinical Cognitive Research consensus statement. *Canadian Journal of Neurological Science* 21:358–64.
Rockwood, K., J. Bowler, T. Erkinjuntti, et al. 1999a. Subtypes of Vascular Dementia. *Alzheimer Disease and Associated Disorders* 13 (Suppl 3):S59–64.
Rockwood, K., K. Howard, C. MacKnight, et al. 1999b. Spectrum of disease in vascular cognitive impairment. *Neuroepidemiology* 18:248–54.
Rockwood, K., C. Wentzel, V. Hachinski, et al. 2000a. Prevalence and outcomes of vascular cognitive impairment. *Neurology* 54:447–51.
Rockwood, K., C. MacKnight,, C. Wentzel, et al. 2000b. The diagnosis of "mixed" de-

mentia in the Consortium for the Investigation of Vascular Impairment of Cognition (CIVIC). *Annals of the New York Academy of Sciences* 903:522–28.

Roman, G.C. 1987. Senile dementia of the Binswanger type: A vascular form of dementia in the elderly. *Journal of the American Medical Association* 258:1782–88.

Roman, G.C. 2000. Binswanger disease: The history of a silent epidemic. *Annals of the New York Academy of Sciences* 903:19–23.

Roman, G.C., T.K. Tatemichi, T. Erkinjuntti, et al. 1993. Vascular dementia: Diagnostic criteria for research studies. Report of the NINDS-AIREN International Workshop. *Neurology* 43:250–60.

Rother, M., T. Erkinjuntti, M. Roessner, et al. 1998. Propentofylline in the treatment of Alzheimer's disease and vascular dementia. *Dementia and Geriatric Cognitive Disorders* 9:36–43.

Ruchoux, M.M., and C.A. Maurage. 1997. CADASIL: Cerebral autosomal dominant arteriopathy with subcortical infarcts and leukoencephalopathy. *Journal of Neuropathology and Experimental Neurology* 56:947–64.

Scheltens, P., D. Leys, F. Barkhof, et al. 1992. Atrophy of medial temporal lobes on MRI in "probable" Alzheimer's disease and normal ageing: Diagnostic value and neuropsychological correlates. *Journal of Neurology, Neurosurgery, and Psychiatry* 55:967–72.

Scheltens, P., T. Erkinjunti, D. Leys, et al. 1998. White matter changes on CT and MRI: An overview of visual rating scales. European Task Force on Age-Related White Matter Changes. *European Neurology* 39:80–89.

Skehan, S.J., M. Hutchinson, and D.P. MacErlaine. 1995. Cerebral autosomal dominant arteriopathy with subcortical infarcts and leukoencephalopathy: MR findings. *American Journal of Neuroradiology* 16:2115–19.

Skoog, I. 1997. The relationship between blood pressure and dementia: A review. *Biomedicine and Pharmacotherapy* 51:367–75.

Skoog, I. 1998. Status of risk factors for Vascular Dementia. *Neuroepidemiology* 17:2–9.

Skoog, I., R.N. Kalaria, and M.M.B. Breteler. 1999. Vascular factors and Alzheimer's disease. *Alzheimer Disease and Associated Disorders* 13 (Suppl. 3):S106–14.

Skoog, I., L. Nilsson, B. Palmertz, et al. 1993. A population-based study on dementia in 85-year-olds. *New England Journal of Medicine* 328:153–58.

Snowdon, D.A., L.H. Greiner, J.A. Mortimer, et al. 1997. Brain infarction and the clinical expression of Alzheimer disease. The Nun Study. *Journal of the American Medical Association* 277:813–17.

Sultzer, D.L., H.S. Levin, M.E. Mahler, et al. 1993. A comparison of psychiatric symptoms in vascular dementia and Alzheimer's disease. *American Journal of Psychiatry* 150: 1806–12.

Suzuki, K., T. Kutsuzawa, K. Takita, et al. 1987. Clinico-epidemiologic study of stroke in Akita, Japan. *Stroke* 18:402–6.

Tatemichi, T.K. 1990. How acute brain failure becomes chronic: A view of the mechanisms and syndromes of dementia related to stroke. *Neurology* 40:1652–59.

Tatemichi, T.K., D.W. Desmond, R. Mayeux, et al. 1992. Dementia after stroke: Baseline frequency, risks, and clinical features in a hospitalized cohort. *Neurology* 42:1185–93.

Tierney, M.C., S.E. Black, J.P. Szalai, et al. 2001. Recognition memory and verbal fluency differentiate probable Alzheimer disease from subcortical ischemic vascular dementia. *Archives of Neurology* 58:1654–59.

Tohgi, H., T. Abe, M. Kimura, et al. 1996.Cerebrospinal fluid acetylcholine and choline in vascular dementia of Binswanger and multiple small infarct types as compared with Alzheimer-type dementia. *Journal of Neural Transmission* 103:1211–20.

van Swieten, J.C., J.H.W. van Den Hout, B.A. van Ketel, et al. 1991. Periventricular lesions in the white matter on magnetic resonance imaging in the elderly: A morphometric correlation with arteriolosclerosis and dilated perivascular spaces. *Brain* 114:761–74.

Wallin, A., and K. Blennow. 1993. Heterogeneity of vascular dementia: Mechanisms and subgroups. *Journal of Geriatric Psychiatry and Neurology* 6:177–88.

Wallin, A., K. Blennow, and C.G. Gottfries. 1989. Neurochemical abnormalities in vascular dementia. *Dementia* 1:120–30.

Wallin, A., K. Blennow, and C.G. Gottfries. 1991. Subcortical symptoms predominate in Vascular Dementia. *International Journal of Geriatric Psychiatry* 6:137–46.

Wentzel, C., K. Rockwood, C. MacKnight, et al. 2001. Progression of impairment in patients with vascular cognitive impairment without dementia. *Neurology* 57:714–16.

Wetterling, T., R.D. Kanitz, and K.J. Borgis. 1994. The ICD-10 criteria for Vascular Dementia. *Dementia* 5:185–88.

Wetterling, T., R.D. Kanitz, and K.J. Borigis. 1996. Comparison of different diagnostic criteria for vascular dementia (ADDTC, DSM-IV, ICD-10, NINDS-AIREN). *Stroke* 27:30–36.

World Health Organization. 1993. *ICD-10 Classification of Mental and Behavioural Disorders: Diagnostic Criteria for Research*. Geneva: World Health Organization.

CHAPTER THIRTEEN

Acquired Immunodeficiency Syndrome Dementia Complex

Richard W. Price, M.D.

Before the advent of combination, highly active antiretroviral therapy (HAART), the acquired immunodeficiency syndrome dementia complex (ADC) was on a trajectory to become one of the most common causes of dementia developing in young and middle-aged people in the United States (Price et al. 1988). Even now, in the advanced therapeutic era, this neurological complication continues to contribute importantly to the morbidity and mortality of human immunodeficiency virus type 1 (HIV) infection. This chapter briefly considers the history of this syndrome, its clinical presentation and diagnosis, laboratory diagnostic studies, pathology and pathogenesis, treatment, and epidemiology. More extensive general reviews can be accessed for detailed consideration of these and other facets of this and related neurological conditions complicating AIDS (Gendelman et al. 1998; Price 1999a, b; Brew 2001a, b).

History and Terminology

Acquired immunodeficiency syndrome dementia complex was identified very early in the AIDS epidemic as a common and novel central nervous system

(CNS) disorder (Gopinathan et al. 1983; Snider et al. 1983), and its salient clinical characteristics and pathological substrate were more clearly defined not long after (Navia et al. 1986; Navia, Jordan, and Price 1986). On the basis of its core clinical features that include impairment of attention and concentration, slowing of mental speed and agility, concomitant slowing of motor speed, and loss of initiative, ADC has been classified among the subcortical dementias (Benson 1987). While a variety of terms have been used to describe this clinical syndrome, including *subacute encephalitis*, *HIV encephalopathy*, *HIV* or *AIDS dementia*, and *HIV-related cognitive motor complex*, I continue to favor the ADC terminology and its associated staging system described below—hence, its use in this chapter (for a more extensive review and discussion of terminology, see Price 1999a, b). Acquired immunodeficiency syndrome dementia complex is one of the most common and clinically important CNS complications of late HIV infection. It is a source of great morbidity and, in its more severe form, is associated with a limited survival (Neaton et al. 1994; Price et al. 1999a. b). Like other major complications of HIV infection, ADC is characteristically a late complication, developing in the setting of depressed helper ($CD4^+$) T cell blood counts and ongoing viremia.

An empirically derived acquired immunodeficiency syndrome dementia complex staging system (also referred to as Memorial Sloan-Kettering, or MSK, staging) has proved a useful instrument in describing functional severity for both clinical and investigative purposes (tab. 13.1) (Price and Brew 1988; Sidtis and Price 1990). This staging is applied once the diagnosis of ADC is made and determined to be the basis for functional incapacity in cognitive and motor activities of work and daily living. Acquired immunodeficiency syndrome dementia complex encompasses both brain and spinal cord dysfunction. However, AIDS patients impaired for other reasons, for example, due to another AIDS-related opportunistic infection like primary CNS lymphoma (PCNSL) or as a result of unrelated CNS disease such as prior head injury, should not be assigned an ADC stage. Likewise, motor or gait impairment caused by peripheral neuropathy rather than brain or spinal cord dysfunction should not contribute to ADC staging. The stage 0.5 designation is useful for classifying patients in whom there are neurological symptoms (equivocal disease) or abnormal findings on examination (subclinical disease) *without functional impairment;* it provides a way to deal with subjects who are neither clearly normal nor functionally impaired. By contrast, stage 1 ADC designates definite dysfunction, although sufficient only to render work or daily living more difficult but without major incapacity. Stages 2–4 are

Table 13.1. Staging of acquired immunodeficiency syndrome dementia complex

Stage	Characteristic
0 (normal)	Normal mental and motor function.
0.5	Either minimal or equivocal symptoms of cognitive or motor dysfunction (equivocal/subclinical) characteristic of ADC, or mild signs (snout response, slowed extremity movements), but without impairment of work or capacity to perform activities of daily living (ADLs). Gait and strength are normal.
1 (mild)	Unequivocal evidence (symptoms, signs, neuropsychological test performance) of functional intellectual or motor impairment characteristic of ADC, but able to perform all but the more demanding aspects of work or ADLs. Can walk without assistance.
2 (moderate)	Cannot work or maintain the more demanding aspects of daily life, but able to perform basic activities of self-care. Ambulatory, but may require a single prop.
3 (severe)	Major intellectual incapacity (cannot follow news or personal events, cannot sustain complex conversation, considerable slowing of all output) or motor disability (cannot walk unassisted, requiring walker or personal support, usually with slowing and clumsiness of arms as well).
4 (end stage)	Nearly vegetative. Intellectual and social comprehension and responses are at a rudimentary level. Nearly or absolutely mute. Paraparetic or paraplegic with double incontinence.

Sources: Price and Brew 1988; Sidtis and Price 1990.

applied to increasingly more severe dysfunction, and establish a degree of neurologic severity sufficient to meet criteria for a clinical AIDS diagnosis (Centers for Disease Control and Prevention 1992). Committees sponsored by the World Health Organization (1990) and American Academy of Neurology (1991) proposed alternative terminologies for ADC which can be readily translated to the ADC staging from which they were derived (Price 1999a, b).

Clinical Presentation and Differential Diagnosis

Although the acquired immunodeficiency syndrome dementia complex presents a similar clinical picture of combined cognitive, motor, and, more variably, behavioral symptoms and signs through the full spectrum of severity, it is useful to separate discussion of its clinical presentation and differential diagnosis into the milder and more severe forms. Of the three affected "spheres" of function, abnormalities in cognition and motor performance are the most helpful in characterizing patients and in defining diagnosis; it is for this reason that they provide the basis of ADC staging which omits behavioral criteria.

Milder Acquired Immunodeficiency Syndrome Dementia Complex

Cognitive impairment usually underlies the earliest symptoms of patients with stage 0.5 or 1 acquired immunodeficiency syndrome dementia complex, and this is the principal thing that leads them or their associates to question if something is wrong. These patients most often have difficulty attending to more complex tasks at work or at home, and they acquire the need to make lists, sometimes very detailed, of the day's activities. They lose track of intended actions (for example, they may get up to go to another room and then forget why they did so) or of conversations in midsentence. Processing unrelated or complex thoughts becomes slower and less facile. While similar lapses can trouble many normal people, especially in the face of fatigue or generalized illness, in the stage 1 ADC patient they intrude on and disrupt smooth daily function to a disturbing degree. Multistaged tasks become difficult: the waiter has trouble accurately relaying orders when he arrives at the kitchen; the computer programmer struggles to recall the line of code she intended to write next and must now outline each step in detail; the avid reader needs to reread paragraphs or pages to the point that an activity that once gave great pleasure is abandoned.

When mild, it may be difficult to substantiate the basis for complaints by bedside examination. Because it was constructed for other conditions, the standard Mini-Mental Status Examination (MMSE; Folstein, Folstein, and McHugh 1975) is often not sensitive enough to distinguish these patients as abnormal. When they do perform abnormally, it is usually on reversals (reversing a five-letter word like *world*, or subtracting serial sevens) or complex sequential tasks (placing the right thumb on the left ear and sticking out the tongue). Notably, even when these and other tasks are performed accurately, the response may be slow and require prompting. Indeed, the examiner should be attentive to these characteristics and not rely solely on accuracy. Folstein and colleagues suggested a verbal adaptation of the Trail Making B test as a screen for the characteristic difficulty in rapid sequential effort (Jones et al. 1993), while Power and colleagues proposed and recently revised a bedside screen that examines some of the salient features of ADC (Power et al. 1995a, b; Davis et al. 2002). For screening and longitudinal evaluations in the context of cohort studies, we have used a combination of either two or four brief quantitative neurological performance tests and a derived mean z-score (either QNPZ-2, which combines scaled scores from the grooved pegboard using the dominant hand [Lezak 1995] and timed gait, or the QNPZ-4, which adds scores of the Digit Symbol Substitution subtest from the WAIS-R [Wechsler 1981] and finger tapping using the nondominant hand [Reitan and Wolfson 1985]) (Price and Sidtis 1990; Price et al. 1999).

Motor symptoms are far less common during this early phase, although individuals relying on rapid or fine coordination sometimes observe a change in performance. Less commonly, clumsiness of handwriting, tying shoes, or buttoning a shirt will be noted. More commonly patients exhibit motor signs on examination in the absence of overt symptoms. These include slowing of rapid opposition of the thumb and forefinger, rotation of the wrist, or tapping of the toe. Slowing of ocular saccades may also be found along with interruption of smooth ocular pursuits. While the gait is generally steady, it may be slowed, and rapid turns may be interrupted by an extra step or performed hesitantly. Reflexes are also often abnormal with hyperactive deep tendon stretch reflexes, including importantly the jaw jerk, although the ankle jerks may be relatively less active when there is concomitant polyneuropathy. Babinski signs may sometimes be present, although more commonly other "pathological" release signs are detected; of these, the snout response is relatively frequent and notably helpful when present in young patients.

The time course and onset of milder acquired immunodeficiency syndrome dementia complex is variable. It mostly is insidious and evolves slowly or even remains static for some period. While phenotypically similar to the more severe disease in its "subcortical" character, it is not entirely certain that this milder form shares the same pathogenesis as more severe ADC. In other patients who are more likely to soon progress further, the onset may be more abrupt and progression more distinct and steady.

The diagnostic exercise in these mild patients often centers on the question of whether indeed they have an "organic" central nervous system affliction. Particularly important is the distinction of ADC from clinical depression, which can produce similar complaints but carries important therapeutic implications. Hypochondriasis and anxiety in those understandably worried about body function may also lead to similar complaints. On the other hand, without proper attention, the presence of stage 0.5 or 1 ADC may be overlooked and erroneously considered by patient and caregiver alike as simply an "expected" manifestation of systemic illness. Eliciting motor slowing and pathological reflexes on neurological examination as discussed above helps to differentiate these, although one must be certain that these signs are not caused by another preexisting or acquired condition. The laboratory studies discussed later in the context of more severe ADC are probably less helpful in this setting. Beyond careful history and examination, more detailed neuropsychological diagnostic testing (beyond the simple screening and longitudinal follow-up tests outlined above) may be particularly helpful to define the presence and pattern of impairment. In some cases neuroimaging may be useful (see below).

More Severe Acquired Immunodeficiency Syndrome Dementia Complex

In patients with stage 2–4 acquired immunodeficiency syndrome dementia complex, the principal diagnostic exercise centers, not on proving the presence of cognitive impairment, but on confirming that abnormal function relates to acquired immunodeficiency syndrome dementia complex rather than to another central nervous system disease. Cognitive function in these subjects is usually clearly abnormal and obviously impairs functional status, although some patients with stage 2 or even 3 ADC may elude recognition by a cursory history and examination when they maintain the civilities of casual conversation and personal interactions. However, careful questioning of both the patient and associates usually makes it very clear that stage 2 patients are too slow or forgetful to work, maintain the household, or, importantly, manage their medications. They may get lost walking or driving and cannot be relied on to prepare meals, much less to balance the checkbook. On examination a broader array of cognitive domains may be afflicted, adding to the core manifestations of mental and motor slowing and poor attention and concentration. The bedside MMSE is now often abnormal (Folstein, Folstein, and McHugh 1975). Surprisingly, in many, although not all, with stage 2 and 3 ADC, judgment remains preserved, and they are able to make or assist with decisions.

Motor abnormalities also become more clearly symptomatic and obvious to others. Walking may be sufficiently unsteady to require a cane. Hyper-reflexia and pathological reflexes are now also virtually always present, and gait instability and slowness is more clearly evident, even on the straightaway. With further progression, ambulation constantly requires support or is entirely precluded (stage 3 or 4). Thinking and speaking also become slower and the content more impoverished. Concomitant behavioral changes may become more evident. Friends say that patients have lost their "sparkle" and that they are duller and less vivacious. They may sit still without spontaneously offering conversation, and only provide brief responses to direct questions. This apathy and poverty of output may be mistaken for depression, but dysphoria is absent in most. Disinterest and lack of initiative are the predominating aspects of behavior without sadness. When patients then progress even further, paraplegia or near quadriplegia may develop, at times in flexion and usually with associated incontinence of bladder and bowel. Complete or nearly complete mutism with only rudimentary cognition characterizes the end result (stage 4) of the disease.

A striking variant that manifests in a small minority of patients includes agitation with features of mania (Navia, Jordan, and Price 1986; Boccellari, Dilley, and Shore 1988; Fernandez and Levy 1993; Sewell et al. 1994; Ellen et al. 1999; Mijch et al. 1999; Ferrando and Wapenyi 2002). While in some this behavioral state may be unrelated, in others it appears to be a manifestation of ADC and carries a similar prognosis. These patients usually exhibit a background of confusion that persists even as the overactivity is controlled by medication. Treatment combines antiretroviral therapy with psychotropic medications targeting the symptoms.

The myelopathic variant of acquired immunodeficiency syndrome dementia complex has a distinct pathological substrate, known as vacuolar myelopathy, and may be clinically distinguishable in some when the gait dysfunction is disproportionally affected in comparison to the intellect (Petito et al. 1985; Dal Pan, Glass, and McArthur 1994; Petito, Vecchio, and Chen 1994). Some of these patients may become wheelchair bound with normal or near normal cognition. In others, the myelopathy is combined with cognitive difficulty. While the lower extremities are more severely affected than the arms, there is no distinct segmental level of spinal cord dysfunction. Rather, there is a gradual caudal increase in abnormality: knee tendon reflexes are more active than those in the arms, and gait is worse than hand coordination or rapid finger movements. Mild sensory loss is common, and is usually worse distally in the feet, with impaired vibration and position sense most common; sensation is usually normal over the trunk and in the upper extremities. Since myelopathy is frequently combined with neuropathy, the cause of sensory loss in individual patients may not always be clear, and one often relies on the ankle tendon jerks to indicate the relative contribution of myelopathy (increased ankle jerks) or neuropathy (decreased ankle jerks) in the presence of increased patellar stretch reflexes. Clinical presentation usually includes an ataxic and, sometimes, spastic gait. As with some other myelopathies, the ataxia may seem worse than can be accounted for by the loss of position sense in the toes and feet. Babinski signs are usually present as well, accompanying the hyperactive deep tendon reflexes. Urinary dysfunction with precipitous micturition may develop early.

Diagnosis of stage 2–4 acquired immunodeficiency syndrome dementia complex is both an inclusionary and exclusionary exercise. The combination of the characteristic cognitive dysfunction and symmetrical motor abnormalities usually readily allows tentative diagnosis on the basis of the history and examination alone, and there are few other conditions that mimic the typical and uncomplicated presentation. However, when signs and symptoms are less clear-cut, a number of other diseases join in the differential diagnosis. A full discussion is beyond the scope of this chapter; they are considered in an algorithmic context elsewhere (Price 1999a, b). They include primary CNS lymphoma (PCNSL), notably when this tumor involves both frontal lobes or their white matter connections to the basal ganglia. Cytomegalovirus (CMV) encephalitis may also cause progressive cognitive and motor abnormalities, although more often this mimics toxic or metabolic encephalopathies that concomitantly alter the level of arousal along with cognitive impairment in contrast to ADC, where consciousness is preserved (Cinque et al. 1992; Cohen 1996). With the aging of the HIV-infected population, Alzheimer disease may enter into the differential, although the early involvement of memory in the absence of motor abnormalities characteristic of this condition usually allows clear distinction of these diagnoses; there may be greater difficulty when the two conditions develop together and synergistically alter cognition. This has not yet been noted as a common problem, but remains a potential future development as AIDS increases in the aging population. An important differential diagnosis of vacuolar myelopathy is the myelopathy caused by another type of retrovirus, HTLV-I or II (Murphy et al. 1997; Izumo, Umehara, and Osame 2000).

The time course of more severe acquired immunodeficiency syndrome dementia complex is also variable (McArthur et al. 1994). While vacuolar myelopathy may be insidious in onset and gradually progressive over many weeks or months, both this and the cognitive impairment of ADC may develop more rapidly and evolve over only one or a few weeks. This rapid onset and progression is the reason that *subacute encephalitis* was introduced as a descriptive term for what was later to be called ADC (Snider et al. 1983).

Laboratory Diagnosis of Acquired Immunodeficiency Syndrome Dementia Complex

Acquired immunodeficiency syndrome dementia complex is a clinical syndrome and, hence, it is a clinical diagnosis without a specific laboratory marker.

Nonetheless, laboratory studies are important in diagnosis, both to support and to exclude alternatives. Among the most useful assessments are general laboratory tests defining the presence and stage of systemic HIV infection, neuroimaging, and cerebrospinal fluid (CSF) analysis. Neuropsychological testing is also useful as noted above, but might be more properly considered an extension and quantitative refinement of the clinical evaluation (Sidtis et al. 1993; Sidtis 1994; Deutsch et al. 2001).

Clinical Context

Since acquired immunodeficiency syndrome dementia complex is a complication of human immunodeficiency virus type 1, its diagnosis includes confirmation of this underlying retroviral infection. Usually this is known when the patient presents but not always, and ADC may be the initial presentation of underlying HIV infection (Navia and Price 1987). In fact, because of the protective effect of HAART, there is likely a selection for ADC presenting in those unaware of their underlying HIV infection. Serological diagnosis of HIV infection is therefore essential in those not yet tested. While obtaining informed consent for testing can be awkward, it is often more difficult for the physician than the patient and there should be no hesitation in obtaining the test in this context. Because stage 2 or greater ADC develops principally, although not exclusively, in patients with more advanced HIV infection, the blood $CD4^+$ lymphocyte count is helpful in assessing ADC risk. Most will have $CD4^+$ counts below 200 cells/µl. This, along with assessment of the blood concentration of HIV RNA (*viral load*), is an essential component in guiding patient care decisions, and both of these laboratory parameters should be measured at the time of diagnosis and subsequently during treatment.

Neuroimaging

Anatomic brain imaging is probably most specific in establishing alternative diagnoses. Thus, PCNSL, progressive multifocal leukoencephalopathy (PML), cerebral toxoplasmosis, and other opportunistic brain infections are usually detected by computerized tomography (CT) or more sensitively and specifically by magnetic resonance imaging (MRI). However, neuroimaging may also more directly support the diagnosis of ADC. Both CT and MRI often reveal cerebral atrophy in ADC patients, and because these patients are relatively young this atrophy is usually readily distinguished from the normal loss of brain volume that occurs with age (Navia, Jordan, and Price 1986; Post, Berger, and Quencer

1991; Dal Pan et al. 1992; Gelman and Guinto 1992). However, brain atrophy is not diagnostically specific and may be found in HIV patients as a consequence of alcohol or drug use, nutritional factors, or other unrelated causes. Of greater interest, MRI may also reveal characteristic signal changes within the brain parenchyma in ADC patients, showing as fluffy or confluent increases in water content prominent on T2-weighted images in the deeper white matter, usually sparing the U-fibers immediately adjacent to the cortex, or diencephalon (Jarvik et al. 1988; Post et al. 1988; Jakobsen et al. 1989; Moeller and Backmund 1990; Power et al. 1993). These changes are distinct enough to be termed *AIDS encephalopathy* by the imaging community; unfortunately, they do not correlate exactly with an ADC diagnosis or its severity and must still be regarded as ancillary. More recently metabolic imaging using magnetic resonance spectroscopy (MRS) has been applied to studies of ADC and revealed patterns of abnormality that may eventually prove of practical use in the clinic and, more particularly, in clinical trials. Among the abnormalities are decreased levels of the neuronal marker, N-acetyl neuraminic acid (NAA) in the later phases of ADC, and increases in choline peaks somewhat earlier (Jarvik et al. 1993; Tracey et al. 1996; Wilkinson et al. 1997; Chang et al. 1999).

Cerebrospinal Fluid

Analysis of cerebrospinal fluid (CSF) is also useful in assessing acquired immunodeficiency syndrome dementia complex patients, although, like neuroimaging, more in excluding alternative diagnoses like cryptococcal meningitis, neurosyphilis, or cytomegalovirus encephalitis than in precise diagnosis of acquired immunodeficiency syndrome dementia complex. The CSF is frequently abnormal in ADC, with elevation of both protein and white blood cells, but unfortunately these abnormalities are also common in asymptomatic HIV-infected patients. With the first application of quantitative HIV nucleic acid hybridization techniques to CSF, it was hoped that this technology would prove diagnostically useful (Brew et al. 1997). However, with further experience, it is clear that HIV RNA can also be increased in the CSF of neurologically normal individuals and is not diagnostically specific (Ellis et al. 1997). Similarly, a number of "markers" of immune activation, including less specific markers of macrophage activation such as neopterin and β-2-microglobulin and some possible pathogenetic mediators including quinolinc acid, several chemokines, metalloproteinases, and others require further work for increased diagnostic specificity (Brew et al. 1990; Griffin, McArthur, and Cornblath 1991; Heyes et al. 1991;

Brew et al. 1992; Kelder et al. 1998; Letendre, Lanier, and McCutchan 1999; Sabri et al. 2001). While it is hoped that a more precise "battery" of these markers might be deployed both for more certain diagnosis of ADC and to assess its activity (i.e., to distinguish ongoing pathology from residual injury), a group of tests that effectively combine for this purpose has not yet been defined (Brew 2001b).

Pathology and Pathogenesis

A detailed discussion of acquired immunodeficiency syndrome dementia complex pathogenesis is beyond the scope of this chapter. However, some understanding of the pathological substrate and current theories of pathogenesis is useful in following the rationale of therapy. A simple distillation of the prevailing theory is that ADC is caused by brain infection by HIV, rather than by some other opportunistic infection but that the manner by which this retrovirus induces brain injury is not by direct cytolysis with simple killing of the "functional" cellular elements of the brain (neurons, oligodendrocytes, and astrocytes). Rather, brain injury is mediated through "indirect" pathways, some of which involve immunopathology and host-coded signals or toxins. The following brief discussion considers the principal elements of pathogenesis: HIV brain infection, immune system participation in ADC, and mechanisms of brain injury.

Human Immunodeficiency Virus Type 1 Brain Infection

Several types of pathology are found in the central nervous system of patients with acquired immunodeficiency syndrome dementia complex. These include multinucleated-cell encephalitis, white matter pallor, and spinal cord vacuolation. Microscopically, there is an increase in macrophages and microglia and astrogliosis, along with astrocytic apoptosis and simplification of neuronal dendritic trees (Navia et al. 1986; Petito et al. 1986; Rosenblum 1990; Budka 1991; Gray et al. 1991; Masliah et al. 1994; Petito and Roberts 1995; Masliah et al. 1996; Petito et al. 1999). Of these changes, multinucleated cell encephalitis is the most distinct marker of HIV Brain infection; it was first documented by nucleic acid blotting shortly after the cause of AIDS was identified (Shaw et al. 1985) and then defined by numerous other techniques (Gabuzda et al. 1986; Koenig et al. 1986; Stoler et al. 1986; Wiley et al. 1986; Pumarole-Sune et al. 1987; Vazeux et al. 1987). However, the correlation between the viral burden in the brain and clinical severity has not always been exact so that some patients may have evidence of active infection but no neurological impairment during life while others may have advanced impairment but no evidence of HIV encephalitis (Brew et al. 1995; Takahashi et al. 1996). The most striking discrepancy has been with vacuolar myelopathy, in which there is no clear evidence of local causative infection, suggesting that this indeed has a different pathogenesis than brain disease (Petito et al. 1985; Rosenblum et al. 1989; Dal Pan, Glass, and McArthur 1994; Petito, Vecchio, and Chen 1994; Tan, Guiloff, and Scaravilli 1995).

A second important consideration is that most of the infection in brain, and likely all of the fully productive infection, takes place in cells of the macrophage lineage (perivascular and parenchymal macrophages and microglia) rather than in neurons, oligodendrocytes, and astrocytes, although the latter can at times support incomplete infection and expression of certain early viral gene products (Saito et al. 1994; Tornatore et al. 1994). How then is the brain injured? One viral factor that may be important is the "type" of virus infecting the brain. Human immunodeficiency virus type 1 isolates are noted to vary in their cell tropism, and those derived from the brain of ADC patients have generally exhibited macrophage tropism (capacity to replicate in macrophages) and utilization of the CCR5 chemokine receptor as their secondary cell receptor (Janssen et al. 1989; O'Brien 1994; Gabuzda et al. 1998; Chan et al. 1999; Gorry et al. 2001). This is consistent with identification of the macrophage as the major productively infected cell in the brain. There may be additional viral characteristics beyond macrophage tropism that confer greater neuropathogenicity, although these are less well defined (Power et al. 1995a, b).

Immune System in Human Immunodeficiency Virus Type 1

The immune system is also an important participant in acquired immunodeficiency syndrome dementia complex pathogenicity, likely in two fundamental ways, one permissive and the other more directly pathogenic. First, restriction of severe ADC to those with advanced systemic disease suggests that immunosuppression has a permissive effect on development on this disorder (Price 2000). This may relate to the loss of defenses against HIV infection within the brain which is needed for "invasive" brain infection to develop. Second, immune cell, and particularly, macrophage activation appears to be a central component of ADC pathogenesis. Most of the CSF markers discussed above that have been found to be elevated in patients with ADC are products of stimulated macrophages.

Brain Injury

The mechanisms of brain injury remain a matter of speculation—perhaps principally because there is a plethora of candidate toxic pathways and it is difficult to segregate their relative contributions. These fall into two general categories: virus-coded and cell-coded signals or toxins (for reviews, see Price et al. 1988; Epstein and Gendelman 1993; Price 1995; Tyor et al. 1995; Kaul, Garden, and Lipton 2001). Among the former, the envelope glycoprotein gp120 and the regulatory protein *Tat* have received the most attention. A larger number of cellular factors have been implicated, including quinolinic acid, NO, platelet activating factor, and others, perhaps all converging on the *N*-methyl-D-aspartate (NMDA) receptor. Most likely these various factors interact and participate in redundant pathways that act together to disturb brain function. Importantly, these indirect mechanisms of injury appear to be driven largely by infection and are at least partially reversible.

Treatment

These concepts of pathogenesis, while still imprecisely defined, provide rationale for the current approaches to treatment which can be divided into two general categories: *antiviral* and *adjuvant* therapies. Unlike most neurodegenerative diseases, treatment of ADC can be directed at the underlying etiology. If indeed the pathogenesis of brain injury is driven by local brain infection, then it should be possible to interrupt the train of disease events (whatever the intermediate steps) by reducing the burden of viral replication with antiviral therapy. While imperfect, a good deal of experience suggests that this is indeed the case. Proof of concept is found in earlier clinical trials, chiefly involving monotherapy with zidovudine (referred to commonly then as AZT) or two-drug treatment with nucleoside antivirals (Pizzo et al. 1988; Schmitt et al. 1988; Portegies et al. 1989; Sidtis et al. 1993; Vago et al. 1993; Gray et al. 1994). Studies of combination drug therapy, which is now the standard approach to treating systemic HIV infection, have proved difficult, largely due to logistical and ethical constraints. However, if one extrapolates from the experience with monotherapy to the greater potency of combination therapy, it is highly likely that contemporary therapy is indicated in ADC. This is supported by the preventative effect of combination therapy (see below) and by case series and common clinical observation of both ADC and CSF antiviral effects (Foudraine et al. 1998; Staprans et al. 1999; Sacktor et al. 2001). Vacuolar myelopathy may respond less well to HAART than cognitive impairment, although some of these patients clearly do improve after treatment (Di Rocco and Tagliati 2000).

By contrast, evidence is less certain that adjuvant therapeutic approaches to acquired immunodeficiency syndrome dementia complex are helpful. The rationale for these therapies is based on the importance of the intermediate steps in ADC pathogenesis discussed above. It has been suggested that brain injury might be reduced by interventions that target these secondary toxic pathways. Based on this concept and findings in cell culture studies, several clinical trials have now tested approaches to blocking secondary neurotoxicity, but none have shown convincing efficacy (Lipton 1991; Navia et al. 1998). It is my opinion that, while these approaches are of interest in dissecting pathogenesis, they are not likely to add much to the effect of antiviral therapy which drives these processes.

On the other hand, symptomatic therapies may be helpful in certain cases—for example, neuroleptics, anticonvulsants, or lithium in the agitated or manic patient or antidepressants in those with superimposed depression (Ferrando and Wapenyi 2002). However, dosing should be cautious in these individuals since they may be particularly sensitive to some drugs, particularly neuroleptics (Sewell et al. 1994). Other supportive measures are also important (Boccellari and Zeifert 1994).

Despite the remarkable achievements in antiviral therapy and their effects on acquired immunodeficiency syndrome dementia complex incidence, there remain a number of important questions. One of these relates to optimal retroviral therapy and the importance of CNS penetration of antiretroviral drugs. If HIV infection is indeed wholly "compartmentalized" within the CNS, then it can be argued that treatment requires fully therapeutic local tissue concentrations to be effective. Since some antiviral drugs, for example, the protease inhibitors, penetrate the CNS relatively poorly because of high protein binding and active transport by P-glycoprotein (Kim et al. 1998; Choo et al. 2000), they might not be as helpful in treating nervous system as systemic infection. Less effective treatment of this reservoir not only might allow this focus of infection to escape therapy, but also could facilitate the development of mutant, drug-resistant viruses that are favored by exposure of infected cells to subtherapeutic drug concentrations. While it is now clear that viruses isolated from CSF or brain can indeed differ from those detected in blood, the extent to which this has an impact on effective treatment remains uncertain. If one uses CSF virus as an index of CNS infection, in most cases therapy which is effective in reducing or eliminating detectable HIV in the blood also effectively eliminates it in the CSF, perhaps because CNS infection is not fully independent and autonomous but depends on continued reseeding by systemic sources (Staprans et al. 1999; Price 2000). Clearly, more work is needed to define optimal treatment of the CNS and the factors that enhance therapeutic success.

Epidemiology

From the time of its recognition, the incidence of acquired immunodeficiency syndrome dementia complex has been controversial. In part this is related to case definitions and ascertainment, and in part to the groups studied. As noted, ADC is a clinical diagnosis without a precise laboratory marker; hence, estimates may be inflated when other causes of cognitive impairment contaminate samples or undercounted when subjects are not carefully examined and neurological impairment is missed. Population studies, which have the advantages of larger and representative sampling, suffer most from these problems of diagnostic accuracy, while smaller studies with more accurate diagnosis often encompass more selected, nonrepresentational populations.

Early estimates based on hospitalized or neurologically referred patients, and hence based on a group with late human immunodeficiency virus type 1 infection, estimated that the majority of patients manifested acquired immunodeficiency syndrome dementia complex (Navia, Jordan, and Price 1986). Other studies focusing on early HIV infection or a broad spectrum of HIV-infected subjects give far lower estimates (Janssen et al. 1989; Janssen et al. 1992; Bacellar et al. 1994; Neaton et al. 1994). In the Multicentered AIDS Cohort Study that followed a selected group of gay men, including a subset that seroconverted during the course of the study, estimated the incidence rate over a five-year period to be 7.3 cases per 100 person years for subjects with $CD4^+$ counts < 100, 3.0 cases in those with counts of 101–200, 1.3 for counts of 201–350, 1.8 for counts of 351–500, and 0.5 for counts > 500 (Bacellar et al. 1994). As in most other studies, this showed the strong relationship between ADC incidence and low $CD4^+$ T-lymphocyte counts. Data from the Community Programs for Clinical Research on AIDS following AIDS patients in a series of treatment protocols show this same association, and additionally that stage 2 or greater ADC is associated with limited survival (Neaton et al. 1994). The 6-month cumulative mortality of 97 ADC patients among an overall group of more than 3000 HIV-1-infected subjects followed in this program was 67%. Other studies have confirmed the association of cognitive impairment in ADC with higher mortality (Price et al. 1999a, b).

The more contemporary incidence of acquired immunodeficiency syndrome dementia complex has been importantly altered by the widespread use of highly active antiretroviral therapy. Like mortality and the severe opportunistic infections characteristic of AIDS, ADC incidence has clearly fallen (Sacktor et al. 2001). However, there is some controversy over how much the incidence has fallen and whether its decrease is proportional to that of other severe complications of ADC (Dore et al. 1999). In my experience the incidence of new cases is markedly decreased and occurs mainly in those who are excluded from care—in patients who are not receiving HAART out of ignorance, choice, or incapacity. These are most often social, economic, or psychiatric outcasts, and their diagnosis and care may be further confounded by these preexisting conditions or circumstances. Among patients with well-treated HIV infection, ADC is far less common, although exact figures are not available. While it is feared that the combination of (a) more protracted survival of those with HIV and (b) continued appreciable (albeit lower) incidence of ADC might lead to a higher prevalence of the disease, in my experience this has not been obvious. This might be surprising given the frequency of "virological failure" in which treatment fails to induce long-term complete suppression of viremia (Deeks 1999). However, it may mean either that incomplete treatment is still effective in preventing ADC (for example, by maintaining the immune system to a point that it does not allow ADC, or by selecting drug-resistant viral variants that are less neuropathogenic). These clinical impressions need to be substantiated (or refuted) by more careful and precise epidemiological information.

Clinical Conclusions

While a number of unresolved issues of diagnosis, epidemiology, pathogenesis, and treatment remain, it is clear that acquired immunodeficiency syndrome dementia complex continues to be both an intriguing and important cause of neurological morbidity. It is a model of viral and immunopathogenesis with lessons for other conditions and, in itself, is an important condition and target for prevention and therapy. While it is hoped that future advances in primary (vaccine) and secondary (antiviral and other strategies) treatments will further reduce ADC, it likely will continue to be an important diagnosis and source of neurological morbidity in the developed world and, even more so, in the underdeveloped nations experiencing an explosive and devastating HIV epidemic.

ACKNOWLEDGMENTS

My work on HIV infection and ADC is supported by NIH grants R01 NS37660 and R01 MH62701.

REFERENCES

American Academy of Neurology, AIDS Task Force. 1991. Nomenclature and research case definitions for neurologic manifestations of human immunodeficiency virus-type 1 (HIV-1) infection. Report of a Working Group of the American Academy of Neurology AIDS Task Force [review]. *Neurology* 41(6):778–85.

Bacellar, H., A. Munoz, E.N. Miller, et al. 1994. Temporal trends in the incidence of HIV-1-related neurologic diseases: Multicenter AIDS Cohort Study, 1985–1992. *Neurology* 44 (10):1892–900.

Benson, D. 1987. The spectrum of dementia: A comparison of the clinical features of AIDS dementia and dementia of the Alzheimer's type. *Alzheimer Disease and Associated Disorders* 14:217–20.

Boccellari, A., and P. Zeifert. 1994. Management of neurobehavioral impairment in HIV-1 infection [review]. *Psychiatric Clinics of North America* 17 (1):183–203.

Boccellari, A., J.W. Dilley, and M.D. Shore. 1988. Neuropsychiatric aspects of AIDS dementia complex: A report on a clinical series. *Neurotoxicology* 9 (3):381–89.

Brew, B J. 2001a. *HIV Neurology.* New York: Oxford University Press.

Brew, B.J. 2001b. Markers of AIDS dementia complex: The role of cerebrospinal fluid assays. *AIDS* 15 (14):1883–84.

Brew, B.J., R. Bhalla, M. Paul, et al. 1990. Cerebrospinal fluid neopterin in human immunodeficiency virus type 1 infection. *Annals of Neurology* 28:556–60.

Brew, B.J., R.B. Bhalla, M. Paul, et al. 1992. Cerebrospinal fluid beta 2-microglobulin in patients with AIDS dementia complex: An expanded series including response to zidovudine treatment. *AIDS* 6 (5):461–65.

Brew, BJ.., M. Rosenblum, K. Cronin, et al. 1995. The AIDS dementia complex and HIV-1 brain infection: Clinical-virological correlations. *Annals of Neurology* 38:563–70.

Brew, B.J., L. Pemberton, P. Cunningham, et al. 1997. Levels of human immunodeficiency virus type 1 RNA in cerebrospinal fluid correlate with AIDS dementia stage. *Journal of Infectious Diseases* 175:963–66.

Budka, H. 1991. Neuropathology of human immunodeficiency virus infection [review]. *Brain Pathology* 1 (3):163–75.

Centers for Disease Control and Prevention. 1992. 1993 revised classification for HIV infection and expanded surveillance case definition for AIDS among adolescents and adults. *Morbidity and Mortality Weekly Report* 41 (RR-17):1–19.

Chan, S.Y., R.F. Speck, C. Power, et al. 1999. V3 recombinants indicate a central role for CCR5 as a coreceptor in tissue infection by human immunodeficiency virus type 1. *Journal of Virology* 73 (3):2350–58.

Chang, L., T. Ernst, M. Leonido-Yee, et al. 1999. Cerebral metabolite abnormalities correlate with clinical severity of HIV-1 cognitive motor complex. *Neurology* 52 (1): 100–108.

Choo, E.F., B. Leake, C. Wandel, et al. 2000. Pharmacological inhibition of P-glycoprotein transport enhances the distribution of HIV-1 protease inhibitors into brain and testes. *Drug Metabolism and Dispositions* 28 (6):655–60.

Cinque, P., L. Vago, M. Brytting, et al. 1992. Cytomegalovirus infection of the central nervous system in patients with AIDS: Diagnosis by DNA amplification from cerebrospinal fluid. *Journal of Infectious Diseases* 166 (6):1408–11.

Cohen, B.A. 1996. Prognosis and response to therapy of cytomegalovirus encephalitis and meningomyelitis in AIDS. *Neurology* 46:444–50.

Dal Pan, G.J., J.D. Glass, and J.C. McArthur. 1994. Clinicopathologic correlations of HIV-1-associated vacuolar myelopathy: An autopsy-based case-control study. *Neurology* 44 (11):2159–64.

Dal Pan, G.J., J.H. McArthur, E. Aylward, et al. 1992. Patterns of cerebral atrophy in HIV-1-infected individuals: Results of a quantitative MRI analysis. *Neurology* 42 (11): 2125–30.

Davis, H.F., R.L. Skolasky, O.A. Selnes, et al. 2002. Assessing HIV-associated dementia: Modified HIV dementia scale versus the grooved pegboard. *AIDS Reader* 12 (1): 29–38.

Deeks, S.G. 1999. Failure of HIV-1 protease inhibitors to fully suppress viral replication. Implications for salvage therapy. *Advances in Experimental Medicine and Biology* 458:175–82.

Deutsch, R., R.J. Ellis, J.A. McCutchan, et al. 2001. AIDS-associated mild neurocognitive impairment is delayed in the era of highly active antiretroviral therapy. *AIDS* 15 (14):1898–99.

Di Rocco, A., and M. Tagliati. 2000. Remission of HIV myelopathy after highly active antiretroviral therapy. (Comment On: Neurology. 2000 Jan. 11;54(1):267–8 UI: 20100127 Comment On: Neurology. 2000 Apr. 11;54(7):1477–82 UI: 20215055). *Neurology* 55 (3):456.

Dore, G.J., P.K. Correll, Y. Li, et al. 1999. Changes to AIDS dementia complex in the era of highly active antiretroviral therapy. *AIDS* 13 (10):1249–53.

Ellen, S.R., F.K. Judd, A.M. Mijch, et al. 1999. Secondary mania in patients with HIV infection. *Australia and New Zealand Journal of Psychiatry* 33 (3):353–60.

Ellis, R.J., K. Hsia, S.A. Spector, et al. 1997. Cerebrospinal fluid human immunodeficiency virus type 1 RNA levels are elevated in neurocognitively impaired individuals with acquired immunodeficiency syndrome. HIV Neurobehavioral Research Center Group. *Annals of Neurology* 42 (5):679–88.

Epstein, LG., and H.E. Gendelman. 1993. Human immunodeficiency virus type 1 infection of the nervous system: Pathogenetic mechanisms. *Annals of Neurology* 33 (5): 429–36.

Fernandez, F., and J.K. Levy. 1993. The use of molindone in the treatment of psychotic and delirious patients infected with the human immunodeficiency virus: Case reports. *General Hospital Psychiatry* 15 (1):31–35.

Ferrando, S.J., and K. Wapenyi. 2002. Psychopharmacological treatment of patients with HIV and AIDS. *Psychiatric Quarterly* 73 (1):33–49.

Folstein, M., S. Folstein, and P. McHugh. 1975. "Mini-Mental State": A practical method for grading the cognitive state of patients for the clinician. *Journal of Psychiatry Research* 12:189–98.

Foudraine, N.A., R.M. Hoetelmans, J.M. Lange, et al. 1998. Cerebrospinal-fluid HIV-1 RNA and drug concentrations after treatment with lamivudine plus zidovudine or stavudine. *Lancet* 351 (9115):1547–51.

Gabuzda, D., D. Ho, S. De La Monte, et al. 1986. Immunohistochemical identification of HTLV-III antigen in brains of patients with AIDS. *Annals of Neurology* 20:289.

Gabuzda, D., J. He, A. Ohagen, et al. 1998. Chemokine receptors in HIV-1 infection of the central nervous system. *Seminars in Immunology* 10 (3):203–13.

Gelman, B., and F.J. Guinto. 1992. Morphometry, histopathology, and tomography of cerebral atrophy in the acquired immunodeficiency syndrome. *Annals of Neurology* 31: 32–40.

Gendelman, H.E., S.A. Lipton, L. Epstein, et al. 1998. *The Neurology of AIDS.* New York: Chapman & Hall.

Gopinathan, G., L. Laubenstein, B. Mondale, et al. 1983. Central nervous system manifestations of the acquired immunodeficiency (AID) syndrome in homosexual men. *Neurology* 33 (Suppl. 2):S105.

Gorry, P.R., G. Bristol, J.A. Zack, et al. 2001. Macrophage tropism of human immunodeficiency virus type 1 isolates from brain and lymphoid tissues predicts neurotropism independent of coreceptor specificity. *Journal of Virology* 75 (21):10073–89.

Gray, F., H. Haug, L. Chimelli, et al. 1991. Prominent cortical atrophy with neuronal loss as correlate of human immunodeficiency virus encephalopathy. *Acta Neuropathologica* 82 (3):229–33.

Gray, F., L. Belec, C. Keohane, et al. 1994. Zidovudine therapy and HIV encephalitis: A 10-year neuropathological survey. *AIDS* 8 (4):489–93.

Griffin, D.E., J.C. McArthur, and D.R. Cornblath. 1991. Neopterin and interferon-gamma in serum and cerebrospinal fluid of patients with HIV-associated neurologic disease. *Neurology* 41 (1):69–74.

Heyes, M.P., B.J. Brew, A. Martin, et al. 1991. Quinolinic acid in cerebrospinal fluid and serum in HIV-1 infection: Relationship to clinical and neurologic status. *Annals of Neurology* 29:202–9.

Izumo, S., F. Umehara, and M. Osame. 2000. HTLV-I-associated myelopathy. *Neuropathology* 20 (Suppl.):S65–68.

Jakobsen, J., C. Gyldensted, B. Brun, et al. 1989. Cerebral ventricular enlargement relates to neuropsychological measures in unselected AIDS patients. *Acta Neurologica Scandinavica* 79:59.

Janssen, R.S., D.R. Cornblath, L.G. Epstein, et al. 1989. Human immunodeficiency virus (HIV) infection and the nervous system: Report from the American Academy of Neurology AIDS Task Force. *Neurology* 39 (1):119–22.

Janssen, R.S., O.C. Nwanyanwu, R.M. Selik, et al. 1992. Epidemiology of human immunodeficiency virus encephalopathy in the United States. *Neurology* 42 (8):1472–76.

Jarvik, J., J. Hesselink, C. Kennedy, et al. 1988. Acquired immunodeficiency syndrome: Magnetic resonance patterns of brain involvement with pathologic correlation. *Neurology* 45:731.

Jarvik, J.G., R.E. Lenkinski, R.I. Grossman, et al. 1993. Proton MR spectroscopy of HIV-infected patients: Characterization of abnormalities with imaging and clinical correlation. *Radiology* 186 (3):739–44.

Jones, B.N., E.L. Teng, M.F. Folstein, et al. 1993. A new bedside test of cognition for patients with HIV infection. *Annals of Internal Medicine* 119 (10):1001–4.

Kaul, M., G.A. Garden, and S.A. Lipton. 2001. Pathways to neuronal injury and apoptosis in HIV-associated dementia. *Nature* 410 (6831):988–94.

Kelder, W., J.C. McArthur, T. Nance-Sproson, et al. 1998. Beta-chemokines MCP-1 and RANTES are selectively increased in cerebrospinal fluid of patients with human immunodeficiency virus-associated dementia. *Annals of Neurology* 44 (5):831–35.

Kim, R.B., M.F. Fromm, C. Wandel, et al. 1998. The drug transporter P-glycoprotein limits oral absorption and brain entry of HIV-1 protease inhibitors. *Journal of Clinical Investigation* 101 (2):289–94.

Koenig, S., H. Gendelman, J. Orenstein, et al. 1986. Detection of AIDS virus in macrophages in brain tissue from AIDS patients with encephalopathy. *Science* 233: 1089–93.

Letendre, S.L., E.R. Lanier, and J.A. McCutchan. 1999. Cerebrospinal fluid beta chemokine concentrations in neurocognitively impaired individuals infected with human immunodeficiency virus type 1. *Journal of Infectious Diseases* 180 (2):310–19.

Lezak, M. 1995. *Neuropsychological Assessment.* New York: Oxford University Press.

Lipton, S.A. 1991. Calcium channel antagonists and human immunodeficiency virus coat protein-mediated neuronal injury. *Annals of Neurology* 30 (1):110–14.

Masliah, E., C.L. Achim, N. Ge, et al. 1994. Cellular neuropathology in HIV encephalitis. *Research Publications—Association for Research in Nervous and Mental Disease* 72:119–31.

Masliah, E., N. Ge, C. Achim, et al. 1996. Patterns of neurodegeneration in HIV encephalitis. *Journal of Neuro-AIDS* 1 (1):161–73.

McArthur, J.C., O.A. Selnes, J.D. Glass, et al. 1994. HIV dementia: Incidence and risk factors. *Research Publications—Association for Research in Nervous and Mental Disease* 72: 251–72.

Mijch, A.M., F.K. Judd, C.G. Lyketsos, et al. 1999. Secondary mania in patients with HIV infection: Are antiretrovirals protective? *Journal of Neuropsychiatry and Clinical Neuroscience* 11 (4):475–80.

Moeller, A.A., and H.C. Backmund. 1990. Ventricle brain ratio in the clinical course of HIV infection. *Acta Neurologica Scandinavica* 81 (6):512–15.

Murphy, E.L., J. Fridey, J.W. Smith, et al. 1997. HTLV-associated myelopathy in a cohort of HTLV-I and HTLV-II-infected blood donors. The REDS investigators. *Neurology* 48:315–20.

Navia, B., and R. Price. 1987. The acquired immunodeficiency syndrome dementia complex as the presenting or sole manifestation of human immunodeficiency virus infection. *Archives of Neurology* 44:65–69.

Navia, B., B. Jordan, and R. Price. 1986. The AIDS dementia complex: I. Clinical features. *Annals of Neurology* 19:517–24.

Navia, B., E.-W. Cho, C. Petito, et al. 1986. The AIDS dementia complex: II. Neuropathology. *Annals of Neurology* 19:525–35.

Navia, B.A., U. Dafni, D. Simpson, et al. 1998. A phase I/II trial of nimodipine for HIV-related neurologic complications. *Neurology* 51 (1):221–28.

Neaton, J., D. Wentworth, F. Rhame, et al. 1994. Methods of studying interventions. Considerations in choice of a clinical endpoint for AIDS clinical trials. *Statistics in Medicine* 13:2107–25.

O'Brien, W. 1994. Genetic and biologic basis of HIV-1 neurotropism. *HIV, AIDS and the Brain.* Editor. New York: Raven Press, pp. 47–70.

Petito, C.K., and B. Roberts. 1995. Evidence of apoptotic cell death in HIV encephalitis. *American Journal of Pathology* 146 (5):1121–30.

Petito, C.K., D. Vecchio, and Y.T. Chen. 1994. HIV antigen and DNA in AIDS spinal cords correlate with macrophage infiltration but not with vacuolar myelopathy. *Journal of Neuropathology and Experimental Neurology* 53 (1):86–94.

Petito, C.K., B. Navia, E. Cho, et al. 1985. Vacuolar myelopathy pathologically resembling subacute combined degeneration in patients with acquired immunodeficiency syndrome (AIDS). *New England Journal of Medicine* 312:874–79.

Petito, C.K., E.-S. Cho, W. Lemann, et al. 1986. Neuropathology of acquired immunodeficiency syndrome (AIDS): An autopsy review. *Journal of Neuropathology and Experimental Neurology* 45:635–46.

Petito, C.K., A.P. Kerza-Kwiatecki, H.E. Gendelman, et al. 1999. Review: Neuronal injury in HIV infection. *Journal of Neurovirology* 5 (4):327–41.

Pizzo, P., J. Eddy, J. Fallon, et al. 1988. Effect of continuous intravenous infusion of zidovudine (AZT) in children with symptomatic HIV infection. *New England Journal of Medicine* 319:889–96.

Portegies, P., J.M. de Gans, M. Derix, et al. 1989. Declining incidence of AIDS dementia complex after introduction of zidovudine treatment. *British Medical Journal* 299: 819–21.

Post, M.J., J.R. Berger, and R.M. Quencer. 1991. Asymptomatic and neurologically symptomatic HIV-seropositive individuals: Prospective evaluation with cranial MR imaging. *Radiology* 178 (1):131–39.

Post, M., L. Tate, R. Quencer, et al. 1988. CT, MR, and pathology in HIV encephalitis and meningitis. *American Journal of Radiology* 151:373.

Power, C., P.A. Kong, T.O. Crawford, et al. 1993. Cerebral white matter changes in acquired immunodeficiency syndrome dementia: Alterations of the blood-brain barrier. *Annals of Neurology* 34 (3):339–50.

Power, C., J.C. McArthur, R.T. Johnson, et al. 1995a. Distinct HIV-1 env sequences are associated with neurotropism and neurovirulence. *Current Topics in Microbiology and Immunology* 202:89–104.

Power, C., O.A. Selnes, J.A. Grim, et al. 1995b. HIV Dementia Scale: A rapid screening test. *Journal of Acquired Immune Deficiency Syndromes and Human Retrovirology* 8 (3): 273–78.

Price, R. 1995. The cellular basis of central nervous system HIV-1 infection and the AIDS dementia complex: Introduction. *Journal of Neuro-AIDS* 1 (1):1–28.

Price, R.W. 1999a. Management of the neurological complications of HIV-1 and AIDS. *The Medical Management of AIDS*. Editor. Philadelphia: W.B. Saunders Co., pp. 217–40.

Price, R.W. 1999b. Neurologic disease. *AIDS Therapy*. Editor. New York: Churchill Livingston, pp. 620–38.

Price, R.W. 2000. The two faces of HIV infection of cerebrospinal fluid. *Trends in Microbiology* 8 (7):387–90.

Price, R.W., and B. Brew. 1988. The AIDS dementia complex. *Journal of Infectious Disease* 158:1079–83.

Price, R.W., and J.J. Sidtis. 1990. Evaluation of the AIDS dementia complex in clinical trials. *Journal of AIDS* 3 (Suppl. 2):S51–60.

Price, R.W., B. Brew, J. Sidtis, et al. 1988. The brain in AIDS: Central nervous system HIV-1 infection and AIDS dementia complex. *Science* 239:586–92.

Price, R.W., C. Yiannoutsos, D. Clifford, et al. 1999. Neurological outcomes in late HIV infection: Adverse impact of neurological impairment on survival and protective effect of antiviral therapy. *AIDS* 13:1677–85.

Pumarole-Sune, T., B. Navia, C. Cordon-Cardo, et al. 1987. HIV antigen in the brains of patients with the AIDS dementia complex. *Annals of Neurology* 21:490–96.

Reitan, R., and D. Wolfson. 1985. *The Halstead-Reitan Neuropsychological Test Battery: Theory and Clinical Interpretation*. Phoenix: Neuropsychology Press.

Rosenblum, M. 1990. Infection of the central nervous system by the human immunodeficiency virus type 1: Morphology and relation to syndromes of progressive encephalopathy and myelopathy in patients with AIDS. *Pathology Annual* 25:117–69.

Rosenblum, M., A. Scheck, K. Cronin, et al. 1989. Dissociation of AIDS-related vacuolar myelopathy and productive human immunodeficiency virus type 1 (HIV-1) infection of the spinal cord. *Neurology* 39:892–96.

Sabri, F., A. De Milito, R. Pirskanen, et al. 2001. Elevated levels of soluble Fas and Fas ligand in cerebrospinal fluid of patients with AIDS dementia complex. *Journal of Neuroimmunology* 114 (1-2):197–206.

Sacktor, N., R.H. Lyles, R. Skolasky, et al. 2001. HIV-associated neurologic disease incidence changes: Multicenter AIDS Cohort Study, 1990–1998. The Multicenter AIDS Cohort Study. *Neurology* 56 (2):257–60.

Saito, Y., L. Sharer, L. Epstein, et al. 1994. Overexpression of nef as a marker for restricted HIV-1 infection of astrocytes in postmortem pediatric central nervous system tissues. *Neurology* 44:474–81.

Schmitt, F., J. Bigleg, R. McKinnis, et al. 1988. Neuropsychological outcome of azidothymidine (AZT) in the treatment of AIDS and AIDS-related complex: A double blind, placebo-controlled trial. *New England Journal of Medicine* 319:1573–78.

Sewell, D.D., D.V. Jeste, L.A. Mcadams, et al. 1994. Neuroleptic treatment of HIV-associated psychosis. *Neuropsychopharmacology* 10 (4):223–29.

Shaw, G., M. Harper, B. Hahn, et al. 1985. HTLV-III infection in brains of children and adults with AIDS encephalopathy. *Science* 227:177–82.

Sidtis, J.J. 1994. Evaluation of the AIDS dementia complex in adults. *Research Publications—Association for Research in Nervous and Mental Disease* 72:273–87.

Sidtis, J.J., and R.W. Price. 1990. Early HIV-1 infection and the AIDS dementia complex [comment]. *Neurology* 40 (2):323–26.

Sidtis, J.J., C. Gatsonis, R.W. Price, et al. 1993. Zidovudine treatment of the AIDS dementia complex: Results of a placebo-controlled trial. AIDS Clinical Trials Group. *Annals of Neurology* 33 (4):343–49.

Snider, W., D. Simpson, S. Nielson, et al. 1983. Neurological complications of acquired immune deficiency syndrome: Analysis of fifty patients. *Annals of Neurology* 14: 403–18.

Staprans, S., N. Inkina, D. Glidden, et al. 1999. Time course of cerebrospinal fluid (CSF) responses to antiretroviral therapy: Evidence for variable compartmentalization of infection. *AIDS* 13:1051–61.

Stoler, M., T. Eskin, S. Benn, et al. 1986. Human T-cell lymphotropic virus type III infection of the central nervous system: Preliminary in situ analysis. *Journal of the American Medical Association* 256:2360–64.

Takahashi, K., S. Wesselingh, D. Griffin, et al. 1996. Localization of HIV-1 in human brain using polymerase chain reaction/in situ hybridization and immunocytochemistry. *Annals of Neurology* 39:705–11.

Tan, S. V., R.J. Guiloff, and F. Scaravilli. 1995. AIDS-associated vacuolar myelopathy. A morphometric study. *Brain* 118:1247–61.

Tornatore, C., R. Chandra, J.R. Berger, et al. 1994. HIV-1 infection of subcortical astrocytes in the pediatric central nervous system. *Neurology* 44 (3 Pt. 1):481–87.

Tracey, I., C.A. Carr, A.R. Guimaraes, et al. 1996. Brain choline-containing compounds are elevated in HIV-positive patients before the onset of AIDS dementia complex: A proton magnetic resonance spectroscopic study. *Neurology* 46 (3):783–88.

Tyor, W., S. Wesselingh, J. Griffin, et al. 1995. Unifying hypothesis for the pathogenesis of HIV-associated dementia complex, vacuolar myelopathy, and sensory neuropathy. *Journal of Acquired Immune Deficiency Syndrome and Human Retrovirology* 9: 379–88.

Vago, L., A. Castagna, A. Lazzarin, et al. 1993. Reduced frequency of HIV-induced brain lesions in AIDS patients treated with zidovudine. *Journal of Acquired Immune Deficiency Syndromes* 6 (1):42–45.

Vazeux, R., N. Brousse, A. Jarry, et al. 1987. AIDS subacute encephalitis: Identification of HIV-infected cells. *American Journal of Pathology* 126:403–10.

Wechsler, D. 1981. *Wechsler Adult Intelligence Scale Revised.* New York: The Psychological Corporation.

Wiley, C., R. Schrier, J. Nelson, et al. 1986. Cellular localization of human immunodeficiency virus infection within the brains of acquired immune deficiency patients. *Proceedings of the National Academy of Sciences USA* 83:7089–93.

Wilkinson, I.D., S. Lunn, K.A. Miszkiel, et al. 1997. Proton MRS and quantitative MRI assessment of the short term neurological response to antiretroviral therapy in AIDS. *Journal of Neurology, Neurosurgery, and Psychiatry* 63 (4):477–82.

World Health Organization. 1990. 1990 World Health Organization consultation on the neuropsychiatric aspects of HIV-1 infection. *AIDS* 4:935–36.

Part IV / Depressive Dementias

CHAPTER FOURTEEN

Depressive Dementia

A "Prepermanent Intermediate-stage Dementia" in a Long-term Disease Course of Permanent Dementia?

V. Olga B. Emery, Ph.D.,
and Thomas E. Oxman, M.D.

This chapter is a theoretical, empirical, clinical, and nosological discussion of the dementia spectrum of depression. The spectrum involves an array of varied but related presentations that form a continuous series. Depressive disorders are associated with cognitive impairment that can range from mild to severe. Mild cognitive impairment as part of major depression generally raises minimal diagnostic or therapeutic uncertainty. However, when cognitive impairment becomes so severe as to dominate the clinical presentation of patients with symptoms of depressive disorder, issues emerge that require a framework for understanding, classifying, and treating combined disturbances of mood and cognition. To date, the conceptual, empirical, and clinical relationships between depression with severe cognitive deterioration and "permanent" degenerative dementia are as yet not adequately understood. Core questions have been whether and how depressive illness itself causes severe cognitive deterioration (i.e., depressive dementia) or, alternatively, whether some form of irreversible degenerative dementia (World Health Organization 1992, 1993; American Psychiatric Association 1994, 2000) already is present. Recent research and emergent explanations indicate that both lines of explanation have some validity

(Emery 1988, 1992, 1999; Alexopoulos 1990, 1998, 2001, in press; Emery and Oxman 1992, 1997, 2000; Devanand et al. 1996; Kindermann et al. 2000; Lockwood et al. 2000; Snowdon 2001), constituting different points on the depression-dementia spectrum.

The empirically based thesis that will be developed in this chapter is that *depressive dementia*, in many cases, constitutes what we are terming a *prepermanent intermediate-stage dementia* in the multiphasic long-term disease course between major depression without dementia and, what is to date, irreversible or permanent degenerative dementia. Accordingly, depressive dementia represents a transitional stage in the conversion of an initially-reversible or prepermanent dementia into a nonreversible or permanent end-stage dementia (e.g., dementia of the Alzheimer type, or DAT).

Definition of Depressive Dementia

The term *depressive dementia* (McHugh and Folstein 1978; Emery 1994, 1996, 1999; Emery and Oxman 1994, 1997, 2000) has been used to reference a subtype of the broader overarching historical category of *pseudodementia*. Accordingly, depressive dementia has comprised a subclass of the superordinate class of "pseudodementia," which refers to a clinical phenotype approximated by a wide variety of underlying disorders, rather than to a singular homogeneous disorder (Emery 1988, 1999) (see chap. 16). Although the prevalence of disorders presenting as "pseudodementia" remains unclear, it is clear depressive dementia, synonymously termed major depression with depressive dementia, dementia syndrome of depression, or depressive pseudodementia, constitutes the majority of cases in case series of "pseudodementia." Further, it has been observed that in the differential diagnosis between dementia and "pseudodementia," depressive dementia has been the single most difficult disorder to distinguish from the "organic" categories, especially degenerative DAT (Kiloh 1961; Kral 1983; Emery 1988, 1992, 1996, 1999; Kral and Emery 1989; Alexopoulos 1990, 1998, 2001; Devanand et al. 1996) (see chaps. 15 and 16).

Pioneering discussions of "pseudodementia" (Kral 1956, 1972, 1983, 1986; Kiloh 1961; Post 1975; McHugh and Folstein 1978; Wells 1979; Caine 1981; Reifler 1982; Emery 1988) have defined the importance of depressive dementia and tended to dichotomize it with parameters of reversibility versus nonreversibility and functional, nonorganic versus structural, organic etiology. Questioning these dichotomies, we examined the relationship between depression and dementia from multiple perspectives and developed a framework using continua to conceptualize illnesses where mood and cognitive disorders coexist. In evaluating the efficacy of the dichotomy versus continuity or spectrum paradigms for understanding the dementia spectrum of depression, it will be argued that the continuity/spectrum paradigm has greater goodness-of-fit and validity for accommodating the organic, pathogenetic underpinnings of the depression-dementia spectrum, which will be discussed later in this chapter. Data will be presented which suggest that depressive dementia has organic substrates and evidences parameters consistent with "real" rather than "pseudo"-dementing disorder. In the context of this chapter, depressive dementia will be reconceptualized and redefined as a *transitional dementia* with the goal of elucidating its possible function as a transitional phase in a long-term, multiphasic disease course involving several clinical presentations of the depression-dementia spectrum.

Historical Background of the Dichotomy Viewpoint

The attempt to differentiate what historically have been considered "reversible" dementialike disorders from nonreversible dementias has a long theoretical and clinical tradition. Historically, dementia has been defined as an acquired, severe, irreversible kind of intellectual deterioration secondary to organic brain disease (Bulbena and Berrios 1986). The diagnostic attempt to distinguish between nonreversible dementias and dementialike presentations that with treatment or passage of time appeared to be "reversed," dates back to at least the 1800s (Mairet 1883). The term *vesanic dementia* was used to describe dementia syndromes that appeared "reversible," until that term was replaced by Wernicke's term *pseudodementia* in the late 1800s (Emery 1988, 1997). The term *vesania* originates from the Latin word *sanus*, which means "sane, sound, healthy" (Burnham 1977, p. 174). Implied, therefore, in both the conceptualization of vesanic dementia and pseudodementia is a functional or nonorganic etiology.

In 1898, Ganser described three victims of accidents who seemed to "mimic" mental weakness (Ganser 1974 [1898]). Subsequently, Ganser syndrome became inaccurately equated with the totality of the category of pseudodementia, thus adding to the confusion surrounding the pseudodementia construct (Emery 1988). "Pseudodementia" is more accurately conceptualized as a historical term, which refers to a superordinate category of which depressive dementia and Ganser syndrome comprised subclasses. Accordingly, the logic of hierarchical classification makes it erroneous to equate any one subclass or subtype with the whole of any superordinate category. To define any one subtype as coextensive with the whole of any superordinate category leads inevitably to lack of construct validity (Emery 1988, 1999, 2000; Emery, Gillie, and Ramdev 1995; Emery, Gillie, and Smith 1996, 2000) (see chaps. 8 and 10). Many series of patients diagnosed with dementia have revealed that a dementialike profile can be presented by patients with a variety of neuropsychiatric disorders other than depressive dementia or Ganser syndrome, including conversion disorder, depersonalization, delirium, dissociative states, hypomania, mania, paraphrenia, schizophrenia, drug use, deafness, epilepsy, and normal-pressure hydrocephalus (Kiloh 1961; Wells 1979; Caine 1981; Carney 1983; Erkinjuntti et al. 1987; Khouzam, Emery, and Reaves 1994; Sachdev and Kiloh 1994; Almeida et al. 1995; Sobin and Sacheim 1997) (see chaps. 15, 16, and 17).

Both historical definitions and present-day case reports of pseudodementia center on two characteristics: (1) appearance of organic deterioration of cognitive function, and (2) reversibility or remission of cognitive symptoms inconsistent with "true" organic neurodegenerative dementia. In sum, historical, as well as current, discussions of pseudodementia in general, and depressive dementia specifically, tend to promulgate a dichotomous perspective whereby cognitive deterioration is regarded as either functional-nonorganic-reversible or structural-organic-irreversible, rather than both in varying degrees at differing times in depression-dementia spectrum disease course.

Empirical Context of the Continuum Viewpoint

The dichotomy between organic and nonorganic cognitive dysfunction was first challenged by Mairet (1883) with his conceptualization of "melancholic dementia" as organic. Mairet presented a series of patients with melancholic dementia who showed both organic brain changes and "reversibility." On autopsy, Mairet observed deterioration of the temporal lobe in these melancholic patients; these melancholic patients would be subsumed under depressive dementia as we are defining it in this chapter. In the same vein, Newton (1948) reported a disproportionate 42% of seventy-six postmortem brains from patients with affective psychosis evidenced the neurofibrillary tangles and neuritic plaques associated with DAT. This was significantly greater than the 25% of twenty-four schizophrenic postmortem brains with tangles and plaques (Newton 1948).

Although depressive dementia has generally been regarded as absolutely distinct from organic irreversible dementias, research suggests that in some cases of depressive dementia, remission of depression results in only partial improvement of cognition, with an irreversible component remaining (Abas, Sahakian, and Levy 1990; Nebes et al. 2000, 2001). Further, longitudinal data reveal that depressed patients with an initially "reversible" dementia are at high risk for developing irreversible neurodegenerative dementia. Accordingly, cognitive improvement for many patients with depressive dementia following treatment or remission of depression is neither complete nor permanent; this is particularly evident with long-term follow-up.

In analyzing outcome data from long-term investigations, it becomes clear that frequency of documented progression of depressive dementia into irreversible degenerative dementia is related in part to length of follow-up. At one-year follow-up, Murphy (1983) found that 3% of 124 elderly patients with depressive dementia had developed degenerative dementia. At 2-year follow-up, it was reported that 12% of older patients with depression had degenerative dementia (Rabins Merchant, and Nestadt 1984). And, in a longitudinal investigation of 23 hospitalized elderly patients with depression, research results indicated that 39% developed irreversible dementia over a median period of 30 months (Alexopoulos et al. 1993). With a 3-year follow-up, Reding, Haycox, and Blass (1985) found that more than 50% of elderly patients with depressive dementia had converted into irreversible degenerative dementia. Further, in the long-term follow-up investigation of 8-year average duration (range, 4–18 years; variability in part function of patient death), Kral and Emery (1989) found that 79% of 44 patients with depressive dementia (mean age, 76.5 years) developed degenerative dementia with an Alzheimerlike profile. The modal pattern of these patients was as follows: (1) several episodes of major depression/ unipolar without significant cognitive impairment; (2) one or more episodes of major depression/unipolar during which cognitive function was significantly impacted with subsequent return to "normal"; (3) an episode of apparent depression during which the patient presented with an Alzheimer-type profile, with cognitive symptoms subsequently appearing to "reverse" (i.e., depressive dementia). And, finally, (4) a presentation with an Alzheimer-type profile without remission of cognitive symptoms, and with subsequent progressive neurodegeneration consistent with DAT. At the beginning of the investigation all forty-four patients had normal brain CT and electroencephalogram values. In the last modal pattern phase, cortical atrophy was identified in brain CT and generalized slowing was found in the electroencephalogram. Where postmortems were permitted (nine patients), neuropathological examination of these nine patients revealed the typical markers of DAT: neuronal loss, neurofibrillary tangles, and neuritic plaques (Kral and Emery 1989) (see chaps. 3, 4, and 6).

Thus, it is suggested that a subset of patients with major depression/unipolar are at risk for depressive dementia, and in turn, the majority of patients with depressive dementia are at risk for developing irreversible dementia. Alexopoulos suggested that the meta-analysis of long-term investigations indicates 9–25% of elderly patients with depression and an initially-reversible dementia develop irreversible dementia each year (see chap. 15).

In a related vein, a recent epidemiological study, using a prospective longitudinal design with follow-up of 1 to 5 years, evaluated the relationship between depression and incidence of dementia of the Alzheimer type in community-dwelling elderly persons (Devanand et al. 1996). This study found that in 478 depressed with no dementia, after 2.54 years of follow-up, depressed mood at baseline was associated with an increased risk of irreversible dementia (relative risk, 2.94; $p = 0.001$). The increased risk related primarily to development of DAT (relative risk, 2.05). This effect remained after study controls for age, gender, education, language of assessment, and "all major clinical risk factors" (p. 180). Further, in the subset of depressed elderly persons in whom the apolipoprotein E genotype was assessed, factoring in the effect of the apolipoprotein E-4 allele did not weaken strength of association between depressed mood and subsequent incident irreversible dementia (Devanand et al. 1996). Similar data resulted from a study of elderly twins, which found that depression was a risk factor for development of irreversible dementia, irrespective of absence or presence of the apolipoprotein E-4 allele (Steffens et al. 1997).

Additional data indicate history of depression is associated with increased incidence of dementia of the Alzheimer type (Jorm et al. 1991; Kokmen et al. 1991; Speck et al. 1995; Geerlings et al. 2000; Jorm 2000) and that depressive symptoms are associated with poorer cognition at study entry and with cognitive deterioration at study follow-up (Bassuk, Berkman, and Wypij 1998; Yaffe et al. 1999). Further, in the ongoing Nun Study, it was suggested that, after holding demographic and environmental variables constant, depression may be associated with the cognitive disintegrity of DAT as well as with shortened life (Snowdon 2001). Additionally, Van Reekum et al. (1999) and Jorm (2000) concluded that depression might be a predictor for irreversible dementia; and Berger et al. (1999) and Geerlings et al. (2000) concluded that depression might constitute a subclinical or prodromal phase for Alzheimer disorder.

In sum, recent investigations converge on the idea that lifetime history of depression increases risk for irreversible dementia, regardless of genetic predisposition or family history (VanDuijn et al. 1994; Devanand et al. 1996; Steffens et al. 1997; Wetherell et al. 1999). As a final example, in an investigation of sixty-five registry-based twin pairs discordant for DAT, it was found that history of psychiatric illness, especially depression, was associated with elevated risk for DAT (Wetherell et al. 1999).

In conclusion, although there has been clinical interest in the differential diagnosis between depressive dementia and the "organic" dementias for many years (e.g., Kiloh 1961; Wells 1979; Emery 1988, 1992, 1996, 1999; McNeil 1999), the idea that some fundamental relationship might exist between these nosologically distinct categories is relatively new and represents a major paradigm shift (Kral 1972, 1983; Emery 1988, 1994, 1996, 1999; Kral and Emery 1989; Emery and Oxman 1992, 1994, 1997, 2000; Alexopoulos et al. 1993; Alexopoulos and Nambudiri 1994; Alexopoulos 1998, in press). Historically, the affective disorders have not been conceptualized as having a connection with "organic" brain syndromes. The association between major depression without dementia, depressive dementia, and neurodegenerative "irreversible" dementia represents a new clinical and research focus. Whether depression without dementia, and its possible devolution into depressive dementia, represents a risk factor for irreversible dementia; or whether the cognitive deficits of depression represent an early preclinical phase of irreversible dementia are questions that bring into focus two sides of a fundamental continuity or spectrum relationship. Two sides of the same coin, one being the obverse of the other; these issues point to a fundamental connection between depression and dementia, which historically was not known, which represents a breakthrough perspective, and which will, accordingly, contribute to better understanding of both.

Continua of Depression and Dementia

Consideration of variability in three different processes associated with aging might help clarify the discrepant historical viewpoints. Although these processes fall along separate continua, we are particularly interested in their co-occurrence or intersection. We therefore describe these three continuous processes of depression, cognitive impairment, and degenerative pathology along with anchor points as context for interaction. Each of these processes can be assessed by a variety of continuous measures. Defining a disorder or disease level is not a dichotomous decision. Most of the continuous measures are associated with cutoff points or scores. However, the presence and degree of disease is not as clear as the cutoff points themselves.

Depressive Axis

For the depressive axis, the separation of depressive symptoms from depressive disorder is problematic, especially in elderly persons (Blazer 1990; Oxman et al. 2000a, b). Depressive symptoms are measured by a variety of instruments. Regardless of the instrument and its cutoff score, most community surveys show about a 15% prevalence rate of depressive symptoms in persons over age 65 (Blazer 1990; Lobo et al. 1995; Oxman et al. 2000a, b). This rate is not significantly different from that found in middle-aged or younger adults (Khandelwal 2001). There has been much debate as to whether depression increases or decreases with old age. Data indicate that when the variables of physical function and illness are controlled, age by itself in elderly persons is not associated with depressive symptomatology (Snowdon 1997a, b).

Crossing the threshold from depressive symptoms to criterial or diagnostic levels of depressive disorder, we see that lifetime risk for major depression in community samples, calculated across adult age, has varied from 10% to 25% for women and from 5% to 12% for men. The point prevalence for major depressive disorder for adults in community samples has varied from 5% to 9% for women and from 2% to 3% for men (American Psychiatric Association 1994, 2000). The "gold standard" for assessing depressive disorder is a clinician-based interview. Surveys using this standard for major depressive disorder (the type of depression most often associated with severe cognitive impairment) show lowest rates in individuals older than 65 years (Carney 1983; Oxman et al. 1987, 2000a; Oxman and Emery 1993). Epidemiological studies, most notably the National Institute of Mental Health Epidemiologic Catchment Area (ECA) surveys, indicate that depression, particularly major depressive disorder, is less common in late life than at other ages. The rate of major depressive disorder in more than 5700 elderly persons located at five sites across the United States was less than 1% (0.4% in men; 1.4% in women); this rate was about one-fourth of that reported for adults ages 18–44 (Weissman et al. 1988).

Looking outside the United States, a prevalence study of depression and dementia in a Spanish city (Lobo et al. 1995) found depressive disorders in 4.8% of people over 65 years of age. In another European epidemiologic study of prevalence of psychiatric disorders in elderly persons, the rate for depressive illness in six centers of the United Kingdom was 10.0% (Saunders et al. 1993). Included in the category of depressive illness, however, were both "depressive psychosis" and "depressive neurosis," the latter overlapping the boundary between depressive symptoms and major depressive disorder, thus increasing the prevalence rate, which when broken down into its components is not dissimilar to rates in the United States. This same stratified study of 5222 people over age 65 found a prevalence rate of 4.7% for organic disorders. Of importance is the finding that the "apparent decline with age observed for depression disappears when organic cases are excluded from analysis" (Saunders et al. 1993, p. 838).

The meaning of these data is still not fully understood. Historically, going back to Galen in the second century (Jackson 1969), it has been commonly believed that the combined assaults of physical deterioration and psychosocial losses of old age predispose to depression. But recent data described in the foregoing (e.g., Oxman et al. 1987, 2000a, b; Weissman et al. 1988; Koenig and Blazer 1992) point to a decreased rate of depression in old age. We can think of several reasons, which can explain some but not all of the variance. Recent cohorts of elderly persons are more affluent, more educated, and healthier than their predecessors (Schaie and Willis 1991; Cattell 1999; Coupland and Coupland 1999; Hamilton 1999). These cohort changes could impact rates of depression. Data show that each of these variables (e.g., health, education) correlates inversely with depression (Fuhrer et al. 1992).

Beyond this, what of the important data suggesting that the statistical effect of decreased depression in late life disappears when organic cases are excluded from analysis (e.g., Saunders et al. 1993)? Possibly depression decreases as dementia increases because dementia is a process of progressive dedifferentiation and desocialization (Emery 1985, 1988, 1999, 2000), which results in loss of identity and selfhood. But core symptoms of depression, such as feelings of worthlessness, guilt, hopelessness, helplessness, suicidality, or self-immolation (American Psychiatric Association 1994, 2000), all require some sense of self and knowledge of identity. Related to this, it has been found that patients with dementia (e.g., DAT) are not fully aware of their depressive symptoms (Chemerinski et al. 2001). There appears to be a threshold for central cholinergic function below which the clinical expression of depression is not possible (see chap. 17). Because degenerative dementia can be defined in part by progressive loss of cholinergic function in the central nervous system (Perry and Perry 1980;

Zubenko et al. 1989), it would follow that major depression would decrease as dementia increases (see chap. 17).

Cognitive Impairment Axis

For the cognitive impairment axis, cross-sectional studies have shown increases of impairment with age (see chaps. 1, 2, and 3). Longitudinal studies suggest that degree of and age at impairment are variable and specific to the particular cognitive process examined (Nesselroade and Reese 1973; Emery 1985, 1988, 1999, 2000; Schaie and Willis 1991; Turner and Troll 1994). As with measures of depression, neuropsychological test batteries and mental status instruments are continuous measures, with normal ranges and cutoff scores suggesting cognitive impairment. When variables of gender, education, and differences in test form are controlled, substantial declines in cognitive function can occur with age even in the absence of systemic disease (Emery 1985, 1986, 1999; Albert 1988; Schaie and Willis 1991; Barresi et al 1999; Hamilton 1999). Also, as with the depression axis, the boundary between age-expected cognitive impairment and early degenerative dementia is not so easily established (Blazer 1990; Gifford and Cummings 1999; Scanlan and Borson 2001) (see chap. 1). Prevalence figures for dementia are highly age-correlated, ranging from 3% at age 65 to 47% at age 86 or older (Blazer 1990; Devanand et al. 1996; Snowdon 2001).

Degenerative-Pathology Axis

Looking at the degenerative-pathology axis, cognitive performance in healthy people correlates with structural and functional measures of brain function (see chap. 1). Age-associated structural changes in normal brains include selective regional neuronal loss, cerebral atrophy, senile plaques, and neurofibrillary tangles (Terry, DeTeresa, and Hansen 1987; Hardy 2000; Khachaturian 2000; Selkoe 2000). Functional changes at the interface between normal aging and dementia include changes in metabolism, hormones, neurotransmitters, inflammation, proteases, and other changes in the brain's microenvironment (Cotman and Anderson 2000; Lynch and Mobley 2000; Nixon 2000; Rogers and Shen 2000; Sapolsky and Finch 2000). These structural and functional changes vary continuously and are seen in both normal aging and dementia. The demarcation between normal aging and dementia is not easily defined. For example, senile plaques are evident in as many as 70% of people over the age of 65; sometimes, although rarely, in quantities comparable to those found in DAT (Crystal et al. 1988; Friedland et al. 2000).

Standards for assessment of neuronal loss, synaptic loss, cerebral atrophy, and neurotransmitter changes are in the beginnings of development or indeterminate (National Institute of Neurological and Communicative Disorders and Stroke 1975; Ball et al. 1985; Carlsson 1985; Albert and Stafford 1988; Terry et al. 1991; Alexopoulos and Nambudiri 1994; Mulsant and Zubenko 1994) (see chaps. 15 and 17); however, several groups have suggested age-correlated cutoff scores for numbers of tangles and plaques required for diagnosis of dementia of the Alzheimer type (Khachaturian 1985; Wisniewski and Merz 1985; Braak and Braak 1991; Mirra et al. 1991, 1993). Recently, diagnostic criteria for neuropathologic assessment of Alzheimer disease were recommended by the National Institute on Aging and Reagan Institute Working Group (1997) that include: (1) use of semiquantitative methods outlined by CERAD (Mirra et al. 1993) for assessment of neuritic plaques and neurofibrillary tangles; (2) use of topographical staging method developed by Braak and Braak (1991) to determine extent of neurofibrillary changes; and (3) examination of hippocampal formation and neocortex for presence of neurofibrillary tangles. To rule out potentially confounding disorders in the diagnosis of Alzheimer disease, microscopic examination of the following brain structures was recommended: (1) areas of neocortex to include inferior parietal lobe, superior temporal gyrus, mid-frontal cortex, occipital cortex including primary visual cortex and association cortex; (2) hippocampal formation at level of lateral geniculate body; (3) hippocampal formation including entorhinal cortex at level of the uncus; and (4) substantia nigra and locus ceruleus. In addition to classical Alzheimer pathology, the National Institute of Aging and Reagan Institute Work Group (1997) diagnostic protocol included assessment and suggested cut-points for major coexisting lesions (e.g., Lewy bodies).

The scope of this chapter does not permit giving equal attention to all types of "irreversible" dementias. As described elsewhere in this book, each type of dementia has its own special issues, all of which cannot be dealt with in one chapter. Accordingly, the main focus of this chapter is on the spectrum of depression and DAT. For data and discussion relating to the spectrum of depression and vascular dementia, see chapters 9 and 15.

We now describe five points along the depression, cognitive-impairment, and degenerative-pathology axes to define five prototype groups: major depression without depressive dementia, depressive dementia, degenerative dementia without depression, degenerative dementia with depression, and the independent co-occurrence of depression and degenerative dementia.

Major Depression without Depressive Dementia

The first basic group in the depression-dementia spectrum is major depression with minimal or subclinical deficits. It would be incorrect to define this prototypical group as depression with no cognitive deficits because most research suggests that depression in persons over age 40 almost always involves some cognitive disadvantage in relation to normal subjects (Emery, 1988, 1992, 1994, 1999; Emery and Breslau 1989; Cassens, Wolfe, and Zola 1990; Karlsson et al. 2000). After investigation of the cognitive and biological correlates of depression, Alexopoulos and Nambudiri (1994) concluded that cognitive dysfunction was an intrinsic part of major depression without dementia (see chap. 15). Other investigators have reached similar conclusions (e.g., Abas, Sahakian, and Levy 1990; Bassuck, Berkman, and Wypij 1998; Yaffe et al. 1999). Indeed, poor performance on cognitive examination, allegedly due to poor effort from apathy and poor concentration (which itself involves cognitive parameters), is part of diagnostic criteria for major depressive disorder (American Psychiatric Association 1994, 2000). Recent data point to the idea that the subclinical cognitive impairments of depression without dementia can constitute a risk factor or initial presentation in a long-term multiphasic disease course culminating in irreversible degenerative dementia (Kral 1956, 1983, 1986; Kiloh 1961; Emery 1988, 1992, 1994, 1999; Kral and Emery 1989; Alexopoulos 1990, 1998, 2001; Devanand et al. 1996; Steffens et al. 1997; Bassuk, Berkman, and Wypij 1998; Berger et al. 1999; Van Reekum et al. 1999; Wetherell et al. 1999; Geerlings et al. 2000; Jorm 2000; Snowdon 2001).

Recent investigations using positron emission tomography (PET) scanning and functional magnetic resonance imaging (fMRI) have defined a potential anatomical abnormality in the prefrontal cortex ventral to the genu in the corpus collosum of patients without dementia but with major depressive disorder, especially in familial cases (Kandel 2000). Activity of this brain region is decreased in depressed patients without dementia, and the decrease appears to be accounted for at least in part by substantial reduction in volume of gray matter in this part of prefrontal cortex (Bench et al. 1992; Kandel 2000). Drevets (2000) also found volume reduction in the subgenual anterior cingulate in familial major depression without dementia. Further, reduction in glia of the subgenual prelimbic anterior cingulate gyrus has been found in patients with major depression/unipolar (Rajkowska, Miguel-Hidalgo, and Wei 1999; Lai et al.

2000). Also, abnormalities in neurons of the dorsolateral prefrontal cortex were found in major depression/unipolar (Ongur, Drevets, and Price 1998; Rajkowska, Miguel-Hidalgo, and Wei 1999). Finally, structural neuroimaging investigations of patients without dementia but with geriatric depression have revealed bilateral white matter hyperintensities significantly greater than found in normal elderly persons (Krishnan, Hays, and Blazer 1997; Kumar 2001). Of importance from the perspective of this chapter is the fact that the above described brain regions of prefrontal cortex have extensive connections with regions of brain involved in cognitive processing; abnormalities in these brain regions seriously compromise ability to reason and make rational decisions; also compromised are ability to experience and respond normatively to certain emotional stimuli (Damasio 1994, 1999; Kandel 2000).

Depressive Dementia

The second prototypical group of the depression-dementia spectrum is major depression with cognitive deficits that reach clinical proportions, in other words, *depressive dementia* (McHugh and Folstein 1978; Emery 1988, 1994, 1999; Emery and Oxman 1994, 1997, 2000). The primary diagnosis is depression, and cognitive deficits are secondary to depression. Thus far it only has been possible to establish depressive dementia retrospectively, after treatment of depression. However, the material of this chapter contributes to the definition of depressive dementia such as to enable tentative diagnosis at time of presentation, especially when the clinician or researcher has long-term information about the patient, and the patient fits the modal pattern of depressive dementia described in an earlier section of this discussion. As noted before, the terms *depressive dementia, depressive pseudodementia, dementia syndrome of depression* (Folstein and McHugh 1978), and *major depression with depressive dementia* are synonymous.

Pioneering in the description of dementia associated with depression, Kral (1956, 1972, 1983, 1986) focused on the posterior hippocampus for explanation; the posterior hippocampus has been shown to be a substrate for the malignant form of memory deterioration integral to degenerative dementia; and, the posterior hippocampus also forms part of Papez's mechanism of emotions (Kral 1956, 1972, 1983). On the basis of clinical and neuropathological data, Kral concluded (1956, 1972, 1983, 1986) that the dementia of depression was at least in part a function of damage to the posterior hippocampus, which is an underlying substrate at the interface between depression and dementia. As described by Folstein and McHugh (1978), depressive dementia involves organic but "reversible" cognitive dysfunction, possibly caused by factors associated with the pathology of mood disorder such as brainstem neuronal dysfunction or biogenic amine deficiency.

There have been very few investigations of the structural and functional substrates underlying depressive dementia per se. This appears to be in part because until just very recently, there has been widespread failure to recognize that a relationship might exist between depression and dementia, at least under some conditions, which have yet to be adequately specified.

On the foreground of research, Alexopoulos (2001) conceptualized a "depression-executive dysfunction syndrome," which appears to be descriptive of at least a subset of patients with late-life depressive dementia (see chap. 15). The syndrome is characterized by impaired activities of daily living, reduced interest in activities, psychomotor retardation, and suspiciousness, and has slow, unstable response to classical antidepressants (Alexopoulos et al. 2000) (see chap. 15). Data from physiological and neuropsychological investigations provide evidence for right hemisphere dysfunction in depression (Alexopoulos 1990). Related to this are findings of impaired executive function in elderly depressed patients with cognitive impairment (Massman, Butters, and Delis 1994; Butters et al. 2000; Nebes et al. 2001). The construct of executive function includes such parameters as planning, organization, foresight, judgment, and control and management of time. Alexopoulos (in press) suggested that the pathogenesis of late-life "depression-executive dysfunction" might stem from frontostriatal dysfunction (see chap. 15).

Even though there have been very few investigations of depressive dementia per se, it becomes clear from what limited data exist that depressive dementia is a heterogeneous syndrome. There appear to be at least two possible modal patterns in which depressive dementia could constitute one phase in a long-term multiphasic disease course. One such possible multiphasic disease course involves a progression from major depression without dementia to depressive dementia, which after some years develops into a degenerative dementia of the Alzheimer phenotype (Murphy 1983; Rabins, Merchant, and Nestadt 1984; Reding, Haycox, and Blass 1985; Kral and Emery 1989). This possible modal pattern crosscuts subcortical and cortical parameters and as part of a possible disease progression initially appears to involve predominantly "subcortical" brain regions; but, with disease progression this modal pattern becomes increasingly "cortical" in brain areas of involvement. A second modal disease pattern appears to be predominantly "subcortical," beginning with depression without dementia and devolving into depressive dementia and later into "irreversible" dementia of a vascular dementia phenotype (see chaps. 9 and 15). The depression-executive dysfunction syndrome introduced by Alexopoulos (2001) appears to fit this second modal pattern (see chap. 15), whereas the first modal pattern is at the core of the data and discussion comprising the present chapter.

Finally, age at first onset of depression is a potentially important characteristic often associated with family history, depressive delusions, treatment response, as well as severity of cognitive decline. Some studies have suggested that late-onset depression or geriatric depression is associated with more medical and neuroanatomic changes as well as with greater risk and severity of cognitive decline or dementia (Jacoby and Levy 1980; Alexopoulos 1990, 2001; Rabins et al. 1991). The evidence, however, is not definitive and there is still controversy as to whether late-onset depression is associated with cognitive impairment greater than that of early-onset depression, especially when the variable of patient age at assessment is controlled. A close look at a number of investigations reveals that in comparisons between early-onset depression and late-onset or geriatric depression, patient age of subjects from the early-onset population is younger. Comparisons of younger depressed patients with old depressed patients leads to numerous confounds where age itself is a core variable in severity of cognitive and other kinds of decline, including neuroanatomic and every other kind of organic deterioration.

Historically, as well as currently, depressive dementia has been categorized as a subtype of the broader phenotype of pseudodementia (Kiloh 1961; Wells 1979; Emery 1988, 1989). It is the position of the authors of this chapter that depressive dementia is not a "pseudo"-dementia, but a real dementia, what we are terming "prepermanent intermediate-stage dementia." Further, it is proposed in this chapter that depressive dementia often appears to be a transitional stage in a long-term disease progression from depression without dementia to some form of irreversible or permanent end-stage dementia, such as DAT. Accordingly, some formal nosologic changes need to be made to accommodate the syndrome of depressive dementia. We argue that the "reversibility" of depressive dementia is often only temporary. Depressive dementia appears to be an initially-reversible transitional stage in a long-term, multiphasic, morphogenetic course of illness. Hence, we are coining the terms *transitional dementia* (Emery and Oxman 1997), *prepermanent dementia*, and *intermediate-stage dementia* as part of the definition and conceptualization of depressive dementia.

Degenerative Dementia without Depression

The third prototypical group of the depression-dementia spectrum is permanent degenerative dementia without depression (see chaps. 2–8). Reported frequencies of permanent degenerative dementia without affective symptoms vary widely across investigations, ranging from 13% to 100% (Rovner et al. 1989; Cooper, Mungas, and Weiler 1990; Lopez et al. 1990; Lobo et al. 2000; Lyketsos et al. 2000; Gauthier and Ferris 2001). This spread is due in large measure to varying criteria for affective symptoms, and other methodological variations, such as sample definition, selection, and exclusion. For example, some dementia investigations exclude depression and other psychiatric disorders as part of research design.

For detailed research data, discussion, and explanation relating to this third prototypical group of, what is to date, irreversible or "permanent" degenerative dementia without depression, see chapters 2 through 11.

Degenerative Dementia with Depression

The fourth major point of reference on the axes of the depression-dementia spectrum is irreversible or permanent dementia with varying degrees of depression. Depression frequently occurs in association with dementia. Estimates of prevalence of depression in patients with DAT range from 0% to 87% (Cooper, Mungas, and Weiler 1990; Lopez et al. 1990; Mulsant and Zubenko 1994) with most estimates around 20% (see chap. 17). As noted in relation to the third prototypical group, such a spread between reported prevalence is due mainly to variations in diagnostic criteria and research design.

A major issue has been whether degenerative diseases of the brain such as dementia of the Alzheimer type cause depression or whether depression is prodromal or a preclinical expression of dementia. In other words, does depression precede dementia or occur as a result of dementia? The answer appears to be that both these relationships exist between depression and dementia, representing different points on the depression-dementia spectrum. In some cases depression precedes dementia, having been a risk factor for dementia and is possibly even prodromal or a preclinical expression of dementia (Rabins, Merchant, and Nestadt 1984; Kral and Emery 1989; Berger et al. 1999; Van Reekum et al. 1999; Geerlings et al. 2000; Jorm 2000). About 30% of depressed patients with DAT have had a history of prior psychiatric disorder (Rovner et al. 1989). Further, 18% of all patients with DAT have had history of depression or paranoia (Agbayewa 1986). This relationship of depression, and in turn, depressive dementia preceding and possibly prodromal for end-stage permanent dementia is the focus of this chapter.

In other cases, depression seems to arise for the first time in association with an already existing dementia (see chap. 17). A number of investigations have found that first-time depression of dementia may result from anatomic damage to the brain (e.g., Boland 2000). Of interest, however, is the finding that first-time depression in the context of dementia is associated with significantly greater family history of depression than is dementia without depression (Pearlson et al. 1990). Forty-one patients with degenerative dementia in their first episode of depression had significantly more first-degree and second-degree relatives with depression than did seventy-one nondepressed patients with degenerative dementia (Pearlson et al. 1990). Thus even though some patients with degenerative dementia and depression appear to lack a personal history of prior depression, a history of prior depression can be found in their family history, pointing again to the relatedness of the two patterns of depression as a prodrome of dementia and dementia as context for depression. The relationship between depression and dementia is best understood using a spectrum approach, which permits resolution of data that would otherwise seem contradictory. Depression preceding dementia, and depression arising in the context of dementia appear to be two points of a continuous spectrum. We briefly look now at pathophysiological substrates underlying degenerative dementia with depression.

For the past thirty-five years, research and theory have implicated the catecholaminergic system in the pathophysiology of depression (Schildkraut 1965; Jimerson 1987; Zubenko et al. 1988, 1990, 1991; Zubenko 1997; Zubenko, Hughes, and Stiffler 1999 a, b). A majority of noradrenergic and dopaminergic neurons are contained in the locus ceruleus and substantia nigra, respectively; and both depression and dementia are associated with abnormalities or degeneration of these nuclei (Boller et al. 1980; Huber, Shuttleworth, and Paulson 1986; Mulsant and Zubenko 1994). Zubenko and Moossy (1988) found that degeneration of either of these nuclei was associated with depression in patients with degenerative dementia (see chap. 17).

Serotonin also seems to serve a function common for both depression and degenerative dementia. There is increasing evidence that a combination of disturbances in cholinergic and serotonergic function may play a role in cognitive impairment in DAT (Meltzer et al. 1999). Even though the role of serotonergic dysfunction in major depression has been well documented (e.g., Meltzer and Arora 1991), investigations of serotonergic function in degenerative dementia are still few in number. In one such investigation, serotonin (5-HT) uptake was determined in blood platelets of patients with DAT with the finding that maximum number of 5-HT uptake sites (Vmax) were significantly increased in patients with mild and moderate Alzheimer disease, but decreased in patients with severe Alzheimer disease (Arora, Emery, and Meltzer 1991). This finding relates to the "curvilinearlike" relationship between depression and dementia that we will propose sometimes exists.

For lack of a better term, we will invoke the term *curvilinearlike* in the following explanation. The relationship between depression and dementia, in some instances, appears to be curvilinearlike because there appears to be a threshold for central cholinergic function below which expression of clinical depression is not possible (see chap. 17). Because degenerative dementia is defined in part by progressive loss of cholinergic function in the central nervous system (Zubenko et al. 1989), it follows that major depression decreases as dementia increases. This curvilinearlike relationship between depression and dementia, which is based on threshold values of central cholinergic function, can explain the research finding, which previously has been so puzzling, that depression decreases as dementia increases (Saunders et al. 1993). Thus, for heuristic purposes, we are proposing that there is a positive correlation between depression and cognitive impairment, possibly until about the spectrum point of depressive dementia, after which the relationship starts to become negative, with depression ceasing clinical expression at the threshold point below which clinical depression can no longer be expressed. In other words, in some cases it appears that as depression increases, cognitive impairment increases to the point where the cognitive impairment itself becomes the most significant presenting feature and classical symptoms of depression become less manifest and then nonmanifest.

This heuristic model we are introducing to explain the spectrum relationship between depression and dementia, concomitantly, helps to explain data that up to now have been hard to understand. For example, in a research monograph comparing patients with major depression/unipolar, depression dementia, and DAT, Emery (1988) found that Hamilton Depression Scale (Hamilton 1967) scores for these populations were 31.3, 25.2, and 12.4, respectively. In contrast, mean correct scores out of a maximum of thirteen correct answers on the Kahn-Goldfarb Mental Status Questionnaire (Kahn et al. 1960) for major depression/unipolar, depressive dementia, and DAT were 11.0, 6.4, and 5.5, respectively. These data demonstrate that as cognitive impairment increases, clinical expression of depression decreases. In the same vein, Reynolds and associates (1988) reported that patients with depressive dementia had higher Hamilton Depression Scale scores than did patients with degenerative dementia. Similarly, the curvilinearlike relationship between depression and dementia we are invoking as explanation was again in evidence in still other research. When comparing depressive dementia to degenerative dementia, it was found that depressive dementia, which is initially reversible and represents a lesser degree of dementia on the continuum of cognitive impairment than irreversible degenerative dementia (Emery 1988, 1992, 1994, 1999; Emery and Oxman 1992, 1994, 2000), involved higher frequency of depressed mood and delusions than did degenerative dementia (Rabins, Merchant, and Nestadt 1984; McAllister and Powers 1994; Mulsant and Zubenko 1994). Also, Lazarus et al. (1987) reported that patients with depressive dementia had higher scores than patients with DAT on assessments of intrapsychic symptoms of depression such as helplessness, hopelessness, and worthlessness. In sum, analysis of data pertaining to the intersecting continua of depression and cognitive impairment reveals a curvilinearlike relationship whereby cognitive impairment increases and manifestation of classical symptoms of depression decrease as one moves from major depression/unipolar to initially-reversible depressive dementia to irreversible degenerative dementia on the continuous depression-dementia spectrum.

Independent Co-occurrence of Degenerative Dementia and Depression

The fifth prototypical group involves the co-occurrence of a degenerative dementing disorder and an independent, usually preexisting and recurrent, depressive disorder. This type confounds causal explanations of dependency between depression and dementia. What argues against simple co-occurrence is that percentages related to depression as a risk factor for dementia (e.g., Alexopoulos 1990, 1998, 2001; Devanand et al. 1996; Steffens et al. 1997; Berger et al. 1999; Van Reekum et al. 1999; Wetherell et al. 1999; Geerlings et al. 2000; Jorm 2000), and percentages related to prepermanent, intermediate-stage depressive dementia devolving into an end-stage permanent dementia (Rabins,

Merchant, and Nestadt 1984; Kral and Emery 1989; Alexopoulos et al. 1993) are disproportionately higher than would be expected from usual prevalence figures for, what is to now, permanent degenerative dementia (e.g., Blazer 1990; Lobo et al. 2000). Even when the high prevalence figures for degenerative dementia from the East Boston Study (Evans et al. 1989; Larson 1989) are used, percentages of patients with initially-reversible depressive dementia that progressed to irreversible or permanent degenerative dementia are still significantly higher than could be expected from simple co-occurrence or random chance.

Discussion

Initially-reversible depressive dementia is the least well understood prototypical group of the depression-dementia spectrum. Because many patients with depressive dementia have cognitive deficits severe enough to meet formal diagnostic criteria for dementia (World Health Organization 1992, 1993; American Psychiatric Association 1994, 2000), the term *depressive dementia* better reflects the reality of the syndrome than does depressive pseudodementia. Most clinical, neuropsychological, and neurobiological research suggests that the cognitive impairments of depressive dementia are real and organic rather than pseudo or simulated. Depressive dementia appears to be a prepermanent intermediate-stage dementia in the long-term disease course of end-stage permanent or nonreversible dementia. Thus, depressive dementia represents a transitional stage in the morphogenesis in presentations across the depression-dementia spectrum.

Whereas there is a fairly large literature on the neuropsychology of major depression without dementia, there are far fewer data relating to the neuropsychology of depressive dementia. What neuropsychological research exists suggests that depressive dementia is closer in both scores and pattern to irreversible degenerative dementia than to major depression without dementia (Emery 1988, 1992, 1999; Emery and Breslau 1989; Cassens, Wolfe, and Zola 1990; Speedie et al. 1990). It is as if the common factor of dementia that crosscuts initially-reversible depressive dementia and irreversible degenerative dementia has more weight and significance than does the common factor of depression in major depression with and without dementia. For example, one investigation of language found no significant differences between demographically equivalent patients with depressive dementia and DAT on language measures of confrontation naming, repetition, auditory word comprehension, sequential commands, complex syntax, and reading commands (Emery 1999). In contrast, patients without dementia but with major depression performed significantly better than their counterparts with dementia on all language measures (Emery 1999). Similarly, Speedie et al. (1990) found that depressed patients without dementia performed significantly better than those with depressive dementia on both number of correct responses and speed of response on confrontation naming, whereas patients with depressive dementia could not be distinguished from those with degenerative dementia. On memory function assessments, data reveal that depressed patients without dementia differ only quantitatively from normal controls, whereas patient groups of depressive dementia and DAT differ qualitatively and quantitatively from normal elderly persons, and are almost indistinguishable from one another (Emery 1988, 1992, 1994, 1999; Poitrenaud et al. 1989). Finally, an investigation of the cognitive domain of abstract reasoning found that patients with depressive dementia scored significantly lower than did patients without dementia but with major depression; the performance of patients with depressive dementia was similar to that of patients with organic dysfunction (Cassens, Wolfe, and Zola 1990). In sum, data converge on the finding that patients with depressive dementia and irreversible degenerative dementia share similar cognitive deficits, and both populations with dementia differ significantly from those with major depression without dementia.

Further, neurobiological data suggest that depressive dementia is associated with organic abnormalities that resemble more those of degenerative dementia than major depression without dementia (see chaps. 15 and 17). Nonetheless, it is clear that depressive dementia and irreversible degenerative dementia are not identical or coterminous. What is at issue is why and how these different disorders sometimes evolve into a common phenotypic presentation. Initially, reversible depressive dementia and nonreversible degenerative dementia appear —sometimes, but not always—to represent two different points of organic deterioration and severity in a long-term, multiphasic disease course. Put another way, depressive dementia often appears to be a prepermanent intermediate-stage dementia in the morphogenesis from depression without dementia to a permanent end-stage degenerative dementia. Heuristically speaking, we would suggest there are a number of ways to arrive at the common end point of nonreversible degenerative dementia. We suggest that depressive dementia involves a diathesis or vulnerability for the final common pathway or presentation of permanent degenerative dementia.

In studying the history of the concept of depressive dementia, one finds an effort dating back several hundred years, to differentiate nonreversible dementias from what on the surface appear to be reversible dementias. Both historical and present-day approaches have tended to dichotomize depressive dementia on parameters of nonorganic-reversible versus organic-nonreversible. We have suggested that such dichotomization obscures the reality of depressive dementia and slows down clinical and research progress relating to depressive dementia. We have concluded that essential questions related to dementialike presentations cannot be resolved using a dichotomy model of dementia-pseudodementia. The perspective of this chapter is a continuity perspective. Organic deterioration is viewed as a continuous quality. Difficult questions begin to yield once it is recognized that a continuum of organic deterioration exists. As a concomitant to the organic degenerative continuum, there appears to be a continuum of reversibility-nonreversibility; degrees of reversibility exist. But also, reversibility must be put in a diachronic context. Thus, depressive dementia might initially appear to be "reversed," but for how long? Reversibility has time-limited variability. Depressive dementia is a disorder that sometimes appears to be initially "reversible" for a period of time, but without reversing completely to premorbid baseline. The initially "reversible" phase of depressive dementia appears to be just that—a phase or stage in a long-term disease course from prepermanent dementia to permanent dementia, in many but not all, cases of depressive dementia. A critical question then becomes—why do some but not all cases of prepermanent depressive dementia convert into permanent end-stage dementia?

In terms of nosology, depressive dementia is better classified as what we have termed *prepermanent dementia* or *intermediate-stage dementia.* Depressive dementia can also be conceptualized as a "transitional dementia" (Emery and Oxman 1997). These terms signify that the disease course resolution or final presentation for any patient with depressive dementia is at that particular time in the disease course unknown. The conceptualizations of prepermanent dementia or intermediate-stage dementia or transitional dementia all denote the changing, multiphasic, long-term morphogenesis that can be part of depressive dementia (and possibly other subtypes of the overarching phenotype historically referred to as pseudodementias) (see chap. 16).

To conclude, we have examined the interrelationships between prototypical groups of the depression-dementia spectrum. Further, we have focused on the least well understood prototypical condition of depressive dementia and have redefined and reconceptualized it as a prepermanent, intermediate-stage dementia with the goal of elucidating its possible function as a transitional stage in a long-term, morphogenetic disease course involving several clinical presentations of the depression-dementia spectrum. Future directions include addressing the core question of why some and not other cases of depression without dementia devolve into depressive dementia, and in turn, why a significant percentage of cases of depressive dementia convert to an end stage of permanent dementia.

Clinical Conclusions

Differential Diagnosis

Precisely because it appears that, in a number of cases, depressive dementia is a transitional, intermediate-stage disorder in a long-term, multiphasic disease course with an end point of irreversible dementia, clinical diagnosis of depressive dementia is very important. To date, the irreversible dementias remain "irreversible." In consequence, in a long-term disease course that consists of several stages, clinical intervention before the end stage of permanent dementia becomes critical. Such clinical intervention also represents a broadened, more hopeful treatment approach to the irreversible dementias. Put another way, if successful clinical intervention of irreversible dementia occurs at an earlier stage of its long-term disease course (i.e., at the stage of depressive dementia), then, by logical extension, the clinician has ipso facto successfully intervened in the context of an irreversible dementia. As shown previously, depressive dementia appears to represent an initially-reversible stage in a long-term devolution into irreversible dementia. However, in an undetermined percentage of cases, depressive dementia does not progress into an irreversible dementia. Why do some and not other cases of depressive dementia turn into irreversible dementia after a number of years? This question may be the most important question. It is these unknown variables which constitute hope for the future of treatment and reversibility of what are presently regarded as irreversible dementias. And it is right here at the heart of this issue that the clinician can intervene with focus and persistence to try to keep an initially-reversible dementia from progressing on the continuum of organic deterioration. Thus, the importance of clinical intervention at the stage of depressive dementia is incontrovertible, but possibly not so easy to accomplish. It has been stated by clinicians quite familiar with depressive dementia (e.g., Kiloh 1961, 1981; Kral 1972, 1983; Wells 1979; Caine 1981; Kral and Emery 1989) that depressive dementia is most difficult to differentiate from irreversible degenerative dementia.

It has been noted previously that for purposes of this chapter we did a computerized search spanning back forty years. In the process of this search, it became evident that the literature on depressive dementia per se was very limited. Further, material pertaining to successful differential diagnostic procedures was even more limited. We now describe several of the differential diagnostic parameters the clinician can use that appear to be at least somewhat reliable.

Cognitive and Vegetative Depressive Symptoms

Behavioral consistency is an important parameter for clinical diagnosis of depressive dementia. The patient with depressive dementia evidences less behavioral consistency than does the patient with irreversible degenerative dementia precisely because depressive dementia is a transitional stage. On the continuum of organic deterioration, depressive dementia is before irreversible degenerative dementia, and concomitantly represents a lesser degree of organic deterioration and irreversibility. An example of the difference in behavioral consistency is that patients with depressive dementia can find their way around a hospital when hungry or looking for a television set, but patients with irreversible degenerative dementia cannot, irrespective of motivation (Wells 1979; Emery 1999). This clinical parameter has been empirically supported by Reynolds and associates (1988), who found that patients with degenerative dementia had significantly more impairment finding their way indoors or on familiar streets than did patients with depressive dementia.

Also, sleep disturbance is an important vegetative symptom of major depression. As degenerative dementia progresses, a breakdown of the sleep-wakefulness cycle also occurs, as indicated by nocturnal wandering (Prinz et al. 1982; Pearlson et al. 1990). Reynolds and colleagues (1988) reported that patients with depressive dementia differ from those with degenerative dementia by having more severe early morning awakening. This can be explained by the continuum concept because depressive dementia is closer or more proximate to major depression on the continuum of organic deterioration than is degenerative dementia, and accordingly would evidence symptoms closer in profile to major depression than would degenerative dementia.

Neuropsychological Features/Memory

In investigations of memory in age-matched patients with depressive dementia, dementia of the Alzheimer type, and major depression without depressive dementia, Emery (1994, 1999) found that greatest discriminant function between depressive dementia and major depression without dementia occurred with measures of orientation and simple general information. But the greatest discriminant function between depressive dementia and DAT was in simple general information and story recall. Thus, the patient with depressive dementia was less oriented and had less information than did depressed patients without dementia, but still could respond with more general information than patients with DAT. The patient with depressive dementia often can still tell you how many days there are in a week, whereas the patient with DAT more often cannot (Emery 1999, 2000). Similarly, Speedie et al. (1990) found that patients with depressive dementia performed worse than depressed patients without dementia on assessments of free recalls and delayed recall but not on delayed visual memory; the patients with depressive dementia did significantly better on delayed visual memory than did patients with degenerative dementia. In a related vein, a recent study (Swainson et al. 2001) found that a visuospatial associative learning test accurately distinguished patients with DAT from patients with major depression but without dementia, as well as from a subgroup with what appears to include patients with depressive dementia. Finally, in a prospective neuropsychological study comparing depressive dementia with DAT (McNeil 1999), it was found that the two groups differed only on assessments of short-term verbal memory, on which depressive dementia performed significantly better. Resolution of depression in patients with depressive dementia resulted in "return to normal levels" for three years on most measures of verbal functioning, but nonverbal abilities remained impaired. The study concluded that treatment of depression in patients with depressive dementia can "buy back" up to three years of cognitive function (McNeil 1999).

Neuropsychological Features/Language

Speedie et al. (1990) found that patients with depressive dementia were indistinguishable from those with degenerative dementia on numbers of items correctly named and speed of response. In the same vein, Emery (1999) found no significant differences between depressive dementia and DAT on language measures of repetition, confrontation naming, auditory word recognition, sequential commands, complex syntax, or reading commands. However, depressive dementia and DAT were successfully discriminated by a response speech task (e.g., "How many months in a year?") and by a simple sentence completion task (e.g., "Roses are red, violets are what?"). Linguistically these two tasks are among the least complex (Emery 2000). On the continuum of progressive organic deterioration, patients with depressive dementia can still manage to answer questions derived from the simplest, least complex linguistic forms significantly better than can patients with DAT (Emery 1988, 1994, 1999).

Neurobiological Features

Discussions of neurobiological features in different prototypes of the depression-dementia spectrum can be found in earlier sections of this chapter (also see chaps. 15 and 17). Several investigations, however, will be discussed in this section, which have especial clinical application.

In one of the few neuroimaging studies that specifically investigated depressive dementia, Pearlson et al. (1989) compared normal subjects with three prototypical groups of the dementia spectrum of depression. Measures of both ventricular size and CT attenuation (density) revealed a consistent pattern of increasing abnormality from normal control subjects through patients with major depression but without dementia through patients with depressive dementia to those with degenerative dementia without depression. Many of these patients had an early onset of depression although at time of assessment all were older than 59 years of age. Research findings included that patients with depressive dementia had ventricular enlargement and radioattenuation numbers not significantly different from patients with DAT. These abnormalities were observed even in patients with depressive dementia who had not developed degenerative dementia after two-year follow-up (Pearlson et al. 1989). Ventricular dilatation and low radioattenuation of the brain may be early signs of a degenerative process that can result in a clinically evident dementia after many years. What all the intervening variables are between atrophy of normal aging, atrophy of depressive disorders, and fully developed degenerative dementia have yet to be identified.

Some neurophysiological data are important in the differential diagnosis of depressive dementia from irreversible dementia. In an EEG investigation, higher REM percentage and phasic REM activity/intensity were observed in depressive dementia when compared to degenerative dementia with depression; more specifically, a greater first REM period duration was found in patients with depressive dementia (Buysse et al. 1988). It was tentatively concluded that these findings reflect significant differences in the cholinergic/monominergic regulation of REM sleep between patients with depressive dementia and those with degenerative dementia (Buysse et al. 1988). Further, EEG segmentation appears to be relevant in the measurement of altered brain function in aging and diseases of the brain (Ihl and Brinkmeyer 1999). A recent EEG study found that depressed patients had more different segments than patients with mild DAT. The study concluded that reduction of number of different segments in DAT compared to depression spectrum patients could be used in differential diagnosis (Ihl and Brinkmeyer 1999).

Finally, patients with dementia of the Alzheimer type may have more apraxia than do patients with depressive dementia (Emery 1988), and patients with dementia of the Alzheimer type appear to have greater olfactory dysfunction than do patients across the spectrum of depression (Solomon et al. 1998).

Treatment

Several implications for clinicians result from the continuum orientation and model of practice. This orientation serves to lower unrealistic expectations of "totally reversible" or "curable" dementia. Further, this orientation discourages the stereotypical equation between concepts of reversibility, treatment, and cure. Instead, it provides a rationale for more aggressive treatment of "excess disability" (Reifler and Sherrill 1990; McAllister and Powers 1994). This model of practice serves to discourage a dichotomous approach to treatment, whereby some patients are considered treatable and others are considered not treatable. Further, the orientation militates against segmentation of biological and psychological treatments. Of great importance for the spectrum approach to treatment is a long-term view and follow-up evaluation of depressed patients. A clinical application of the continuum/spectrum model of practice requires that treatment of depression include arrangements for longer-term monitoring (e.g., "med-checks"), not only of affective symptomatology, but of cognitive stability and function as well. This approach to treatment of the spectrum of depression requires added focus on longer-term consequences of treatments on cognitive function (e.g., use and duration of anticholinergic antidepressants). Related to this concern, Patterson and Clarfield (see chap. 3) have created a table listing common medications that can result in cognitive impairment. The clinician's task in weighing and balancing positive and negative treatment effects would now include some refocusing as to possible long-term cognitive side effects of treatments.

To conclude, the clinician's role in the long-term multiphasic presentations of the depression-dementia spectrum is of paramount importance in terms of both differential diagnosis and rationally based treatments. We have attempted to point to some areas of clinical diagnosis and treatment where the clinician can intervene successfully in the multifaceted disease course of depressive dementia.

REFERENCES

Abas, M., B. Sahakian, and R. Levy. 1990. Neuropsychological deficits and CT scan in elderly depressives. *Psychological Medicine* 20:507–20.

Agbayewa, M. 1986. Earlier psychiatric morbidity in patients with Alzheimer's disease. *Journal of the American Geriatrics Society* 34:561–64.

Albert, M.S. 1988. Cognitive function. In *Geriatric Neuropsychology*, edited by M.S. Albert and M. Moss. New York: Guilford, pp. 33–53.

Albert, M.S., and J. Stafford. 1988. Computed tomographic studies. In *Geriatric Neuropsychology*, edited by M.S. Albert and M. Moss. New York: Guilford, pp. 211–27.

Alexopoulos, G. 1990. Clinical and biological findings in late-onset depression. In *Review of Psychiatry*, vol. 9, edited by A. Tasman, S. Goldfinger, and C. Kaufman. Washington, D.C.: American Psychiatric Press, pp. 249–62.

Alexopoulos, G. 1998. The assessment and treatment of depressed-demented patients. In *Geriatric Psychopharmacology*, edited by J.C. Nelson. New York: Marcel Dekker, pp. 223–43.

Alexopoulos, G. 2001. The depression-executive dysfunction syndrome of late life: A target for D3 receptor agonists. *American Journal of Geriatric Psychiatry* 9:1–8.

Alexopoulos, G. In press. Late life mood disorders. *Comprehensive Review of Geriatric Psychiatry*. Washington, D.C.: American Psychiatric Press.

Alexopoulos, G., and D. Nambudiri. 1994. Depressive dementia. In *Dementia: Presentations, Differential Diagnosis, and Nosology*, edited by V.O. B. Emery and T.E. Oxman. Baltimore: Johns Hopkins University Press, pp. 321–36.

Alexopoulos, G., B. Meyers, R. Young, et al. 1993. The course of geriatric depression with "reversible dementia": A controlled study. *American Journal of Psychiatry* 150: 1693–99.

Alexopoulos, G., B. Meyers, R. Young, et al. 2000. Executive dysfunction and risk for relapse and recurrence of geriatric depression. *Archives of General Psychiatry* 57: 285–90.

Almeida, O., R. Howard, R. Levy, et al. 1995. Cognitive features of psychotic states arising in late life. *Psychological Medicine* 25:685–98.

American Psychiatric Association. 1994. *Diagnostic and Statistical Manual of Mental Disorders*. 4th ed. Washington, D.C.: American Psychiatric Association.

American Psychiatric Association. 2000. *Diagnostic and Statistical Manual of Mental Disorders*. 4th ed., text revision. Washington, D.C.: American Psychiatric Association.

Arora, R., V.O.B. Emery, and H. Meltzer. 1991. Serotonin uptake in the blood platelets of Alzheimer disease patients. *Neurology* 41:1307–9.

Ball, M., M. Fishman, V. Hachinski, et al. 1985. A new definition of Alzheimer's disease: A hippocampal dementia. *Lancet* 1:14–16.

Barresi, B., L. Obler, R. Au, et al. 1999. Language-related factors influencing naming in

adulthood. In *Language and Communication in Old Age*, edited by H. Hamilton. New York: Garland, pp. 77–91.
Bassuk, S., L. Berkman, and D. Wypij. 1998. Depressive symptomatology and incident cognitive decline in an elderly community sample. *Archives of General Psychiatry* 55: 1073–81.
Bench, C., K. Friston, R.G. Brown, et al. 1992. The anatomy of melancholia: Focal abnormalities of cerebral blood flow in major depression. *Psychological Medicine* 22: 607–15.
Berger, A., L. Fratiglioni, Y. Forsell, et al. 1999. The occurrence of depressive symptoms in the preclinical phase of AD: A population-based study. *Neurology* 53:1998–2002.
Blazer, D. 1990. Epidemiology of late-life depression and dementia: A comparative study. In *Review of Psychiatry*, vol. 9, edited by A. Tasman, S. Goldfinger, and C. Kaufman. New York: Guilford, pp. 210–19.
Boland, R. 2000. Depression in Alzheimer's disease and other dementias. *Current Psychiatry Reports* 2:427–33.
Boller, F., T. Mizutani, U. Roessmann, et al. 1980. Parkinson's disease, dementia, and Alzheimer's disease: Clinicopathological correlations. *Annals of Neurology* 7:329–35.
Braak, H., and E. Braak. 1991. Neuropathological staging of Alzheimer-related changes. *Acta Neuropathologica* 82:239–69.
Bulbena, A., and G. Berrios. 1986. Pseudodementia: Facts and figures. *British Journal of Psychiatry* 148:87–94.
Burnham, J. 1977. Paracelsus, Theophrastus Phillippus Aureolus Bombastus Von Hohenheim (c. 1493–1541). In *International Encyclopedia of Psychiatry, Psychology, Psychoanalysis, and Neurology*, edited by B. Wolman. New York: Aesculapius Publishers, p. 174.
Butters, M.A., J. Becker, R.D. Nebes, et al. 2000. Changes in cognitive functioning following treatment of late-life depression. *American Journal of Psychiatry* 157:1949–54.
Buysse, D., C. Reynolds, D. Kupfer, et al. 1988. Electroencephalographic sleep in depressive pseudodementia. *Archives of General Psychiatry* 45:568–75.
Caine, E. 1981. Pseudodementia: Current concepts and future directions. *Archives of General Psychiatry* 38:1359–64.
Carlsson, A. 1985. Neurotransmitter changes in the aging brain. *Danish Medical Bulletin* 32:40–43.
Carney, M. 1983. Pseudoproblems: Pseudodementia. *British Journal of Hospital Medicine* 29:312–18.
Cassens, G., L. Wolfe, and M. Zola. 1990. The neuropsychology of depressions. *Journal of Neuropsychiatry* 2:202–13.
Cattell, M. 1999. Elders' complaints: Discourses on old age and social change in rural Kenya and urban Philadelphia. In *Language and Communication in Old Age: Multidisciplinary Perspectives*, edited by H. Hamilton. New York: Garland, pp. 295–319.
Chemerinski, E., P. Sabe, J. Kremer, et al. 2001. The specificity of depressive symptoms in patients with Alzheimer's disease. *American Journal of Psychiatry* 158:68–72.
Cooper, J., D. Mungas, and P. Weiler. 1990. Relation of cognitive status and abnormal behaviors in Alzheimer's disease. *Journal of the American Geriatrics Society* 38:867–87.
Cotman, C., and A. Anderson. 2000. The brain's microenvironment, early functional loss, and the conversion to Alzheimer's disease. *Annals of the New York Academy of Sciences* 924:112–17.

Coupland, N., and J. Coupland. 1999. Ageing, ageism, and antiageism: Moral stance in geriatric medical discourse. In *Language and Communication in Old Age: Multidisciplinary Perspectives,* edited by H. Hamilton. New York: Garland, pp. 177–209.
Crystal, H., D. Dickson, P. Fuld, et al. 1988. Clinicopathologic studies in dementia: Nondemented subjects with pathologically confirmed Alzheimer's disease. *Neurology* 38:1682–87.
Damasio, A. 1994. *Descartes' Error.* New York: Avon Books.
Damasio, A. 1999. *The Feeling of What Happens: Body and Emotion in the Making of Consciousness.* New York: Harcourt, Brace.
Devanand, D., M. Sano, M. Tang, et al. 1996. Depressed mood and the incidence of Alzheimer's disease in the elderly living in the community. *Archives of General Psychiatry* 53:175–82.
Drevets, W. 2000. Neuroimaging studies of mood disorders. *Biological Psychiatry* 48: 813–19.
Emery, V.O. B. 1985. Language and aging. *Experimental Aging Research* 11:3–62.
Emery, V.O.B. 1986. Linguistic decrement in normal aging. *Language and Communication* 6:47–62.
Emery, V.O. B. 1988. *Pseudodementia: A Theoretical and Empirical Discussion.* Cleveland: Case Western Reserve University School of Medicine.
Emery, V.O. B. 1992. Interaction of language and memory in major depression and senile dementia of Alzheimer's type. In *Memory Functioning in Dementia,* edited by L. Backman. Amsterdam: Elsevier, pp. 175–204.
Emery, V.O.B. 1994. Memory and language interaction in depressive dementia. In *Dementia: Presentations, Differential Diagnosis, and Nosology,* edited by V.O.B. Emery and T.E. Oxman. Baltimore: Johns Hopkins University Press, pp. 298–320.
Emery, V.O.B. 1996. Language functioning. In *The Cognitive Neuropsychology of Alzheimer-type Dementia,* edited by R. Morris. Oxford: Oxford University Press, pp. 166–93.
Emery, V.O.B. 1997. Depressive symptomatology in Alzheimer's patients. In *Postgraduate Dementia Course: Heterogeneity of Alzheimer's Disease,* edited by Paul Janssen Medical Institute. Amsterdam: Reed Elsevier, pp. 5–7.
Emery V.O.B. 1999. On the relationship between memory and language in the dementia spectrum of depression, Alzheimer syndrome, and normal aging. In *Language and Communication in Old Age: Multidisciplinary Perspectives,* edited by H. Hamilton. New York: Garland, pp. 25–62.
Emery, V.O.B. 2000. Language impairment in dementia of the Alzheimer type: A hierarchical decline? *International Journal of Psychiatry in Medicine* 30:145–64.
Emery, V.O.B., and L. Breslau. 1989. Language deficits in depression: Comparisons with SDAT and normal aging. *Journal of Gerontology* 44:85–92.
Emery, V.O.B. and T.E. Oxman. 1992. Update on the dementia spectrum of depression. *American Journal of Psychiatry* 149:305–17.
Emery, V.O.B., and T.E. Oxman. 1994. The spectrum of depressive dementia. In. *Dementia: Presentations, Differential Diagnosis, and Nosology,* edited by V.O.B. Emery and T.E. Oxman. Baltimore: Johns Hopkins University Press, pp. 251–77.
Emery, V.O.B., and T.E. Oxman. 1997. Depressive dementia: A "transitional dementia"? *Clinical Neuroscience* 4:23–30.

Emery, V.O.B. and T.E. Oxman. 2000. Depressive dementia: A transitional stage between major depression/unipolar and degenerative dementia? *Psychosomatics* 41:161.

Emery, V.O.B., E.X. Gillie, and P. Ramdev. 1995. Noninfarct vascular dementia. In *Treating Alzheimer's and Other Dementias*, edited by M. Bergener and S. Finkel. New York: Springer, pp. 184–203.

Emery, V.O.B., E.X. Gillie, and J. Smith. 1996. Reclassification of the vascular dementias: Comparisons of infarct and noninfarct vascular dementias. *International Psychogeriatrics* 8:33–61.

Emery, V.O.B., E.X. Gillie, and J. Smith. 2000. Interface between vascular dementia and Alzheimer syndrome: Nosologic redefinition. *Annals of the New York Academy of Sciences* 903:229–38.

Erkinjuntti, T., R. Sulkava, J. Kovanen, et al. 1987. Suspected dementia: Evaluation of 323 consecutive referrals. *Acta Neurologica Scandinavica* 76:359–64.

Evans, D., H. Funkenstein, M.S. Albert, et al. 1989. Prevalence of Alzheimer's disease in a community population of older persons. *Journal of the American Medical Association* 262:2551–56.

Folstein, M., and P. McHugh. 1978. Dementia syndrome of depression. In *Alzheimer's Disease: Senile Dementia and Related Disorders: Aging*, edited by R. Katzman, R. Terry, and K. Bick. New York: Raven Press, pp. 87–93.

Friedland, R., J. Shi, J. LaManna, et al. 2000. Prospects for noninvasive imaging of brain amyloid B in Alzheimer's disease. *Annals of the New York Academy of Sciences* 903: 123–29.

Fuhrer, R., T. Antonucci, M. Gagnon, et al. 1992. Depressive symptomatology and cognitive functioning: An epidemiological survey in an elderly community sample in France. *Psychological Medicine* 22:159–72.

Ganser, S. 1974 [1898]. A peculiar hysterical state. In *Themes and Variations in European Psychiatry*, edited by S. Hirsh and M. Shepard. Charlottesville: University Press of Virginia, pp. 170–77.

Gauthier, S., and S. Ferris. 2001. Outcome measures for probable vascular dementia and Alzheimer's disease with cerebrovascular disease. *International Journal of Clinical Practice* 120:29–39.

Geerlings, M., B. Schmand, A. Braam, et al. 2000. Depressive symptoms and risk of Alzheimer's disease in more highly educated older people. *Journal of the American Geriatrics Society* 48:1092–97.

Gifford, D., and J. Cummings. 1999. Evaluating dementia screening tests. Methodologic standards to rate their performance. *Neurology* 52:224–27.

Hamilton, H. 1999. Language and communication in old age: Some methodological considerations. In *Language and Communication in Old Age: Multidisciplinary Perspectives*, edited by H. Hamilton. New York: Garland, pp. 3–25.

Hamilton, M. 1967. Development of a rating scale for primary depressive illness. *British Journal of Social and Clinical Psychology* 6:278–96.

Hardy, J. 2000. Pathways to primary neurodegenerative disease. *Annals of the New York Academy of Sciences* 924:29–35.

Huber, S., E. Shuttleworth, and G. Paulson. 1986. Dementia in Parkinson's disease. *Archives of Neurology* 43:987–95.

Ihl, R., and J. Brinkmeyer. 1999. Differential diagnosis of aging, dementia of the Alzheimer type and depression with EEG-segmentation. *Dementia and Geriatric Cognitive Disorders* 10:64–69.

Jackson, S. 1969. Galen on mental disorders. *Journal of History of the Behavioral Sciences* 5:365.

Jacoby, R., and R. Levy. 1980. Computed tomography in the elderly 3: Affective disorder. *British Journal of Psychiatry* 136:270–75.

Jimerson, D. 1987. Role of dopamine mechanisms in the affective disorders. In *Psychopharmacology: The Third Generation of Progress,* edited by H. Meltzer. New York: Raven Press, pp. 505–11.

Jorm, A. 2000. Is depression a risk factor for dementia or cognitive decline? *Gerontology* 46:219–27.

Jorm, A., C. van Duijn, V. Chandra, et al. 1991. Psychiatric history and related exposures as risk factors for Alzheimer's disease: A collaborative re-analysis of case-controlled studies. *International Journal of Epidemiology* 20 (Suppl. 4):S43–47.

Kahn, R., A. Goldfarb, M. Pollack, et al. 1960. Brief objective measures for determination of mental status in the aged. *American Journal of Psychiatry* 117:326–28.

Kandel, E. 2000. Disorders of mood: Depression, mania, and anxiety disorders. In *Principles of Neural Science,* edited by E. Kandel, J. Schwartz, and T. Jessell. New York: McGraw Hill, pp. 1209–27.

Karlsson, I., J. Godderis, C. DeMendonca Augusto, et al. 2000. A randomized, double-blind comparison of the efficacy and safety of citalopram compared to mianserin in elderly, depressed patients with or without mild to moderate dementia. *International Journal of Geriatric Psychiatry* 15:295–305.

Khachaturian, Z. 1985. Diagnosis of Alzheimer's disease. *Archives of Neurology* 42: 1097–1105.

Khachaturian, Z. 2000. Toward a comprehensive theory of Alzheimer's disease: Challenges, caveats, and parameters. *Annals of the New York Academy of Sciences* 924:184–94.

Khandelwal, Z. 2001. Depressive disorders in old age. *Journal of the Indian Medical Association* 99:42–44.

Khouzam, H., P. Emery, and B. Reaves. 1994. Secondary mania in late life. *Journal of the American Geriatrics Society* 42:85–87.

Kiloh, L. 1961. Pseudodementia. *Acta Psychiatrica Scandinavica* 37:336–51.

Kiloh, L. 1981. Depressive illness masquerading as dementia in the elderly. *Medical Journal of Australia* 2:550–53.

Kindermann, S., B. Kalayam, G. Brown, et al. 2000. Executive functions and P300 latency in elderly depressed patients and control subjects. *American Journal of Geriatric Psychiatry* 8:57–65.

Koenig, H., and D. Blazer. 1992. Epidemiology of geriatric affective disorders. *Clinics in Geriatric Medicine* 8:235–51.

Kokmen, E., C. Beard, V. Chandra, et al. 1991. Clinical risk factors for Alzheimer's disease: A population-based case-control study. *Neurology* 41:1393–97.

Kral, V. 1956. The amnestic syndrome. *Monatschrift für Psychiatry und Neurology* 132: 65–80.

Kral, V. 1972. Depression in the aged and their treatment. *Psychiatry Digest* 33:49–56.

Kral, V. 1983. The relationship between senile dementia (Alzheimer type) and depression. *Canadian Journal of Psychiatry* 28:304–6.

Kral, V. 1986. Differential diagnosis of the dementias of unknown origin: A clinician's view. *Canadian Journal of Neurological Sciences* 13:381–82.
Kral, V., and V.O.B. Emery. 1989. Long-term follow-up of depressive pseudodementia of the aged. *Canadian Journal of Psychiatry* 34:445–47.
Krishnan, K., J. Hays, and D. Blazer. 1997. MRI-defined vascular depression. *American Journal of Psychiatry* 154:497–500.
Kumar, A. 2001. Neuroanatomy of late-life mood disorders. *Economics of Neuroscience* 3: 44–48.
Lai, T.-J., M. Payne, C. Byrum, et al. 2000. Reduction of orbital frontal cortex volume in geriatric depression. *Biological Psychiatry* 48:971–75.
Larson, E. 1989. Alzheimer's disease in the community. *Journal of the American Medical Association* 262:2591–92.
Lazarus, L., N. Newton, B. Cohler, et al. 1987. Frequency and presentation of depressive symptoms in patients with primary degenerative dementia. *American Journal of Psychiatry* 144:41–45.
Lobo, A., P. Saz, G. Marcos, et al. 1995. The prevalence of dementia and depression in the elderly community of a Southern European population. *Archives of General Psychiatry* 52:497–506.
Lobo, A., L. Launer, L. Fratiglioni, et al. 2000. Prevalence of dementia and major subtypes in Europe: A collaborative study of population-based cohorts. *Neurology* 54 (Suppl. 5):S4–9.
Lockwood, K., G. Alexopoulos, T. Kakuma, et al. 2000. Subtypes of cognitive impairment in depressed older adults. *American Journal of Geriatric Psychiatry* 8:201–8.
Lopez, O., F. Boller, J. Becker, et al. 1990. Alzheimer's disease and depression: Neuropsychological impairment and progression of the illness. *American Journal of Psychiatry* 147:855–60.
Lyketsos, C., J. Sheppard, C. Steele, et al. 2000. Randomized, placebo-controlled, double blind clinical trial of sertraline in the treatment of depression complicating Alzheimer's disease: Initial results from the Depression in Alzheimer's Disease Study. *American Journal of Psychiatry* 157:1686–89.
Lynch, C., and W. Mobley. 2000. Comprehensive theory of Alzheimer's disease: The effects of cholesterol on membrane receptor trafficking. *Annals of the New York Academy of Sciences* 924:104–12.
Mairet, A. 1883. *De le Demence Melancholique: Contribution a l'Etude des Localisations Cerebrales d'Ordre Psychique.* Paris: Masson.
Massman, P., N. Butters, and D. Delis. 1994. Some comparisons of the verbal learning deficits in Alzheimer dementia, Huntington disease, and depression. In *Dementia: Presentations, Differential Diagnosis, and Nosology*, edited by V.O. B. Emery and T.E. Oxman. Baltimore: Johns Hopkins University Press, pp. 232–49.
McAllister, T., and R. Powers. 1994. Approaches to the treatment of dementing illness. In *Dementia: Presentations, Differential Diagnosis, and Nosology*, edited by V.O. B. Emery and T.E. Oxman. Baltimore: Johns Hopkins University Press, pp. 355–84.
McHugh, P., and M. Folstein. 1978. Psychopathology of dementia: Implications for neuropathology. *Research Publication for the Association for Research in Nervous and Mental Diseases* 57:17–30.
McNeil, J.K. 1999. Neuropsychological characteristics of the dementia syndrome of de-

pression: Onset, resolution, and three-year follow-up. *Clinical Neuropsychologist* 13: 136–46.

Meltzer, C.C., G. Smith, S. DeKosky, et al. 1999. Serotonin in aging, late-life depression, and Alzheimer's disease: The emerging role of functional imaging. *Neuropsychopharmacology* 21:321–22.

Meltzer, H., and R. Arora. 1991. Platelet serotonin studies in affective disorders: Evidence for a serotonergic abnormality? In *5-Hydroxytryptamine in Psychiatry: A Spectrum of Ideas*, edited by M. Sandler, A. Coppen, and S. Hartnett. Oxford: Oxford University Press, pp. 50–89.

Mirra, S., M. Hart, and R. Terry. 1993. Making the diagnosis of Alzheimer's disease: A primer for the practicing pathologist. *Archives of Pathology and Laboratory Medicine* 117:132–44.

Mirra, S., A. Heyman, D. McKeel, et al. 1991. The Consortium to Establish a Registry for Alzheimer's Diseases (CERAD): Part II: Standardization of the neuropathologic assessment of Alzheimer disease. *Neurology* 41:479–86.

Mulsant, B., and G. Zubenko. 1994. Clinical, neuropathologic, and neurochemical correlates of depression and psychosis in primary dementia. In *Dementia: Presentations, Differential Diagnosis, and Nosology*, edited by V.O.B. Emery and T.E. Oxman. Baltimore: Johns Hopkins University Press, pp. 336–52.

Murphy, E. 1983. The prognosis of depression in old age. *British Journal of Psychiatry* 142:111–19.

National Institute on Aging and Reagan Institute Working Group on Diagnostic Criteria for the Neuropathological Assessment of Alzheimer's Disease. 1997. Consensus recommendations for the postmortem diagnosis of Alzheimer's disease. *Neurobiology of Aging* 18 (Suppl. 3):S1–2.

National Institute of Neurological and Communicative Disorders and Stroke. 1975. A classification and outline of cerebrovascular disease II. *Stroke* 6:564–616.

Nebes, R., M. Butters, B. Mulsant, et al. 2000. Decreased working memory and processing speed mediate cognitive impairment in geriatric depression. *Psychological Medicine* 30:679–91.

Nebes, R., M. Butters, P. Houck, et al. 2001. Dual-task performance in depressed geriatric patients. *Psychiatry Research* 102:139–51.

Nesselroade, J., and H. Reese. 1973. *Life-Span Developmental Psychology*. New York: Academic Press.

Newton, R. 1948. The identity of Alzheimer's disease and senile dementia and their relation to senility. *Journal of Mental Science* 94:225–49.

Nixon, R. 2000. A "protease activation cascade" in the pathogenesis of Alzheimer's disease. *Annals of the New York Academy of Sciences* 924:117–32.

Ongur, D., W. Drevets, and J. Price. 1998. Glial reduction in the prefrontal cortex in mood disorders. *Proceedings of the National Academy of Sciences USA* 95:13290–95.

Oxman, T.E., and V.O.B. Emery. 1993. Dr. Emery and Dr. Oxman Reply. *American Journal of Psychiatry* 150:352–53.

Oxman, T.E., J.E. Barrett, J. Barrett, et al. 1987. Psychiatric symptoms in the elderly in a primary care practice. *General Hospital Psychiatry* 9:167–73.

Oxman, T.E., J.E. Barrett, A. Sengupta, et al. 2000a. The relationship of aging and dysthymia in primary care. *American Journal of Geriatric Psychiatry* 8:318–26.

Oxman, T.E., N. Korsen, D. Hartley, et al. 2000b. Improving the precision of primary care physician self-report of antidepressant prescribing. *Medical Care* 38:771–76.

Pearlson, G., P. Rabins, W. Kim, et al. 1989. Structural brain CT changes and cognitive deficits in elderly depressives with and without reversible dementia ("pseudodementia"). *Psychological Medicine* 19:573–84.

Pearlson, G., C. Ross, W. Lohr, et al. 1990. Association between family history of affective disorder and the depressive syndrome of Alzheimer's disease. *American Journal of Psychiatry* 147:452–56.

Perry, E., and R. Perry. 1980. The cholinergic system in Alzheimer's disease. In *Biochemistry of Dementia*, edited by P. Roberts. New York: John Wiley, pp. 135–83.

Poitrenaud, J., F. Moy, A. Girousse, et al. 1989. Psychometric procedures for analysis of memory losses in the elderly. *Archives of Gerontology and Geriatrics* 1:173–83.

Post, F. 1975. Dementia, depression, and pseudodementia. In *Psychiatric Aspects of Neurological Disease*, edited by F. Benson and D. Blumer. New York: Grune and Stratton, pp. 165–74.

Prinz, P., E. Peskind, M. Vitaliano, et al. 1982. Changes in sleep and waking EEGs of nondemented and demented elderly subjects. *Journal of the American Geriatrics Society* 30:86–93.

Rabins, P., A. Merchant, and G. Nestadt. 1984. Criteria for diagnosing reversible dementia caused by depression: Validation by two-year follow-up. *British Journal of Psychiatry* 144:488–92.

Rabins, P., G. Pearlson, E. Aylward, et al. 1991. Cortical magnetic resonance imaging changes in elderly inpatients with major depression. *American Journal of Psychiatry* 148:617–20.

Rajkowska, G., L. Miguel-Hidalgo, and J. Wei. 1999. Morphometric evidence for neuronal and glial prefrontal cell pathology in major depression. *Biological Psychiatry* 45: 1085–98.

Reding, M., J. Haycox, and J. Blass. 1985. Depression in patients referred to a dementia clinic. *Archives of Neurology* 42:894–96.

Reifler, B. 1982. Arguments for abandoning the term pseudodementia. *Journal of the American Geriatrics Society* 30:665–68.

Reifler, B., and K. Sherrill. 1990. Dementias: Reversible and irreversible. In *Review of Psychiatry*, vol. 9, edited by A. Tasman, S. Goldfinger, and C. Kaufman. Washington, D.C.: American Psychiatric Press, pp. 220–31.

Reynolds, C.F., D. Kupfer, P. Houck, et al. 1988. Reliable discrimination of elderly depressed and demented patients by electroencephalographic sleep data. *Archives of General Psychiatry* 45:258–64.

Rogers, J., and Y. Shen. 2000. A perspective on inflammation in Alzheimer's disease. *Annals of the New York Academy of Sciences* 924:132–36.

Rovner, B., J. Broadhead, M. Spencer, et al. 1989. Depression and Alzheimer's disease. *American Journal of Psychiatry* 146:350–53.

Sachdev, P., and L. Kiloh. 1994. The nondepressive pseudodementias. In *Dementia: Presentations, Differential Diagnosis, and Nosology*, edited by V.O.B. Emery and T.E. Oxman. Baltimore: Johns Hopkins University Press, pp. 277–98.

Sapolsky, R., and C. Finch. 2000. Alzheimer's disease and some speculations about the evolution of its modifiers. *Annals of the New York Academy of Sciences* 924:99–104.

Saunders, P., J. Copeland, M. Dewey, et al. 1993. The prevalence of dementia, depression, and neurosis in late life: The Liverpool MRC-ALPHA study. *International Journal of Epidemiology* 22:838–47.

Scanlan, J., and S. Borson. 2001. The Mini-Cog: Receiver operating characteristics with expert and naïve raters. *International Journal of Geriatric Psychiatry* 16:216–22.

Schaie, K., and S. Willis. 1991. *Adult Development and Aging*. New York: HarperCollins.

Schildkraut, J. 1965. The catecholamine hypothesis of affective disorders: A review of supporting evidence. *American Journal of Psychiatry* 122:509–22.

Selkoe, D. 2000. Toward a comprehensive theory for Alzheimer's disease: Hypothesis: Alzheimer's disease is caused by the cerebral accumulation and cytotoxicity of amyloid B-protein. *Annals of the New York Academy of Sciences* 924:17–26.

Snowden, J. 1997a. Epidemiologic questions on mood disorders in old age. *Clinical Neuroscience* 4:3–7.

Snowden, J. 1997b. Diagnosis and treatment of depression in old age. *Modern Medicine of Australia* 40:52–57.

Snowdon, D. 2001. *Aging with Grace*. New York: Bantam Books.

Sobin, C., and H. Sacheim. 1997. Psychomotor symptoms of depression. *American Journal of Psychiatry* 154:4–17.

Solomon, G., W. Petrie, J. Hart, et al. 1998. Olfactory dysfunction discriminates Alzheimer's dementia from major depression. *Journal of Neuropsychiatry and Clinical Neurosciences* 10:64–67.

Speck, C., W. Kukull, D. Brenner, et al. 1995. History of depression as a risk factor for Alzheimer's disease. *Epidemiology* 6:366–69.

Speedie, L., P. Rabins, G. Pearlson, et al. 1990. Confrontation naming deficit in dementia of depression. *Journal of Neuropsychiatry* 2:59–63.

Steffens, D., B. Plassman, M. Helms, et al. 1997. A twin study of late-onset depression and apolipoprotein E epsilon 4 as risk factors for Alzheimer's disease. *Biological Psychiatry* 41:851–56.

Swainson, R., J. Hodges, C. Galton, et al. 2001. Early detection and differential diagnosis of Alzheimer's disease and depression with neuropsychological tasks. *Dementia and Geriatric Cognitive Disorders* 12:265–80.

Terry, R., R. DeTeresa, and L. Hansen. 1987. Neocortical cell counts in normal human adult aging. *Annals of Neurology* 21:530–39.

Terry, R., E. Masliah, D. Salmon, et al. 1991. Physical basis of cognitive alterations in Alzheimer's disease: Synapse loss is the major correlate of cognitive impairment. *Annals of Neurology* 30:572–80.

Turner, B., and L. Troll. 1994. *Women Growing Older*. Thousand Oaks, Calif.: Sage.

VanDuijn, C., D. Clayton, V. Chandra, et al. 1994. Interaction between genetic and environmental risk factors for Alzheimer's disease: A reanalysis of case-control studies. *Genetic Epidemiology* 11:539–51.

Van Reekum, R., M. Simard, D. Clarke, et al. 1999. Late-life depression as a possible predictor of dementia: Cross-sectional and short-term follow-up results. *American Journal of Geriatric Psychiatry* 7:151–59.

Weissman, M., P. Leaf, G. Tischler, et al. 1988. Affective disorders in five United States communities. *Psychological Medicine* 18:141.

Wells, C.E. 1979. Pseudodementia. *American Journal of Psychiatry* 136:895–900.

Wetherell, J., M. Gatz, B. Johansson, et al. 1999. History of depression and other psychiatric illness as risk factors for Alzheimer disease in a twin sample. *Alzheimer Disease and Associated Disorders* 13:47–52.

Wisniewski, H.M., and G. Merz. 1985. Neuropathology of the aging brain and dementia of the Alzheimer type. In *Aging 2000: Our Health Care Destiny*, edited by C. Gaitz and T. Samorajski. New York: Springer-Verlag, pp. 231–43.

World Health Organization. 1992. *The ICD-10 Classification of Mental and Behavioral Disorders: Clinical Descriptions and Diagnostic Guidelines.* Geneva: World Health Organization.

World Health Organization. 1993. *The ICD-10 Classification of Mental and Behavioral Disorders: Diagnostic Criteria for Research.* Geneva: World Health Organization.

Yaffe, K., T. Blackwell, R. Gore, et al. 1999. Depressive symptoms and cognitive decline in nondemented elderly women: A prospective study. *Archives of General Psychiatry* 56: 425–30.

Zubenko, G.S. 1997. Molecular neurobiology of Alzheimer's disease (syndrome?). *Harvard Review of Psychiatry* 5:1–37.

Zubenko, G.S., and J. Moossy. 1988. Major depression in primary dementia: Clinical and neuropathologic correlates. *Archives of Neurology* 45:1182–86.

Zubenko, G.S., H. Hughes, and J. Stiffler. 1999a. Clinical and neurobiological correlates of D10S1423 genotype in Alzheimer's disease. *Biological Psychiatry* 46:740–49.

Zubenko, G.S., H. Hughes, and J. Stiffler. 1999b. Neurobiological correlates of a putative risk allele for Alzheimer's disease on chromosome 12q. *Neurology* 52:725–32.

Zubenko, G.S., J. Moossy, I. Hanin, et al. 1988. Bilateral symmetry of cholinergic deficits in Alzheimer's disease. *Archives of Neurology* 45:225–29.

Zubenko, G.S., J. Moossy, A. Martinez, et al. 1989. A brain regional analysis of morphologic and cholinergic abnormalities in Alzheimer's disease. *Archives of Neurology* 46:634–38.

Zubenko, G.S., P. Sullivan, J. Nelson, et al. 1990. Brain imaging abnormalities in mental disorders of late life. *Archives of Neurology* 47:1107–11.

Zubenko, G.S., J. Moossy, J. Martinez, et al. 1991. Neuropathologic and neurochemical correlates of psychosis in primary dementia. *Archives of Neurology* 48:619–24.

CHAPTER FIFTEEN

Depressive Dementia

Cognitive and Biological Correlates and Course of Illness

George S. Alexopoulos, M.D.

Depressed elderly patients often present with a syndrome of dementia that subsides after remission of depressive symptomatology (Emery 1988). The concept of reversible dementia can be traced to at least the mid-nineteenth century (Berrios 1985; Emery 1988). Later, Madden, Luban, and Kaplan (1952) used the term *pseudodementia* to describe what appeared to be reversible disturbances in orientation, recent memory, calculation, and judgment that occurred as part of depression, involutional psychosis, and other disorders. The concept of "pseudodementia" came into increased focus when Kiloh (1961) described ten cases in which reversible dementia was associated with psychiatric syndromes, including Ganser state, reactive depression with hysteric features, melancholic depression, hypomania, atypical psychosis, paraphrenia, catatonia, depersonalization, and malingering. Currently, pseudodementia is conceptualized as a heterogeneous syndrome of cognitive impairment, occurring in the context of various psychiatric disorders, which follows a variable course.

Psychiatric Manifestations of Reversible Dementias

The psychiatric symptoms and signs of patients with reversible dementia depend on the age of the patient, the underlying psychiatric disorder, and the setting in which the patient is treated (Wells 1979; Kiloh 1981; Rabins, Merchant, and Nestadt 1984; Alexopoulos 1990; Emery and Oxman 1992). A previous history of psychiatric illness with apparent recovery, recent and abrupt onset of current illness, and a normal electroencephalogram appeared to be associated with the varied disorders classified as reversible dementia ("pseudodementia") in Kiloh's series (1961). A frequently cited clinical series (Wells 1979) suggested that patients with dementia that developed as part of their psychiatric disorders expressed complaints and distress about their cognitive loss. These patients were able to identify precisely the onset of their illness and to describe its course. When faced with cognitive tests, however, these same patients often said they did not know the correct answers, even when the task was clearly within their capabilities. In addition, the patients showed marked variability in their performance on tasks of similar difficulty and over-dramatized their cognitive loss. These observations were based on a series of middle-aged patients examined in the setting of a consultation-liaison service. Most of these cases had psychiatric diagnoses other than mood disorders. Therefore, their clinical presentation may not be applicable to geriatric patients with depression and reversible dementia.

The psychiatric presentation of older patients with reversible dementia is different than that of younger adults. Depressive disorders are the most frequent psychiatric conditions associated with dementialike syndromes in elderly persons ("depressive dementia"). Depressed elderly patients do not express excessive cognitive complaints or "I don't know" responses (Young, Manly, and Alexopoulos 1985; Emery 1988; Meyers 1992). A study of hospitalized geriatric patients with major depression showed that patients with depressive dementia had a later age of illness onset when compared to patients with major depression alone (Alexopoulos et al. 1993). Hospitalized elderly patients with depressive dementia also appeared to have more motor retardation, depressive delusions, hopelessness, and helplessness than either elderly patients with depression without dementia or elderly patients with depression and irreversible dementia (Alexopoulos and Abrams 1991). In a sample of elderly inpatients and outpatients with depressive dementia, the syndrome was associated with more psychic and somatic anxiety, early morning awakening, and loss of libido than was primary degenerative dementia complicated by depression (Reynolds et al. 1986).

Focusing on reversible depressive dementia (see chaps. 14 and 19), Post (1975) suggested that the symptoms of depression preceded those of cognitive dysfunction in depressive dementia. In contrast, depressive symptoms occurring in the context of neurologic dementing disorders usually follow the development of cognitive loss. However, clinical examination and laboratory tests often are unable to establish the diagnosis of depressive dementia that will subside after remission of depression. Even in typical cases (e.g., an elderly patient who first develops mild dementia after the onset of a severe episode of late-onset depression characterized by retardation and depressive delusions), the outcome of dementia is difficult to predict. Appropriate antidepressant treatment is necessary both in order to help depression and characterize the dementia syndrome as reversible or not. Dementia work-up also needs to be pursued at this point in order to exclude treatable causes of dementia.

Cognitive Impairment in Reversible Depressive Dementias

An analysis of reported cases suggested that the dementia syndrome of depressed elderly patients is clinically similar to the dementia syndrome of neurologic dementing disorders (McAllister 1983). In contrast, the dementialike presentation of younger patients is often a caricature or an imitation of dementia, as most of these patients have personality disorders with histrionic characteristics (Wells 1979).

The cognitive disturbance of depressive dementia during its early stages is not severe (Caine 1981; Rabins, Merchant, and Nestadt 1984; Reynolds et al. 1986; Alexopoulos et al. 1993) and has prominent features of impaired attention and free recall. Calculation, orientation, and spatial functions are less impaired (Alexopoulos and Abrams 1991). Presence of mild dementia, inability to recall four objects in four to five minutes, and preserved ability to perform simple calculations discriminated patients with reversible depressive dementia from geriatric patients with irreversible dementia who also met the criteria for major depression in 85% of cases. Depressed elderly patients with reversible dementia had naming abnormalities similar to those of patients with irreversible dementia (Speedie et al. 1990).

Emery (1988) performed a study in which selected memory and language tests were used to compare the performance of four groups of elderly subjects:

(1) those with major depression without dementia, (2) those with reversible depressive dementia, (3) those with Alzheimer disease (AD); and (4) control subjects without depression or dementia. Apraxia and calculation were also tested. Significant differences were observed among the four groups on all measures of memory and language, and all three patient groups had more memory dysfunction than did normal subjects. Memory tests also distinguished the depressed group without dementia from the group with Alzheimer dementia. Memory performance in reversible depressive dementia, however, was similar to that in AD on all tests except story recall and information. When within-sample patterns of memory deficits were compared, the pattern of depressive dementia was comparable to the AD pattern. Analysis of language tests suggested that tests of lesser complexity (Emery 1985, 1986) (such as naming) are most useful for discriminating depressive dementia from AD, whereas more complex measures (i.e., syntactic processing and reading comprehension) discriminated depressive dementia from depression without dementia and from normal aging. Calculation tests were helpful in differentiating depressive dementia and AD from depression without dementia, whereas tests of apraxia distinguished depressive dementia from AD.

It should be emphasized that even depressed elderly patients without dementia have cognitive dysfunction. Depressed elderly persons without dementia have deficits in effortful processes, while patients with AD have deficits in semantic encoding and retrieval as well as in automatic processes (Hasher and Zacks 1979; Cohen et al. 1982). Elderly patients without dementia but with recurrent major depression had equivalent impairment of short-term memory but less impairment of conditional associative learning than patients with early dementia of the Alzheimer type (Abas, Sahakian, and Levy 1990). Impairment was found in approximately 70% of the depressed group without dementia in this study and was particularly seen in memory and in measures of latency. Qualitative differences were found between the two groups, however. The depressed group showed a different pattern of errors and a consistently prolonged latency of response that was independent of delay in a matching-to-sample test compared with early-stage AD. Differences in cognitive performance have also been observed between elderly patients with depression and those with diseases associated with syndromes of subcortical dementia (Sahakian 1991). Subcortical dementia is characterized by slowing of cognition, memory impairment, visuospatial abnormalities, and mood disturbance. Delayed matching-to-sample performance may be qualitatively different in major depression compared with

Parkinson disease (Sahakian et al. 1988; Abas, Sahakian, and Levy 1990), which often develops into a subcortical dementia.

Outcome of Depression with an Initially-reversible Dementia

An integral part of the original concept of depressive dementia was its reversibility ("pseudodementia") after successful treatment of the underlying psychiatric disorder (Kiloh 1961; Wells 1979). Although clinicians often consider depressive dementia as completely distinct from irreversible dementias, studies suggest that in some cases of depressive dementia (see chaps. 14 and 19) alleviation of depression results in a partial improvement of cognition while an irreversible component persists (Reifler 1982; Abas, Sahakian, and Levy 1990; Nebes et al. 2000, 2001). This observation has led to the view that depressive pseudodementia is often superimposed on the cognitive dysfunction of patients with early-stage dementing disorders (Reifler 1982). Therefore, the early term *pseudodementia* was considered misleading, because it implied a completely reversible syndrome.

With some exceptions (Rabins, Merchant, and Nestadt 1984; Pearlson et al. 1989), follow-up studies suggest that geriatric patients with depression and an initially-reversible dementia are at high risk for developing irreversible dementia. A longitudinal study of twenty-three hospitalized elderly patients with depression and an initially-reversible dementia found that 39% developed irreversible dementia over a median period of thirty months (Alexopoulos et al. 1993). These patients initially met DSM-III criteria for both major depression and dementia and had total Mini-Mental State Examination (MMSE) scores in the dementia range (i.e., total scores were 23 or less) (Folstein, Folstein, and McHugh 1975). After alleviation of depressive symptomatology, however, total MMSE scores improved by at least 3 points and reached a final score of 24 or above for each patient. Similar findings were reported in earlier studies. In a community sample of twenty-one patients with initially-reversible depressive dementia, 24% developed dementia and 28% developed cognitive dysfunction but did not fully meet criteria for dementia (Copeland et al. 1992). In a mixed inpatient-outpatient sample of geriatric patients with depression and an initially-reversible dementia, 50% developed irreversible dementia over a follow-up period of two years (Reding, Haycox, and Blass 1986). Reding, Haycox, and Blass (1985) observed that 57% of geriatric outpatients with depression and memory complaints developed irreversible dementia over an average follow-up of three years; these patients sought evaluation in a dementia clinic but did not meet criteria for dementia during the initial evaluation. A lengthier follow-up study demonstrated that 79% of elderly patients with depressive pseudodementia developed irreversible dementia over an average period of eight years (Kral and Emery 1989). At entry to this study, all patients had normal brain CT and electroencephalographic values. When the irreversible dementia became apparent, cortical atrophy was identified in brain CT and generalized slowing appeared in the electroencephalogram. Where brain autopsy was obtained, neuropathological findings were consistent with AD. The value of this study lies in the finding that patients with depressive dementia are at high risk for the development of irreversible dementia, even after many years of apparent recovery from previous depression-dementia episodes. Taken together, these studies suggest that 9–25% of elderly patients with depression and an initially-reversible dementia develop irreversible dementia each year.

Three studies have reported low rates of irreversible dementia in patients with depression and an initially-reversible dementia syndrome (Alexopoulos et al. 1993). In a 2-year longitudinal study of 18 elderly subjects who initially met the criteria for both depression and dementia, 17% continued to have dementia during the follow-up period despite improvement of depression (Rabins, Merchant, and Nestadt 1984). Another study showed that only 1 out of 11 depressed elderly patients with a reversible dementia syndrome developed irreversible dementia over a 2-year follow-up (Pearlson et al. 1989). A third study noted that only 1 out of 19 elderly patients originally diagnosed as depression with "reversible dementia" developed an irreversible dementia syndrome within 10 years (Sachdaw et al. 1990). However, 10.5% of subjects refused in-person evaluation and 42% died during the study period. Despite methodological limitations, the above 3 studies suggest that a population exists among elderly depressed persons with reversible dementia which remains cognitively intact at least for a few years after resolution of the dementia syndrome.

The above differences in the course of cognitive dysfunction in depressed patients with an initially-reversible dementia suggest that this syndrome is heterogeneous. In some patients, cognitive dysfunction at baseline may be due to decreased reserve cognitive capacity that is exacerbated by the disturbances of the depressive syndrome. Therefore, some depressed persons with an initially-reversible dementia may already be suffering from an early-stage dementing disorder (Alexopoulos in press). This view is supported by recent studies suggesting that depression is a prodrome of dementing disorders. History of depression is associated with increased incidence of AD (Jorm et al. 1991; Kokmen et al. 1991; Speck et al. 1995). Depressive symptoms were associated with poorer cognitive function at baseline and with cognitive decline during follow-up (Devanand et al. 1996; Bassuk, Berkman, and Wypij 1998; Yaffe et al. 1999). Depressive symptoms are common in elderly individuals who later develop dementia. Among elderly individuals with subclinical cognitive dysfunction, those who developed dementia three years later had more depressive symptoms (Ritchie et al. 1999). As subjects were progressing to dementia, they exhibited fewer affective symptoms and more agitation and psychomotor slowing. These changes paralleled reduction of cerebral blood flow in the left temporal region.

Another possibility is that depression predisposes toward dementing disorders. This assertion is supported by observations suggesting high rates of previous psychiatric illness in patients with AD. Approximately 30% of depressed patients with AD have had history of previous psychiatric illness (Rovner et al. 1989), while 18% of all patients with AD were found to have history of depression or paranoia (Agbayewa 1986). Lifetime history of depression may increase the risk of AD, regardless of presence or absence of family history of dementing disorders (van Duijn et al. 1994). In elderly twins, depression was one of risk factors for the development of dementia, regardless of the presence or absence of an ApoE4 allele (Steffens et al. 1997). Depressive symptoms and diagnoses were found to be associated with cognitive decline and high risk for AD (Geerlings et al. 2000). Depressive symptoms occurring more than ten years before the onset of dementia were found to be a risk factor for AD (Speck et al. 1995). In a meta-analytic study, history of depression was associated with onset of AD after age 70 only when depressive symptoms had appeared within ten years before the onset of dementia (Jorm et al. 1991). However, depression with onset more than ten years before the diagnosis of dementia was associated with onset of AD at any age. These observations suggest that depression can sometimes represent a predisposing factor in some patients and a prodromal expression of a dementing disorder in others (Alexopoulos in press).

Several explanations may account for the identification of reversible dementia in depressed elderly patients who remain cognitively intact on follow-up. Disturbances in attention and motivation may interfere with the examination of high intellectual functions in severely depressed elderly patients. Another possibility is that the cognitive dysfunction of depression may be prominent in patients with asymptomatic nonprogressive brain lesions (e.g., silent stroke).

Such patients may develop a dementia syndrome only during depression but not develop dementia during follow-up. The concept of depression-lesion interaction is supported by the observation that neurological symptoms and signs are exacerbated when patients become depressed (Fogel and Sparadeo 1985).

Another possibility may be that severe cognitive dysfunction is an integral part of severe geriatric depression. There is evidence suggesting that cognitive dysfunction is a direct expression of the pathophysiology of depression rather than a behavioral consequence of the affective symptoms. Neuropsychological and physiological experiments have given evidence of right hemisphere dysfunction in depression (Alexopoulos 1990). Memory and executive dysfunction often occur in depressed elderly patients (Butters et al. 2000; Kinderman et al. 2000; Lockwood et al. 2000; Nebes et al. 2001). Memory and executive functions improve when geriatric depression subsides but sometimes do not completely recover (Butters et al. 2000; Nebes et al. 2001). Dysnomia has been noted in depressed elderly patients compared to controls (Speedie et al. 1990). Positron emission tomography studies show reduced glucose metabolism in the basal ganglia and the prefrontal areas (Drevets 2000) of depressed patients, while MRI studies observed reduced volumes of the putamen (Hussain et al. 1991) and the caudate (Krishnan et al. 1992) in depressed patients compared to normal controls. These observations suggest that the spectrum of clinical manifestations of depression includes a wide range of cognitive impairments that may account for some of the subjects with reversible dementia who did not deteriorate on follow-up.

The "Depression-Executive Dysfunction" Syndrome of Late Life

While early literature focused on cognitive outcomes of depression with initially-reversible dementia, recent literature suggests that cognitive impairment not meeting criteria for depression influences the course of affective symptomatology. Abnormal scores in initiation/perseveration and in response inhibition (neuropsychological expressions of frontostriatal dysfunction) were reported to predict poor or delayed antidepressant response of geriatric major depression, while memory impairment did not influence the response to antidepressants (Kalayam and Alexopoulos 1999; Alexopoulos et al. 2000). Poor or slow antidepressant response was also associated with psychomotor retardation, a behavioral disturbance that may result from frontostriatal dysfunction. White matter hyperintensities were found to predict chronicity of geriatric depression (Hickie et al. 1995). In elderly persons, white matter abnormalities were found associated with executive dysfunction (Boone et al. 1992), perhaps related to disruption of frontostriatal pathways. In addition to chronicity, abnormal scores of initiation/perseveration and response inhibition have been found to predict early relapse of geriatric major depression and residual depressive symptomatology (Alexopoulos et al. 2000; Alexopoulos 2001a, b). Neither memory impairment, nor disability, medical burden, social support, or number of previous episodes influenced the course of geriatric depression in this study. While replication of these findings is needed, the relationship of executive dysfunction to chronicity, relapse, and recurrence of geriatric depression appears to be specific to this disturbance.

The relationship of frontostriatal dysfunction to the course of geriatric depression suggests that this dysfunction contributes to the pathogenesis of at least some late-life depressive syndromes. Basic research as well as clinical observations, pathology findings, and structural and functional neuroimaging studies support this view (Alexopoulos in press).

The frontal lobe is connected to the basal ganglia through five contiguous, nonoverlapping parallel zones (corticostriatopallidocortical pathways). Three corticostriatopallidocortical pathways may be relevant to depression as damage of these pathways leads to behavioral abnormalities that resemble in part the depressive syndrome (George, Ketter, and Post 1994). Damage of the orbitofrontal circuit may lead to disinhibition, irritability, and diminished sensitivity to social cues. Damage of the anterior cingulate may result in apathy and reduced initiative. Damage of the dorsolateral circuit may result in difficulties in set shifting, learning, and word list generation.

Clinical studies have demonstrated that patients with disorders of subcortical structures often develop depression (Sobin and Sacheim 1997). Moreover, the executive abnormalities of depressed elderly patients are similar to those of patients with basal ganglia disorders (Masserman et al. 1992).

Neuropathological studies identified abnormalities in frontal structures. Reduction in glia of the subgenual prelimbic anterior cingulate gyrus has been demonstrated in unipolar depressed patients (Rajkowska, Miguel-Hidalgo, and Wei 1999; Lai et al. 2000). Abnormalities in neurons of the dorsolateral prefrontal cortex have also been documented in unipolar disorder (Ongur, Drevets, and Price 1998; Rajkowska, Miguel-Hidalgo, and Wei 1999).

Structural neuroimaging studies of depressed elderly patients have revealed abnormalities consistent with frontostriatal impairment. Volume reduction in the subgenual anterior cingulate has been reported in familial major depression (Drevets et al. 1997). Bilateral white matter hyperintensities are prevalent in geriatric depression (Krishnan, Hays, and Blass 1997; Kumar 2001) and mainly occur in subcortical structures and their frontal projections. Lesions localized in the basal ganglia and their frontal projections (Robinson and Paradiso 2001) are associated with high incidence of depression.

Functional neuroimaging studies suggest that depression is associated with abnormal metabolism (mostly increased) in limbic regions, including the amygdala, the pregenual and subgenual anterior cingulate, and the posterior orbital cortex, as well as the posterior cingulate and the medial cerebellum (Drevets 2000). In contrast, the lateral and dorsolateral prefrontal cortex, the dorsal anterior cingulate (located posteriorly to the pregenual cingulate), and the caudate have reduced blood flow during depression (Drevets et al. 1992). Bilateral activation of the dorsal anterior cingulate and the hippocampus has been reported in severely depressed elderly patients without dementia performing a word activation task (de Asis et al. 2001). Similarly, younger patients with mood disorders, when challenged with the Stroop response interference task, demonstrated blunted activation of the left anterior cingulate and minimal activation of the right anterior cingulate gyrus compared to normal controls (Rogers et al. 1998). Patients with mood disorders showed increased activity in the left dorsolateral prefrontal and visual cortex. These findings underscore the importance of subcortical neural systems in mediating development of depression.

The mechanisms underlying the relationship of frontostriatal dysfunction to poor outcome of geriatric depression are not well understood. However, metabolic changes in frontostriatal structures occur during changes in depressive symptomatology (Alexopoulos et al. in press a). Remission of depression is associated with metabolic increases in dorsal anterior cingulate, posterior cingulate, and dorsolateral cortex (Drevets 2000). In contrast, decreases in subgenual cingulate and some limbic and paralimbic structures occur during remission (Mayberg 2001). Persistence of elevated metabolism of the amygdala during remission of depression was associated with high risk for relapse of depression (Drevets 1999). Hypometabolism of the rostral anterior cingulate is associated with treatment-resistant depression in younger adults, while cingulate hypermetabolism is a predictor of favorable response (Mayberg 2001). A preliminary study noted that microstructural abnormalities in white matter lateral to the anterior cingulate (medial frontal lobe) were found to predict poor or slow antidepressant response to citalopram. This effect was specific to this site, as microstructural white matter abnormalities in other frontal areas or in a temporal area were not related to antidepressant response. White matter disruption in this area may lead to a "disconnection syndrome" interfering with the reciprocal regulation between ventral limbic and dorsal neocortical structures and inhibiting response to antidepressant treatment.

Based on these findings, a "depression-executive dysfunction syndrome" has been described and conceptualized as an entity with pronounced frontostriatal dysfunction (Alexopoulos 2001a, b). The syndrome is characterized by psychomotor retardation, reduced interest in activities, suspiciousness, and impaired instrumental activities of daily living, but less-pronounced middle insomnia and diurnal mood variation (Alexopoulos et al. in press c). The syndrome has slow and unstable response to classical antidepressants (Kalayam and Alexopoulos 1999; Alexopoulos et al. 2000). On a clinical level, identification of the depression-executive dysfunction syndrome may help clinicians in determining the prognosis of their patients and making appropriate plans for treatment and follow-up. On a theoretical level, the depression-executive dysfunction syndrome provides the rationale for development of novel treatment approaches. Pharmacological agents modifying the function of neurotransmitter systems of the frontostriatal circuitry may have antidepressant action. These include the dopamine, acetylcholine, and opiate systems. Drugs influencing these agents are available for human use and include selective dopamine receptor agonists, cholinesterase inhibitors, muscarinic and nicotinic receptor agonists, and opiate receptor agonists and antagonists. The depression-executive dysfunction syndrome of late life appears to be an appropriate target for monotherapy or augmentation therapy with these agents. Behavioral approaches aimed at both symptoms of depression and executive dysfunction can improve the short- and long-term outcomes of patients with the depression-executive dysfunction syndrome of late life. Combining problem-solving techniques with structure of activities and probes to initiate behavior may improve the outcome of patients with the depression-executive dysfunction syndrome. Besides a potential impact on the course of depressive symptomatology, behavioral interventions may improve the function of these patients. In patients without dementia, depression appears to contribute to behavioral disability mainly in the context of executive dysfunction, while the impact of depression is relatively mild in patients with unimpaired executive functions (Kiosses, Alexopoulos, and Murphy 2000; Kiosses et al. 2001).

Clinical Conclusions

Diagnostic Concepts

When presented with a depressed elderly patient with cognitive impairment, the clinician needs to evaluate both the psychiatric symptoms and signs and the cognitive impairment. The diagnosis of depression and dementia should be made independently of each other rather than assuming that one causes the other (Alexopoulos 1998). This view is based on the complex associations between depression and dementia syndromes that do not permit safe assignment of a single diagnosis during a cross-sectional examination. In some cases, the syndromes of depression and dementia are caused by the same disorders (e.g., vascular dementias, Parkinson disease, Alzheimer disease, hypothyroidism, autoimmune diseases, steroid encephalopathy, etc.). Nonetheless, even in such cases, the clinician may suspect but not safely establish that the two syndromes have a common etiology. In other cases, depression and dementia may be relatively independent of each other and simply coexist. For example, a patient with a recurrent or chronic depression since early life who develops dementia in old age may have two independent disorders. However, even in this case, the assumption that depression and dementia are independent of each other is not safe. Early-onset depression does not protect from later development of dementia and may even be a risk factor for dementia (Sheline et al. 1999). Therefore, the same patient may have depressive episodes of different etiology across the life span (e.g., a depressive episode in late life may be an early expression of a dementing disease, while depressive episodes in early life have a different etiology).

Assessment of the Dementia Syndrome

Characterizing the syndrome of cognitive impairment of depressed cognitively impaired elderly patients has important clinical implications. Depressed elderly patients with cognitive impairment should be examined for inattention, fluctuating state of consciousness, and sleep-wake disturbances. Elderly patients often develop delirium in response to drug side effects, dehydration, infections, and other toxic or metabolic factors. Depressed elderly patients are likely to develop delirium, especially when they become malnourished or dehydrated, or when treated with anticholinergic antidepressants. It should be emphasized that making the diagnosis of delirium does not exclude the diagnosis of dementia. Dementia does not protect from delirium but rather predisposes to it. Delirious patients should be reexamined to exclude an underlying dementing disorder that becomes easier to identify after the resolution of delirium.

Identifying treatable causes of dementia is critical. Dementia due to drug intoxication, hypothyroidism and other endocrinopathies, B_{12} deficiency, organ failure, and space-occupying lesion may be reversed to varying degrees. Therefore, appropriate laboratory work-up is necessary for persons with dementia regardless of the presence or absence of depression.

The clinical presentation of a dementia syndrome has implications for diagnosis and treatment planning. At least three dementia syndromes may be relevant to the evaluation of patients in whom depression and dementia are considered:

1. *Subcortical dementia.* The prominent symptoms of this syndrome are significant memory impairment, executive dysfunction, and psychomotor retardation. Subcortical dementia syndromes are the dementia syndromes most likely to be complicated by depression. They are usually caused by vascular dementia, Parkinson disease, or Lewy body dementia. Each of these disorders requires rather specific treatment (e.g., vascular dementia often is treated with aspirin and antioxidants; Parkinson disease with L-dopa preparations, dopamine receptor agonists, and anticholinergic agents; and Lewy body dementia with cholinesterase inhibitors and avoidance of neuroleptics).
2. *Cortical dementia.* These patients have a broader spectrum of impairments, including memory impairment, apraxia resulting in disheveled appearance, language impairment leading to paraphasic errors, and construction problems (e.g., inability to draw a clock). The most common cause of cortical dementia is AD, a condition treated with cholinesterase inhibitors at least during the early and middle phases.
3. *Frontal lobe dementia.* The most prominent behavioral aspects of this syndrome are apathy, socially inappropriate behavior, and disinhibition that may be expressed as irritability. These symptoms may be prominent when the memory impairment is still mild. Frontal lobe dementia may have a variety of causes, including frontotemporal dementia, early-stage AD, stroke, and so forth.

Evaluation of cognitive dysfunction is important even in depressed elderly patients who do not have dementia. Patients with psychomotor retardation, reduced interest in activities, suspiciousness, and disability are likely to have executive dysfunction. Depression with executive dysfunction may have a poor and unstable response to antidepressants (Kalayam and Alexopoulos 1999; Alexopoulos et al. 2000). For this reason, patients with the depression-executive dysfunction syndrome of late life require a careful, planned psychopharmacological treatment of sequential trials and augmentation strategies. Nonpharmacological interventions need to be added, including problem-solving therapy and rehabilitation approaches aimed at remedying their behavioral deficits.

Evaluation of the syndrome of depression in persons with dementia is complicated by the symptomatologic overlap with dementia, the instability of depressive manifestations over time, and the poor ability of elderly patients to report their symptoms. Rather than seeking to identify the etiology of each symptom, it is clinically helpful to examine whether the patient meets the criteria for depression or dementia independently. If the criteria for one of the depressive syndromes are met or approximated, the clinician should consider an antidepressant treatment trial. There are two reasons for this recommendation. First, depressed patients should have the opportunity to receive a potentially effective treatment, regardless of whether or not they have dementia. Second, improvement or remission of the depressive syndrome can increase the clinician's ability to evaluate the severity of the dementing disorder and have a clearer idea of the prognosis.

Once the decision for an antidepressant treatment trial is made, attention is needed to the duration and intensity of antidepressant treatment. Recently developed Expert Consensus Guidelines recommend that for an older patient with major depression and mild to moderate dementia, the treatment of choice is a combination of an antidepressant with psychosocial intervention. Antidepressant medication alone is another option (Alexopoulos et al. in press b). Among the antidepressants, the experts considered citalopram, sertraline, and venlafaxine first-line choices. Among psychosocial interventions, caregiver-focused treatment and supportive psychotherapy were favored. The minimal length of antidepressant trial should be three to four weeks and the maximum length should be six to seven weeks before switch to another antidepressant or an augmentation agent is used.

Variability in the course of depression with initially-reversible dementia mandates that these patients have careful follow-up, since these patients are likely to have a relapse or a recurrence of the depressive syndrome. A considerable subgroup of these patients is expected to meet the criteria for a dementing disorder within two years after the resolution of the initially-reversible dementia syndrome. Early treatment for the dementing disorder may increase the time during which the patient can function independently and allow the patient and family to make appropriate plans for the future.

ACKNOWLEDGMENTS

This work was supported by National Institute of Mental Health grants RO1 MH42819, RO1 MH51842, P30 MH49762, T32 MH19132, the Sanchez Foundation, and the Dr. I Foundation.

REFERENCES

Abas, M.A., B.J. Sahakian, and R. Levy. 1990. Neuropsychological deficits and CT scan changes in elderly depressives. *Psychological Medicine* 20:507–20.

Agbayewa, M.O. 1986. Earlier psychiatric morbidity in patients with Alzheimer's disease. *Journal of the American Geriatrics Society* 34:561–64.

Alexopoulos, G.S. 1990. Clinical and biological findings in late-onset depression. In *American Psychiatric Press Review of Psychiatry*, edited by A. Tasman, S.M. Goldfinger, and C.A. Kaufmann. 9:249–62.

Alexopoulos, G.S. 1998. The assessment and treatment of depressed-demented patients. In *Geriatric Psychopharmacology*, edited by J.C. Nelson. New York: Marcel Dekker, pp. 223–43.

Alexopoulos, G.S. 2001a. The depression-executive dysfunction syndrome of late life: A target for D3 receptor agonists. *American Journal of Geriatric Psychiatry* 9:1–8.

Alexopoulos, G.S. 2001b. Executive dysfunction and course of geriatric depression. Paper presented at the annual meeting of the American Association of Geriatric Psychiatry, San Francisco.

Alexopoulos, G.S. In press. Late life mood disorders. In *Comprehensive Review of Geriatric Psychiatry*. Washington, D.C.: American Psychiatric Press.

Alexopoulos, G.S., and R.C. Abrams. 1991. Depression in Alzheimer's disease. *Psychiatric Clinics of North America* 14:327–40.

Alexopoulos, G.S., R.C. Young, and B.S. Meyers. 1993. Geriatric depression: Age of onset and dementia. *Biological Psychiatry* 34:164–69.

Alexopoulos, G.S., B.S. Meyers, R.C. Young, et al. 1988. Brain changes in geriatric depression. *International Journal of Geriatric Psychiatry* 3:157–61.

Alexopoulos, G.S., B.S. Meyers, R.C. Young, et al. 1993. The course of geriatric depression with "reversible dementia": A controlled study. *American Journal of Psychiatry* 150:1693–99.

Alexopoulos, G.S., B.S. Meyers, R.C. Young, et al. 2000. Executive dysfunction and risk for relapse and recurrence of geriatric depression. *Archives of General Psychiatry* 57: 285–90.

Alexopoulos, G.S., K. Buckwalters, C. Wainscott, et al. In press a. Aging and comorbidity in geriatric depression. *Biological Psychiatry.*

Alexopoulos, G.S., I.R. Katz, C.F. Reynolds III, et al. In press b. The Expert Consensus Guideline Series: Pharmacotherapy of late life depression. *Postgraduate Medicine.*

Alexopoulos, G.S., D.N. Kiosses, B. Kalayam, et al. In press c. Clinical presentation of the "depression-executive dysfunction syndrome" of late life. *American Journal of Geriatric Psychiatry.*

Bassuk, S.S., L.F. Berkman, and D. Wypij. 1998. Depressive symptomatology and incident cognitive decline in an elderly community sample. *Archives of General Psychiatry* 55:1073–81.

Berrios, G.E. 1985. "Depressive pseudodementia" or "melancholic dementia": A nineteenth century view. *Journal of Neurology, Neurosurgery and Psychiatry* 48:393–400.

Boone, K.B., B.L. Miller, I.M. Lesser, et al. 1992. Neuropsychological correlates of white matter lesions in healthy elderly subjects. *Archives of Neurology* 49:549–54.

Butters, M.A., J.T. Becker, R.D. Nebes, et al. 2000. Changes in cognitive functioning following treatment of late-life depression. *American Journal of Psychiatry* 157: 1949–54.

Caine, E. 1981. Pseudodementia: Current concepts and future directions. *Archives of General Psychiatry* 38:1359–64.

Cohen, R.M., H. Weingartner, S.A. Smallberg, et al. 1982. Effort and cognition in depression. *Archives of General Psychiatry* 39:593–97.

Copeland, J.R.M., I.A. Davidson, M.E. Dewey, et al. 1992. Alzheimer's disease, other dementias, depression and pseudodementia: Prevalence, incidence and three year outcome in Liverpool. *British Journal of Psychiatry* 161:230–39.

de Asis, J.M., E. Stern, G.S. Alexopoulos, et al. 2001. Hippocampal and anterior cingulate activation deficits in patients with geriatric depression. *American Journal of Psychiatry* 158:1321–23.

Devanand, D.P., M. Sano, M.X. Tang, et al. 1996. Depressed mood and the incidence of Alzheimer's disease in the elderly living in the community. *Archives of General Psychiatry* 53:175–82.

Drevets, W.C. 1999. Prefrontal cortical-amygdalar metabolism in major depression. *Annals of the New York Academy of Science* 877:614–37.

Drevets, W.C. 2000. Neuroimaging studies of mood disorders. *Biological Psychiatry* 48: 813–19.

Drevets, W.C., T.O. Videen, J.L. Price, et al. 1992. A functional anatomical study of unipolar depression. *Journal of Neuroscience* 12:3628–41.

Drevets, W.C., J.L. Price, J.R. Simpson, et al. 1997. Subgenual prefrontal cortex abnormalities in mood disorders. *Nature* 386:824–27.

Emery, V.O.B. 1985. Language and aging. *Experimental Aging Research Monographs* 11(1).

Emery, V.O.B. 1986. Linguistic decrement in normal aging. *Language and Communication* 6:47–64.

Emery, V.O.B. 1988. *Pseudodementia: A Theoretical and Empirical Discussion.* Cleveland: Case Western Reserve University School of Medicine.

Emery V.O., and T.E. Oxman. 1992. Update on the dementia spectrum of depression. *American Journal of Psychiatry* 149:305–17.

Fogel, B., and F.R. Sparadeo. 1985. Focal cognitive deficits accentuated by depression. *Journal of Nervous and Mental Disease* 173:120–23.

Folstein, M.F., S.E. Folstein, and P.R. McHugh. 1975. "Mini-Mental State": A practical method for grading the cognitive state of patients for the clinician. *Journal of Psychiatric Research* 12:189–98.

Geerlings, M.I., R.A. Schoevers, A.T. Beekman, et al. 2000. Depression and risk of cognitive decline and Alzheimer's disease. Results of two community-based studies in the Netherlands. *British Journal of Psychiatry* 176:568–75.

George, M.S., T.A. Ketter, and R.M. Post. 1994. Prefrontal cortex dysfunction in clinical depression. *Depression* 2:59–72.

Hasher, L., and R.T. Zacks. 1979. Automatic and effortful processes in memory. *Journal of Experimental Psychology: General* 108:356–88.

Hickie, I., E. Scott, P. Mitchell, et al. 1995. Subcortical hyperintensities on magnetic resonance imaging: Clinical correlates and prognostic significance in patients with severe depression. *Biological Psychiatry* 37:151–60.

Hussain, M.M., W.M. McDonald, P.M. Doraiswamy, et al. 1991. A magnetic resonance imaging study of putamen nuclei in major depression. *Psychiatry Research* 40:95–99.

Jorm, A.F., C.M. van Duijn, V. Chandra, et al. 1991. Psychiatric history and related exposures as risk factors for Alzheimer's disease: A collaborative re-analysis of case-control studies. *International Journal of Epidemiology* 20 (Suppl. 2):S43–47.

Kalayam, B., and G.S. Alexopoulos. 1999. Prefrontal dysfunction and treatment response in geriatric depression. *Archives of General Psychiatry* 56:713–18.

Kiloh, L. 1961. Pseudo-dementia. *Acta Psychiatrica Scandinavica* 37:336–51.

Kiloh, L. 1981. Depressive illness masquerading as dementia in the elderly. *Medical Journal of Australia* 2:550–53.

Kindermann, S.S., B. Kalayam, G.G. Brown., et al. 2000. Executive functions and P300 latency in elderly depressed patients and control subjects. *American Journal of Geriatric Psychiatry* 8:57–65.

Kiosses, D.N., G.S. Alexopoulos, and C. Murphy. 2000. Symptoms of striatofrontal dysfunction contribute to disability in geriatric depression. *International Journal of Geriatric Psychiatry* 15:992–99.

Kiosses, D.N., S. Klimstra, C. Murphy, et al. 2001. Executive dysfunction and disability in elderly patients with major depression. *American Journal of Geriatric Psychiatry* 9:269–74.

Kokmen, E., C.M. Beard, V. Chandra, et al. 1991. Clinical risk factors for Alzheimer's disease: A population-based case-control study. *Neurology* 41:1393–97.

Krishnan, K.R.R., J.C. Hays, and D.G. Blazer. 1997. MRI-defined vascular depression. *American Journal of Psychiatry* 154:497–500.

Krishnan, K.R.R., W.M. McDonald, P.R. Escalona, et al. 1992. Magnetic resonance imaging of the caudate nuclei in depression: Preliminary observations. *Archives of General Psychiatry* 49:553–57.

Kral, V.A., and V.O.B. Emery. 1989. Long term follow-up of depressive pseudodementia of the aged. *Canadian Journal of Psychiatry* 34:445–47.

Kumar A. 2001. Neuroanatomy of late-life mood disorders. *Economics of Neuroscience* 3:44–48.

Lai, T.-J., M.E. Payne, C.E. Byrum, et al. 2000. Reduction of orbital frontal cortex volume in geriatric depression. *Biological Psychiatry* 48:971–75.

Lockwood, K.A., G.S. Alexopoulos, T. Kakuma, et al. 2000. Subtypes of cognitive impairment in depressed older adults. *American Journal of Geriatric Psychiatry* 8:201–8.

Madden, J., J. Luban, and L. Kaplan. 1952. Non-dementing psychosis in older persons. *Journal of the American Medical Association* 150:1567–72.

Masserman, P. J., D.C. Delis, N. Butters, et al. 1992. The subcortical dysfunction hypothesis of memory deficits in depression: Neuropsychological validation in a subgroup of patients. *Journal of Clinical Experiential Neuropsychology* 14:687–706.

Mayberg, H.S. 2001. Depression and frontal-subcortical circuits. Focus on prefrontal-limbic interactions. In *Frontal-Subcortical Circuits in Psychiatric and Neurological Disorders*, edited by D.C. Lichter and J.L. Cummings. New York: Guilford Press, pp. 177–206.

McAllister, T.W. 1983. Overview: Pseudodementia. *American Journal of Psychiatry* 140: 528–33.

Meyers, B.S. 1992. Adverse cognitive effects of tricyclic antidepressants in the treatment of geriatric depression: Fact or fiction? In *Psychopharmacological Treatment Complications in the Elderly*, edited by C. Shamoian. Washington, D.C.: American Psychiatric Press, pp. 1–16.

Nebes, R., M.A. Butters, B.H. Mulsant, et al. 2000. Decreased working memory and processing speed mediate cognitive impairment in geriatric depression. *Psychological Medicine* 30:679–91.

Nebes, R.D., M.A. Butters, P.R. Houck, et al. 2001. Dual-task performance in depressed geriatric patients. *Psychiatry Research* 102:139–51.

Ongur, D., W.C. Drevets, and J.L. Price. 1998. Glial reduction in the prefrontal cortex in mood disorders. *Proceedings of the National Academy of Sciences USA* 95:13290–95.

Pearlson, G.D., P.V. Rabins, W.S. Kirn, et al. 1989. Structural brain CT changes and cognitive deficits in elderly depressives with and without reversible dementia ("pseudodementia"). *Psychological Medicine* 19:573–84.

Post, F. 1975. Dementia, depression, and pseudodementia. In *Psychiatric Aspects of Neurological Disease*, edited by F. Benson and D. Blumer. New York: Grune & Stratton, pp. 98–110.

Rabins, P., A. Merchant, and G. Nestadt. 1984. Criteria for diagnosing reversible dementia caused by depression: Validation by two-year follow-up. *British Journal of Psychiatry* 144:488–92.

Rajkowska, G., L.L. Miguel-Hidalgo, and J. Wei. 1999. Morphometric evidence for neuronal and glial prefrontal cell pathology in major depression. *Biological Psychiatry* 45:1085–98.

Reding, M., J. Haycox, and J. Blass. 1985. Depression in patients referred to a dementia clinic: A three-year prospective study. *Archives of Neurology* 42:894–96.

Reifler, B.V. 1982. Arguments for abandoning the term pseudodementia. *Journal of the American Geriatrics Society* 30:665–68.

Reynolds, C.F., III, D.J. Kupfer, C.C. Hoch, et al. 1986. Two year follow-up of elderly patients with mixed depression and dementia: Clinical and electroencephalographic sleep findings. *Journal of the American Geriatrics Society* 34:793–99.

Reynolds, C.F., III, C.C. Hoch, D.J. Kupfer, et al. 1988a. Bedside differentiation of depressive pseudodementia from dementia. *American Journal of Psychiatry* 145: 1099–1103.

Reynolds, C.F., III, D.J. Kupfer, P.R. Houck, et al. 1988b. Reliable discrimination of elderly depressed and demented patients by electroencephalographic sleep data. *Archives of General Psychiatry* 45:258–64.

Ritchie, K., C. Gilman, B. Ledesert, et al. 1999. Depressive illness, depressive symptomatology, and regional cerebral blood flow in elderly people with subclinical cognitive impairment. *Age and Ageing* 28:385–91.

Robinson, R.G., and S. Paradiso. 2001. Psychiatric aspects of vascular disorders. In *Psychiatric Treatment of the Medically Ill*, edited by R.G. Robinson and W.R. Yates. New York: Marcel Decker, pp. 299–338.

Rogers, M.A., J.L. Bradshaw, C. Pantelis, et al. 1998. Frontostriatal deficits in unipolar major depression. *Brain Research Bulletin* 47:297–310.

Rovner, B.W., J. Broadhead, M. Spencer, et al. 1989. Depression and Alzheimer's disease. *American Journal of Psychiatry* 146:350–53.

Sachdaw, P.S., J.S. Smith, H. Angus-Lepan, et al. 1990. Pseudodementia twelve years on. *Journal of Neurology, Neurosurgery and Psychiatry* 53:254–59.

Sahakian, B.J. 1991. Depressive pseudodementia in the elderly. *International Journal of Geriatric Psychiatry* 6:453–58.

Sahakian, B.J., R.G. Morris, J.L. Evenden, et al. 1988. A comparative study of visuospatial memory and learning in Alzheimer-type dementia and Parkinson's disease. *Brain* 111:695–718.

Sheline, Y.I., M. Sanghavi, M.A. Mintun, et al. 1999. Depression duration but not age predicts hippocampal volume loss in medically healthy women with recurrent major depression. *Journal of Neuroscience* 19:5034–43.

Sobin, C., and H.A. Sacheim. 1997. Psychomotor symptoms of depression. *American Journal of Psychiatry* 154:4–17.

Speck, C.E., W.A. Kukull, D.E. Brenner, et al. 1995. History of depression as a risk factor for Alzheimer's disease. *Epidemiology* 6:366–69.

Speedie, L., P. Rabins, G. Pearlson, et al. 1990. Confrontation naming deficit in dementia of depression. *Journal of Neuropsychiatry* 2:59–63.

Steffens, D.C., B.L. Plassman, M.J. Helms, et al. 1997. A twin study of late-onset depression and apolipoprotein E epsilon 4 as risk factors for Alzheimer's disease. *Biological Psychiatry* 41:851–56.

van Duijn, C.M., D.G. Clayton, V. Chandra, et al. 1994. Interaction between genetic and environmental risk factors for Alzheimer's disease: A reanalysis of case-control studies. *Genetic Epidemiology* 11:539–51.

Wells, C.E. 1979. Pseudodementia. *American Journal of Psychiatry* 136:895–900.

Yaffe, K., T. Blackwell, R. Gore, et al. 1999. Depressive symptoms and cognitive decline in nondemented elderly women: A prospective study. *Archives of General Psychiatry* 56: 425–30.

Young, R.C., M. Manley, and G.S. Alexopoulos. 1985. "I don't know" responses in elderly depressives and in dementia. *Journal of the American Geriatrics Society* 33:253–57.

CHAPTER SIXTEEN

The Nondepressive Pseudodementias

Perminder Sachdev, M.D., Ph.D., FRANZCP,
and Sharon Reutens, M.B.B.S., FRANZCP

The use of the term *pseudodementia* in this chapter requires some clarification. The history of this concept has been detailed elsewhere and will not be discussed here (see chaps. 14 and 15) (Wells 1979; Caine 1981; Berrios 1985, 1986; Bulbena and Berrios 1986; Emery 1988). Kiloh (1961) conceptualized pseudodementia as a purely descriptive term for patients with a clinical presentation mimicking dementia but for whom this diagnosis was subsequently abandoned because of the course of illness. Pseudodementia was seen as a copy of dementia, or as its caricature, and not as a category of dementia or a diagnostic entity in itself. Inherent in this distinction was the understanding that dementia has a basis in (thus far) irreversible degenerative brain disease. Therefore, pseudodementia frequently gave itself away when the cognitive dysfunction reversed or proved to be inconsistent. Kiloh (1981) recognized that the picture of pseudodementia was produced by a number of psychiatric disorders, of which depression was by far the most common. Hence, the plural term *pseudodementias* will be used, signifying the multiplicity of disorders that can result in this presentation.

The definition of pseudodementia as well as the clinical and research utility of such a definition have been debated extensively over the past three decades

Table 16.1. Should the term pseudodementia *be retained?*

Pro	Con
Suggests that a primary nonorganic psychiatric disorder is responsible for the clinical picture.	The concept of dementia no longer incorporates as a necessary feature reversibility, therefore cannot be an argument for pseudodementia.
Encourages efforts at diagnostic work-up and effective therapy.	*The cognitive deficit in some psychiatric disorders, notably depression, is "genuine" with a basis in brain pathophysiology.*
Suggests a nonprogressive and reversible course.	*Dementia is not always a cortical phenomenon but may be "subcortical." Depressive "pseudodementia" shares many features with "subcortical dementia."*
Provides the clinician with a descriptive term for a range of disorders that have a common presentation.	*Depression is a common and under-recognized part of the dementia syndrome. A diagnosis of "pseudodementia" may miss the underlying dementia.*
Communicates parsimoniously both the understanding of features of the clinical presentation and what it is not caused by.	Pseudodementia is largely a negative concept, with no single accepted definition or characteristic pattern of symptoms.

(Reifler 1982; Mahendra 1984; Folstein and Rabins 1991). Some of the arguments both for and against the use of this term are presented in table 16.1. The term continues to be applied clinically, however, and its use has proven to be robust in the face of criticism. The main appeal is its utility as a descriptor for a variety of clinical situations, communicating the main features of both what the patient's condition is and is not. Although criticism of the term has come from many quarters, the main thrust has been from researchers of the neuropsychological aspects of depression who argue that cognitive impairment in depression is "genuine" and the term *pseudodementia* is misleading. Furthermore, they argue that the term discourages research into the pathophysiological basis of such impairment. This argument is essentially a semantic one, and we are willing to go along with the editors of this book in separating "depressive dementia" from the "pseudodementias" for the purpose of our discussion here. It does, however, create some conceptual difficulties.

The definition of pseudodementia we have generally used is of a clinical picture of dementia (however defined) with the absence of evidence of specific, irreversible degenerative factors of sufficient severity to cause the disturbance, and the presence of strong cross-sectional or historical evidence of a primary psychiatric disorder that could account for the current problem (Sachdev et al. 1990). If depression is excluded from this category (as in this book), this conceptualization immediately runs into difficulty. Should such an exclusion also apply to schizophrenia, mania, and so forth as causes of pseudodementia? If we exclude these, then we are left with pseudodementia as a simulation of dementia, emphasizing its parodylike nature rather than its primary psychiatric disorder etiology. We believe that the original definition of pseudodementia (which includes depression in its rubric) may prove to be more useful clinically. Because cognitive impairment caused by depression has been discussed extensively in other chapters, however, we limit our discussion to other primary psychiatric disorders associated with pseudodementia.

We propose that these disorders can be divided into two basic types. The first includes disorders simulating dementia, either conscious and intentional (such as malingering and factitious disorder) or unconscious (such as hysteria or dissociative and conversion disorders). The second type includes other primary, axis-I (DSM-IV) psychiatric disorders that can result in severe cognitive impairment but are not necessarily progressively degenerative or irreversible, such as depressive disorders, mania, schizophrenia, obsessive-compulsive disorder, and generalized anxiety disorder. The Ganser syndrome is an interesting anomaly that overlaps both types.

Pseudodementia as a Simulation of Dementia

The literature suggests that simulation of dementia is uncommon and that competent simulation is a difficult task rarely carried out with conviction and consistency (Anderson, Trethowan, and Kenna 1959; Lishman 2000). The literature may not reflect the exact extent of this problem, however, as anyone with forensic and medicolegal psychiatric experience would testify (Gilandas and Touyz 1983). The recent increase in the public awareness of dementing disorders makes it likely that simulated dementia might become more common in the future.

Simulation may be entirely conscious (intentional) or it may be presumed to be an unconscious process. Very often, a clinical decision on the *degree* of voluntariness involved in the process is extremely difficult and, unless the patient admits to the simulation, is at best an educated guess. Not uncommonly, simulation is suspected to be the cause of a gross exaggeration of neuropsychological deficits. When conscious simulation is clearly motivated by external incentives, malingering is diagnosed; external incentives include obtaining financial compensation or drugs; avoiding military duty, criminal prosecution, or work in general; or securing better living conditions. When the intentional production or feigning of symptoms occurs in the absence of external incentives and results from the psychological need to assume the "sick" role, factitious disorder with psychological symptoms is the diagnosis. In hysterical pseudodementia, the simulation is unconsciously determined and is suggestive of emotional conflicts with the person. Some differences in the presentation of these disorders will be discussed later.

Is Competent Simulation of Dementia Possible?

In many clinical situations, the judgment that cognitive deficits are not genuine can be made when adequate information is available, although this is not always the case. The nature of symptoms in simulated dementia depends to some extent on the medical and psychological sophistication of the subject. In most cases, genuine dementia is hard to simulate. The history of sudden onset of rapid progression inconsistent with neurological and neuroradiological findings may help, but sometimes the onset is after a head injury or similar cerebral insult that is difficult to quantify. In most cases, a discrepancy between the duration of illness and the severity of brain injury, as well as the extent of neuropsychological symptoms, will alert the clinician to the possibility of simulation. The setting of the production of symptoms, if it provides motivation to simulate or suggests an underlying severe personality disorder or emotional conflict, may be a further indicator for the correct diagnosis.

Even when the experienced clinician is alerted to the possibility of simulation by the setting, background, or history of deficits, the role of the formal mental state examination remains crucial for the diagnostic decision. Careful examination and observation can reveal much that is inconsistent with genuine cognitive impairment. The simulated dementia is essentially the patient's notion of the disorder he or she wishes to portray, and is therefore limited by the patient's lack of knowledge (Bluglass 1976). Simulated symptoms are often severe rather than complex. Examination may be significantly curtailed owing to muteness, monosyllabic answers, or evasiveness and uncooperativeness of the patient. Often, the patient is likely to present with gross impairment of a single function, such as speech or memory. Inconsistencies usually become apparent on detailed examination (Wells 1979). The patient may fail a relatively simple task, yet go on to perform a cognitively more complex task (Emery 1988); thus, the simulated performance may not relate to a hierarchy of the difficulty of tasks. Such patients may fail on tasks that are usually affected only in severest dementia. Patients may appear theatric and make unconvincing displays of noncomprehension or even insanity (Caine 1981). They may give "near-miss" or "bizarre" answers to questions, but lack convincing evidence of perseveration or concrete thinking (Lishman 2000). The degree of deficits on formal examination is not reflected in the general behavior of the patient in the ward or at home. Standards of dress, personal hygiene and self-care, social judgments, and spatial orientation may be preserved. In fact, these may be remarkably competent in contrast to the gross deficits on formal testing.

A few exceptional reports of the simulation of dementia have been published. Some of the earliest work was by Jung (1903) using the word-association test. Hubner (1919) attempted to train naïve normal subjects to simulate psychiatric disorders, including pseudodementia, and Lowenstein (1924) attempted the same for neurological disorders and found that with practice, subjects adopted a consistent symptom. Bender (1938) used her Gestalt Test to assess the performance of normal subjects who were asked to simulate mental defect and found they were unable to inhibit essential gestalt principles conformable to maturation level. World War II saw the publication of a number of papers on malingering and simulation, but none added substantially to the theoretic understanding.

A subsequent experiment by Anderson, Trethowan, and Kenna (1959), however, is notable for its thoroughness. The performance of eighteen psychology students simulating dementia was compared with that of twenty-five patients with organic dementia and ten patients with hysteric (or dissociative) dementia. All three groups differed on some aspects of performance. All gave "near-miss" answers, but these were most common in the hysteric pseudodementia group. Transposition and reversal errors (e.g., of given digits, order of months) were made by all groups. However, perseveration was prominent in the organic group and rare in the other groups. Length and thoroughness of examination were important in revealing the spuriousness of simulation. Fatigue in the simulating group tended to produce more normal answers, whereas the patients with hysteric pseudodementia tended to become more uncooperative. The authors concluded that consciously simulated dementia was qualitatively different from both organic and hysteric pseudodementia.

Some studies have examined whether neuropsychological tests can distinguish between genuine and simulated deficits. Benton (1945) used the Rorschach test because the unfamiliar, seemingly irrational task typically aroused the malingerer's suspicions and defenses, resulting in slow, sparse, and constricted responses. Benton and Spreen (1961) reported that on visual-memory tasks, simulators made more errors of distortion than did brain-damaged patients and fewer errors of omission, perseveration, and size. Heaton et al. (1978) compared the results of sixteen volunteer malingerers and sixteen uncooperative nonlitigating patients with head trauma on the Wechsler Adult Intelligence Scale, Halstead-Reitan Battery, and Minnesota Multiphasic Personality Inventory. With discriminant function analysis of the test results, 100% and 94%, respectively, of subjects were correctly classified into the two groups.

Goebel (1983), however, cautioned against concluding from these results that simulation and genuine impairment are readily distinguishable, arguing that because there were more variables than subjects, these findings might result from chance variation. Goebel asked normal subjects to fake lateralized and diffuse cognitive deficits, then compared their performance to those of normal and brain-damaged samples. Goebel concluded that normal individuals of at least average intelligence could not adjust their performance to appear brain-damaged and that patterns of lateralized impairment across language, memory, motor, and sensory functions were beyond their abilities to produce. Hayward et al. (1987) similarly concluded that their knowledgeable group of informed simulators had great difficulty reproducing the test performance of persons with left frontotemporal impairment. Porch, Friden, and Porec (1971) tested the ability of normal subjects to simulate aphasia on the Porch Index of Communicative Ability, and they found (as predicted) that the simulators had lower scores on the easier end because of their inability to judge the level of task difficulty.

The Minnesota Multiphasic Personality Inventory and other similar tests have incorporated scales and formulas to detect conscious malingering and other test-taking variables that might affect the validity of the test (Osborne 1970). There is some evidence that performance on the Minnesota inventory might help identify persons with neurologic complaints of nonorganic origin. Shaw and Mathews (1965) used seventeen of its items to devise the Pseudo-Neurologic Scale, designed to identify persons who had neurologic complaints in the absence of abnormalities on neurologic examination. Shaw and Mathews reported that this scale correctly classified 81% of patients with brain damage without neurologic signs but misclassified 25% of those with unequivocal neurologic deficits. Cross-validation studies, while still significant, have been somewhat less impressive in terms of the percentages correctly classified through use of the Pseudo-Neurologic Scale.

Although evidence suggests that neuropsychological deficits are difficult to simulate convincingly, examining the individual patient to reach a clinical decision can be extremely difficult. Lezak (1983) provided a guide for the practitioner attempting such differential diagnosis, recommending the following tests, depending on the clinical situation:

— Bender-Gestalt
— Benton Visual Retention Test
— Halstead-Reitan Battery
— Minnesota Multiphasic Personality Inventory
— Porch Index of Communicative Ability
— Rorschach Projective Test

The possibility of simulation can be further investigated with tests devised by Rey (1941, 1964): memorization of fifteen items, dot counting (grouped and ungrouped dots), and word recognition. An additional test, recommended by Pankratz (1979), requires the patient to make 100 forced-choice decisions of a simple, two-alternative problem involving the patient's symptom or complaint. By chance alone, approximately 50% of the patient's choices will be correct. A correct score of below 40% suggests simulation. Table 16.2 summarizes the differences between simulated and degenerative dementia.

Malingering

While the world wars focused attention on malingering, it continues to be of interest in civilian life, especially in the medicolegal context. Differential diagnosis between malingering and dissociation is difficult, but some guidelines might help. Malingerers convey the impression of being aware of what they are doing, and they appear to be working toward a preconceived goal. Malingerers therefore are likely to be on guard lest they give themselves away. Malingerers usually are cooperative until detailed probing comes close to the truth, at which time they become uncooperative and evasive, and will attempt to defeat the purpose of the investigation. If discrepancies in symptoms are pointed out, there is

Table 16.2. Comparison between simulated and true dementia

Characteristic	Simulated Dementia	True Dementia (Alzheimer Type)
History		
Onset	Often sudden, may follow minor cerebral insult	Slow and insidious
Progression	May be rapid	Usually gradual
Setting	Litigation, incarceration, interpersonal conflict, and so on	No special setting
Age	Often young	Usually > 60 years
Past history of conversion, multiple hospitalizations, litigation, and so on	More likely	Less likely
History of disrupted family background	More likely	Less likely
Family history of dementia	Less likely	More likely
Mental State		
Consistency with duration of illness	Symptoms not consistent	Symptoms consistent
Nature of symptoms	Reflect patient's notion of dementia	Well-recognized syndrome
	More severe than complex	Complex, and may be severe
	May be grossly incoherent, or mute	Grossly incoherent only in the very late stages
	"Near-miss" or "bizarre" answers	These are rare
	Perseverations absent	Often present
	Concreteness usually absent	Usually absent
Behavior during interview	May appear theatric	Usually serious and undramatic
	Unconvincing display	Easy to emphasize with
	May be very suggestible and performance may vary	Performance not modified by suggestion
	May become totally uncooperative and evasive	Uncooperative only if psychotic or lacking insight
General behavior	Usually maintains standards of dress, hygiene, and self-care	These are often neglected

Table 16.2. Continued

Characteristic	Simulated Dementia	True Dementia (Alzheimer Type)
	Usually maintains social judgment	May be impaired
	Often maintains spatial orientation	Often disturbed
	May be competent in tasks of daily life in the presence of gross deficits on testing	These are commensurate with each other
Neuropsychological testing		
Inconsistencies in performance	Usually present	Usually absent
Effects of fatigue	Becomes uncooperative, or improves	Worsens
Perseveration	Usually absent	Often present
Rorschach test	Slow, sparse, and constricted responses suggesting defensiveness	"Organic" responses
Bender gestalt test	General gestalt principles observed	Not observed
Visual memory tasks	More errors of distortion	More errors of omission, perseveration, and size
Lateralized dysfunction	Poor and inconsistent performance	Consistent performance
Tests for aphasia	Lower scores on easier as well as severe end	A gradient of scores related to severity
Personality inventories	Low scores on validity scales	Usually not so
Rey tests (1964)	Poor performance	Good performance
Forced-choice decisions	Performance below chance level	Higher than chance level
Investigations		
Neuroanatomic studies (CT, MRI)	Normal (or minimally abnormal)	Usually abnormal
Functional-imaging studies		
EEG	Normal	Usually abnormal, may be normal in mild cases
SPECT	Normal	Often abnormal
PET	Normal	Often abnormal

a tendency for them to react with anger or become upset (Kraupl-Taylor 1966). This is unlike the dissociative patient, who may show little emotional concern for the inconsistencies and may in fact present with easily identifiable inconsistencies that are apparent even to the layman. Also unlike the dissociative, the malingerer is not readily suggestible. Malingering often occurs in the context of a personality disorder, with an emphasis on antisocial traits.

These difficulties do not always help to distinguish malingering from dissociation, and many clinical situations remain ambiguous. The clinical evaluation may suggest elements of both conscious and unconscious simulation. Malingering (occurring on the background of personality psychopathology) is likely to mobilize some unconscious processes. In deceiving others, the malingerer often partially deceives the self. Gain is present in both malingering and dissociation, although the gain for the malingerer is more obvious, external, and materially substantial. Even a confession of simulation might not completely settle the issue, because such confessions have also been reported in degenerative dementia and dissociative pseudodementia (Kennedy and Neville 1957). Malingering can be differentiated from somatoform disorders (e.g., conversion disorder) by the intentional production of symptoms, and the malingerer is less likely to present symptoms symbolically related to any underlying emotional conflict. Malingering differs from factitious disorder in that motivation for symptom production in the former is external and material, whereas the motivation in factitious disorder stems from an intrapsychic need for hospitalization (Wassersug 1982; Carney 1983; Axen 1986). Table 16.3 systematically compares malingering, factitious disorder, and dissociative pseudodementia on core dimensions.

Factitious Disorder

Most patients with factitious disorder have physical symptoms, corresponding to the classic portrayal of Munchausen syndrome, but patients with only cognitive or psychological symptoms have been described (Goldstein 1998). Although symptoms in factitious disorder are voluntarily feigned, the purpose is to assume the role of the patient rather than obtain any material gain. The presentation is usually pansymptomatic, and the attitude may be one of marked suggestibility or, on the other hand, negativism and uncooperativeness. The features overlap with the other simulated dementias (tab. 16.3) and with Ganser syndrome. "Approximate" answers (Moeli 1888; Ganser 1898) may be present. There is almost always a background of severe personality disorder, and often

Table 16.3. Comparison of the simulated dementias

Characteristic	Dissociative (Hysteric)	Malingering	Factitious
Process	Unconscious	Conscious	Conscious
Underlying emotional conflicts	Present	Absent	Present
Motivation	Primary gain	Material gain	Hospitalization
Past history	Pseudoneurologic symptoms	Antisociality or litigation	Multiple hospitalizations and medical interventions
Onset	After emotional trauma or following fugue or minor cerebral injury	After minor cerebral injury or material desire or frustating circumstance	After emotional conflict
Attitude to symptoms	La belle indifference	Inconsistent and concerned	Appears concerned until hospitalized
Attitude to examiner	Cooperative and suggestible, usually	Evasive and on guard, usually	May be suggestible and uncooperative
Presentation	Often dramatic and histrionic	Not usually dramatic	May be dramatic
Response to confrontation	Appears unconcerned, uses denial	Evasive or angry	Disbelief or anger, and escape from hospital

a history of past hospitalizations is available. Two broad categories of patients have been described. The first generally presents after an acute stress with a disorder that does not require invasive intervention. These patients are less likely to have "classic" features of frequent and dramatic presentations, wandering to hospitals, and self-harm behavior. The prognosis of these patients is more positive than that of the second, chronic group of patients who rarely identify a stressor before presentation. When confronted with the appropriate diagnosis, patients usually react with disbelief and anger, or a quiet escape from the hospital only to present to another institution.

Why the hospital has such significance for these patients is not known. Some researchers have suggested that it may be related to neglect, abuse, or abandonment in childhood (Wassersug 1982). Others have proposed that an early hospital experience may have provided more warmth and caring than was otherwise experienced by the patient (Wassersug 1982; Axen 1986). Whatever the historical reasons, patients with factitious disorder willingly submit to extensive and often painful hospitalization for illnesses they have fabricated (Axen 1986).

Dissociative (Hysteric) Pseudodementia

The presumption of unconscious simulation is fraught with pitfalls, as many follow-up studies of "hysteria" have shown (Tissenbaum, Harter, and Friedman 1951; Slater 1965; Merskey and Buchrich 1975). The problem is compounded by the tendency of many physicians to diagnose "hysteria" when they fail to understand the disorder rather than when clear evidence for an emotional disorder exists. The approach taken by recent classificatory systems to drop the term *hysteria* in favor of *somatoform* and *dissociative disorders* (e.g., DSM-IV), although welcome, for some reasons further complicates use of the terms to describe this syndrome and evaluate it historically.

The nature of the deficits in dissociative pseudodementia is similar to that of the intentionally simulated pseudodementias. Usually, the associated features distinguish between dissociative pseudodementia and the intentional simulations of dementia. The patient will often give a past history of pseudoneurologic symptoms, such as sensory loss, paralysis, and blindness, or dissociative symptoms, such as amnesia or fugue states. The patient may show a detached affect or lack of concern for the deficits ("la belle indifference") and appear sullen or paradoxically cheerful. In general, emotional responses are superficial and unconvincing. The history usually suggests personality disturbance with histrionic traits or marked dependency (Wells 1979), and suggestibility is an important feature. Emotional precipitants may be elicitable, and these often relate to interpersonal conflicts or psychosexual difficulties. Onset may be abrupt after an emotional trauma, or it may begin with a fuguelike state, after which the patient presents with intellectual impairment. A relatively minor head trauma may be followed by complaints of severe deficit. Symptoms can be relatively isolated (e.g., amnesia) (Kennedy and Neville 1957) or may involve multiple cognitive processes. In rare cases, the patient may regress to a state of helpless infancy, lying curled up in bed, incontinent and unable to articulate. This has been called *hysterical puerilism* or *hysterical infantilism* (Bleuler 1924). Some symptom relief may be obtained through hypnosis or an amobarbital interview.

Dissociative mechanisms may sometimes occur in the context of other psychiatric disorders, such as depression or Ganser syndrome, or may exacerbate an underlying degenerative dementia. Dissociative pseudodementia is usually of short duration, but symptoms can also become chronic and resistant to any intervention, especially in cases that involve compensable injury or other secondary gain (Freud 1963 [1905]). Table 16.3 summarizes the main differences between the three subtypes of simulated dementia.

Ganser Syndrome

Pseudodementia is sometimes equated with Ganser syndrome, but there is little justification for this, as Ganser syndrome is only one of the pseudodementias. Ganser syndrome is a heterogeneous disorder exhibiting considerable overlap with the simulated dementias, schizophrenia, delirium, and "true" dementia. It therefore is important to briefly review the history of this concept to understand the context of usage of the term over the years.

The three patients originally described by Ganser (1898) were prisoners whose mental status was characterized by what Ganser called *vorbeireden* or "talking past the point" or "approximate answers." This symptom, which had been described earlier by Moeli (1888), later came to be referred to as the *Ganser symptom* and has attracted considerable attention since its first description. Apart from this symptom, Ganser's patients also manifested visual and auditory hallucinations, illusions, clouding of sensorium, "hysterical" stigmata of various kinds, transient excitement, anxiety, and an air of uncertainty. These symptoms subsided in a few days, leaving the patients with amnesia for the duration of the disorder. In fact, the picture was of an acute confusional psychosis that cleared in a short period. Two of Ganser's patients had had a head injury, and the third was recovering from typhus fever. Other cases were associated with a prison setting, which led Wertham to comment that the Ganser state was "hysterical pseudostupidity that occurs almost exclusively in jails and in old-fashioned German textbooks" (in Whitlock 1967). Similar cases were described later in civilian life (May, Voegele, and Paolino 1960; Kiloh 1961; Arieti and Bemporad 1974). Although the disorder was rare, interest in Ganser syndrome grew.

The symptoms of the approximate answer have held a particular fascination for clinicians. Such answers may be so close to the correct ones that they betray knowledge of the correct answer (Emery 1988) or they may be so absurd as to totally contradict all facts. Yet, the approximate answer is given with apparent seriousness. At times there may be a compulsive quality to the answers. The symptom is interspersed with accurate answers. Many responses so labeled are not truly approximate but are characterized by randomness and the impression that the patient understands the correct answer (Whitlock 1967).

Scott (1965) emphasized the distinction between the Ganser symptom and Ganser syndrome, with the latter referring to the original description of *vorbeireden* (approximate answers) in the context of a clouding of the consciousness, sudden termination of most symptoms, and amnesia for the duration of the episode (Whitlock 1967). In contrast, the Ganser symptom is associated with a number of disorders, including depression, schizophrenia, emotional trauma, head injury, stroke, early dementia, and acute confusional states because of drugs, alcohol, and other causes. It therefore is difficult to clarify the nosological status of the symptom.

Ganser himself was impressed with the genuineness of the disorder that was subsequently named after him. He believed the disorder was caused in part, but not entirely, by dissociative mechanisms. The organic component, however, must still be emphasized. The typical case presents with alteration of consciousness and amnesia or frontal-executive deficits. It is possible that organic dysfunction facilitates dissociative mechanisms without which the characteristic symptoms would not appear. The Ganser symptom can also be conceptualized as a failure of self-monitoring by the subject in his responses to questions, owing to frontal lobe dysfunction. While the patient can process at least part of the information in the question, and can access a response in the same category, the mechanisms of selection of the correct response, and feedback if the response is incorrect, are dysfunctional. If this is correct, Ganser-like responses should be seen in acute frontal lobe lesions, with the likelihood that such responses will disappear as the lesion becomes chronic.

Pseudodementia as Part of Other Primary Psychiatric Disorders

Manic Pseudodementia

A number of cases have been reported in which mania was mistakenly diagnosed as dementia or in which the latter figured prominently in the differential diagnosis (Kiloh 1961; Chiles and Cohen 1979; Smith and Kiloh 1981; Summers 1983; Koenigsberg 1984; Thase and Reynolds 1984; Casey and Fitzgerald 1988; Wright and Silove 1988). This may seem surprising, because hypomania and mania are often thought of as characterized by alacrity of mind and an impression of brilliance. Manic persons are also distractible, however, and severe mania results in disorganization of thinking and memory processes (Kiloh 1961; Smith and Kiloh 1981). The clinical picture is often that of delirium, which may in turn be mistakenly equated with dementia.

The history of acute delirious mania goes back to the mid-nineteenth century (Bell 1849), and since then many authors have provided descriptions of delirious mania (Kraepelin 1921; Carlson and Goodwin 1973; Bond 1980). The term has not entered general usage for two reasons: (1) with early intervention the severe form of mania is uncommon, and (2) delirium generally has been regarded in the psychiatric literature as requiring search for other medical etiologies.

Carlson and Goodwin (1973) provided an eloquent account of the manifestations of severe mania. The illness begins with the more usual manic symptoms of increased psychomotor activity, pressure of speech, euphoria or grandiosity, increased sexual activity, and reduced need for sleep. The authors tracked their patients over a period of days to a stage where activity becomes totally disorganized, hallucinations appear, delusions are no longer mood congruent, affect becomes dysphoric, and the patient becomes disoriented and is unable to acquire new information. At this stage, when the patient appears confused, a delirium (or in some cases dementia) might be mistakenly diagnosed. Answers may be so random as to create the impression of gross memory defect, while answers to formal mental state cognitive examinations might suggest gross intellectual failure. Family and personal histories, chronology of the development of symptoms, presence of manic symptoms, and the absence of other definitive organic factors help in the diagnosis. Response to treatment (lithium salts in particular) also aids in diagnosis. The presence of delirious mania or manic pseudodementia does not seem to indicate a more or less favorable outcome compared with less severe forms of mania (Carlson and Goodwin 1973), at least in the short run. More extended longitudinal investigation is required to address this issue systematically.

Mania in elderly people is particularly likely to be mistakenly diagnosed as delirium or dementia (Carney 1983; Summers 1983; McDonald 2000). The incoherence, poor concentration, and poor memory may suggest an organic process. The physical deterioration may further reinforce this impression. Hyperactivity may be mistaken for agitation, and sexual and other indiscretions may be taken for disinhibition of the frontal lobe type that occurs in Pick disease, frontal lobe tumors, neurosyphilis, and so forth (see chaps. 3 and 7). The occurrence of manic disorders secondary to central nervous system and systemic disorders creates a further difficulty for the differential diagnosis between manic pseudodementia and primary degenerative dementia, especially because patients who have mania secondary to an organic cause often have mild cognitive impairment (Krauthammer and Klerman 1978).

Recent research has challenged the assumption that the cognitive features of affective illness are exclusively state-related. Cognitive dysfunction has been identified in both the manic and the euthymic phases of bipolar disorder in mixed-age groups, although such dysfunction is not severe enough for dementia to be diagnosed. In the manic phase, widespread deficits, including executive functioning, episodic memory, and spatial span performance, have been identified (Sweeny, Kmiec, and Kupfer 2000), while several researchers have identified deficits in executive function (Van Gorp et al. 1998; Ferrier et al. 1999; Rossi et al. 2000) and declarative memory (Van Gorp et al. 1998, 1999) in the euthymic phase of bipolar disorder. However, the relationship between cognitive dysfunction and clinical outcome remains unclear. Van Gorp and colleagues (1998) found an association between poor performance on measures of declarative memory and frontal lobe function with both number and duration of manic and depressive episodes. In contrast, Ferrier and colleagues (1999) were unable to find any association between clinical outcome and cognitive impairment.

Neuroimaging of patients with bipolar disorders has shown evidence for structural abnormalities, particularly deep white matter hyperintensities on MRI. These abnormalities have been identified in both young and older subjects and appear to be more prevalent in patients with poor illness outcome (Moore et al. 2001). However, deep white matter hyperintensities are not specific for bipolar disorder and have been reported in schizophrenia (Sachdev et al. 1999) and depressive disorders (Hickie et al. 1995, 1997).

In conclusion, mild cognitive deficits are seen in patients with bipolar disorder that seem to persist in the euthymic phase. In severe mania, however, disorganization of thinking and memory processes may be severe enough to mimic a picture of delirium or dementia that is state-dependent.

Schizophrenic Pseudodementia

Schizophrenia is important in the discussion of pseudodementia for a variety of reasons. First, as with mania, an acute schizophrenic episode can result in considerable concentration problems, disorganized behavior and thinking, poor judgment, and impaired memory. In some cases when the onset is acute, clouding of consciousness may be present and the diagnosis of delirium considered. When acute psychosis occurs in an older patient against a background of some organic damage resulting from past trauma, alcohol or drug use, or some other cause, the picture may become very unclear. Treatment with antipsychotic medications can help in the differential diagnostic process, but it must be remembered that psychotic symptoms (irrespective of their cause) will often respond to antipsychotic drugs (Sarason and Sarason 1989).

Second, a patient with chronic residual schizophrenia may present in a disheveled state, showing obvious personal neglect, and on examination may show poverty of thought, poor abstraction, memory deficit, and little knowledge of current events or general information. This state may be difficult to distinguish from a primary degenerative dementia. Schneiderian first-rank symptoms (a key feature of schizophrenia) will often not be forthcoming, and characteristic schizophrenic thought disorder may be absent. If the patient is observed closely, however, it will be seen that the ability to carry out many basic day-to-day activities is maintained. The patient will often surprise the diagnostician with the ability to retain significant information with minimal effort, even in such a disorganized state.

Another, and perhaps best, example of a schizophrenia as a pseudodementia is the so-called *buffoonery syndrome* (Bleuler 1924). The patient with this syndrome presents with a failure on very simple cognitive tasks as well as bizarre and dramatic behavior. The patient may be facetious and jocular in a fatuous manner and may give approximate answers. If a longitudinal history is unavailable, the picture may be mistaken for a simulated dementia rather than schizophrenia. We have suggested earlier that dissociative mechanisms in the setting of psychosis produce this picture.

Paraphrenia or late-onset schizophrenia is another aspect of schizophrenia and pseudodementia. Although the studies of Roth (1955), Kay and Roth (1961), and Post (1966) distinguished paraphrenia from "senile," "arteriosclerotic," and "confusional" psychoses (Kraepelin 1919), paraphrenia still remains a heterogeneous disorder, and it includes patients who progress to dementia. The follow-up of Kraepelin's original cases by Mayer-Gross (1932) supported this notion, and recent research continues to argue for the organic basis of much of what is diagnosed as paraphrenia. Holden (1987) found in a sample of thirty-seven patients with a diagnosis of paraphrenia in a major London teaching hospital that thirteen progressed to dementia in three years. However, recent work suggests that outcome of late paraphrenia is similar to early-onset schizophrenia, at least in the short term (Roth and Kay 1998). An international consensus statement on paraphrenia concluded that similar cognitive impairments were seen in late- and early-onset schizophrenia, with late onset being associated with milder cognitive deficits. The group concluded that there was no evidence for an association with dementing processes (Howard et al. 2000).

Brain imaging in paraphrenia has tended to yield results similar to early-onset schizophrenia, with affected subjects found to have larger lateral and third ventricles and smaller left temporal lobes (Sachdev and Brodaty 1999; Howard et al. 2000; Sachdev et al. 2000). Structural lesions are detected in a minority of patients with paraphrenia (Jacoby, Levy, and Bird 1981; Flint, Rifat, and Eastwood 1991; Miller et al. 1991; Sachdev and Brodaty 1999). Hence, it can be argued that although only some patients with paraphrenia show evidence of progressive degenerative deterioration, many others show evidence of an underlying organic deficit. It is also possible that the presence of psychosis in individuals with some brain impairment may lead to further deterioration of cognitive processing, thus resulting in a picture much resembling dementia. It therefore is imperative to consider a diagnosis of late-life schizophrenia when presented with a dementia-like picture and psychotic symptoms.

Is There a Schizophrenic Dementia?

The evidence for organic brain abnormalities in schizophrenia is compelling (Halliday 2001; Shenton et al. 2001). The evidence for dysfunction of intellect and other cognitive processes is also substantial (Rund 1998; De Vries et al. 2001), although there is debate concerning whether these deficits are static or progressive. Some cross-sectional studies have suggested that cognitive and especially executive function appear to decline at a faster rate in schizophrenia compared to the normal population (Davidson et al. 1995; Fucetola et al. 2000), while others have found no difference in the rate of decline (Heaton et al. 1994; Mockler, Riordan, and Sharma 1997; Zorilla et al. 2000). In comparison, longitudinal studies have consistently failed to report any progression of cognitive deficits (Rund 1998). An association between early onset of illness, negative symptoms, and cognitive decline has been consistently cited in the literature, but the nature of the cognitive impairment has continued to be poorly characterized. This probably reflects the heterogeneous nature of schizophrenic illness, variation in subject ages and duration of illness, and the differing tests used. Deficits in working memory, global IQ, and executive function have been identified, indicating a frontotemporal pattern of impairment.

Recent advances in histological techniques have led to the discovery of subtle abnormalities in the brains of people with schizophrenia. The most consistent reported findings are decreased gray matter in the hippocampus, amygdala, parahippocampus, superior temporal gyrus, and thalamus. The changes in the frontotemporal cortex are characterized by increased neuronal density but decreased neuronal cell size, in contrast to consistent findings of neuronal loss in the anterior, medial, and dorsal thalamic nuclei. However, it has been pointed out that similar changes have been noted in chronic alcoholics and that alcohol may have a significant confounding role (Halliday 2001).

The large body of neuroimaging data reporting consistent structural abnormalities in schizophrenia has aided the advances in neuropathological research in schizophrenia. A comprehensive review of MRI studies in schizophrenia found strong evidence for larger lateral and third ventricles, smaller medial temporal lobe structures, and smaller superior temporal lobe gyri compared to healthy controls (Shenton et al. 2001). Some longitudinal studies have demonstrated ongoing reductions in temporal lobe volume (Gur et al. 1998) and ventricular enlargement (DeLisi 1997) that are consistent with a progressive illness.

Another consistent MRI finding in psychiatric patients is of white matter hyperintensities, which have also been reported in early- and late-onset schizophrenia. White matter hyperintensities are thought to result from a number of white matter pathologies, including vascular and degenerative conditions (Rivkin et al. 2000) and, as mentioned above, are not specific for a particular psychiatric disorder. Comparisons of early- and late-onset schizophrenia with healthy controls have not found any significant difference in the volume of deep white matter hyperintensities (Sachdev et al. 1999; Rivkin et al. 2000) and their significance in the pathogenesis and phenotypic expression of the disorder remains uncertain. The presence of deep white matter hyperintensities, widened ventricles, and smaller frontal and temporal lobes has led to the observation that schizophrenia bears similarities to normal aging. Positron emission tomography (PET) studies of schizophrenia have found decreased metabolism in the frontal and temporal regions, a finding also observed in normal aging (Buchsbaum and Hazlett 1997). In contrast with normal aging, similar abnormalities are seen in first-episode and chronically ill patients (Kim et al. 2000), suggesting that these changes are static. Further studies using a longitudinal design should examine if age-related changes are accelerated in schizophrenia.

All of the research findings taken together seem to argue for frontal and temporal lobe disturbance in schizophrenia. Berman and Weinberger (1986) likened these deficits to subcortical dementia as described in progressive supranuclear palsy, Huntington disease, Parkinson disease, and other subcortical disorders (see chap. 9). Certainly, schizophrenia shares some features with subcortical dementia (e.g., forgetfulness, mood and personality changes, slowness of thought processing, and deficits in manipulating acquired information) (see chaps. 9 and 13). Patients with subcortical dementias, however, have more consistent neuropsychological deficits. Moreover, their deficits lead to greater functional impairment, and they often have a progressive course. Similarly, more consistent neuropathologic correlates of cognitive deficits are demonstrable. In schizophrenia, even when cognitive deficits are present, their functional importance over and above the impact of psychotic symptoms is often difficult to discern. One must therefore conclude that patients with schizophrenia have a neurocognitive dysfunction that possibly occurs early in the developmental process. The neurocognitive deficit in schizophrenia appears to have significant but nonlinear anatomic and physiologic correlates, and it produces dysfunction that is difficult to quantify and appears to be nonprogressive. Whether this should be called dementia is a matter more concerned with the definition of dementia itself.

Other Psychiatric Disorders Uncommonly Associated with Pseudodementia

Other psychiatric disorders, especially when severe in intensity, may sometimes present with a picture of dementia. A patient with severe obsessive compulsive disorder may be so debilitated by the symptoms that self-neglect and a deteriorated state result. Performance on cognitive tests may be poor because of interference from obsessive compulsive symptoms, the usual manifestation being marked slowing on most tests. Kiloh (1961) reported a 51-year-old man who performed poorly on reading and memory tasks because of his obsessional ritual of checking each individual word to see if it had been spelled correctly.

Similarly, a patient with severe anxiety can present with memory complaints and test poorly on formal examination (Kiloh 1961; Wells 1979). If depersonalization occurs in the setting of anxiety, it can further create the impression of dementia (Kiloh 1961). Persons with dysthymic disorder also may complain of cognitive difficulties, but they usually do not present with major diagnostic problems. When dissociative symptoms accompany the disorder, however, a pseudodementing picture may be produced.

Finally, the difficulties of diagnosing pseudodementia in persons with limited intellectual ability have been commented on briefly elsewhere. Pseudodementia has been reported in a mentally retarded individual, with a discussion of some of the differential diagnostic difficulties that result from the clinical picture (Myers and Pueschel 1987).

Summation

There is controversy over the use of the term *pseudodementia.* Because depression historically has been considered a main cause of pseudodementia, the decision to classify "depressive dementia" outside the defining parameters of pseudodementia creates a need for redefinition of the syndrome of pseudodementia. In the process of reworking the concept, we again are struck by the heterogeneity of the syndrome; hence, the use of the term *the pseudodementias.* Pseudodementia as simulated dementia emerges as the most important entity for discussion. The presentations of both consciously and unconsciously simulated dementias are discussed and contrasted, and the Ganser syndrome is treated as a syndrome distinct from hysteric pseudodementia because of its heterogeneity and its not-uncommon basis in psychosis and organicity. The status of the dementia produced by schizophrenia is examined, and although a pseudodementia can be produced by schizophrenia, the cognitive deficits associated with schizophrenia remain a genuine problem for taxonomy and nosology.

Clinical Conclusions

Although many clinicians use the terms *pseudodementia* and *depressive dementia* synonymously, the concept of pseudodementia has evolved considerably and its clinical usage should be carefully considered. We recommend its continuing usage as a descriptive term to describe cognitive deficits and a dementialike picture secondary to a psychiatric disorder.

Cognitive deficits, both real and apparent, can be caused by many primary psychiatric disorders (e.g., depression, mania, schizophrenia, factitious disorder, malingering, dissociative disorder, and anxiety disorders), and each should be considered in the differential diagnosis. A careful examination of the nature of the deficits is of assistance in this process. The presence of a psychiatric disorder considered to be primary does not mean that the cognitive disorder is trivial or not worthy of attention.

In some disorders (e.g., major depression, bipolar disorder, and schizophrenia), some cognitive deficits may persist even after the illness has sufficiently remitted.

ACKNOWLEDGMENTS

This work was supported in part by a grant from the National Health and Medical Research Council of Australia, the Brain and Ageing Program of the University of New South Wales, and Eli Lilly Fellowship to Sharon Reutens and the NSW Institute of Psychiatry.

REFERENCES

Anderson, E.W., W.H. Trethowan, and J.C. Kenna. 1959. An experimental investigation of simulation and pseudo-dementia. *Acta Psychiatrica et Neurologica Scandinavica* 34 (Suppl. 132):S1–42.

Arieti, S., and J. Bemporad. 1974. Rare, unclassified and collective psychiatric syndromes. In *American Handbook of Psychiatry*, edited by S. Arieti and E. Brody. New York: Basic Books, pp. 710–22.

Axen, M. 1986. Chronic factitious disorders. *Journal of Psychosocial Nursing* 24:19–27.

Bell, L. 1849. On a form of disease resembling some advanced stages of mania and fever, but so contradistinguished from any ordinarily observed or described combination of symptoms as to render it probable that it may be an overlooked and hitherto unrecorded malady. *American Journal of Insanity* 6:97–127.

Bender, L. 1938. *A Visual Motor Gestalt Test and Its Clinical Use.* New York: American Orthopsychiatric Association.

Benton, A.L. 1945. Rorschach performance of suspected malingerers. *Journal of Abnormal and Social Psychology* 40:94–96.

Benton, A.L., and O. Spreen. 1961. Visual memory test: The simulation of mental incompetence. *Archives of General Psychiatry* 4:79–83.

Berman, K.F., and D.R. Weinberger. 1986. Schizophrenic dementia. In *Neuropsychiatric Dementias*, edited by D.V. Jeste. Washington, D.C.: American Psychiatric Association, pp. 44–72.

Berrios, G.E. 1985. Pseudodementia or melancholic dementia: A nineteenth-century view. *Journal of Neurology, Neurosurgery and Psychiatry* 48:393–400.

Berrios, G.E. 1986. Dementia during the seventeenth and eighteenth centuries: A conceptual history. *Psychological Medicine* 17:829–37.

Bleuler, E.P. 1924. *Textbook of Psychiatry.* New York: Macmillan.

Bluglass, R. 1976. Malingering. In *Encyclopaedic Handbook of Medical Psychology* edited by S. Krauss. London: Butterworths, pp. 280–81.

Bond, T.C. 1980. Recognition of acute delirious mania. *Archives of General Psychiatry* 37: 553–54.
Buchsbaum, M.S., and E.A. Hazlett. 1997. Functional brain imaging and aging in schizophrenia. *Schizophrenia Research* 27:129–41.
Bulbena, A., and G. Berrios. 1986. Pseudodementia: Facts and figures. *British Journal of Psychiatry* 148:94–97.
Caine, E. 1981. Pseudodementia. *Archives of General Psychiatry* 38:1359–64.
Carlson, G.A., and F.K. Goodwin. 1973. The stages of mania: A longitudinal analysis of the manic episode. *Archives of General Psychiatry* 28:221–28.
Carney, M. 1983. Pseudo-problems pseudodementia. *British Journal of Hospital Medicine* 29:312–18.
Casey, D., and B. Fitzgerald. 1988. Mania and pseudodementia. *Journal of Clinical Psychiatry* 49:73–74.
Chiles, J.A., and D. Cohen. 1979. Pseudodementia and mania. *Journal of Nervous and Mental Disease* 167:357–58.
Coffman, J.A., and H.A. Nasrallah. 1986. Magnetic resonance brain imaging in schizophrenia. In *The Neurology of Schizophrenia*, edited by H.A. Nasrallah and D.R. Weinberger. New York: Elsevier Science Publishers, pp. 251–66.
Davidson, M., P.D. Harvey, P. Powchik, et al. 1995. Severity of symptoms in chronically institutionalized geriatric schizophrenic patients. *American Journal of Psychiatry* 152: 197–207.
DeLisi, L.E. 1997. Is schizophrenia a lifetime disorder of brain plasticity, growth and aging? *Schizophrenia Research* 23:119–29.
DeLisi, L.E., A. Alexandropoulos, and N. Colter. 1988. Reduced temporal lobe area: A study of siblings with schizophrenia. *Schizophrenia Research* 1:169–70.
De Vries, P.J., W.G. Honer, P.M. Kemp, et al. 2001. Dementia as a complication of schizophrenia. *Journal of Neurology, Neurosurgery and Psychiatry* 70:588–96.
Emery, V.O.B. 1988. *Pseudodementia: A Theoretical and Empirical Discussion*. Cleveland: Case Western Reserve University School of Medicine.
Ferrier, I.N., B.R. Stanton, T.P. Kelly, et al. 1999. Neuropsychological function in euthymic patients with bipolar disorder. *British Journal of Psychiatry* 175:246–51.
Flint, A.J., S.L. Rifat, and M.R. Eastwood. 1991. Late-onset paranoia: Distinct from paraphrenia? *International Journal of Geriatric Psychiatry* 6:103–9.
Folstein, M.F., and P.V. Rabins. 1991. Replacing pseudodementia. *Neuropsychiatry, Neuropsychology, and Behavioral Neurology* 4:36–40.
Freud, S. 1963 [1905]. *Dora: An Analysis of a Case of Hysteria*. New York: Macmillan.
Fucetola, R., L.J. Seidman, W.S. Kremen, et al. 2000. Age and neuropsychologic function in schizophrenia: A decline in executive abilities beyond that observed in healthy volunteers. *Biological Psychiatry* 48:137–46.
Ganser, S.J.M. 1898. Ueber Eigen Eigenartigen Hyusterischen Daemmerzustand. *Archiv für Psychiatrie und Nervenkrankheiten* 30:633–40. (Translated by C.E. Schorer, in *British Journal of Criminology*, 1965, 5:120–26.)
Gilandas, A.J., and S.W. Touyz. 1983. Forensic neuropsychology: A selective introduction. *Journal of Forensic Sciences* 28:713–23.
Goebel, R.A. 1983. Detection of faking on the Halstead-Reitan Neuropsychological Test Battery. *Journal of Clinical Psychology* 39:731–41.
Goldstein, A.B. 1998. Identification and classification of factitious disorders: An analysis

of cases reported during a ten year period. *International Journal of Psychiatry in Medicine* 28:221–24.

Gur, R.E., P. Cowel, B.I. Turetsky, et al. 1998. A follow-up magnetic resonance imaging study of schizophrenia: Relationship of neuroanatomical changes to clinical and neurobehavioural measures. *Archives of General Psychiatry* 55:145–52.

Halliday, G. 2001. Schizophrenia: A review of the neuropathology of schizophrenia. Proceedings of the Australian neuroscience society symposium. *Clinical Pharmacology and Physiology* 28:64–65.

Hayward, L., W. Hall, M. Hunt, et al. 1987. Can localised brain impairment be simulated on neuropsychological test profiles? *Australian and New Zealand Journal of Psychiatry* 21:87–93.

Heaton, R.K., H.H. Smith, Jr., R.A.W. Lehman, et al. 1978. Prospects of faking believable deficits on neuropsychological testing. *Journal of Consulting and Clinical Psychology* 46:892–900.

Heaton, R., J. Paulsen, L.A. McAdams, et al. 1994. Neuropsychological deficits in schizophrenia: Relationship to age, chronicity and dementia. *Archives of General Psychiatry* 51:469–76.

Hickie, I., E. Scott, P. Mitchell, et al. 1995. Subcortical hyperintensities on magnetic resonance imaging: Clinical correlates and prognostic significance in patients with severe depression. *Biological Psychiatry* 37:151–60.

Hickie, I., E. Scott, K. Wilhelm, et al. 1997. Subcortical hyperintensities on magnetic resonance imaging in patients with severe depression: A longitudinal evaluation. *Biological Psychiatry* 42:367–74.

Holden, N.L. 1987. Late paraphrenia or the paraphrenias?: A descriptive study with a 10-year follow-up. *British Journal of Psychiatry* 150:635–39.

Howard, R., P.V. Rabins, M.V. Seeman, et al. 2000. Late-onset schizophrenia and very-late-onset schizophrenia-like psychosis: An international consensus. *American Journal of Psychiatry* 157:172–78.

Hubner, A.H. 1919. Weitere Versuche und Beobachtungen zur Simulations/Rage. *Deutsche Medizinische Wochenschrift* 45:95–97.

Jacoby, R.J., R. Levy, and J.M. Bird. 1981. Computed tomography and the outcome of affective disorder: A follow-up study of elderly patients. *British Journal of Psychiatry* 139:288–92.

Jung, C.G. 1903. Uber Simulation von Geistesstorung. *Journal of Psychologie und Neurologie* II:181–201.

Kay, D.W., and M. Roth. 1961. Environmental and hereditary factors in the schizophrenias of old age ("late paraphrenia") and their bearing on the general problem of causation in schizophrenia. *Journal of Mental Science* 107:146–58.

Kennedy, A., and J. Neville. 1957. Sudden loss of memory. *British Medical Journal* 2: 428–33.

Kiloh, L.G. 1961. Pseudodementia. *Acta Psychiatrica Scandinavica* 37:336–51.

Kiloh, L.G. 1981. Depressive illness masquerading as dementia in the elderly. *Medical Journal of Australia* 2:550–53.

Kim, J.J., S. Mohamed, N.C. Andreasen, et al. 2000. Regional neural dysfunctions in chronic schizophrenia studied with positron emission tomography. *American Journal of Psychiatry* 157:542–48.

Koenigsberg, H.J.W. 1984. Manic pseudodementia. *Journal of Clinical Psychiatry* 45: 132–34.

Kraepelin, E. 1919. *Dementia Praecox and Paraphrenia.* Edinburgh: Livingstone.

Kraepelin, E. 1921. *Manic-Depressive Insanity and Paranoia.* Edinburgh: Livingstone.

Kraupl-Taylor, F. 1966. *Psychopathology: Its Causes and Symptoms.* London: Butterworths.

Krauthammer, C., and G.L. Klerman. 1978. Secondary mania. *Archives of General Psychiatry* 138:837–38.

Lewis, S.W. 1990. Computerised tomography in schizophrenia 15 years on. *British Journal of Psychiatry* 157:16–24.

Lezak, M.D. 1983. *Neuropsychological Assessment.* New York: Oxford University Press.

Lishman, A.W. 2000. *Organic Psychiatry: The Psychological Consequences of Cerebral Disorder.* Oxford: Blackwell Scientific Publications.

Lowenstein, O. 1924. Cited in: Anderson, E.W., W.H. Trethowan, and J.C. Kenna. 1959. An experimental investigation of simulation and pseudo-dementia. *Acta Psychiatrica et Neurologica Scandinavica* 31 (Suppl. 132):S1–42.

McDonald, W.M. 2000. Epidemiology, etiology and treatment of geriatric mania. *Journal of Clinical Psychiatry* 61 (Suppl. 13):S3–11.

Mahendra, B. 1984. Pseudodementia: Abandon the term? *American Journal of Psychiatry* 141:471–72.

May, R.H., G.E. Voegele, and A.F. Paolino. 1960. The Ganser Syndrome: A report of 3 cases. *Journal of Nervous and Mental Disease* 130:331–39.

Mayer-Gross, W. 1932. Die Schizophrenie. In *Bumke Handbuch der Geisterkrankheiten,* edited by S. Spez. Berlin: Springer, pp. 69–81

Merskey, H., and N.A. Buhrich. 1975. Hysteria and organic brain disease. *British Journal of Medical Psychology* 48:359–66.

Miller, B.L., I.M. Lesser, K.B. Boone, et al. 1991. Brain lesions and cognitive function in late-life psychosis. *British Journal of Psychiatry* 158:76–82.

Mockler, D., J. Riordan, and T. Sharma. 1997. Memory and intellectual deficits do not decline with age in schizophrenia. *Schizophrenia Research* 26:1–7.

Moeli, C. 1888. Ueber ihre Verbrecher. In *Some Uncommon Psychiatric Syndromes,* edited by M.D. Enoch, W.H. Trethowan, and J.C. Barker, 1967. Bristol: John Wright, pp. 101–8

Moore, P.B., D.J. Shepherd, D. Eccleston, et al. 2001. Cerebral white matter lesions in bipolar affective disorder: Relationship to outcome. *British Journal of Psychiatry* 178: 172–76.

Myers, B.A., and S.M. Pueschel. 1987. Pseudodementia in the mentally retarded. *Clinical Pediatrics* 26:275–77.

Nasrallah, H.A. 1990. Brain structure and function in schizophrenia: Evidence for fetal neurodevelopmental impairment. *Current Opinion in Psychiatry* 3:75–78.

Osborne, D.A. 1970. A moderate variable approach to MMPI validity. *Journal of Clinical Psychology* 26:486–90.

Pankratz, L. 1979. Symptom validity testing and symptom retraining: Procedures for the assessment and treatment of functional sensory deficits. *Journal of Consulting and Clinical Psychology* 47:409–10.

Porch, B.E., T. Friden, and J. Porec. 1971. Objective differentiation of aphasic vs. nonorganic patients. Paper presented at the Fifth Annual Meeting of the International Neuropsychological Society, Santa Fe, New Mexico.

Post, F. 1966. *Persistent Persecutory States of the Elderly.* Oxford: Pergamon Press.

Raz, S., and N. Raz. 1990. Structural brain abnormalities in the major psychoses: A quantitative review of the evidence from computerized imaging. *Psychological Bulletin* 108: 93–108.

Reifler, B.V. 1982. Arguments for abandoning the term pseudodementia. *Journal of the American Geriatrics Society* 30:665–68.

Rey, A. 1941. L'examen psychologique dans les cas d'encephalopathie traumatique. *Archives de Psychologie* 28:126–39.

Rey, A. 1964. *L'examen clinique en psychologie.* Paris: Presses Universitaires de France.

Rivkin, P., M. Kraut, P. Barta, et al. 2000. White matter hyperintensity volume in late-onset and early-onset schizophrenia. *International Journal of Geriatric Psychiatry* 15: 1085–89.

Roberts, G.W. 1991. Schizophrenia: A neuropathological perspective. *British Journal of Psychiatry* 158:8–17.

Rossi, A., L. Arduini, E. Daneluzzo, et al. 2000. Cognitive function in euthymic bipolar patients, stabilized schizophrenia patients and health controls. *Journal of Psychiatric Research* 34:333–39.

Roth, M. 1955. The natural history of mental disorder in old age. *Journal of Mental Science* 101:281–301.

Roth, M., and D.W. Kay. 1998. Late paraphrenia: A variant of schizophrenia manifest in late life or an organic clinical syndrome? A review of recent evidence. *International Journal of Geriatric Psychiatry* 13:755–84.

Rund, B.R. 1998. A review of longitudinal studies of cognitive functions in schizophrenia patients. *Schizophrenia Bulletin* 24:425–35.

Sachdev, P., and H. Brodaty. 1999. Quantitative study of signal hyperintensities on T2-weighted magnetic resonance imagining in late-onset-schizophrenia. *American Journal of Psychiatry* 156:1958–67.

Sachdev, P.S., J.S. Smith, H. Angus-Lepan, et al. 1990. Pseudodementia twelve years on. *Journal of Neurology, Neurosurgery, and Psychiatry* 53:254–59.

Sachdev, P.S., H. Brodaty, N. Rose, et al. 1999. Schizophrenia with onset after age 50 years: 2: Neurological, neuropsychological and MRI investigation. *British Journal of Psychiatry* 175:416–21.

Sachdev P., H. Brodaty, D. Cheang, et al. 2000. Hippocampus and amygdala volumes in elderly schizophrenic patients as assessed by magnetic resonance imaging. *Psychiatry and Clinical Neuroscience* 54:105–12.

Sarason, I.G., and B.R. Sarason. 1989. *Abnormal Psychology.* Englewood Cliffs, N.J.: Prentice-Hall.

Scott, P.D. 1965. The Ganser syndrome. *British Journal of Criminology* 5:127–31.

Shaw, D.J., and C.G. Mathews. 1965. Differential MMPI performance of brain-damaged versus pseudo-neurologic groups. *Journal of Clinical Psychology* 21:405–8.

Shelton, R.C., and D.R. Weinberger. 1986. X-ray computerized tomography studies in schizophrenia: A review and synthesis. In *The Neurology of Schizophrenia,* edited by H.A. Nasrallah and D.R. Weinberger. New York: Elsevier Science Publishers, pp. 207–50.

Shenton, M.R., C.C. Dickey, M. Frumin, et al. 2001. A review of MRI findings in schizophrenia. *Schizophrenia Research* 49:1–52.

Slater, E. 1965. Diagnosis of 'hysteria.' *British Medical Journal* 1:1395–99.
Smith, J.S., and L.G. Kiloh. 1981. The investigation of dementia: The result of 200 consecutive admissions. *Lancet* 1:824–27.
Summers, W.K. 1983. Mania with onset in the eighth decade: Two cases and a review. *Journal of Clinical Psychiatry* 44:141–43.
Sweeny, J.A., J.A. Kmiec, and D.J. Kupfer. 2000. Neuropsychologic impairments in bipolar and unipolar mood disorders on the CANTAB neurocognitive battery. *Biological Psychiatry* 48:674–85.
Thase, M.E., and C.F. Reynolds. 1984. Manic pseudodementia. *Psychosomatics* 25:256–60.
Tissenbaum, M.J., H.M. Harter, and A.P. Friedman. 1951. Organic neurological syndromes diagnosed as functional disorders. *New England Journal of Medicine* 147: 1519–21.
Van Gorp, W.G., L. Altshuler, D.C. Theberge, et al. 1998. Cognitive impairment in euthymic bipolar patients with and without prior alcohol dependence: A preliminary study. *Archives of General Psychiatry* 55:41–46.
Van Gorp, W.G., L. Altshuler, D.C. Theberge, et al. 1999. Declarative and procedural memory in bipolar disorder. *Biological Psychiatry* 46:525–31.
Waddington, J.L., E. O'Callaghan, C. Larkin, et al. 1990. Magnetic resonance imaging and spectroscopy in schizophrenia. *British Journal of Psychiatry* 157:56–65.
Wassersug, J.P. 1982. Deceptive patients—wise physicians. *Consultant* 21 (December):97–108.
Wells, C.E. 1979. Pseudodementia. *American Journal of Psychiatry* 136:895–900.
Whitlock, F.A. 1967. The Ganser syndrome. *British Journal of Psychiatry* 113:19–29.
Wright, J.M., and D. Silove. 1988. Pseudodementia in schizophrenia and mania. *Australian and New Zealand Journal of Psychiatry* 22:109–14.
Zorilla, L.T., R.K. Heaton, L.A. McAdams, et al. 2000. Cross-sectional study of older outpatients with schizophrenia and health comparison subjects: No differences in age-related cognitive decline. *American Journal of Psychiatry* 157:1324–26.

CHAPTER SEVENTEEN

Neurobiology of Major Depression in Alzheimer Disease

George S. Zubenko, M.D., Ph.D.

The original catecholamine hypothesis of affective disorders focused largely on the role of the noradrenergic components of the central nervous system (CNS) in the etiology of depression and mania (Bunney and Davis 1965; Schildkraut 1965). Additional evidence from clinical, pharmacological, and physiological studies has emerged since the original hypothesis was proposed and generally supports the view that clinically significant depression may result from a dysfunction of CNS mechanisms employing the catecholamine neurotransmitters, norepinephrine and dopamine (Jimerson 1987; Siever 1987). Neurochemical studies of serotonin (5-HT) receptors and 5-hydroxyindoleacetic acid (5-HIAA) in spinal fluid or brain tissue have also suggested an alteration in serotonergic components of the CNS in both idiopathic major depression and suicide (Lloyd et al. 1974; Brikmayer and Riederer 1975; Mendlewicz, Vanderheyden, and Noel 1981; Stanley and Mann 1983; Crow et al. 1984). In contrast to these hypotheses, which suggest that depression may result from the decreased function of one or more central aminergic systems, the cholinergic hypothesis of affective disorders (Janowsky and Risch 1987) predicts that idiopathic depression may be associated with the hyperfunctioning of cholinergic systems. This last prediction is especially interesting in the context of Alzheimer disease (AD), since the progression of the central cholinergic deficit that occurs in this disorder may interact with the pathophysiology of depression to limit the prevalence of major depression in later stages of this disorder.

The pigmented nuclei of the brainstem contain the cell bodies of the majority of the catecholaminergic neurons in the brain. The locus ceruleus and the substantia nigra are the largest of these nuclei, and they project noradrenergic afferents to the forebrain and dopaminergic afferents to the striatum, thalamus, and amygdala (Carpenter 1985; Foote and Morrison 1987). Studies in primates and humans indicate that the brainstem raphe nuclei contain predominantly serotonergic cell bodies that likewise project to the forebrain and subcortical structures (Felten and Sladek 1983; Foote and Morrison 1987). Finally, the basal nucleus of Meynert is an important source of the cholinergic innervation of the cortex (Whitehouse et al. 1982). Since AD is often associated with degenerative changes in these nuclei (Boller et al. 1980; Mayeux et al. 1981; Whitehouse et al. 1982; Bondareff and Mountjoy 1986; Huber, Shuttleworth, and Paulson 1986) as well as concurrent depression, we present evidence supporting the hypothesis that degeneration of one or more of these nuclei is associated with the occurrence of major depression in patients with this multifocal brain disease.

Neuropathologic and Neurochemical Correlates of Major Depression in Alzheimer Disease

Five published postmortem studies have addressed the neuropathologic and neurochemical correlates of major depression in Alzheimer disease. Table 17.1 compares the study designs and methods. Sample sizes of AD cases have ranged from three to fifty-two (fifty with complete data). All employed prospective behavioral assessments of patients with dementia who were enrolled in longitudinal studies of AD and related dementias, as well as neuropathologically determined diagnoses of dementia. Our initial studies included 81% with AD, 19% with Parkinson disease, and 14% with multiple infarctions. The remaining studies included patients with autopsy-confirmed AD, although it is uncertain whether patients with the Lewy body variant of AD or concurrent brain diseases were excluded.

In all studies, patients with concurrent diagnoses of Alzheimer disease "with depression" fulfilled the DSM-III or DSM-III-R symptom criteria for a major

Table 17.1. Methodologic comparison of four neuropathologic studies of major depression in Alzheimer disease

	Zubenko et al. 1988, 1990	Zweig et al. 1988	Chan-Palay 1990	Forstl et al. 1992
Sample size, *n*	37	21–25	3	50–52
Prospective behavioral assessments	yes	yes	unknown	yes
Neuropathologic diagnoses of dementia	81% AD, 20% PD, 14% infarcts	100% AD*	100% AD	100% AD*
Symptom criteria for depression	DSM-III Major depressive episode	DSM-III Major depressive episode	DSM-III-R Major depressive episode	DSM-III-R Major depressive episode
Depressed; *n* (%)	14 (39%)	8 (38%)	1 (33%)	14 (27%)
Family history assessment of major depression	yes	no	no	no
Analyses blind to clinical information	yes	yes	unknown	yes
Characterization of aminergic nuclei	five cyto/histo-pathologic features	cell loss	cell loss	cell loss
Measurement of neurotransmitters/choline acetyltransferase (ChAT)	yes	no	no	no
Multivariate statistics	yes	no	no	yes

*May have included Lewy body variant of AD.

depressive episode. In the context of dementia, depressed mood was required to serve as one of these symptoms. According to these criteria, 27–39% of patients developed an episode of major depression during their follow-up assessments. This proportion is higher than expected based on the reported 15–25% estimates of the comorbidity of major depression and AD among individuals who present for evaluation and treatment at geriatric outpatient clinics. This observation has suggested that major depression may be a risk factor for mortality among patients with AD. In a recently completed prospective study of 196 patients with clinically diagnosed AD, the severity of depressive symptoms as measured by the seventeen-item Hamilton Depression Rating Scale score was an independent predictor of mortality (Zubenko et al., in preparation). Our results in this regard are consistent with those of Hoch and co-workers (1989), who found that survivorship in a two-year study of patients with AD and concurrent depression was predicted by abnormalities of REM latency and the presence of sleep-disordered breathing, functions whose anatomic substrates are also thought to reside in the brainstem.

In three of the studies, neuropathological and neurochemical assessments were reported to have been performed by investigators who were blind to demographic and clinical information. Neuropathological evaluations of the aminergic nuclei in our studies included five indices of neurodegeneration; in the remaining studies, neuron counts served as the sole index of neurodegeneration. In our published neurochemical study, the levels of aminergic neurotransmitters, their metabolites, and choline acetyltransferase-specific activity were measured in eight regions (four cortical, four subcortical) to which these aminergic nuclei project. In only two studies were the samples of sufficient size to support multivariate statistical approaches that minimize the number of comparisons needed to test a hypothesis and to control for the effects of potentially confounding variables.

Table 17.2 summarizes and compares the major findings of these studies. Neither age at onset nor duration of dementia differentiated AD patients with or without major depression in any of these studies. In our initial study, 43% of patients with dementia and major depression had a family history of major depression, while the corresponding value for patients with dementia but without depression was 9% (exact $p = 0.02$, one-tailed). These results are consistent with those previously reported by Pearlson and co-workers (1990).

All of the existing neuropathologic studies have reported increased degeneration of the locus ceruleus associated with the emergence of major depression

Table 17.2. Clinical, neuropathological, and neurochemical correlate of major depression in Alzheimer disease

	Zubenko et al. 1988, 1990	Zweig et al. 1988	Chan-Palay 1990	Forstl et al. 1992
Clinical features				
Age at onset of dementia	No effect	No effect	—	No effect
Duration of dementia	No effect	No effect	—	No effect
Family history of major depression	↑	—	—	—
Neuropathologic features				
LC	↑ Degeneration	↑ Degeneration	↑ Degeneration	↑ Degeneration
SN	↑ Degeneration	—	—	No effect
DR	—	↑ Degeneration	—	—
bnM	—	—	—	Preservation
Cortical SP	No effect	—	—	No effect
Cortical NFT	No effect	—	—	—
Neurochemical features				
NE	↓ esp. in cortex	—	—	—
DA	No consistent effect	—	—	—
5-HT/5-HIAA	Modest ↓ all regions	—	—	—
ChAT	Preservation, esp. in subcortical region		—	— —

Notes: Associations not addresses in a study are indicated by a dash. LC = locus ceruleus (noradrenergic); SN = substantia nigra (dopaminergic); DR = dorsal raphe (serotonergic); bnM = basal nucleus Meynert (cholinergic); SP = senile plaques; NFT = neurofibrillary tangles; NE = norepinephrine; DA = dopamine; 5-HT = serotonin; 5-HIAA = 5-hydroxyindoleacetic acid (serotonin metabolite); ChAT = choline acetyltransferase.

in Alzheimer disease. This has been a robust finding, considering that these studies have involved four geographically disparate populations of patients with AD with differing mean durations of illness at the time of autopsy and varying laboratory methods. Consistent with these observations, patients with dementia who have this behavioral complication have been reported to manifest substantial reductions of norepinephrine levels in the cortex.

Patients with dementia and major depression in our initial study also exhibited increased degeneration of the substantia nigra, a result that was not found in the study of Forstl and colleagues (1992). This difference may be attributable to the inclusion of patients with Parkinson disease or Lewy body variant of AD in our study population and highlights the importance of diagnostic homogeneity in investigations of biological correlates of behavioral complications of dementia. Corresponding neurochemical measurements revealed an increased dopamine level in the entorhinal cortex that did not reach statistical significance after correction for multiple comparisons and no consistent pattern of change in the levels of this neurotransmitter in the remaining seven brain regions.

Increased degeneration of the serotonergic raphe nuclei was associated with major depression in the study reported by Zweig and co-workers (1988), a finding that has not yet been reexamined. However, this association is supported by several additional lines of evidence. The development of major depression in primary dementia was accompanied by consistent modest reductions in both 5-HT and 5-HIAA in eight projection areas of the dorsal raphe (Zubenko, Moossy, and Kopp 1990). In addition, the highly selective 5-HT reuptake blocker citalopram has been demonstrated to significantly outperform placebo in the treatment of depression in a double-blind, placebo-controlled study of ninety-eight patients with Alzheimer-type or vascular dementia (Gottfries, Karlsson, and Nyth 1992).

In our study of primary dementia, choline acetyltransferase-specific activity was measured as a proxy for degeneration of the basal nucleus of Meynert, whose anatomic boundaries make reproducible morphometric analyses difficult. In this neurochemical study, major depression was associated with the relative preservation of choline acetyltransferase activity, especially in subcortical areas. Consistent results from the study of Forstl and co-workers (1992) indicate that major depression in AD is likewise accompanied by the preservation of the basal nucleus of Meynert.

The relative preservation of basal nucleus of Meynert and choline acetyltransferase activity in depressed patients with dementia suggests that there is a threshold for central cholinergic function below which the clinical expression of depression is not possible. Since primary degenerative dementia is associated with a progressive loss of cholinergic function in the central nervous system (Davies and Maloney 1976; Perry and Perry 1980; Zubenko et al. 1989), this interpretation suggests that the prevalence of major depression in primary dementia may decrease as dementia progresses. Several groups of investigators have observed such a clinical relationship among patients with primary degenerative dementia of the Alzheimer type (Reifler, Larson, and Hanley 1982; Reifler et al. 1989; Fischer, Simanyi, and Danielczyk 1990; Zubenko et al. 1992; Forsell et al. 1993). Interestingly, this relationship may have some specificity for AD, since it was not observed in patients with vascular dementia (Fischer, Simanyi, and Danielczyk 1990). The existence of such a threshold might also explain the high rate of induction of depression (five of seven cases) during the treatment of patients with AD with oxotremorine, a potent cholinergic agonist (Davis et al. 1987).

Mechanism of Neuronal Death in Alzheimer Disease

Neuronal death in the brains of patients with Alzheimer disease appears to occur by mechanisms of both necrosis and apoptosis. While these pathways may overlap to some extent, they are typically triggered by different events, are manifested by distinguishable cytologic and biochemical features, and have somewhat different outcomes (Kerr, Wylie, and Curie 1972). Necrosis usually results from physical injury, is not genetically controlled, is typified by the destruction of organelles and the plasma membrane, and results in the release of cellular debris that often stimulates a local inflammatory response. In contrast, apoptosis, or programmed cell death, represents a genetically controlled response to specific developmental or environmental stimuli. Cells undergoing apoptosis manifest shrinkage, membrane blebbing, chromatin condensation, and DNA fragmentation. The last two characteristics have commonly been used to identify apoptotic cells in formalin-fixed, paraffin-embedded sections of brain tissue. Apoptotic cells and their fragments undergo phagocytosis by microglia and do not stimulate an inflammatory response.

Several lines of evidence have implicated apoptosis in the loss of neurons from vulnerable brain areas in Alzheimer disease. Increased oxidative damage, disturbances of calcium homeostasis, reductions in neurotrophic factors, deposition of β-amyloid aggregates, and reduced energy metabolism are all characteristic of the central neurodegeneration that occurs in AD (Zubenko 1997) and all of these conditions induce or stimulate apoptosis in cultured neuronal cell lines (for review, see Cotman and Su 1996). DNA fragmentation labeling techniques have been used to identify substantial numbers of cells in vulnerable cortical regions (frontal, temporal, hippocampus) that appear to have initiated the apoptosis pathway in AD victims, a process that occurs to a substantially lesser extent in normal aging (Su et al. 1994; Dragunow et al. 1995; Lassmann et al. 1995; Smale et al. 1995; Thomas et al. 1995). These observations do not appear to result from DNA damage that occurs during the postmortem interval or due to agonal factors (Anderson, Su, and Cotman 1996; Cotman and Su 1996) and is consistent with evolving research on one of the regulatory functions of the presenilin genes (Vita, Lacana, and D'Adamio 1996; Wolozin et al. 1996). Our data also implicate apoptotic events in cell loss from the brainstem aminergic nuclei in AD, and invite an exploration of the role of apoptosis in the increased degeneration of these nuclei associated with the emergence of major depression.

Discussion

In the context of Alzheimer disease, these studies suggest that major depression describes a clinically and pathologically distinct subgroup of patients who have degenerative changes in the brainstem aminergic nuclei (especially the locus ceruleus) that are disproportionate to those that occur in the cerebral cortex and relative preservation of the basal nucleus of Meynert. Whether there are important pathogenetic differences between these patients and those who do not develop major depression, or whether they represent merely extremes of the distributions of degenerative changes in these structures that occur in all patients with AD cannot be determined from available data. Furthermore, these results do not exclude the potential importance of degenerative changes other than those measured or psychosocial factors that were not assessed in the pathogenesis of major depression in patients with AD.

Our published studies provide considerable evidence that the neuropathological and neurochemical correlates of major depression in primary dementia have specificity. Patients with dementia with or without major depression included in our studies and that of Forstl and colleagues (1992) did not differ with respect to mean age at onset, age at death, duration of illness, or brain weight, or in the mean densities of senile plaques or neurofibrillary tangles in the cortex. Therefore, the emergence of major depression did not appear to result from greater global brain degeneration. Furthermore, the profile of neurochemical changes associated with major depression differed qualitatively from that for dementia (Zubenko, Moossy, and Kopp 1990; Zubenko et al. 1991). The relative preservation of cholinergic neurons in the basal nucleus of Meynert and of choline acetyltransferase activity in its projection areas in patients with depression and major depression was the most dramatic example of this. Finally, two reports failed to find an association of increased degeneration of the locus ceruleus with psychosis (delusions or hallucinations) in AD (Zweig et al. 1988; Bierer et al. 1990), and the profiles of neurochemical changes associated with major depression and psychosis appear to be qualitatively and topographically distinct (Zubenko, Moossy, and Kopp 1990; Zubenko et al. 1991). This evidence further suggests that the observed neuropathological and neurochemical correlates of major depression are not nonspecifically related to all behavioral complications of AD.

The patients with dementia with or without major depression in our previous study were similar with respect to a variety of potentially important covariates, including sex ratio, age at onset, age at death, duration of illness, and postmortem interval, and in terms of their medication history at or near the time of death, supporting the specificity of the observed neurochemical correlates of major depression in dementia. These medications were grouped into one of eight classes: antibiotic, anticonvulsant, antidepressant, antiparkinson, cardiovascular, analgesic, steroid, and other. After corrections for multiple comparisons were made, none of these classes of medications was associated with significant or consistent effects on any of the neurochemical measurements made. Similar negative results have been reported by investigators at the Mt. Sinai ADRC (Bierer et al. 1990, personal communication) and may reflect (a) the true inability of some medications to modulate the neurochemical variables studied, (b) compensatory mechanisms that blunt acute effects of medications over time, (c) the reduced responsiveness of these neurochemical measures to medication effects in the context of neurodegeneration, or (d) a combination of these.

The pathophysiology of major depression may not be identical in dementias of differing etiology. The importance of achieving diagnostic homogeneity in studies of the biological correlates of major depression in AD was illustrated in the previous section. For this reason, patients with AD and Lewy body variant of AD should be analyzed separately in future clinicopathologic studies. While the nomenclature of the Lewy body variant of AD has been somewhat inconsistent and controversial, the distinguishing features of this subgroup of AD patients is the presence of Lewy bodies in addition to an age-specific increase in the density of senile plaques in the neocortex (Hansen et al. 1990). Historically, this subtype of AD has been under-recognized due to the difficulty in visualizing neocortical Lewy bodies, which require immunolabeling with antiubiquitin antibodies for reliable detection. Pathologically, the Lewy body variant of AD is associated with fewer cortical neurofibrillary tangles (Hansen et al. 1990, 1993; Lippa, Smith, and Swearer 1994) and greater degeneration of the brainstem aminergic nuclei than AD alone (Hansen et al. 1990; Langlais et al. 1993). Retrospective clinical-correlative studies suggest that, as a group, patients with the Lewy body variant are more likely to develop clinically significant depression, psychotic symptoms, fluctuations in cognitive impairment, extrapyramidal symptoms, and increased sensitivity to neuroleptic medications compared to patients with AD alone (Hansen et al. 1990; McKeith et al. 1992). Estimates of the proportion of AD cases that have cortical Lewy bodies have varied widely (Joachim, Morris, and Selkoe 1988; Hansen et al. 1990, 1993; Kazee and Han 1995; Victoroff et al. 1995). The Lewy body variant of AD may be associated with both greater degeneration of the brainstem aminergic nuclei and a higher prevalence of major depression than patients with AD alone. Such a finding would provide additional support for an etiologic relationship between degeneration of these nuclei and major depression in AD.

The etiopathogenesis of major depression seems likely to be heterogeneous across the age spectrum as well as within particular age strata. The results described in the preceding sections are largely consistent with preexisting neurochemical hypotheses of major depression that emerged from studies of young and middle-aged adults. However, these individuals are likely to develop depression through dysfunctions of one or more of these systems by mechanisms that are more subtle than neuronal loss (for reviews, see Hyman and Nestler 1993; Nemeroff et al. 1996). In contrast, normal aging is accompanied by progressive neuronal loss in the brainstem aminergic nuclei (McGeer, McGeer, and Suzuki 1977; Vijayashankar and Brody 1977; Mann, Yates, and Hawkes 1983), a process that may have relevance to the pathogenesis of late-onset depression among elderly persons with normal cognition. Two characteristics of depressed patients with AD appear to distinguish them as a group from elderly depressed patients with normal cognition. Most estimates of the prevalence of a major depressive syndrome among outpatients with AD have been in the range of 15–25%. These prevalence estimates are substantially higher than the 1.4% figure reported by the Epidemiology Catchment Area study of community-dwelling elders without dementia (Weissman et al. 1991). Second, Pearlson and co-workers (1990) reported that a family history of major depression was significantly higher among first-degree relatives with patients with AD and major depression than those who did not develop this behavioral complication, and our preliminary data support this finding. This latter result suggests that the development of major depression in AD may rely on an interaction of specific degenerative events with one or more familial (possibly inherited) factors that confer a constitutional vulnerability to the development of this mood disorder. This observation also distinguishes major depression in AD from late-onset major depression in older patients with normal cognition, a disorder that is rarely familial (for review, see Greenwald and Kramer-Ginsberg 1988). If confirmed, these results suggest that the pathophysiologic events that lead to major depression in these two contexts may overlap but are not identical.

Considerable evidence implicates elements of the programmed cell death pathway in the loss of neurons from the neocortex, hippocampus, and brainstem aminergic nuclei in Alzheimer disease. However, the process that affects mature neurons in the CNS during normal aging and AD appears to differ in important ways from most examples of apoptosis. The time course from the initiation of apoptosis until cell death (and resumption in vivo) is typically measured in hours (Wyllie 1992). In AD, neurons that manifest chromatic condensation and DNA fragmentation appear to be in a state of dynamic and extended competition between progression toward cell death and compensatory (potentially restorative) processes that include the upregulation of the antiapoptotic Bcl-2 protein and the DNA repair enzyme Ref-1 (Satou, Cummings, and Cotman 1995; Anderson, Su, and Cotman 1996; Cotman and Su 1996; Su et al. 1996). Moreover, the association of Bcl-2 upregulation with greater disease severity in AD (Satou, Cummings, and Cotman 1995) suggests that postmortem studies provide an appropriate time window within which to study this phenomenon.

The apparent biomodality in the frequency histograms showing the number of locus ceruleus neurons in Alzheimer disease with or without depression suggests that the loss of neurons from this nucleus does not result from a stochastic process. Instead, it suggests that the subset of patients with AD who develop major depression have increased susceptibility to neuronal loss from the locus

Table 17.3. Phenotypic characterization of six susceptibility alleles in fifty autopsied cases of Alzheimer disease

	Clinical Features		Histopathologic Features*		Neurochemical Features**	
Allele	AAO	AAD	SP	NFT	NE	DA
APOE E4	0	0	+	+	0	0
D12S1045 91bp	—	—	0	+	0	—
D10S1423 234bp	0	0	0	0	+	—
DXS1047 202bp	0	0	0	0	+	−tr
D1S518 195bp	0	0	0	−tr	0	0
D1S547 286bp	0	0	0	0	0	0

Notes: + = positive association; − = negative association; −tr = negative trend; o = no association. AAO = age at onset; AAD = age at death; SP = senile plaque density; NFT = neurofibrillary tangle density; NE = norepinephrine levels; DA = dopamine levels.

*None of the alleles manifested an association with cerebral amyloid angiopathy.

**None of the alleles manifested an association with cortical choline acetyltransferase activities or serotonin levels.

ceruleus (and possibly the dorsal raphe and substantia nigra). At least some of the variability in the susceptibility of aminergic neurons to degeneration in AD may be attributable to genetic heterogeneity in the pathophysiology of this disorder. We reported the results of a genome survey that identified five novel AD susceptibility loci in addition to the ApoE locus (Zubenko et al. 1998). Alleles at three of these loci, D10S1423, D12S1045, and DXS1047, appear to modulate the cortical levels of both norepinephrine and dopamine (Zubenko, Hughes, and Stiffler 1999a, b, c) in patients with AD, as shown in table 17.3 (Zubenko 2000). Specifically, the D10S1423 234bp allele, the D12S1045 91bp allele, and the DXS1047 202 bp allele were associated with greater loss of cortical DA levels and relative preservation of cortical norephinephrine levels among fifty autopsy-confirmed cases of AD. These three alleles did not modulate cortical levels of 5-HT or choline acetyltransferase, and none of the remaining AD risk alleles detected by our genomic survey (D1S518 195bp, D1S547 286 bp, APOE ε4) affected any of these neurochemical indices. Whether these alleles influence the emergence of depression, other behavioral symptoms/syndromes, or parkinsonian features among patients with AD remains to be determined. Interestingly, recent evidence suggestive of linkage between D10S1423 and schizophrenia, another disorder whose pathophysiology may include disturbances of the dopaminergic nervous system, has been reported by the National Institute of Mental Health Genetics Initiative and Millennium Consortium (Faraone et al. 1998).

Implications for Research and Treatment

Degeneration of the aminergic nuclei is associated with the development of major depression in primary dementia. Histo/cytopathologic features in the locus ceruleus seem most strongly associated with depression in pure AD, while those in the substantia nigra are also associated with depression in Lewy body diseases (Lewy body variant of AD, Parkinson disease). Pharmacologic evidence also suggests a role for the serotonergic dorsal raphe in the pathogenesis of depression in these neurodegenerative disorders. Cytochemical and immunocytochemical evidence of apoptotic features is apparent in the locus ceruleus, substantia nigra, and dorsal raphe of patients who die with these disorders. One interpretation of these observations is that such neurons are in a dynamic state of extended competition between progression toward cell death and compensatory, potentially restorative processes. The bimodality in the distribution of surviving neurons in the locus ceruleus of patients who die with AD suggests that the subset of patients who develop major depression have increased susceptibility to neuronal loss in this region and possibly other brain regions. At least some of this variability in the susceptibility of aminergic neurons to degeneration in AD may be attributable to genetic heterogeneity in the pathophysiology of this disorder. Alleles at these recently described AD risk loci appear to modulate the cortical levels of dopamine and norepinephrine in patients with this disorder. Whether these alleles influence the emergence of depression, other behavioral symptoms/syndromes, or parkinsonian features among patients with AD remains to be determined. The overlap between the genetic region targeted by D10S1423 and the susceptibility of developing AD and schizophrenia raise the interesting possibility that particular genetic loci may contribute to the pathophysiology of more than one neuropsychiatric disorder (Zubenko 2000).

Clinical Conclusions

Major depression in patients with Alzheimer disease presenting in specialty settings is more common than in community samples. There appears to be a threshold for cholinergic function below which the clinical expression of depression is not possible. This suggests that the prevalence of major depression in AD and other dementias may decrease as the degenerative process progresses in specific brain nuclei. Neither age at onset nor duration of dementia differentiates these patients. However, family history of major depression may be more common and major depression appears to be a risk factor for mortality in patients with both AD and major depression.

ACKNOWLEDGMENTS

This work was supported by research grants MH43261 and MH/AG47346, and Independent Scientist Award MH00540 from the National Institute of Mental Health and the National Institute on Aging. An earlier version of this chapter appeared in *International Psychogeriatrics* 12 (Suppl. 1, 2000):S217–35; used with permission of the International Psychogeriatric Association.

REFERENCES

Anderson, A.J., J.H. Su, and C.W. Cotman. 1996. DNA damage and apoptosis in Alzheimer's disease: Colocalization with c-Jun immunoreactivity, relationship to brain area, and effect of postmortem delay. *Journal of Neuroscience* 16:1710–19.

Bierer, L.M., V. Haroutunian, D. Perl, et al. 1990. Relationship of non-cognitive behavioral disturbances to neuropathologic and neurochemical indices in brain specimens of patients with Alzheimer's disease. American College of Neuropsychopharmacology, 29th annual meeting, San Juan, Puerto Rico.

Boller, F., T. Mizutani, U. Roessmann, et al. 1980. Parkinson's disease, dementia, and Alzheimer's disease: Clinicopathological correlations. *Annals of Neurology* 7:329–35.

Bondareff, W., and C.Q. Mountjoy. 1986. Number of neurons in nucleus locus ceruleus in demented and non-demented patients: Rapid estimation and correlated parameters. *Neurobiology of Aging* 7:297–300.

Brikmayer, W., and P. Riederer. 1975. Biochemical post-mortem findings in depressed patients. *Journal of Neural Transmission* 37:95–109.

Bunney, W.E., and J. Davis. 1965. Norepinephrine in depressive reactions: A review of supporting evidence. *Archives of General Psychiatry* 13:483–97.

Carpenter, M.B. 1985. *Core Text of Neuroanatomy*. 3rd ed. Baltimore: Williams & Wilkins.

Cotman, C.W., and J.H. Su. 1996. Mechanisms of neuronal death in Alzheimer's disease. *Brain Pathology* 6:493–506.

Crow, T.J., A.J. Cross, S.J. Cooper, et al. 1984. Neurotransmitter receptors and monoamine metabolites in the brains of patients with Alzheimer-type dementia and depression, and suicides. *Neuropharmacology* 23:1561–69.

Davies, P., and A.J. Maloney. 1976. Selective loss of cholinergic neurons in Alzheimer's disease. *Lancet* 2:1403.

Davis, K.L., E. Hollander, M. Davidson, et al. 1987. Induction of depression with oxotremorine in patients with Alzheimer's disease. *American Journal of Psychiatry* 144: 468–71.

Dragunow, M., R.L.M. Fauli, P. Lawlor, et al. 1995. *In situ* evidence for DNA fragmentation in Huntington's disease striatum and Alzheimer's disease temporal lobes. *NeuroReport* 6:1053–57.

Faraone, S.V., T. Matise, D. Svrakic, et al. 1998. Genome scan of European-American Schizophrenia Pedigrees: Results of the NIMH Genetics Initiative and Millennium Consortium. *American Journal of Medical Genetics* 81:290–95.

Felten, D.L., and J.R. Sladek. 1983. Monoamine distribution in primary brain vs. monoaminergic nuclei: Anatomy, pathways and local organization. *Brain Research Bulletin* 10:171–284.

Fischer, P., M. Simanyi, and W. Danielczyk. 1990. Depression in dementia of the Alzheimer type and in multi-infarct dementia. *American Journal of Psychiatry* 147:1484–87.

Foote, S.L., and J.H. Morrison. 1987. In *Current Topics in Developmental Biology*, edited by A.A. Moscona and A. Monroy. New York: Academic Press, pp. 391–423.

Forsell, Y., A.F. Jorm, L. Fratiglioni, et al. 1993. Application of *DSM-III-R* criteria for major depressive episode to elderly subjects with and without dementia. *American Journal of Psychiatry* 150:1199–1202.

Forstl, H., A. Burns, R. Levy, et al. 1992. Neurologic signs in Alzheimer's disease. Results of a prospective clinical and neuropathologic study. *Archives of Neurology* 49:1038–42.

Gottfries, C.G., I. Karlsson, and A. Nyth. 1992. Treatment of depression in elderly patients with and without dementia disorders. *International Clinical Psychopharmacology* 5:55–64.

Greenwald, B.S., and E. Kramer-Ginsberg. 1988. Age at onset of geriatric depression: Relationship to clinical variables. *Journal of Affective Disorders* 15:61–68.

Hansen, L., D. Salmon, D. Galasko, et al. 1990. The Lewy body variant of Alzheimer's disease: A clinical and pathologic entity. *Neurology* 40:1–8.

Hansen, L.A., E. Masliah, D. Galasko, et al. 1993. Plaque-only Alzheimer's disease is usually the Lewy body variant, and vice versa. *Journal of Neuropathology and Experimental Neurology* 52:648–54.

Hoch, C.C., C.F. Reynolds, P.R. Houch, et al. 1989. Predicting mortality in mixed depression and dementia using EEG sleep variables. *Journal of Neuropsychiatry and Clinical Neurosciences* 1:366–71.

Huber, S.J., E.C. Shuttleworth, and G.W. Paulson. 1986. Dementia in Parkinson's disease. *Archives of Neurology* 43:987–95.

Hyman, S.E., and E.J. Nestler. 1993. *The Molecular Foundations of Psychiatry*. Washington, D.C.: American Psychiatric Press.

Janowsky, D.S., and S.C. Risch. 1987. Role of acetylcholine mechanisms in the affective disorders. In *Psychopharmacology: The Third Generation of Progress*, edited by H.Y. Meltzer. New York: Raven Press, pp. 527–53.

Jimerson, D.C. 1987. Role of dopamine mechanisms in the affective disorders. In *Psychopharmacology: The Third Generation of Progress*, edited by H.Y. Meltzer. New York: Raven Press, pp. 505–11.

Joachim, C.L., J.H. Morris, and D.J. Selkoe. 1988. Clinically diagnosed Alzheimer's disease: Autopsy results in 150 cases. *Annals of Neurology* 24:50–56.

Kazee, A.M., and L.Y. Han. 1995. Cortical Lewy bodies in Alzheimer's disease. *Archives of Pathology Laboratory Medicine* 119:448–53.

Kerr, J.F., A.H. Wylie, and A.R. Currie. 1972. Apoptosis: A basic biological phenomenon with wide-ranging implications in tissue kinetics. *British Journal of Cancer* 26: 239–57.

Langlais, P.J., L. Thal, L. Hansen, et al. 1993. Neurotransmitters in basal ganglia and cortex of Alzheimer's disease with and without Lewy bodies. *Neurology* 43:1927–34.

Lassmann, H., C. Bancher, H. Breitschopf, et al. 1995. Cell death in Alzheimer's disease evaluated by DNA fragmentation in situ. *Acta Neuropathology* 89:35–41.

Lippa, C.F., T.W. Smith, and J.M. Swearer. 1994. Alzheimer's disease and Lewy body disease: A comparative clinicopathological study. *Annals of Neurology* 35:81–88.

Lloyd, K.J., I.J. Farley, J.H.N. Deck, et al. 1974. Serotonin and 5-hydroxyindoleacetic acid in discrete areas of brainstem of suicide victims and control patients. *Advanced Biochemical Psychopharmacology* 11:387–97.

Mann, D.M.A., P.O. Yates, and J. Hawkes. 1983. The pathology of the human locus ceruleus. *Clinical Neuropathology* 2:1–7.

Mayeux, R., Y. Stern, J. Rosen, et al. 1981. Depression, intellectual impairment, and Parkinson disease. *Neurology* 31:645–50.

McGeer, P.L., E.G. McGeer, and J.S. Suzuki. 1977. Aging and extrapyramidal function. *Archives of Neurology* 34:33–35.

McKeith, I.G., R.H. Perry, A.F. Fairbairn, et al. 1992. Operational criteria for senile dementia of Lewy body type (SDLT). *Psychological Medicine* 22:911–22.

Mendlewicz, J., J.E. Vanderheyden, and G. Noel. 1981. Serotonin and dopamine in patients with unipolar depression and parkinsonism. *Advanced Experiments in Medical Biology* 133:753–67.

Nemeroff, C.B., D.S. Charney, D.L. Evans, et al. 1996. The role of specific neurotransmitter systems in the pathophysiology and treatment of depression: Implications for serotonin-norepinephrine reuptake inhibitors. Secausus, N.J.: Churchill Communications North America, Inc.

Perry, E.K., and R.H. Perry. 1980. The cholinergic system in Alzheimer's disease. In *Biochemistry of Dementia*, edited by P.J. Roberts. New York: John Wiley & Sons, pp. 135–83.

Reifler, B.V., E. Larson, and R. Hanley. 1982. Coexistence of cognitive impairment and depression in geriatric outpatients. *American Journal of Psychiatry* 139:623–26.

Reifler, B.V., L. Teri, M. Raskind, et al. 1989. Double-blind trial of imipramine in Alzheimer's disease patients with and without depression. *American Journal of Psychiatry* 146:45–49.

Satou, T., B.J. Cummings, and C.W. Cotman. 1995. Immunoreactivity for Bcl-2 protein within neurons in the Alzheimer's disease brain increases with disease severity. *Brain Research* 697:35–43.

Schildkraut, J.J. 1965. The catecholamine hypothesis of affective disorders: A review of supporting evidence. *American Journal of Psychiatry* 122:509–22.

Siever, L.J. 1987. Role of noradreneric mechanisms in the etiology of the affective disorders. In *Psychopharmacology: The Third Generation of Progress*, edited by H.Y. Meltzer. New York: Raven Press, pp. 493–504.

Smale, G., N.R. Nichols, D.R. Brady, et al. 1995. Evidence for apoptotic cell death in Alzheimer's disease. *Experimental Neurology* 133:225–30.

Stanley, M., and J.J. Mann. 1983. Increased serotonin-2 binding sites in frontal cortex of suicide victims. *Lancet* 1:214–16.

Su, J.H., A.J. Anderson, B.J. Cummings, et al. 1994. Immunohistochemical evidence for apoptosis in Alzheimer's disease. *NeuroReport* 5:2529–33.
Su, J.H., T. Satou, A.J. Anderson, et al. 1996. Up-regulation of Bcl-2 is associated with neuronal DNA damage in Alzheimer's disease. *NeuroReport* 7:437–40.
Thomas, L.B., D.J. Gates, E.K. Richfield, et al. 1995. DNA end labeling (TUNEL) in Huntington's disease and other neuropathological conditions. *Experimental Neurology* 133:265–72.
Victoroff, J., W.J. Mack, S.A. Lyness, et al. 1995. Multicenter clinicopathological correlation in dementia. *American Journal of Psychiatry* 152:1476–84.
Vijayashankar, N., and H. Brody. 1977. Aging in the human brain stem: A study of the nucleus of the trochlear nerve. *Acta Anatomica* 99:169–72.
Vita, P., E. Lacana, and L. D'Adamio. 1996. Interfering with apoptosis: Ca^{2+}-binding protein ALG-2 and Alzheimer's disease gene ALG-3. *Science* 271:521–25.
Weissman, M.M., M.L. Bruce, P.J. Leaf, et al. 1991. Affective disorders. In *Psychiatric Disorders in America: The Epidemiologic Catchment Area Study*, edited by L.N. Robins and D.A. Regier. New York: The Free Press, pp. 53–80.
Whitehouse, P.J., D.L. Price, R.G. Struble, et al. 1982. Alzheimer's disease and senile dementia: Loss of neurons in the basal forebrain. *Science* 215:1237–39.
Wolozin, B., K. Iwasaki, P. Vito, et al. 1996. Participation of presenilin 2 in apoptosis: Enhanced basal activity conferred by an Alzheimer mutation. *Science* 274:1710–13.
Wyllie, A.H. 1992. Apoptosis and the regulation of cell numbers in normal and neoplastic tissues: An overview. *Cancer Metastasis Review* 11:95–103.
Zubenko, G.S. 1997. Molecular neurobiology of Alzheimer's disease (syndrome?). *Harvard Review of Psychiatry* 5:1–37.
Zubenko, G.S. 2000. Do susceptibility loci contribute to the expression of more than one mental disorder?: A view from the genetics of Alzheimer's disease. *Molecular Psychiatry* 5:131–36.
Zubenko, G.S., H.B. Hughes, and J.S. Stiffler. 1999a. Clinical and neurobiological correlates of D10S1423 genotype in Alzheimer's disease. *Biological Psychiatry* 46:740–49.
Zubenko, G.S., H.B. Hughes, and J.S. Stiffler. 1999b. Clinical and neurobiological correlates of DXS1047 genotype in Alzheimer's disease. *Biological Psychiatry* 46:173–81.
Zubenko, G.S., H.B. Hughes, and J.S. Stiffler. 1999c. Neurobiological correlates of a putative risk allele for Alzheimer's disease on chromosome 12q. *Neurology* 52:725–32.
Zubenko, G.S., J. Moossy, and U. Kopp. 1990. Neurochemical correlates of major depression in primary dementia. *Archives of Neurology* 47:209–14.
Zubenko, G.S., J. Moossy, A.J. Martinez, et al. 1989. A brain regional analysis of morphologic and cholinergic abnormalities in Alzheimer's disease. *Archives of Neurology* 46:634–38.
Zubenko, G.S., P. Sullivan, J. Nelson, et al. 1991. Brain imaging abnormalities in mental disorders of late life. *Archives of Neurology* 47:1107–11.
Zubenko, G.S., J. Rosen, R.A. Sweet, et al. 1992. Impact of psychiatric hospitalization on behavioral complications of Alzheimer's disease. *American Journal of Psychiatry* 149:1484–91.
Zubenko, G.S., H.B. Hughes, J.S. Stiffler, et al. 1998. A genome survey for novel Alzheimer's disease risk loci: Results at 10cM resolution. *Genomics* 50:121–28.
Zweig, R.M., C.A. Ross, J.C. Hedreen, et al. 1988. The neuropathology of aminergic nuclei in Alzheimer's disease. *Annals of Neurology* 24:233–42.

Part V / Conclusions and Future Directions

Approaches to the Treatment of Dementing Illness

Thomas E. Oxman, M.D.,
and Robert B. Santulli, M.D.

Many illnesses have clearly defined approaches to treatment that most clinicians can master. Chronic, progressive diseases, such as dementia, without cures are often frustrating. Nevertheless, dementia is treatable, even if the underlying etiology is not (Reifler and Sherrill 1990). As with other chronic diseases, such as emphysema, diabetes, or metastatic cancer, the clinician can aggressively identify and treat *excess disability*, optimizing physiological and mental status so that no excess dysfunction impairs the quality of life for persons with dementia or their caregivers (Holmes, Ory, and Teresi 1994; McAllister and Powers 1994). Excess disability has four general causes: chemical and structural brain changes caused by the disease (Mulsant and Zubenko 1994); patient and caregiver reactions to the disease (Cummings et al. 1987); superimposed medical comorbidity (Larson et al. 1985; Levkoff et al. 1996); and environmental stressors (Holmes, Ory, and Teresi 1994; Radebaugh, Buckholtz, and Khachaturian 1996).

Thus far, excess disability in dementia has referred to secondary symptoms and pathophysiology. The most common presentations of excess disability include problem behaviors, delirium, psychosis, and depression. Our understanding of the primary pathophysiologies of the dementias is expanding, and treatment of excess disability has begun to focus on primary pathophysiology.

Nosologically, it is not always easy to distinguish secondary presentations of excess disability from the primary features of dementia. Dementia is characterized by three primary features: cognitive impairment, functional impairment, and neuropathology (see chap. 2). Although cognitive impairment is the sine qua non of dementing disorders, functional impairment is a key element that has a greater impact on the need for treatment and use of health care. Primary functional impairment is not merely a consequence of cognitive impairment, but has a different natural history and pathophysiology (Mortimer et al. 1992; Niederehe and Oxman 1994; Albert et al. 1996; Levy et al. 1996). Differentiating primary dementia pathophysiology from secondary excess disability as the cause of psychiatric symptoms and syndromes in dementia can be difficult. Currently, however, the treatment modalities of reducing medical comorbidity, behavioral and environmental modification, and judicious use of pharmacotherapy are analogous for both causes.

Treatment of the person with dementia requires: (1) diagnosis and documentation of deficits; (2) careful medical management; (3) monitoring and restructuring the environment; (4) pharmacological manipulations; (5) support of caregivers; and (6) communication among all persons participating in treatment. The treatment plan should focus on maintaining the patient's function, comfort, and safety. Revision will probably be necessary frequently to account for new deficits or intercurrent medical problems. Each patient is different and will require a variable mixture of each of the six interventions. However, supervision and communication are essential to all management strategies. This chapter will outline the principles of such treatment. It will not focus exclusively on the pharmacological approaches to reversing cognitive decline in dementia, as this is only a component of a comprehensive treatment approach.

Diagnostic Issues

The initial step in treatment is to confirm the presence of a dementing syndrome. This is accompanied by documentation or completion of a reasonable search for etiologies that could be reversed, such as metabolic or endocrinologic abnormalities (see chap. 3). Even if reversible etiologies are not found, there may be interventions to halt or slow the progression of the illness. For example, the discovery of significant cerebrovascular disease with subsequent vascular dementia will highlight the need for aggressive control of blood pressure and other risk factors. Family concerns should be identified and incorporated into the treatment plan for prioritizing target symptom goals. Confirmation and acceptance of the diagnosis by the primary caregivers and the family is a necessary first step of treatment.

Target symptoms in Alzheimer disease (and other dementias) include three clusters: (1) cognition, (2) noncognitive symptoms, (3) quality of life (usually assessed by caregivers and including overall function). The last usually encompasses judgments on the restrictiveness of the living environment, the capacity to engage in age-appropriate, noninstitutional activities, and the perceived amount of distress manifested by the patient. Specific challenging behaviors, such as hyperactivity, wandering, sleep disturbance, affective instability, aggression, and psychotic symptoms, such as delusions, often factor prominently in the perception of the patient's level of distress. Any therapeutic intervention should have objective, reliable documentation to help assess treatment response and the need for modification. Continued use of potentially toxic and expensive medications is indicated only when clinical response meets or exceeds target symptom goals without adding side effects or costs that outweigh the improvement.

Treatment of Cognitive Impairment in Alzheimer Disease

Therapeutic interventions for dementia attempt to restore depleted neurotransmitters, reverse neuronal dysfunction, or slow neuronal damage. It is not within the scope of this section to discuss potential cognitive drug therapies for every form of dementia; rather, we will focus on Alzheimer disease (AD).

Cholinomimetic Agents

Although multiple neurotransmitter pathways are damaged in Alzheimer disease, cholinergic system damage appears to occur earlier and consistently. Thus, drugs affecting the cholinergic system have received the greatest deal of attention in AD. Cholinomimetic drugs act at several levels: (1) increase of precursor substances (Bartus et al.1982; Canter, Hallett, and Growdon 1982), (2) increase of acetylcholine in synapses (Cahn et al. 1988; Hiersemenzel, Dietrick, and Hermann 1988; Passeri et al. 1988), (3) slowing of degradation of acetylcholine in the synapse (Summers et al. 1986; Mohs and Davis 1987; Nordgren and Holmstedt 1988; Eagger-Sarah, Levy, and Sahakian 1991; Farlow et al. 1992), (4) direct activation of the postsynaptic receptor (Christie et al. 1981; Davidson et al. 1991), and (5) deactivation of inhibiting impulses on cholinergic systems (Hollander et al. 1987; Sarter 1991). Although several drugs have been considered at each level, the cholinesterase inhibitors are currently the only ones FDA-approved, with four available drugs (tacrine, donepezil, rivastigmine, galantamine). Studies with tacrine, a synthetic cholinesterase inhibitor that crosses the blood-brain barrier, yielded controversial but generally positive results. Higher doses were associated with better outcomes, but hepatotoxicity and multiple dosing were troublesome features (Summers et al. 1986; Farlow et al. 1992; Cummings 2000). The three newer agents are safer and in increasingly wide use.

Choline acetyltransferase and acetylcholinesterase, enzymes of synthesis and degradation of acetylcholine, are markedly reduced in brains of persons with Alzheimer disease. In contrast, butylcholinesterase, another enzyme that catabolizes acetylcholine, is markedly increased in AD and may play a role in the development of neuritic plaques (Perry et al. 1978; Mesulam and Guela 1994; Guillozet et al. 1997). The available inhibitors differ in their selectivity for actetylcholinesterase versus butylcholinesterase and in their pharmacokinetics (tab. 18.1). All four drugs have been shown in double-blind multicenter studies to slow the decline in cognitive function and functional impairment compared to placebo (Knapp et al. 1994; Corey-Bloom et al. 1998; Burns et al. 1999; Tariot et al. 2000). In addition, they also can reduce neuropsychiatric symptoms such as agitation and related problem behaviors (Knapp et al. 1994; Corey-Bloom 1998; Rogers et al. 1998; Tariot et al. 2000).

There are theoretical reasons why one of these drugs might be preferable over another. Examples include interference with plaque maturation by butylcholinesterase inhibition or drug interactions because of cytochrome P-450 interactions. To date, however, there is insufficient evidence to support such theoretical claims. In general, persons with early to mid-stage AD are most likely to benefit. Little improvement is documented for persons with end-stage disorder. The benefits seen are usually a slowing of decline rather than a clinically meaningful improvement in cognition or function. This distinction and its implication for long-term drug costs and long-term care versus home care should be explained and discussed with patients and caregivers.

There is some evidence that these agents are helpful in some non-Alzheimer dementias, specifically vascular dementia (Doody et al. 2001) and dementia with Lewy bodies (McKeith et al. 2000). It remains unclear how often positive responses are related to the presence of comorbid AD (Knopman 2001).

Table 18.1. Cholinesterase inhibitors

	Tacrine	Donepezil	Rivastigmine	Galantamine
Brand name	Cognex	Aricept	Exelon	Reminyl
Year available	1993	1997	2000	2001
Inhibits				
Acetylcholinesterase	yes	yes	yes	yes
Butylcholinesterase	yes	no	yes	no
Maximum dose	160 mg/d	10 mg/d	12 mg/d	24 mg/d
Dose frequency	q.i.d.	q.d.	b.i.d.	b.i.d.
Metabolism	P-450	P-450	renal	P-450/renal

Other Agents

The American Association of Neurology Subcommittee (Doody et al. 2001) recommends as a guideline that use of vitamin E (1000 I.U. PO BID) be considered for the treatment of Alzheimer disease, given evidence that it may slow the progression of the disease. Conversely, they recommend as a standard that estrogen not be considered for the treatment of AD (Mulnard et al. 2000), although some reports suggest estrogen replacement therapy may reduce the risk of AD (Honjo et al. 1993; Paganini-Hill and Henderson 1994, 1996; Birge 2000). Similarly, there is epidemiological and animal evidence suggesting that nonsteroidal anti-inflammatory drugs may prevent or prolong the development of AD (Veld et al. 2001;Weggen et al. 2001). However, there are no randomized controlled trials (RCTs) of prevention yet and no evidence of benefit in already diagnosed AD. The risk of side effects further mitigates against current use.

Other treatment options include consideration of different antioxidants, selegiline, and other proposed disease-modifying agents. However, the subcommittee cautions that there is a risk of significant side effects without comparable evidence of demonstrated efficacy. Reports of the effectiveness of Gingko biloba are variable (see Oken, Storzbach, and Kaye 1998; LeBars et al. 2000 for reviews) with some reports of modest benefit, depending on the study population, type of cognitive measures employed, and dosing.

Noncognitive Disturbances

The hallmark of a dementia syndrome is the deterioration in cognitive function, particularly memory. This should not obscure the dramatic changes in personality and the array of behavioral problems that are a significant part of the clinical picture. Troublesome behavior occurs in high percentages of both institutionalized and noninstitutionalized persons with dementia (Rabins, Mace, and Lucas 1982; Merriam et al. 1988; Swearer et al. 1988; Teri, Larson, and Reifler 1988; Wragg and Jeste 1989; Mendez et al. 1990). Along with deficits in self-care, these disturbances often predict institutionalization, as well as the consumption of nursing care once institutionalization occurs.

The impact of these behaviors on the caregivers of persons with dementia is dramatic and includes fatigue, anger, depression, family conflict, loss of friends, and loss of personal time (U.S. Congress OTA 1985; Levine and Lawlor 1991; Chappell and Novak 1994; Schulz et al. 1995). Although most studies have focused on the problems associated with AD, those that have looked at demented populations of mixed etiology have found few differences on caregiver impact between groups (Rabins, Mace, and Lucas 1982; Swearer et al. 1988). The evaluation and treatment of these different behavioral syndromes can be a most productive and gratifying component of dementia treatment.

Problem Behaviors

Problem behaviors are a broad category of symptoms, such as wandering, pacing, agitation, vocalizations, and aggression. Although these behaviors occur in both community and institutionalized persons with dementia, they appear to occur more frequently in persons with moderate to severe dementia (Winger, Schirm, and Stewart 1987; Jost and Grossberg 1996; Lyketsos et al. 2000b). For example, Cohen-Mansfield, Marx, and Rosenthal (1989) found that 93% of more than 400 nursing home residents manifested one or more of these symptoms at least once per week. The most common included general restlessness, pacing, cursing, constant requests for attention, and repetitive sentences or questions. Rates in community dwelling residents are lower, but substantial, ranging between 20% and 80% (Rubin et al. 1987; Terri, Larson, and Reifler 1988; Reisberg et al. 1989; Albert et al. 1996; Lyketsos et al. 2000b).

As with behavioral disturbances in other brain disorders, a number of classes of drugs are capable of decreasing the frequency and intensity of a variety of behaviors in persons with Alzheimer and other dementing disorders. Agents used include the full range psychotropic drugs: neuroleptics, anxiolytics, anticonvulsants, sedative-hypnotics, and antidepressants. The typology of behavioral disturbances usually groups disturbances of thinking and perception (psychotic symptoms) with less well-categorized behaviors like agitation, aggression, and wandering. This may account for some of the ambiguous or modest treatment responses reported for various regimens (Tune, Steele, and Cooper 1991).

In addition to medication approaches, psychoeducational approaches directed to the caregivers (including behavioral approaches, environmental manipulation, and community support) should be considered because of the added benefit of reducing caregiver burden and depression as well as problem behaviors in the person with dementia, without the side effects of medications (Mittelman et al. 1996; Rovner et al. 1996; Teri et al. 1997; Buckwalter et al. 1999; McCallion, Toseland, and Freeman 1999; Proctor et al. 1999; Hepburn et al. 2001).

Depression

In 1989 Wragg and Jeste reviewed eighteen studies to determine the relationship of prevalence and predictors of depressive symptomatology in dementia. They found that depression rates ranged from 0% to 86%, with a median of 19%. As is true in the community (Blazer, Hughes, and George 1987) and primary care medical sector (Magruder, Schulberg, and Oxman 1996), isolated symptoms of depression were two to three times more frequent than diagnosable disorders. Wragg and Jeste also identified several methodological problems contributing to the wide variability, including case definition, source of subjects, subject selection, and sample size. Nevertheless, newer studies with improvements in case definition, subject selection, and sample size have replicated both the variability of rates and prominence of symptoms over syndromes (Bungener, Jouvent, and Derouesne 1996; Jost and Grossberg 1996; Levy et al. 1996). For example, Levy et al. (1996) found a 50% one-year prevalence of depressive symptoms, while Bungener, Jouvent, and Derouesne (1996) found a 0% rate of major depressive disorder.

Depression appears to decline as cognitive impairment increases (Wragg and Jeste 1989; Zubenko et al. 1992; Forsell, Jorm, and Winblad 1994; Bungener, Jouvent, and Derouesne 1996). Depression also contributes to functional impairment (Fitz and Teri 1994). With mild cognitive impairment, depression contributes to instrumental activities of daily living (ADLs), while in moderate cognitive impairment depression contributes to basic ADLs. Thus, treatment of depression is clearly important.

Psychosis

Psychosis in dementia is primarily the occurrence of delusions and hallucinations rather than the occurrence of psychiatric syndromes. Nevertheless, as with depression, the prevalence is highly variable, with a range of 0% to 73%. Wragg and Jeste (1989) reviewed twenty-two studies and reported a median cross-sectional prevalence of 34% for delusions or hallucinations. The number of persons experiencing delusions or hallucinations at any time during the course of illness is much higher (Drevets and Rubin 1989; Rosen and Zubenko 1991; Jost and Grossberg 1996). Paranoid delusions appear to be the most common form of reported psychotic symptoms (Wragg and Jeste 1989).

Psychotic symptoms may be associated with a more rapid rate of cognitive decline (Stern et al. 1987; Drevets and Rubin 1989; Rosen and Zubenko 1991; Levy et al. 1996), but documentation of the benefits of treatment and its relationship to improved function is lacking. Caregivers report that psychotic symptoms affect the quality of life for both the patient and themselves (Rabins and Folstein 1982). Particularly distressing for spouse caregivers is when the person with dementia does not recognize the spouse (an agnosia more than a delusion) or experiences fear of the spouse with delusions that the spouse is an unwanted intruder. Delusional symptoms in dementia are more frequently associated with aggression than are hallucinations (Gilley et al. 1997; Bassiony et al. 2000; Rapoport et al. 2001).

It is important to distinguish psychotic symptoms from confabulation. Not uncommonly, patients with marked memory disturbances will make false statements that are typically inconsistent and not maintained for any length of time. These usually do not need to be treated. Only in the event that the false beliefs are consistently maintained over a period of days to weeks should they be considered delusions. This distinction is important because the treatment of psychotic phenomena in the person with dementia can be difficult and should be seriously considered only when the symptoms are causing a significant degree of distress to the patient or caregivers (e.g., there is a link between the paranoid delusion and aggressive or assaultive behavior).

Psychopharmacologic Treatment of Noncognitive Disturbances

General Principles

Before starting a psychopharmacologic agent for the treatment of a noncognitive disturbance in dementia, three questions should be asked. First, does the symptom cause significant impairment or reduction in quality of life for the patient or to those persons around him or her on a regular basis? A symptom does not necessarily need treatment just because it is present. Hallucinations and depressed mood, for example, are often transient, and unless they have an impact on daily life, the cost, potential toxicity, and adherence problems of treatment may outweigh any benefits. Second, are there any other treatable medical problems that might be the cause of the target symptom? Most commonly the use of multiple medications can lead to delirium, and urinary tract infections or other intercurrent illnesses often lead to mental status changes in persons with dementia. Treatment of these conditions should take priority over adding a psychopharmacological agent. Third, are there any reversible, environmental stimuli which are causing or contributing to the behavior? Changes in daily routines, increased or decreased social contacts, or a move to an unfamiliar environment can all lead to changes in behaviors. When possible, altering these environmental conditions should precede addition of a drug.

Once it is determined that a psychopharmacologic agent might be of benefit, four general principles should guide an empiric trial. The first is to try to identify a psychiatric syndrome which can help select the best class of medication. Frequently this is not possible, particularly when agitation or aggression is the predominant presentation. The second principle is to begin with the most benign class of drug, with the agent having the least incidence of side effects. This entails knowing the patient's medical history. For example, neuroleptics might be avoided initially for aggression in someone with Parkinson disease, or carbamazepine or clozapine might be avoided in someone with leukopenia (fig. 18.1).

The third principle is to select a method of quantifying the target symptom in order to assess the efficacy of a treatment. Depending on the symptom, the method might be a brief questionnaire, a global rating, or a periodic frequency count. The fourth principle is to institute drug trials systematically. Single drugs are preferred over combinations of drugs. A trial period should be defined based on the nature of the symptom and the pharmacodynamics and pharmacokinetics of the agent selected. Lower starting doses, longer titration intervals, and lower final doses are generally the rule.

Antipsychotic Drugs

Previously, in meta-analyses antipsychotics had shown only modest effects (Schneider, Pollock, and Lyness 1990; Lanctot et al. 1998) and had been cautiously recommended for use in dementia (McAllister and Powers 1994). With the advent of "atypical" antipsychotic drugs such as risperidone, olanzapine, and

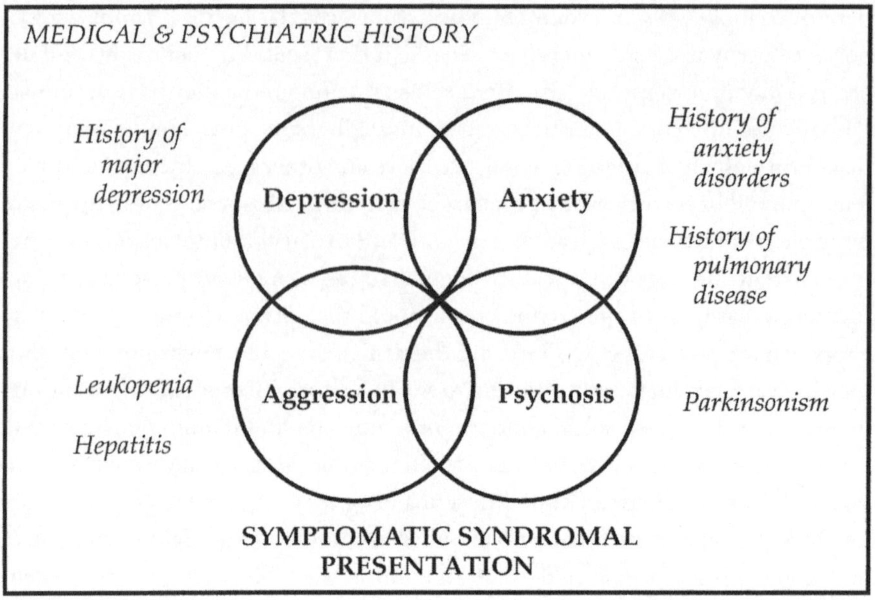

Figure 18.1. Identification of psychiatric syndromes in the context of medical history to aid in the selection or avoidance of psychotropic drugs in the management of noncognitive symptoms in dementia

quetiapine, there has been a resurgence of interest in the use of these drugs specifically for either aggression or psychosis associated with dementia. In large, double-blind, randomized controlled studies, these drugs have been significantly more effective than placebo and have less side effects than older neuroleptics (De Deyn et al. 1999; Katz et al. 1999; Bhana and Spencer 2000; Street et al. 2000). There appears to be a therapeutic window in which modest, not low or high, doses, provide the best outcomes, for example, 1mg of risperidone rather than 0.5 or 2.0 mg and 5 mg of olanzapine rather than 2.5 or 10 mg.

Although rare, consideration of the neuroleptic malignant syndrome should be considered whenever mental status changes and autonomic instability occur after using neuroleptics (Carbone 2000). For persons with Parkinson disease or dementia of the Lewy body type, it appears that the paradigm atypical agent clozapine remains most effective without aggravating extrapyramidal symptoms (Goetz et al. 2000). However, it is uncommonly used in clinical practice because of the risk of agranulocytosis and the need for regular white cell count monitoring.

Benzodiazepines and Other Anxiolytics

Benzodiazepines are one of the most common agents used for the treatment of agitation, particularly in nursing homes. The use of this class of drugs is frequently disparaged because of potential side effects, including falls and oversedation. Several studies have shown an association between falls and benzodiazepine (Passaro et al. 2000; Wang et al. 2001), while others have not (Ebly, Hogan, and Fung 1997; Eto et al. 1998; Schwab et al. 1999; Pierfitte et al. 2001). In general, benzodiazepines with moderate to short half-lives, such as oxazepam and lorazepam, are preferable. It may be that dose is more important than half-life in predicting falls (Cumming 1998). Other psychotropic agents are also associated with falls (Passaro et al. 2000). The effectiveness of benzodiazepines has not been well studied in dementia, but there are open studies suggesting benefits from both short- (Christensen and Benfield 1998) and long-acting benzodiazepines (Calkin et al. 1997).

In addition to alleviating anxiety or agitation, there is some evidence that benzodiazepines modulate acetylcholine release (Sarter 1994; Chain, Ighanian, and Boon 2000) and thus could even have a protective effect in Alzheimer disease (Fastbom, Forsell, and Winblad 1998; Lokensgard et al. 1998) and other dementias (Polc 1995; Messmer and Reynolds 1998).

Buspirone is a serotonin-1A receptor partial agonist which has shown some benefit in reducing agitation and aggression in dementia (Sakauye, Camp, and Ford 1993; Cantillon et al. 1996). It is well tolerated without sedation and has few drug interactions. However, the rare serotonin syndrome has been reported in persons with dementia on buspirone, usually added to other serotonerigic drugs, and should be considered when one or more of the following symptoms occur, usually within initiation or change in medication: confusion, agitation, diaphoresis, tachycardia, myoclonus, and hyperreflexia (Goldberg and Huk 1992; Fischer 1995; Mason, Morris, and Balcezak 2000; Lantz 2001). Although similar in presentation to the neuroleptic malignant syndrome, the serotonin syndrome is more related to toxicity than an idiosyncratic response (Carbone 2000) and does not have pronounced extrapyramidal signs.

Although trazodone was initially released as an antidepressant, in lower doses it has probably received far more use as an anxiolytic or hypnotic. It has been associated with both reduction of problem behaviors and oversedation and occasional orthostasis (Lebert, Pasquier, and Petit 1994). A consensus panel of geriatric psychiatrists has recommended its use as a first-line agent for mild symptoms of aggression (Expert Consensus Panel 1998).

Anticonvulsants

Based on trials of treating aggression in younger persons, anticonvulsants have been used in several double-blind studies in persons with dementia and agitation or aggression (Tariot, Schneider, and Katz 1995; Grossman 1998). In a double-blind placebo controlled study, carbamazepine improved agitation in dementia and the agitation worsened when carbamazepine was withdrawn (Tariot et al. 1999). Valproic acid is generally better tolerated than carbamazepine with fewer drug interactions. Valproic acid has also significantly improved agitation in both open label and now double-blind, placebo controlled studies (Lott, McElroy, and Kelp 1995; Porsteinsson et al. 2001). Valproic acid can cause a dose-related elevation in liver enzymes and an increase in blood ammonia without an increase in liver enzymes (Coulter and Allen 1980; Zaccara et al. 1987). The latter can sometimes be reversed with the dietary supplement carnitine (Komatsu et al. 1987; Raby 1997) or lactulose (Miyaji et al. 1997). As with other medications, lower doses of valproic acid are often sufficient (e.g., 125 mg t.i.d. and blood levels below 50 ng/mL). Gabapentin and lamotrigine are newer anticonvulsants that have also been used for treating agitation in dementia but not in controlled trials as of yet (Goldenberg et al. 1998; Devarajan and Dursun 2000).

Antidepressants

In outpatients with dementia and depression, good clinical management appears to be as effective as tricyclic antidepressants (Reifler et al. 1989) and to cause less cognitive impairment. There are a variety of theoretical reasons to suggest SSRIs would be superior to tricyclics for the treatment of depressive syndromes in dementia (Oxman 1996) (see chap. 17). SSRIs have not been used in a sufficient number of randomized controlled trials with a placebo (as opposed to another antidepressant), but preliminary evidence is promising in outpatients with dementia with clearly diagnosed major depressive disorder (Lyketsos et al. 2000a). The value of SSRIs in later-stage nursing home patients is less certain (Magai et al. 2000). Because of the association of locus ceruleus lesions causing norepinephrine deficits, the monamine oxidase inhibitor moclobemide has received specific attention in persons with dementia and depression (Chan-Palay 1992; Roth, Mountjoy, and Amrein 1996). Moclobemide is a reversible, specific inhibitor of MAO-type A, the major norepinephrine metabolizing enzyme in the locus ceruleus. The drug is well tolerated and does not have the dietary or drug restrictions of less-specific MAO inhibitors.

SSRIs have also been recommended for use in managing mild aggression (Expert Consensus Panel 1998). A multisite, double-blind, randomized controlled study is currently under way comparing olanzapine, quetiapine, risperidone, citalopram, and placebo (Schneider et al. 2001).

Iatrogenic Excess Disability

A note of caution is necessary in promoting psychopharmacologic treatment of excess disability, particularly in nursing homes. Psychotropic medications are useful for treating depression, psychosis, and some forms of problem behaviors. However, psychotropic drugs also increase the risk of falls (Thapa et al. 1995), neuroleptic malignant syndrome (Kimura and Yoshida 1994), and serotonin syndrome (Goldberg and Huk 1992; Fischer 1995). Behavioral and environmental techniques can be successfully used to reduce behavioral problems for many persons with dementia (Avorn et al. 1992; Ray et al. 1993). Accordingly, it is valuable to have experts in geriatric mental health involved in evaluations and decisions about the use of psychotropic medications in dementia.

Nonpharmacologic Interventions

Medication approaches are important but should not be emphasized to the exclusion of psychosocial, interpersonal, environmental, and psychoeducational interventions. A variety of psychosocial approaches have been described in persons with dementia of varying degrees. Treatment needs to involve primary caregivers, whether family or institutional staff, in a mixture of individual, family, and systems approaches (Lewin and Lundervold 1990; Schmid 1990; Deutsch and Rovner 1991; Levine and Lawlor 1991; Teri and Gallagher-Thompson 1991).

General Principles

Guiding themes underlie the application of nonpharmacological interventions to persons with dementia. The first is that behaviors usually come from understandable feelings and reactions that are not inappropriate in themselves but seem inappropriate because of the situation or the frequency with which they are expressed. For example, when looking at disturbing, repetitive verbal or motor behavior judged by an outside observer to be inappropriate, several alternative interpretations can be made. The behavior itself may be appropriate, but what is inappropriate is the frequency, such as constant pacing or questions suggesting anxiety about a situation. Sometimes the inappropriateness is the location of the behavior rather than the behavior itself, such as undressing in public. When recognized, the emotions may be appropriate, such as anger, but the target of the emotion may be inappropriate, such as self-abuse. Recognizing the emotion as appropriate and trying to alter the situation can be beneficial (Cohen-Mansfield and Billig 1986). A related issue is that the physical and social environment affect behaviors. For example, if the environment is too large or confusing, overstimulation can result in agitation or even aggression. Changing the environment or instituting a set routine in that environment can be effective ways of diminishing problem behaviors. Persons with dementia benefit from a calm, simple, secure, predictable environment that minimizes psychological stress and lessens the risk of injury (Robert and Algase 1988). For patients living at home, the caregiver needs to structure the home schedule, remove dangerous objects, and secure exits for the confused person (Brawley, 1997).

The second theme is that individuals with dementia have residual strengths and interests which can be tapped. Identifying these, usually long-standing, interests and strengths can be used to recommend activities to divert attention from more disruptive and aggressive behaviors. The activities should be pleasurable and not tax the remaining abilities of the person with dementia (Baltes et al. 1987; Baltes and Baltes 1993). Thus, maintaining pastimes or chores should be done by simplifying choices and activities, providing reminders and positive feedback, and emphasizing participation or completion rather than quality.

A third important theme is that caregivers are part of an integral unit for a person with dementia. It will thus be important that any psychosocial intervention have a clearly communicated plan before implementation. The treatment team should determine what specific target symptom(s) is to be treated, and how this symptom will be documented. As with pharmacologic interventions, the end point for the therapeutic intervention needs to be clearly stated and the method of measuring this end point determined.

Caregiver distress and burden is another form of excess disability in dementia. High levels of burden are identified in nearly all studies of dementia caregivers (Schultz et al. 1995). As with studies of psychiatric symptoms or syndromes in persons with dementia, rates of depression in caregivers are variable because of methodological differences. In studies using structured interviews, the prevalence of depressive disorders in caregivers ranges between 15% and 30%, while rates of anxiety disorders are somewhat more consistent at approximately 10% (Schultz et al. 1995).

Caregiver burden contributes to use of health services by both the caregiver and the person with dementia. Spousal caregivers of persons with dementia are hospitalized more often than spouses of persons without cognitive impairment (Cohen et al. 1990; Vitaliano et al. 1991; Moritz, Kasl, and Ostfeld 1992). Problem behaviors of persons with dementia are the most frequent predictor of caregiver distress (Mortimer et al. 1992; Schultz et al. 1995). In turn, caregiver burden is a better predictor of the use of long-term care services than any measure of a patient's cognitive or physical functional abilities (Potter 1993). Clinicians need to be attuned to the condition of the caregiver as well as to that of the person with dementia.

Problem Solving

To implement these themes and develop solutions to difficult behaviors in dementia, a behavioral problem solving approach is recommended (Nezu, Nezu, and Arean 1991; Hegel, Barrett, and Oxman 2000). Caregivers should be taught and helped to approach problem behaviors in a systematic, stepwise process. In the first step, the problem is defined and broken into smaller parts that seem easier to solve. Caregivers should be encouraged to become observers and ask themselves the following questions: What is the likely emotion displayed by the person with dementia? When does the problem occur? What seems to trigger the problem? What can be changed in the environment? At the same time, caregivers should be advised to avoid arguing, rationalizing, condescending, or bossing. The clinician should help the caregiver develop this attitude of information gathering with an awareness that it is an ongoing process and that solutions will change.

Once the problem is defined and broken down, caregivers need to brainstorm and think of several possible solutions and then weigh the pros and cons, likelihood of success, and costs to them and others for each solution. Based on this analysis, one solution is selected, attempted, and then evaluated. If the solution works, its implementation is continued and the caregiver moves on to the next problem. If it does not work, the caregiver should then try to assess whether that solution was adequately implemented or whether to move on to the next solution. This approach helps to diminish guilt or feelings of failure in caregivers.

When coupled with some kind of record keeping, caregivers may see that solutions actually work at least partially even if they don't eliminate the behavior.

Education and Support

Education of both the patient and the family is critical. Support groups can serve not only as a source of psychological assistance, but as an important mechanism for getting information about the disease and community treatment resources. Structured psychoeducational programs probably provide even more in the way of knowledge, and a sense of competence and independence in coping with the enormous stresses of caring for someone with a dementing syndrome (Chiverton and Caine 1989; Deutsch and Rovner 1991; Levine and Lawlor 1991). Efforts directed toward improving the knowledge base, health, and sense of well-being of the primary caregiver usually translate directly into better care of the patient (Mittelman et al. 1996; Teri et al. 1997; Buckwalter et al. 1999; McCallion, Toseland, and Freeman 1999; Proctor et al. 1999; Hepburn et al. 2001).

The combination of advancing age, shortened life span, and progressive cognitive decline mandates that patients and their families be routinely counseled with respect to issues such as durable powers of attorney and living wills (Hirsh 1990). It may be helpful to deal explicitly (although not immediately after diagnosis) with the patient's feelings about participation in experimental treatment protocols and issues related to institutional care, should that become necessary.

Institutionalization

Long-term care is the single most expensive item of health services used by persons with dementia. There is evidence that treatment of excess disability can postpone or reduce the rate of institutionalization. Mittelman et al. (1996) randomly assigned spousal caregivers of persons with AD to either a treatment of individual and family counseling or a control group of routine support. The rate of institutionalization in the intervention group was less than half that in the control group during the first year. In long-term follow-up from baseline, the median time to nursing home placement was 329 days longer for the intervention group than the control group. The intervention consisted of six sessions over four months focusing on physical assistance and emotional support for both the caregiver and the family. The family was prompted to give respite to the spouse, and both the spouse and family were advised and helped to use local resources. In general, this and other studies (Hu, Huang, and Cartwright 1986; Hay and Ernst 1987) suggest that community-based care is effective at reducing both caregiver burden and institutionalization. It is not clear whether the total costs of effective home-based care are actually any less than institutionalization. In addition, for some caregivers, preventing institutionalization may worsen, not improve their overall quality of life. Sensitivity to the needs of caregivers and appropriate recommendation and support of nursing home placement is thus frequently an appropriate and important nonpharmacologic intervention.

Discussion

Excess disability is an important aspect of dementia that profoundly influences quality of life and use of health services. The presentations and prevalence of the forms of excess disability are highly variable. A variety of psychopharmacologic and behavioral treatments have at least a modest impact on reducing excess disability. Psychotropic medications must be used cautiously with careful monitoring to avoid iatrogenic excess disability. Geriatric psychiatrists and other behavioral specialists play an important role in implementing and educating other clinicians about the appropriate use and integration of psychotropic medications and behavioral therapies. It is imperative always to include the family as part of the treatment plan. Focus on caregivers may have the greatest impact on reducing excess disability.

Currently, issues of cost containment dominate the policy debate regarding the use of health services for persons with dementia and their caregivers. Outcomes should consider more than survival or institutionalization. Individuals with dementia have residual strengths that can be augmented. Quality-of-life assessment can become a useful tool in evaluating the effectiveness of treatment for excess disability, if not the treatment of dementia in general. Outcome indicators for successful treatment of excess disability should thus include quality of life and be deliberately chosen to reflect problems of social concern and for which improvement is sought.

Clinical Conclusions

The treatment of a dementia syndrome is a complex but potentially rewarding endeavor. Several principles should be borne in mind:

— Relatively safe cholinesterase inhibitors are available. These agents may temporarily improve cognitive symptoms and, more likely, slow the progression of AD and possibly other dementias.
— Although a dementia syndrome may not be reversible, it is treatable. A variety of profound, debilitating behavioral syndromes often accompany dementing syndromes and are responsible for most of the distress experienced by caregivers. Presence of these syndromes predicts institutionalization and the need for more frequent use of nursing care in the institutions.
— Psychotic symptoms including delusions and hallucinations occur in a large number of persons with dementia. When persistent, impairing function, and not reversible by alleviating identifiable environmental or medical conditions, treatment involves the judicious use of modest doses of neuroleptics.
— Agitation is a major cluster of problematic behaviors. A variety of agents, including neuroleptics, benzodiazepines, other sedative-hypnotics, and anticonvulsants, have been used with modest success. It is currently not possible to predict which patients will benefit from which agent. Pharmacologic treatment should include empiric trials defined by target symptoms and goals with systematic monitoring that balances improvement with side effects. Nonpharmacologic interventions are particularly important in managing agitation in dementia.
— Regardless of the associated behavioral disturbance, treatment should include counseling of the patient and family, formal psychoeducational interventions, environmental modifications, and assessment of the need for legal consultation.

REFERENCES

Albert, S.M., C. Del Castillo-Castaneda, M. Sano, et al. 1996. Quality of life in patients with Alzheimer's disease as reported by patient proxies. *Journal of the American Geriatrics Society* 44:1342–47.

Avorn, J., S.B. Soumerai, D.E. Everitt, et al. 1992. A randomized trial of a program to reduce the use of psychoactive drugs in nursing homes. *New England Journal of Medicine* 327:168–73.

Baltes, M.M., T. Kindermann, R. Reisenzein, et al. 1987. Further observational data on the behavioral and social world of institutions for the aged. *Psychology and Aging* 2: 390–403.

Baltes, P.B., and M.M. Baltes. 1993. Psychological perspectives on successful aging: The model of selective optimization with compensation. In *Successful Aging*, edited by P.B. Baltes and M.M. Baltes. Cambridge: Cambridge University Press, pp. 1–34.

Bartus, R.T., R.L. Dean, B. Beer, et al. 1982. The cholinergic hypothesis of geriatric memory dysfunction. *Science* 217:408–17.

Bassiony, M.M., M.S. Steinberg, A. Warren, et al. 2000. Delusions and hallucinations in Alzheimer's disease: Prevalence and clinical correlates. *International Journal of Geriatric Psychiatry* 15:99–107.

Bhana, N., and C.M. Spencer. 2000. Risperidone: A review of its use in the management of the behavioral and psychological symptoms of dementia. *Drugs and Aging* 16:451–71.

Birge, S.J. 2000. HRT and cognition: What the evidence shows. *OBG Management* 12 (10):40–59.

Blazer, D., D. Hughes, and L. George. 1987. The epidemiology of depression in an elderly community population. *Gerontologist* 27:281–87.

Brawley, E.C. 1997. *Designing for Alzheimer's Disease: Strategies for Creating Better Care Environments.* New York: John Wiley & Sons.

Buckwalter, K.C., L. Gernder, F. Kohout, et al. 1999. A nursing intervention to decrease depression in family caregivers of persons with dementia. *Archives of Psychiatric Nursing* 13:80–88.

Bungener, C., R. Jouvent, and C. Derouesne. 1996. Affective disturbances in Alzheimer's disease. *Journal of the American Geriatrics Society* 44:1006–71.

Burns, A., M. Rossor, J. Hecker, et al. 1999. The effects of donepezil in Alzheimer's disease: Results from a multinational trial. *Dementia and Geriatric Cognitive Disorders* 10: 237–44.

Cahn, R., P. Charles, M.G. Borzeix, et al. 1988. Effect of acetyl-L-carnitine on a step-down response in post-ischemic gerbils. In *Senile Dementias*, edited by A. Gnolie, J. Cahn, N. Lessen, et al. Paris: John Libbey Eurotext, pp. 379–82.

Calkin, P.A., M.E. Kunik, C.A. Orengo, et al. 1997. Tolerability of clonzepam in demented and non-demented geropsychiatric patients. *International Journal of Geriatric Psychiatry* 12:745–49.

Canter, N.L., M. Hallett, and J.H. Growdon. 1982. Lecithin does not affect EEG spectral analysis of P300 in Alzheimer's disease. *Neurology* 32:1260–66.

Cantillon, M., R. Brunswick, D. Molina, et al. 1996. Buspirone vs. haloperidol: A double-blind trial for agitation in a nursing home population with Alzheimer's disease. *American Journal of Geriatric Psychiatry* 4:263–67.

Carbone, J.R. 2000. The neuroleptic malignant and serotonin syndromes. *Emergency Medicine Clinics of North America* 18 (2):317–25.

Chain, D.P., K. Ighanian, and F. Boon. 2000. Individual and combined manipulation of muscarinic, NMDA, and benzodiazepine receptor activity in the water maze task: Implications for a rat model of Alzheimer dementia. *Behavioural Brain Research* 111: 125–37.

Chan-Palay, V. 1992. Depression and senile dementia of the Alzheimer type: A role for moclobomide. *Psychopharmacology* 106 (Suppl.):S137–39.

Chappell, N.L., and M. Novak. 1994. Caring for institutionalized elders: Stress among nursing assistants. *Journal of Applied Gerontology* 13:299–315.

Chiverton, P., and E.D. Caine. 1989. Education to assist spouses in coping with Alzheimer's disease: A controlled trial. *Journal of the American Geriatrics Society* 37:593–98.

Christensen, D.B., and W.R. Benfield. 1998. Alprazolam as an alternative to low-dose haloperidol in older, cognitively impaired nursing facility patients. *Journal of the American Geriatrics Society* 46:620–25.

Christie, J.E., A. Shering, J. Ferguson, et al. 1981. Physostigmine and arecoline: Effects of intravenous infusions in Alzheimer presenile dementia. *British Journal of Psychiatry.* 138:46–50.

Cohen, D., D. Luchins, C. Eisdorfer, et al. 1990. Caring for relatives with Alzheimer's disease: The mental health risks to spouses, adult children, and other family caregivers. *Behavior, Health, and Aging* 1:171–82.

Cohen-Mansfield, J., and N. Billig. 1986. Agitated behaviors in the elderly: I. A conceptual review. *Journal of the American Geriatrics Society* 34:711–21.

Cohen-Mansfield, J., M.S. Marx, and A.S. Rosenthal. 1989. A description of agitation in a nursing home. *Journal of Gerontology* 44:77–84.

Corey-Bloom, J., R. Anand, J. Veach, et al. 1998. A randomized trial evaluating the efficacy and safety of ENA 713 (rivastigmine tartrate), a new acetylcholinesterase inhibitor, in patients with mild to moderately severe Alzheimer's disease. *International Journal of Geriatric Psychopharmacology* 1:55–65.

Coulter, D.L., and R.J. Allen. 1980. Secondary hyperammonaemia: A possible mechanism for valproate encephalopathy [letter]. *Lancet.* 1 (8181):1310–11.

Cumming, R.G. 1988. Epidemiology of medication-related falls and fractures in the elderly. *Drugs and Aging* 12:43–53.

Cummings, J.L. 2000. Cholinesterase inhibitors: A new class of psychotropic compounds. *American Journal of Psychiatry* 157 (1):4–15.

Cummings, J.L., B. Miller, M.A. Hill, et al. 1987. Neuropsychiatric aspects of multi-infarct dementia and dementia of the Alzheimer type. *Archives of Neurology* 44:389–93.

Davidson, M., R.G. Stern, L.M. Bierer, et al. 1991. Cholinergic strategies in the treatment of Alzheimer's disease. *Acta Psychiatrica Scandinavica* 366 (Suppl.):S47–51.

De Deyn, P.P., K. Rabheru, A. Rasmussen, et al. 1999. A randomized trial of risperidone, placebo, and haloperidol for behavioral symptoms of dementia. *Neurology* 53:946–55.

Deutsch, L.H., and B.W. Rovner. 1991. Agitation and other noncognitive abnormalities in Alzheimer's disease. *Psychiatric Clinics of North America* 14:341–51.

Devarajan, S., and S.M. Dursun. 2000. Aggression in dementia with lamotrigine treatment *American Journal of Psychiatry.* 157:1178.

Doody, R.S., J.C. Stevens, C. Becn, et al. 2001. Practice parameter: Management of dementia (an evidence-based review) report of the quality standards subcommittee of the American Academy of Neurology. *Neurology* 56:1154–66.

Drevers, W.C., and E.H. Rubin. 1989. Psychotic symptoms and the longitudinal course of senile dementia of the Alzheimer type. *Biological Psychiatry* 25:39–48.

Eagger Sarah, A., R. Levy, and B.J. Sahakian. 1991. Tacrine in Alzheimer's disease. *Lancet* 337:889–92.

Ebly, E.M., D.B. Hogan, and T.S. Fung. 1997. Potential adverse outcomes of psychotropic and narcotic drug use in seniors. *Journal of Clinical Epidemiology* 50:657–63.

Eto, F., I. Saotome, T. Furuichi, et al. 1998. Effects of long-term use of benzodiazepines on gait and standing balance in the elderly. *Annals of the New York Academy of Sciences* 860:543–45.

Expert Consensus Panel for Agitation in Dementia. 1998. Treatment of agitation in older persons with dementia. *Postgraduate Medicine* April, Special No.:1–88.

Farlow, M., S.I. Gracon, L.A. Hershey, et al. 1992. A controlled trial of tacrine in Alzheimer's disease. The Tacrine Study Group. *Journal of the American Medical Association* 268:2523–29.

Fastbom, J., Y. Forsell, and B. Winblad. 1998. Benzodiazepines may have protective effects against Alzheimer disease. *Alzheimer Disease and Associated Disorders* 12:14–17.

Fischer, P. 1995. Serotonin syndrome in the elderly after antidepressive monotherapy [letter]. *Journal of Clinical Psychopharmacology* 15:440–42.

Fitz, A.G., and L. Teri. 1994. Depression, cognition, and functional ability in patients with Alzheimer's Disease. *Journal of the American Geriatrics Society* 42:186–91.

Forsell, Y., A. Jorm, and B. Winblad. 1994. Association of age, sex, cognitive dysfunction and disability with major depressive symptoms in an elderly sample. *American Journal of Psychiatry* 151:1600–1605.

Gilley, D.W., R.S. Wilson, L.A. Beckett, et al. 1997. Psychotic symptoms and physically aggressive behavior in Alzheimer's disease. *Journal of the American Geriatrics Society* 45:1074–79.

Goetz, C.G., L.M. Blasucci, S. Leurgans, et al. 2000. Olanzapine and clozapine: Comparative effects on motor function in hallucinating PD patients. A randomized controlled trial. *Neurology* 55:789–84.

Goldberg, R.J., and M. Huk. 1992. Serotonin syndrome from trazodone and buspirone [letter]. *Psychosomatics* 33:235–36.

Goldenberg, G., K. Kahaner, N. Basavaraju, et al. 1998. Gabapentin for disruptive behaviour in an elderly demented patient. *Drugs and Aging* 13:183–84.

Grossman, F. 1998. A review of anticonvulsants in treating agitated demented elderly patients. *Pharmacotherapy* 18:600–606.

Guillozet, A.L., J.F. Smiley, D.C. Mash, et al. 1997. Butyrylcholinesterase in the life cycle of amyloid plaques. *Annals of Neurology* 42:909–18.

Hay, J.W., and R.L. Ernst. 1987. The economic costs of Alzheimer's disease. *American Journal of Public Health* 77:1169–75.

Hegel, M., J. Barrett, and T. Oxman. 2000. Training United States therapists in problem-solving treatment of depression in primary care (PST-PC): Lessons learned from the Treatment Effectiveness Project. *Families, Systems and Health* 18 (4):423–35.

Hepburn, K.W., J. Tornatore, B. Center, et al. 2001. Dementia family caregiver training: Affecting beliefs about caregiving and caregiver outcomes. *Journal of the American Geriatrics Society* 49:450–57.

Hiersemenzel, R., B. Dietrick, and W.M. Hermann. 1988. Therapeutic and EEG effects of acetyl-L-carnitine in elderly outpatients with mild to moderate cognitive decline: Results of two double-blind placebo controlled studies. In *Senile Dementias*, edited by A. Agnoli, J. Cahn, N. Lassen, et al. Paris: John Libbey Eurotext, pp. 427–31.

Hirsh, H.L. 1990. Legal and ethical considerations in dealing with Alzheimer's disease. *Legal Medicine* 261–26.

Hollander, E., M. Davidson, R.C. Mohs, et al. 1987. RS 86 in the treatment of Alzheimer's disease: Cognitive and biological effects. *Biological Psychiatry* 22:1067–78.

Holmes, D., M.G. Ory, and J.A. Teresi (Eds.). 1994. Special dementia care: Research, policy, and practice issues. *Alzheimer's Disease and Related Disorders* 8 (Suppl.):S1–433.
Honjo, H., Y. Ogino, K. Tanaka, et al. 1993. An effect of conjugated estrogen to cognitive impairment in women with senile dementia-Alzheimer's type: A placebo-controlled double-blind study. *Journal of the Japanese Menopause Society* 1:167–71.
Hu, T., L. Huang, and W.S. Cartwright. 1986. Evaluation of the costs of caring for the senile demented elderly: A pilot study. *Gerontologist* 26:158–63.
Jost, B.C., and G.T. Grossberg. 1996. The evolution of psychiatric symptoms in Alzheimer's disease: A natural history study. *Journal of the American Geriatrics Society* 44: 1078–81.
Katz, I.R., D.V. Jeste, J.E. Mintzer, et al. 1999. Risperidone Study Group. Comparison of risperidone and placebo for psychosis and behavioral disturbances associated with dementia: A randomized, double-blind trial. *Journal of Clinical Psychiatry* 60:107–15.
Kimura, T., and H. Yoshida. 1994. Clinical study of neuroleptic malignant syndrome in demented patients: Examination of our case and reported cases. *No To Shinkei* 46: 859–62.
Knapp, M.J., D.S. Knopman, P.R. Solomon, et al., for the Tacrine Study Group. 1994. A 30-week randomized controlled trial of high-dose tacrine in patients with Alzheimer's disease. *Journal of the American Medical Association* 271:985–91.
Knopman D.S. 2001. An overview of common non-Alzheimer dementias. *Clinics in Geriatric Medicine* 17:281–301.
Komatsu, M., S. Kodama, S. Yokoyama, et al. 1987. Valproate-associated hyperammonemia and DL-carnitine supplement. *Kobe Journal of Medical Sciences* 33 (3):81–87.
Lanctot, K.L., T.S. Best, N. Mittmann, et al. 1998. Efficacy and safety of neuroleptics in behavioral disorders associated with dementia. *Journal of Clinical Psychiatry* 59: 550–61.
Lantz, M.S. 20001. Serotonin syndrome. A common but often unrecognized psychiatric condition. *Geriatrics* 56 (1):52–53.
Larson, E.B., B.V. Reifler, S.M. Sumi, et al. 1985. Diagnostic evaluation of 200 elderly outpatients with suspected dementia. *Journal of Gerontology* 40:536–43.
Le Bars, P.L., M. Kieser, and K.Z. Itil. 2000. A 26-week analysis of a double-blind, placebo-controlled trial of the ginkgo biloba extract EGb 761 in dementia. *Dementia and Geriatric Cognitive Disorders* 11:230–37.
Lebert, F., F. Pasquier, and H. Petit. 1994. Behavioral effects of trazodone in Alzheimer's disease. *Journal of Clinical Psychiatry* 55:536–38.
Levine, J., and B.A. Lawlor. 1991. Family counseling and legal issues in Alzheimer's disease. *Psychiatric Clinics of North America* 14 (2):385–96.
Levkoff, S.E., B. Liptzin, P.D. Cleary, et al. 1996. Subsyndromal delirium. *American Journal of Geriatric Psychiatry* 4:320–29.
Levy, M.L., J.L. Cummings, L.A. Fairbanks, et al. 1993. Longitudinal assessment of symptoms of depression, agitation, and psychosis in 181 patients with Alzheimer's disease. *American Journal of Psychiatry* 153:1438–43.
Lewin, L.M., and D.A. Landervold. 1990. Behavioral analysis of separation individuation conflict in the spouse of an Alzheimer's disease patient. *The Gerontologist* 30:703–5.
Lokensgard, J.R., C.C. Chao, G. Gekker, et al. 1998. Benzodiazepines, glia, and HIV-1 neuropathogenesis. *Molecular Neurobiology* 18:23–33.
Lott, A.D., S.L. McElroy, and M.A. Keys. 1995. Valproate in the treatment of behav-

ioral agitation in elderly patients with dementia. *Journal of Neuropsychiatry and Clinical Neurosciences* 7:314–19.

Lyketsos, C., J.M. Sheppard, C.D. Steele, et al. 2000a. Randomized, placebo-controlled, double-blind clinical trial of sertraline in the treatment of depression complicating Alzheimer's disease: Initial results from the Depression in Alzheimer's Disease Study. *American Journal of Psychiatry* 157:1686–89.

Lyketsos, C., M. Steinberg, J.T. Tschanz, et al. 2000b. Mental and behavioral disturbances in dementia: Findings from the Cache County Study on Memory in Aging. *American Journal of Psychiatry* 157:708–14.

Magai, C., G. Kennedy, C.I. Cohen, et al. 2000. A controlled clinical trial of sertraline in the treatment of depression in nursing home patients with late-stage Alzheimer's disease. *American Journal of Geriatric Psychiatry* 8:66–74.

Magruder, K.M., H.C. Schulberg, and T.E. Oxman. 1996. Measurement and meaning of disablement in primary care [editorial]. *International Journal of Psychiatry in Medicine* 26:1–8.

Mason, P.J., V.A. Morris, and T.J. Balcezak TJ. 2000. Serotonin syndrome. Presentation of 2 cases and review of the literature. *Medicine* 79 (4):201–9.

McAllister, T.W., and R. Powers. 1994. Approaches to the treatment of dementing illness. In *Dementia: Presentations, Differential Diagnosis, and Nosology*, edited by V.O. Emery and T.E. Oxman. Baltimore: Johns Hopkins University Press, pp. 355–83.

McCallion, P., R.W. Toseland, and K. Freeman. 1999. An evaluation of a family visit education program. *Journal of the American Geriatrics Society* 47:203–14.

McKeith, I., T. Del Ser, P.F. Spano, et al. 2000. Efficacy of rivastigmine in dementia with Lewy bodies: A randomised, double-blind, placebo-controlled international study. *Lancet* 356:2031–36.

Mendez, M.F., R.J. Martin, K.A. Smyth, et al. 1990. Psychiatric symptoms associated with Alzheimer's disease. *Journal of Neuropsychiatry and Clinical Neurosciences* 2 (1):28–33.

Merriam, A.E., M.K. Aronson, P. Daston, et al. 1988. The psychiatric symptoms of Alzheimer's disease. *Journal of the American Geriatrics Society* 36:7–12.

Messmer, K., and G.P. Reynolds. 1998. Increased peripheral benzodiazepine binding sites in the brain of patients with Huntington's disease. *Neuroscience Letters* 241:53–56.

Mesulam, M.M., and C. Geula. 1994. Butyrylcholinesterase reactivity differentiates the amyloid plaques of aging from those of dementia. *Annals of Neurology* 36:722–27.

Mittleman, M.S., S.G. Ferrus, E. Shulman, et al. 1996. A family intervention to delay nursing home placement of patients with Alzheimer disease: A randomized controlled trial. *Journal of the American Medical Association* 276 (21):1756–57.

Miyaji, H., S. Ito, T. Azuma, et al. 1997. Effects of helicobacter pylori eradication therapy on hyperammonaemia in patients with liver cirrhosis. *Gut* 40:726–30.

Mohs, R.C., and K.L. Davis. 1987. The experimental pharmacology of Alzheimer's disease and related dementias. In *Psychopharmacology: The Third Generation of Progress*, edited by H.Y. Meltzer. New York: Raven Press, pp. 921–28.

Moritz, D.J., S.V. Kasl, and A.M. Ostfeld. 1992. The health impact of living with a cognitively impaired elderly spouse. *Journal of Aging and Health* 4:244–67.

Mortimer, J.A., B. Ebbitt, S.P. Jun, et al. 1992. Predictors of cognitive and functional progression in patients with probable Alzheimer's disease. *Neurology* 42:1689–96.

Mulnard, R.A., C.W. Cotman, C. Kawas, et al., for the Alzheimer's Disease Cooperative Study. 2000. Estrogen replacement therapy for treatment of mild to moderate Alzheimer disease. *Journal of the American Medical Association* 283:1007–15.

Mulsant, B.H., and G.S. Zubenko. 1994. Clinical, neuropathologic, and neurochemical correlates of depression and psychosis in primary dementia. In *Dementia: Presentations, Differential Diagnosis, and Nosology*, edited by V.O.B. Emery and T.E. Oxman. Baltimore: Johns Hopkins University Press, pp. 336–52.

Nezu, C., A. Nezu, and P. Arean. 1991. Assertiveness and Problem-Solving Training for mildly mentally retarded persons with dual diagnoses. *Research in Developmental Disabilities.* 12:371–86.

Niederehe, G.T., and T.E. Oxman. 1994. The spectrum of dementias: Construct and nosologic validity. In *Dementia: Presentations, Differential Diagnosis, and Nosology*, edited by V.O.B. Emery and T.E. Oxman. Baltimore: Johns Hopkins University Press, pp. 19–45.

Nordgren, I., and B. Holmstedt. 1988. Metrifonate: A review. In *Current Research in Alzheimer Therapy*, edited by E. Giacobini and E. Becker. New York: Taylor and Francis, pp. 281–88.

Oken, B.S., D.M. Storzbach, and J.A. Kaye. 1998. The efficacy of Ginkgo biloba on cognitive function in Alzheimer disease. *Archives of Neurology* 55:1409–15.

Oxman, T.E. 1996. Antidepressants and cognitive impairment in the elderly. *Journal of Clinical Psychiatry* 57 (Suppl. 5):S38–44.

Paganini-Hill, A., and V.W. Henderson. 1994. Estrogen deficiency and the risk of Alzheimer's disease in women. *American Journal of Epidemiology* 140:256–22.

Paganini-Hill, A., and V.W. Henderson. 1996. Estrogen replacement therapy and risk of Alzheimer's disease. *Archives of Internal Medicine* 156:2213–17.

Passaro, A., S. Volpato, F. Romagnoni, et al. 2000. Benzodiazepines with different half-life and falling in a hospitalized population: The GIFA study. Gruppo Italiano di Farmacovigilanza nell'aAnziano. *Journal of Clinical Epidemiology* 53 (12):1222–29.

Passeri, M., M. Iannuccilli, G. Ciotti, et al. 1988. Mental impairment in aging: Selection of patients, methods of evaluation and therapeutic possibilities of acetyl-L-carnitine. *International Journal of Clinical Pharmacology Research* 8:367–76.

Perry, E.K., B.E. Tomlinson, G. Blessed, et al. 1978. Correlation of cholinergic abnormalities with senile plaques and mental test scores in senile dementia. *British Medical Journal* 2:1457–59.

Pierfitte, C., G. Macouillard, M. Thicoipe, et al. 2001. Benzodiazepines and hip fractures in elderly people: Case-control study. *British Medical Journal* 322 (7288):704–8.

Polc, P. 1995. Involvement of endogenous benzodiazepine receptor ligands in brain disorders: Therapeutic potential for benzodiazepine antagonists. *Medical Hypotheses* 44: 439–46.

Porsteinsson, A.P., P.N. Tariot, R. Erb, et al. 2001. Placebo-controlled study of divalproex sodium for agitation in dementia. *American Journal of Geriatric Psychiatry* 9: 58–66.

Potter, J.F. 1993. Comprehensive geriatric assessment in the outpatient setting: Population characteristics and factors influencing outcome. *Experimental Gerontology* 28: 447–57.

Proctor, R., A. Burns, H.S. Powell, et al. 1999. Behavioural management in nursing and residential homes: A randomized controlled trial. *Lancet* 354 (9712):26–29.

Rabins, P.V., and M.F. Folstein. 1982. Delirium and dementia: Diagnostic criteria and fatality rates. *British Journal of Psychiatry* 140:149–53.
Rabins, P.V., N.L. Mace, and M.J. Lucas. 1982. The impact of dementia on the family. *Journal of the American Medical Association* 248:333–35.
Raby, W.N. 1997. Carnitine for valproic acid-induced hyperammonemia [letter]. *American Journal of Psychiatry* 154 (8):1168–69.
Radebaugh, T.S., N. Buckholtz, and Z.S. Khachaturian (Eds.). 1996. Behavioral approaches to the treatment of Alzheimer's disease: Research strategies. *International Psychogeriatrics* 8 (Suppl. 1):S5–144.
Rapoport, M.J., R. van Reekum, M. Freedman, et al. 2001. Relationship of psychosis to aggression, apathy and function in dementia. *International Journal of Geriatric Psychiatry* 16:123–30.
Ray, W.A., J.A. Taylor, K.G. Meador, et al. 1993. Reducing antipsychotic drug use in nursing homes: A controlled trial of provider education. *Archives of Internal Medicine* 153 (6):713–21.
Reifler, B., and K. Sherrill. 1990. Dementias: Reversible and irreversible. In *Review of Psychiatry*, vol. 9, edited by A. Tasman, S. M. Goldfinger, and C. A. Kaufman. Washington, D.C.: American Psychiatric Press, pp. 220–31.
Reifler, B.V., L. Teri, M. Raskind, et al. 1989. Double-blind trial of imipramine in Alzheimer's disease patients with and without depression. *American Journal of Psychiatry* 146:45–49.
Reisberg, B., E. Franssen, S.G. Sclan, et al. 1989. Stage specific incidence of potentially remediable behavioral symptoms in aging and Alzheimer's disease: A study of 120 patients using the BEHAVE-AD. *Bulletin of Clinical Neuroscience* 54:95–112.
Robert, B.L., and D.L. Algase. 1988. Victims of Alzheimer's disease and the environment. *Nursing Clinics of North America* 23:83–93.
Rogers, S.L., M.R. Farlow, R.S. Doody, et al. 1998. A 24-week, double-blind, placebo-controlled trial of donepezil in patients with Alzheimer's disease for the Donepezil Study Group. *Neurology* 50:136–45.
Rosen, J., and G.S. Zubenko. 1991. Emergence of psychosis and depression in the longitudinal evaluation of Alzheimer's disease. *Biological Psychiatry* 29:224–32.
Roth, M., C.Q. Mountjoy, and R. Amrein. 1996. Moclobemide in elderly patients with cognitive decline and depression: An international double-blind, placebo-controlled trial. *British Journal of Psychiatry* 68:149–57.
Rovner, B.W., C.D. Steele, Y. Shumuely, et al. 1996. A randomized trial of dementia care in nursing homes. *Journal of the American Geriatrics Society* 44:7–13.
Rubin, E.H., J.C. Morris, M. Storandt, et al. 1987. Behavioral changes in patients with mild senile dementia of the Alzheimer's type. *Psychiatry Research* 21:55–62.
Sakauye, K.M., C.J. Camp, and P.A. Ford. 1993. Effects of buspirone on agitation associated with dementia. *American Journal of Geriatric Psychiatry* 1:82–84.
Sarter, M. 1991. Taking stock of cognition enhancers. *Tip Reviews* 12:456–61.
Sarter, M. 1994. Neuronal mechanisms of the attentional dysfunctions in senile dementia and schizophrenia: Two sides of the same coin? *Psychopharmacology* 114:539–50.
Schmid, A.H. 1990. Dementia, related disorders, and old age: Psychodynamic dimensions in diagnosis and treatment. *American Journal of Psychoanalysis* 50:253–62.
Schneider, L.S., V.E. Pollock, and S.A. Lyness. 1990. A metaanalysis of controlled tri-

als of neuroleptic treatment in dementia. *Journal of the American Geriatrics Society* 38: 553–63.

Schneider, L.S., P.N. Tariot, C.G. Lyketsos, et al. 2001. National Institute of Mental Health Clinical Antipsychotic Trials of Intervention Effectiveness (CATIE): Alzheimer Disease Trial Methodology. *American Journal of Geriatric Psychiatry* 9:346–60.

Schulz, R., A.T. O'Brien, J. Bookwala, et al. 1995. Psychiatric and physical morbidity effects of dementia: Prevalence, correlates, and causes. *Gerontologist* 35:771–91.

Schwab, M. F. Roder, S. Ammon, et al. 1999. Increased number of hip fractures [letter; comment]. *Lancet* 353 (9170):2160.

Stern, Y., R. Mayeuex, M. Sano, et al. 1987. Predictors of disease course in patients with probable Alzheimer's disease. *Neurology* 37:1649–53.

Street, J.S., W.S. Clark, K.S. Gannon, et al. 2000. HGEU Study Group. Olanzapine treatment of psychotic and behavioral symptoms in patients with Alzheimer disease in nursing care facilities: A double-blind, randomized, placebo-controlled trial. *Archives of General Psychiatry* 57:968–76.

Summers, W.K., L.V. Majovski, G.M. Marsch, et al. 1986. Oral tetrahydroaminoacridine in long-term treatment of senile dementia, Alzheimer type. *New England Journal of Medicine* 315:1241–45.

Swearer, J.M., D.A. Drachman, B.F. O'Donnell, et al. 1988. Troublesome and disruptive behaviors in dementia: Relationships to diagnosis and disease severity. *Journal of the American Geriatrics Society* 36:784–90.

Tariot, P.N., L.S. Schneider, and I.R. Katz. 1995. Anticonvulsant and other non-neuroleptic treatment of agitation in dementia. *Journal of Geriatric Psychiatry and Neurology* 8 (Suppl. 1):S28–39.

Tariot, P.N., L.J. Jakimovich, R. Erb, et al. 1999. Withdrawal from controlled carbazepine therapy followed by further carbamazepine treatment in patients with dementia. *Journal of Clinical Psychiatry* 60:684–89.

Tariot, P.N., P.R. Solomon, J.C. Morris, et al. 2000. A five-month, randomized, placebo-controlled trial of galantamine in AD. *Neurology* 54:2269–76.

Teri, L., and D. Gallagher-Thompson. 1991. Cognitive-behavioral interventions for treatment of depression in Alzheimer's patients. *The Gerontologist* 31:413–26.

Teri, L., E.B. Larson, and B.V. Reifler. 1988. Behavioral disturbance in dementia of the Alzheimer's type. *Journal of the American Geriatrics Society* 36:1–6.

Teri, L., R.G. Logsdon, J. Uomoto, et al. 1997. Behavioral treatment of depression in dementia patients: A controlled clinical trial. *Journals of Gerontology Series B, Psychological Sciences and Social Sciences* 52:P159–66.

Thapa, P.B., P. Gideon, R.L. Fought, et al. 1995. Psychotropic drugs and risk of recurrent falls in ambulatory nursing home residents. *American Journal of Epidemiology* 142: 202–11.

Tune, L.E., C. Steele, and T. Cooper. 1991. Neuroleptic drugs in the management of behavioral symptoms of Alzheimer's disease. *Psychiatric Clinics of North America* 14 (2): 353–73.

U.S. Congress, Office of Technology Assessment. 1985. *Technology and Aging in America*, Publication No. OTA-B A-264. Washington, D.C.: U.S. Government Printing Office.

Veld, B.A., A. Ruitenberg, A. Hofman, et al. 2001. Nonsteroidal antiinflammatory drugs and the risk of Alzheimer's disease. *New England Journal of Medicine* 345:1515–21.

Vitaliano, P.P., J. Russo, H.M. Young, et al. 1991. Predictors of burden in spouse caregivers of individuals with Alzheimer's disease. *Psychology and Aging* 6:392–402.

Wang, P.S. R.L. Bohn, R.J. Glynn, et al. 2001. Hazardous benzodiazepine regimens in the elderly: Effects of half-life, dosage, and duration on risk of hip fracture. *American Journal of Psychiatry* 158 (6):892–98.

Weggen, S., J.L. Eriksen, P. Das, et al. 2001. A subset of NSAIDs lower amyloidogenic A-beta42 independently of cyclooxygenase activity. *Nature* 414:212–16.

Winger, J., V. Schirm, and D. Stewart. 1987. Aggressive behavior in long-term care. *Journal of Psychosocial Nursing Mental Health Services* 25:28–33.

Wragg, R.E., and D.V. Jeste. 1989. Overview of depression and psychosis in Alzheimer's disease. *American Journal of Psychiatry* 146:577–87.

Zaccara, G.R., Campostrini, M. Paganini, et al. 1987. Long-term treatment with sodium valproate: Monitoring of venous ammonia concentrations and adverse effects. *Therapeutic Drug Monitoring* 9 (1):34–40.

Zubenko, G.S., J. Rosen, R.A. Sweet, et al. 1992. Impact of psychiatric hospitalization on behavioral complications of Alzheimer's disease. *American Journal of Psychiatry* 149:1484–91.

CHAPTER NINETEEN

The Spectra of the Dementias

V. Olga B. Emery, Ph.D.,
and Thomas E. Oxman, M.D.

This volume has advanced a spectrum approach to the dementias, whereby each dementing disorder has been understood as part of a spectrum or distribution of varied but related presentations that constitute continua on various parameters. The Alzheimer-type dementias, vascular dementias, depressive dementias and nondepressive pseudodementias, frontotemporal dementias, and other cortical and frontosubcortical dementias have been discussed within the context of a spectrum framework. The ambiguous transitions between normal aging and the dementias, cortical and subcortical dementias, diffuse/generalized diseases and focal diseases, dementias and pseudodementias have been examined from the perspectives of a continuity paradigm. Despite an ever-increasing interest in the boundaries between normal aging and the dementias, as well as among the various categories of dementia, understanding of the relationships between these constructs has been inadequate. The distinguished authors of this volume have used empirical, clinical, theoretical, and nosological material to illuminate the complex interrelationships between different disease categories. There also has been delineation of the hierarchical relationships between overarching categories of dementias and their subtypes. In addition to using the spectrum concept as an organizational principle for this volume, the authors have developed nosology into a critical tool for furthering explanation and treatment of the dementias. This final chapter uses issues of presentations and differential diagnosis of dementia to challenge current nosology, highlights some of the explicit and implicit challenges to current concepts made by our pioneering authors, and underscores paradigm shifts that have been developed as part of this volume. There might be valid objections to some of our suggestions and challenges; our goal in this chapter is heuristic in that we wish to provoke others to address and improve the validity and reliability of current paradigms and nosology that guide, but also circumscribe, our comprehension and treatment of the spectra of the dementias.

Normal Aging

Life Expectancy and Life Span

Normal aging can be conceptualized as the orderly or typical progression of changes in the organism and its behavior that occur as a function of age (see chap. 1). It has been estimated that in the 4500 years from the Bronze Age to the year 1900, human life expectancy increased twenty-seven years, and that in the significantly shorter period from 1900 to 2000, life expectancy yet again increased by at least that much (Rowe and Kahn 1998; National Academy on an Aging Society 2000).

At the turn of the twentieth century in the United States, for example, about 4% of the population was over 65 years of age, whereas today that proportion has risen close to 14%. Life expectancy from birth in the United States has increased from 47 years in 1900 to more than 76 years today (Rowe and Kahn 1998; National Academy on an Aging Society 2000). And worldwide, it is projected that the United States and other developed nations will continue "graying" well into the twenty-first century.

The term *life span* differs from life expectancy in that life span refers to a genetic characteristic of a given species and can be defined as the maximal age or outer limit of life for any given species (Cunningham and Brookbank 1988). Despite the continued increase in human life expectancy in developed nations, it does not appear that genetically determined human life span has changed during the same time intervals; the maximal age or outer limit of human life span appears to remain at about 120 years of age (Cutler 1976; Cunningham and

Brookbank 1988; Rowe and Kahn 1998). For each species, genetically programmed biological aging appears to play a significant role in many bodily changes associated with aging. As life expectancy moves closer to life span in humans, survivorship has improved through lowered numbers of deaths caused by diseases, accidents, and infant mortality; this has resulted in the "rectangularization" of the survivorship curve (Cunningham and Brookbank 1988). For each species, one can plot the logarithm of the probability of death as a function of chronological age; the slope of this line is called the age-specific death rate. This mathematical expression was first introduced by Gompertz in 1825; currently, the Gompertz function illustrates that in the human species, after age 35, the probability of death doubles every seven years (Sacher 1975; Cutler 1976; Cunningham and Brookbank 1988; Rowe and Kahn 1998).

Aging in the Context of Entropy

Normal aging occurs in a number of combined and interacting contexts, including those of personal variables, biological variables, sociocultural variables, species-programmed genetic variables, and variables from the domain of physics. For example, our comprehension of processes of normal and abnormal aging can be informed by the Second Law of Thermodynamics pertaining to entropy, whereby the maintenance of organized systems becomes increasingly improbable across time. Organized systems, such as a human organism, tend toward disorganization with time in the context of molecular randomness and other parameters of entropy. One view of aging might be that aging involves an ever-increasing energy shortage or crisis, as energy required to maintain an organized system gets used up in the increase of random motion of atoms that is part of entropy.

Accordingly, successful aging could be defined as the maintenance of normative baseline parameters in an organized system, as that system struggles to maintain itself as long as possible in its approach to maximal life span. In theory, therefore, maximally successful aging at one level could consist of staving off the disorganization and disintegrity of entropy in the process of having actual chronological age coterminous with species-programmed life span. Thus, in this theoretic model of aging, the human being could maintain its organismic integrity or viability until the age of about 120 years.

However, in reality at the current time in the United States, for example, life expectancy is a little over 74 years of age for men and a little over 78 years of age for women, for the average life expectancy of about 76 years (National

Academy on an Aging Society 2000). While the total U.S. population has tripled since 1900, the absolute number of elderly persons, currently more than 33 million, has increased elevenfold (Rowe and Kahn 1998). And although centenarians were rare in 1900, their numbers have increased to about 70,000 currently (National Academy on an Aging Society 2000). Despite this great increase in life expectancy over the past century, there is still quite a way to go before life expectancy is such that a significant proportion of the population attains species life span.

Changes of Normal Aging

On the parameter of maintaining organismic organization and integration in the context of entropy and other extraorganismic and intraorganismic factors, a critical question becomes whether systematic or regular changes occur with normal aging in the absence of and independently of disease. A well-replicated finding is that even optimally healthy persons between ages 65 and 91 evidence significantly slower psychomotor speed than do young adults (chap. 1). This age-related psychomotor slowing in the absence of any disease has been found to have a negative impact on cognitive measures that require fast response (Birren, Woods, and Williams 1980; Salthouse 1985; Schaie and Willis 1991). And there is evidence of slowing of electrical activity of the brain or EEG changes underlying psychomotor slowing of normal aging (chap. 1). Numerous other changes of normal aging do not, by definition, interfere significantly with social or occupational function (chap. 2). Some such age changes include metabolic slowing (Rowe and Kahn 1998); decrements in vision, hearing, and other sensory processing (Schaie and Willis 1991; Kandel, Schwartz, and Jessell 2000); decline of fluid intelligence (Schaie and Willis 1991); decrements in Piagetian conservation (Emery 1985; Emery and Breslau 1987; Schaie and Willis 1991); decrements in complex language processing (Emery 1985, 1988, 1999, 2000; Snowdon 2001); and decrements in memory (chaps. 1 and 8).

On the positive side, normal aging can result in important increases in overall emotional maturity, psychological integration, psychosocial generativity, and wisdom (Schaie and Willis 1991; Rowe and Kahn 1998; Snowdon 2001). Further, the authors of chapter 1 bring into focus important emerging evidence from studies of neurogenesis that the human adult brain might have potential for regeneration and neural recruitment, both of which may be associated with successful cognitive aging and recovery from brain insults. New evidence suggests that functional brain reorganization may help preserve cognition during the aging process (Shihabuddin et al. 2000). Critically, psychosocial factors appear able to trigger these biological changes. Psychosocial factors that might contribute to successful cognitive aging include optimism, good coping skills, social involvement, diet, exercise, restricted alcohol intake, no other substance abuse (e.g., illegal drugs, prescription drugs), and, importantly, new learning and constancy in use of the brain (e.g., learning new skills, reading, doing crossword puzzles) (Emery 1985, 1988; Schaie and Willis 1991; Baltes 1993; Rowe and Kahn 1998; Nicolas et al. 2001; Snowdon 2001) (chaps. 1, 3, and 8).

Normal Aging and Mild Cognitive Impairment

Currently, there is a redefinition of normal aging such that on the continuum of normal aging and dementia, a segment of aged persons previously considered normal are now redefined as having mild cognitive impairment (MCI) (chaps. 1 and 2). The recent construct of MCI as a diagnostic entity has helped clarify an early stage in the transition from normal aging to dementia. Mild cognitive impairment has been used to describe a group of elderly persons who have greater than expected memory impairment for their age, but do not meet criteria for dementia (Peterson 2000). Current estimates indicate conversion rates from MCI to dementia of the Alzheimer type (DAT) of between 6% and 25% per year (chap. 1).

In conclusion, a critical set of questions in this volume revolves around the ambiguous boundaries between normal aging and dementia. As suggested in chapters 1, 2, and 3, a first step in the differential diagnosis between normal aging and dementia is to determine whether any form of dementia is present. This is essentially a diagnostic choice between normality and abnormality. The appropriate validity questions here are generic; for example, in cases in which a diagnosis of dementia is made, will some evidence of cognitive impairment, functional impairment, neuropathology, neurophysiology, and disease progression be found that validates the accuracy of the diagnostic decision? Cognitive impairment, functional impairment, and neuropathology constitute a central or first-order triad in diagnostic criteria for dementia (chaps. 2 and 3). Second-order modifiers center around disease progression and severity of illness. The exact demarcation between the normal and abnormal is elusive and varies from population to population. The transition between normal aging and dementia can be understood as a threshold phenomenon, as described by authors of chapters 1, 2, 14, and 17. Once the clinician or researcher determines that a diagnosis of dementia is consistent with clinical, neuropsychological, neuropathological, and neuroimaging, and other data, differential diagnosis between the various types and subtypes of dementia is the next step.

Alzheimer Dementias

Nosology and Definition

The most superordinate, overarching, hierarchic classificatory category of this volume is dementia. The next hierarchic level of classification consists of major forms of the overarching category of dementia, such as the Alzheimer dementias, vascular dementias, Pick complex, dementia due to Parkinson disease, HIV/AIDS dementia, dementia due to Creutzfeld-Jakob disease, depressive dementias, and so forth. In turn, the major forms of dementia constituting this second nosologic tier comprise spectra.

Dementia of the Alzheimer type is a syndrome, a final common pathway, and not a singular, homogeneous disease entity. Put another way, DAT is a phenotype or an end-point presentation. More kinds of assault to the human organism appear to exist than there are ways for the human organism to respond or present. We are introducing here the concept of a *limited or finite response medical model;* there are only so many ways in which the human organism can respond to an unlimited or infinite number of assaults, diseases, injuries, or stresses. Hence, a final end-point presentation, such as DAT, can be arrived at through multiple routes (i.e., multiple kinds of assault to the organism). Accordingly, DAT is characterized by heterogeneity and has subtypes, which form a third tier of the nosologic hierarchy of dementia (chaps. 6, 7, 10, 14, and 17). It can be noted here that the terms Alzheimer dementia(s), Alzheimer-type dementia(s), dementia(s) of the Alzheimer type, Alzheimer disease(s), Alzheimer disorder(s), primary degenerative dementia(s) of the Alzheimer type, and Alzheimer syndrome are considered coextensive in this volume.

The defining feature of the overarching, superordinate category of dementia is development of multiple cognitive deficits that include memory impairment as a necessary but not sufficient symptom, and at least one other of the following cognitive disturbances: aphasia, apraxia, agnosia, or disturbance in executive function. The cognitive deficits must be sufficiently severe to cause impairment in social or occupational function and must represent a decline from a previously higher level of function (World Health Organization 1993; American Psychiatric Association 2000). Thus, diagnostic criteria for DAT include, first, all criteria of the superordinate category of dementia. Beyond the generic criteria for dementia, diagnostic criteria for DAT specify that the disease course is characterized by gradual onset and continuing or progressive decline (American Psychiatric Association 2000). Finally, exclusionary criteria exist.

The diagnosis of dementia of the Alzheimer type is made clinically with varying degrees of certainty. Although validity of clinically made diagnosis has increased significantly in recent years, confirmation of diagnosis, to date, is contingent on neuropathological postmortem examination (see chaps. 3–7 and 12).

Characteristic Brain Neuropathology

Dementia of the Alzheimer type is a neurodegenerative disorder characterized by progressive dementia associated with widespread encephalopathy. Brain pathology in DAT is characterized by a broad spectrum of changes, including accumulation of fibrillar beta-amyloid in plaques and vessels, neurofibrillary degeneration, and synaptic and neuronal loss. In chapter 4, data are presented that indicate, neuropathologically, DAT involves a slowly progressive encephalopathy defined by deposition of fibrillar beta-amyloid in plaques and vessels, with region-specific neurofibrillary degeneration and neuronal loss beginning in transentorhinal/entorhinal cortex, and spreading over time to the amygdala, hippocampus, temporal cortex, association and sensory cortices, and finally, to the cerebellum. In chapter 4, Wegiel and colleagues present new data that help us comprehend a pathologic process that begins many years before a later-stage diagnosis of DAT. This process begins with abnormal processing of amyloid precursor protein (APP) and depositions of beta-amyloid fibrils. Amyloid precursor protein consists of more than 700 amino acids, and in neurons is present in vesicles of the cell body, axon, dendrites, and synaptic sites (chap. 4). Beta-amyloid peptides are the product of proteolytic cleavage of APP. Amyloid-beta 1-40 amino acid and amyloid-beta 1-42 amino acid are the products of intracellular processing of APP with beta-secretases and gamma-secretases in the endoplasmic reticulum, trans-Golgi network, and endosomal-lysosomal system (chap. 4). The authors of chapter 4 point out that even though there is a relative paucity of amyloid-beta 1-42 amino acid production, this amino acid is nevertheless the predominant kind found in fibrillar plaques. In terms of intracellular accumulation of amyloid-beta peptides, amyloid-beta 1-42 amino acid accumulates in the perikaryon of pyramidal neurons as discrete granules suggestive of lysosomes or lysosome-derived structures; these deposits precede plaque formation by decades. Further, racemized amyloid-beta peptides are involved in neurofibrillary degeneration (chap. 4).

Wegiel et al. point to the role of abnormal phosphorylation of tau, and possibly other proteins, in initiating formation of neurofibrillary tangles. Neurofibrillary pathology can result from a number of pathologic conditions. It appears that conditions leading to abnormal processing of APP (and formation of beta-amyloid fibrils) might also be implicated in abnormal phosphorylation of tau, with resulting formation of neurofibrillary tangles. This sequence of causal events suggests that DAT, at some point in the neuropathologic process, is a function of beta-protein amyloidosis.

Several reports have suggested that secretion of a soluble form of beta-amyloid protein is possibly a nonpathologic event for a number of cells (Rydel et al. 1992; Selkoe 1992, 2001). If the production of a soluble form of this peptide is nonaberrant, then it could follow that the pathologic production of beta-amyloid protein in DAT results from modifications of normal metabolism. A possible confound of these studies reporting that soluble beta-amyloid protein is a normative metabolic event, is that the cells used in some of these studies were transfected with an extra APP gene, thus creating a non-normative cell analogue.

There has been long-standing controversy as to whether beta-amyloid and neuritic plaques, or tau and neurofibrillary tangles are the primary pathology of dementia of the Alzheimer type (Lee 2001). Chapter 4 contributes heavily to a new understanding of the mechanisms connecting these two kinds of Alzheimer pathology, thereby obviating an either/or perspective. The two kinds of pathology are interrelated.

Genetics of Alzheimer Dementia

The past few years have resulted in exponential growth in genetic research related to dementia of the Alzheimer type. In the majority of cases, DAT is classified as sporadic with late onset. Late-onset DAT is as yet without a definitive link to any genetic markers (chap. 4). However, it does appear that inheritance of the apolipoprotein-E4 allele encoded by a gene on chromosome 19 might increase risk for late-onset DAT (Corder et al. 1993).

In contrast, about 5–10% of familial cases of dementia of the Alzheimer type appear to be transmitted as a pure autosomal dominant trait with high age-dependent penetrance (chap. 4). More than half of early-onset familial cases of

DAT are related to mutations in the presenilin 1 gene on chromosome 14; a small percentage are related to mutations in presenilin 2 gene on chromosome 1 and the amyloid-beta protein precursor gene on chromosome 21 (chaps. 4 and 17). Emerging research suggests that defects on each of these chromosomes might have the common effect of altering production or deposition of amyloid-beta in the brain (Selkoe 2001) (chaps. 2 and 17).

Alzheimer Dementia and Down Syndrome

The overexpression of amyloid precursor protein, overproduction of amyloid-beta, and early intracellular accumulation of amyloid-beta going back to childhood in some cases could be the precondition for both early onset of amyloidosis-beta and neurofibrillary degeneration in adults with Down syndrome (chap. 4). These factors could also represent a common denominator for the process of Alzheimer-type dementing in both the general population and the population of Down syndrome.

Extended life expectancy, from around 9 years of age to more than 50 years of age, has brought into focus increased risk of dementia of the Alzheimer type in adults with Down syndrome (chap. 4). Adults with Down syndrome invariably develop beta-amyloidosis, neurofibrillary degeneration, and often, the cognitive decline associated with DAT (Lemere et al. 1996). Virtually all persons with Down syndrome, who have three copies of the APP gene due to trisomy 21, are affected by accelerated aging and develop Alzheimer-type neuropathology by around 40 years of age (Wisniewski, Wegiel, and Popovitch 1994). This brings into sharp focus the function of the extra copy of the chromosome encoding APP in the overproduction of amyloid-beta and extracellular deposition of fibrillar amyloid in cored plaques and vascular walls (chap. 4). Further, the smaller neuronal "reserve" associated with developmental deficits could contribute, additionally, to increased risk of dementia in Down syndrome (Kuchna et al. 2001).

It is important to note that in both the general population with dementia of the Alzheimer type and the population of dementia of the Alzheimer type with Down syndrome, abnormal processing of amyloid precursor protein and depositions of amyloid-beta fibrils begin many years before the actual diagnosis of dementia of the Alzheimer type (chaps. 4 and 17). This neuropathological finding is consistent with empirical and clinical findings of the Nun Study (Snowdon 2001), in which it was found that a significant number of nuns, who in late life had severe cognitive deficits of the Alzheimer type, already had demonstrated at the early entry age into the convent, lesser complexity of language processing and forms. and lesser idea density.

Heterogeneity, Age of Onset, and Nosology

Although the clinical and neuropathologic aspects of Alois Alzheimer's description (1907) still appear valid today, extensive investigation by this volume's authors indicates that there exists clinical, neuropsychological, genetic, and neuropathological heterogeneity in the Alzheimer-type dementing process so as to give dementia of the Alzheimer type a syndromic character. Alzheimer syndrome appears to be an end-point phenotypic presentation or final common pathway (see chaps. 4–7, 9–11, 14, and 17).

The term *Alzheimer disease* (AD) was used originally to describe a progressive dementia in patients with presenile or early onset of symptoms (before 65 years of age). Since the 1960s, primarily because of histopathological observations that neurofibrillary tangles and senile plaques are found in brains of patients with both early- and late-onset symptomatology, these disorders came to be regarded as a single, homogeneous disease entity. Recently, however, because neuropsychological symptoms, neurochemical deficits, and neuropathological changes appear more severe, or more accurately, have an accelerated disease course in early-onset as compared to late-onset AD, some investigators are questioning the scientific basis for combining these disorders (see chap. 6). Careful analysis of studies that claim no significant difference exists between early- and late-onset AD often reveals a methodological error whereby symptom "severity" has been compared out of the context of disease course (see chap. 2). The configuration of symptoms characterizing DAT appears to be more virulent and accelerated in early-onset than late-onset AD (chap. 6) (Emery and Breslau 1987; Mortimer et al. 1992; Lucca et al. 1993). One can take the point of view that greater acceleration of pathology is involved when a 55-year-old evidences the cognitive deficits of DAT than when a very old person near the end of life does so. The existence of neurofibrillary tangles and neuritic plaques in both early- and late-onset AD is not a sufficient basis for a combined nosologic construction because tangles and plaques are found also in normal elderly persons (see chaps. 1 and 2). Because the quantitative parameter of degree in relation to tangles and plaques is used to separate "normal aging" from DAT, reliable degree differences should also serve to keep nosologically distinct early-onset from late-onset AD. The quantitative variable of degree, when recast in the framework of temporality, becomes disease course acceleration. Thus greater acceleration is equivalent to greater degree.

Subtypes and Nomenclature

In chapter 6, Sjögren, Wallin, and Blennow question the validity of combining early- and late-onset Alzheimer disease, and provide evidence for two distinct subgroups of sporadic Alzheimer disease that differ significantly on several parameters, including the core variable of age at onset. The early-onset subgroup is characterized by onset before 65 years of age, severe memory disturbances, predominant parietal symptoms (e.g., apraxia, visual agnosia, sensory dysphasia), low frequency of vascular factors, relatively normal blood-brain barrier, and low frequency of white matter changes on computed tomography. Chapter 6 further provides evidence that the early-onset subgroup involves greater language disturbances, such as impaired spontaneous speech, verbal comprehension, object naming, writing, as well as decreased survival. The second clinical subgroup is defined around late-onset and is characterized by onset age of 65 or more years, global decline of cognitive functions, milder parietal symptoms, high frequency of episodes of confusion, greater impairment of blood-brain barrier, and high frequency of white matter changes on computed tomography. The authors of chapter 6 provide neurochemical evidence validating the subgrouping of DAT on the basis of age at onset. For example, choline acetyltransferase activity is significantly lower in a number of brain areas in early-onset than in late-onset DAT. Also, there is greater loss of noradrenergic locus ceruleus neurons in early-onset than in late-onset DAT. Very recent neurochemical studies have found differences in structural proteins measured in cerebrospinal fluid. Sjögren and colleagues (2000) found that cerebrospinal fluid level of light neurofilament protein is highly increased in the late-onset subtype of DAT but at normal levels in the early-onset subtype. Evidence for significant differences in population based on age at onset comes also from histopathological investigations; for example, some histopathological studies have suggested quantitative differences in density of senile plaques and neurofibrillary tangles between early-onset and late-onset subtypes of DAT, with higher density found in the early-onset population (chap. 6). Sjögren, Wallin, and Blennow do point out there is also heterogeneity within the late-onset population, and that although many patients with late-onset disorder fit the late-onset subgroup description outlined above, a subset of patients with late-onset disorder have a better goodness-of-fit with the early-onset profile. Finally, chapter 6 produces evidence for heterogeneity within familial AD, with a discussion of differing genetic determinants.

In sum, it seems clear that there exist significant differences between early-onset and late-onset subgroups of dementia of the Alzheimer type that should not be ignored or washed out in the combining of the two subgroups into a conjoint nosologic construction. It is critical that it be recognized that DAT is not a homogeneous, singular disease entity, but rather, that it is comprised of subgroups and represents an end-point phenotypic presentation and final common pathway. This heterogeneity makes diagnosis difficult and creates a need for disease markers. However, the heterogeneity itself obstructs identification of positive disease markers (chap. 6). The authors of chapter 6 demonstrate that a practicable solution is to find markers that are specific for subgroups or subtypes of patients with AD rather than for the whole Alzheimer population. At issue is the fact that as long as DAT is perceived as a singular disease entity, the workable approach of finding subgroup disease markers will not happen. This is an illustration of how conceptualization can precede, influence, and limit research and treatment approaches.

Subtype of Mixed Alzheimer Dementia and Vascular Dementia

The early-onset subtype of dementia of the Alzheimer type corresponds more closely than late-onset to the "classical" or "pure" form or type that Alzheimer himself (1907) described (chap. 6). Late-onset subtype of DAT appears to involve significantly more vascular factors than early-onset and interfaces with vascular dementia (VaD). The argument can be made that the late-onset population represents what we will term an "alzheimerized" or "Alzheimer-type" subtype of VaD, or, at the very least, a mixed Alzheimer-VaD subtype (chap. 10). The late-onset AD subtype conceptualized by authors of chapter 6, in our view, is part of the Alzheimer-VaD spectrum.

Future research imperatives should include focus on the interface between the dementias of the Alzheimer type and vascular dementias. Whereas Sjögren, Wallin, and Blennow (chap. 6) identified a late-onset subgroup of patients with AD with a highly vascular profile, Emery, Gillie, and Smith (1996, 2000) (chap. 10) came to this interface from the other direction. Starting with a wide spectrum of patients with vascular disorder, a subgroup was identified that appears to have an "Alzheimer-type VaD" (chap. 10).

Epidemiologic studies report that dementia of the Alzheimer type is the most prevalent of dementing disorders (chaps. 1 and 2). However, it is our experience as well as that of other investigators (chaps. 4, 6, 10, 14, and 17) that it is difficult to find cases of "pure" AD over the age of 80. These older patients with so-called DAT inevitably have significant vascular components. We conclude that the most prevalent subtype of DAT is a mixed Alzheimer-vascular subtype. Because of this typologic frequency, more investigations should focus on this mixed type. Emergent characteristics and pathogenic factors of this mixed type exist that have not yet been described but will help illuminate the process of degenerative dementing. Whether this subtype will eventually be most validly classified under the broader category of Alzheimer dementias or vascular dementias is a fundamental issue awaiting resolution. Valid prevalence figures for DAT have contingency on the resolution of this issue.

Other Parameters for Subtypes of Alzheimer Disorder

Wegiel et al. (chap. 4) provide evidence for the subtype of dementia of the Alzheimer type of Down syndrome. Data and argument are presented which make the point that the superimposition of DAT on Down syndrome is best understood as a separate subtype.

In chapter 7, Kirshner describes atypical patterns of dementia of the Alzheimer type that mimic focal brain disorders. These atypical "focal" presentations provide potential parameters for other subtypes of DAT. Kirshner provides evidence and discussion relating to the spectrum of the more "typical" presentation of DAT and several "focal-onset" patterns, including presentations with clinically obvious aphasia, visuospatial deficits ordinarily associated with right hemisphere dysfunction, prosopagnosia (failure to recognize faces), myoclonus, and extrapyramidal signs. The spectrum of focal and diffuse lesions is in the foreground of chapter 7; the ambiguity of the transitions and boundaries between focal and diffuse lesions stands out in bold relief.

Zubenko (chap. 17), in discussing his recent work on the neurobiology of major depression in the context of the Alzheimer neurodegenerative process, concludes that major depression describes a clinically and pathologically distinct subtype of patients with dementia of the Alzheimer type. This subtype evidences degenerative changes in brainstem aminergic nuclei, especially the locus ceruleus, which are disproportionate to those that occur in cerebral cortex. Further, the subtype of DAT with depression also evidences a relative preservation of the basal nucleus of Meynert (chap. 17). In exploring the dementia-depression spectrum, Zubenko develops the concept of a threshold for central cholinergic function below which the expression of clinical depression is not possible. A subtyping of Alzheimer syndrome by the presence or absence of depression underscores the ambiguities inhering in the depression-dementia spectrum, which will be addressed further in this chapter in the section on depressive dementia.

The work of this volume's authors leaves little doubt that accurate diagnostics and effective, rationally based treatment for persons with dementia has great contingency on improved validity and widespread recognition of the construct of Alzheimer disorder as representing a heterogeneous disorder comprised of subtypes.

Neural Inflammatory Mechanisms in Alzheimer Syndrome

McGeer and McGeer (chap. 5) bring into focus new material indicating that neural inflammation mechanisms perform a major function in the conversion of dementia of the Alzheimer type from a relatively benign pathology into a malignant inflammatory disorder. Immunohistochemical investigations show that many inflammatory markers newly appear or are upregulated in affected brain regions in persons with DAT. Postmortem data evidence a state of chronic inflammation in these affected regions in the brains of persons with DAT. McGeer and McGeer point out that more than twenty epidemiological investigations indicate that taking nonsteroidal anti-inflammatory drugs (NSAIDs) significantly reduces the incidence of DAT and that NSAIDs might slow the Alzheimer dementing process.

McGeer and McGeer introduce a distinction between autoimmune disorders and "autotoxicity disorders." Dementia of the Alzheimer type is an autotoxicity disorder. Autotoxicity is a pathomechanism of the phylogenetically more primitive innate immune system, whereas autoimmunity is a pathomechanism of the phylogenetically later-to-develop adaptive immune system. Chapter 5 proposes that autotoxicity is a critical variable in the pathogenesis of DAT; autotoxicity describes self-attack by the innate immune system. The innate immune system is more primitive and less able to process complex inputs; the innate immune system appears to more readily confuse self and foe. Chapter 5 describes the function of a chronically activated complement system in the membrane attack complex, which inserts into viable cells, causing death. The overall complement system cascade identifies, opsonizes, and destroys its target; the tangles and plaques of DAT are clearly marked with opsonizing complement system components. When the concentration of membrane attack complex exceeds the defensive ability of its host tissue, then self-attack can occur in a process called bystander lysis. Chapter 5 describes bystander lysis as the smoking gun of autodestruction in DAT, as neurites are progressively eliminated by self-attack.

Zubenko (chap. 17) also discusses mechanisms of neuronal death in dementia of the Alzheimer type, concluding that there appear to be at least two such mechanisms: necrosis and apoptosis. Zubenko argues that, although the pathways of these two mechanisms may overlap to some extent, they are typically triggered by different events, are manifested by distinguishable cytologic and biochemical features, and may have different outcomes. Necrosis usually results from injury, is not genetically controlled, is typified by the destruction of organelles and plasma membrane, and results in release of cellular debris that often stimulates a local inflammatory response. In contrast, apoptosis or programmed cell death represents a genetically controlled response to specific developmental or environmental stimuli. Apoptotic cells and their fragments undergo phagocytosis by microglia but do not stimulate an inflammatory response (chap. 17).

To conclude this section, both chapters 5 and 8 describe the process of Alzheimer dementing as occurring in the context of phylogenetic retrogression. In chapter 8, the term *retrophylogenesis* is introduced to define key components of the memory deficits of DAT.

Memory Impairment of Alzheimer Dementia

The concepts presented in chapter 8 were developed in response to the lack of goodness-of-fit between current memory frameworks in use and data related to the nature and patterns of memory in dementia of the Alzheimer type. It is suggested that a key problem with memory frameworks commonly in use is that they are uninformed by the dimension of development across time; one and all fail to reflect the phylogenetic reality that memory is an evolved organ of adaptation. Chapter 8 points out that memory is a critical adaptational tool enabling an organism to retain information so every minute of existence won't require a de novo response to same or similar challenges. Memory is a multitiered, multidimensional, hierarchically organized "organ" of adaptation laid down in many places of the organism, with redundancy and superimposition as features reflective of phylogenetics, having evolved over millions of years.

Chapter 8 introduces a new synthesis of memory in dementia of the Alzheimer type: a three-tiered evolutionary memory framework, the origins of which represent differing times in evolutionary history: motor memory, emotional memory, and higher cortical memory. In terms of the phyletic scale, the phylogenesis of movement, as well as memory for motor information and programmed motor sequences, preceded phylogenesis of emotion. In turn, phylogenesis of both movement and emotion preceded phylogenesis of the neocortex and its functions, one of which is neocortical or higher cortical memory (Darwin 1955 [1859]; Dobzhansky 1964; Guyton 1981, 2000; Udalova and Karas 1996).

Memory deterioration as part of the Alzheimer-type dementing process undergoes a *retrophylogenesis* in that higher cortical memory deteriorates first, followed by deterioration of emotional memory. Motor or movement memory, the first to have evolved in the origin of the species, appears the best preserved and last to deteriorate as part of DAT. This is consistent with the data of chapter 9 in which motor (procedural) memory is found to be more intact than higher cortical memory (e.g., recall) in DAT. Chapter 8 provides a context for understanding the "primitivization" the person with DAT suffers as part of progression of illness. Finally, chapter 8 provides data to support the idea that the person with DAT also undergoes *retroontogenesis* within higher cortical memory (i.e., things learned first in ontogenetic development deteriorate last).

Vascular Dementias

Nosology and Hierarchic Relations

Vascular dementias are subsumed under the superordinate category of dementia, and are on the same hierarchic level as the Alzheimer dementias, Pick complex, dementia due to Parkinson disease, human immunodeficiency virus/acquired immunodeficiency syndrome dementia, depressive dementias, and others. This is consistent with nosologic categories of DSM-IV-TR (American Psychiatric Association 2000). In turn, the category of vascular dementias also has subtypes comprising it (e.g., multiinfarct dementia, Binswanger disease). It is a goal of this volume to redefine the category of vascular dementias such that noninfarct vascular dementias would be recognized as one of its subtypes (chap. 10). And then, as part of the next classificatory tier, noninfarct vascular dementias would also have subtypes, possibly including noninfarct vascular dementia due to collagen disease (vasculitis), "Alzheimer-type (alzheimerized) vascular dementia," and others not yet typologically defined (chap. 10).

Noninfarct Vascular Dementia

For more than thirty years, there has been an equation between the terms *vascular dementia* (VaD) and *multiinfarct dementia* (MID). One purpose in this volume is to redefine VaD so that the category will include, but not be limited to, MID.

Data from this volume suggest that a wide variety of vascular disorders result in cognitive deterioration (chaps. 10–12). It follows that VaD is neither coextensive with MID nor a homogeneous single disease entity. Vascular dementia appears to be a dementia syndrome caused by a number of underlying vascular mechanisms. Put another way, VaD is an end point, a common final pathway for a spectrum of vascular disorders.

In chapter 10, the nosologic construct of vascular dementia is reconceptualized and broadened to include what the authors have termed *noninfarct vascular dementia:* vascular dementia caused by underlying vascular factors other than cerebral infarction (Emery, Gillie, and Smith 1996, 2000). Data are presented that indicate vascular disease without cerebral infarction results in a continuum of cognitive impairment, with one end of this continuum of cognitive impairment represented by the concept of noninfarct VaD.

Distal Causality of Arteriosclerosis and Abnormal Blood Pressure

The concept of vascular dementia has been too delimited by the cerebral infarct concept. During the mid-1900s, sclerosis of brain arteries was considered the main causal factor in VaD (American Psychiatric Association 1952, 1968). Based on data from several investigations comparing vascular patients with and without cerebral infarction, Emery, Gillie, and Smith (chap. 10) conclude it was an error to completely eliminate the arteriosclerotic explanation in favor of the multiinfarct construct. Arteriosclerosis crosscuts both cerebral infarct and cerebral noninfarct patient groups and is thus implicated in the causal chain of vascular events related to cognitive decline in both populations (Emery, Gillie, and Ramdev 1995; Emery, Gillie, and Smith 1996, 2000). Arteriosclerosis is a major vascular variable in the distal causality of a large percentage of VaD cases (chap. 10). Nosologically, this could be expressed as vascular dementia due to arteriosclerosis, with codes for with cerebral infarction and without cerebral infarction.

This same kind of chain of pathogenic vascular events applies to abnormalities of blood pressure. Kobayashi (chap. 11) found that hypertension was a critical factor in the vascular chain of pathogenic events leading to dementia, with or without actual cerebral infarction. Furthermore, hypotension as well as hypertension is implicated in severe cognitive impairment and dementia (e.g., in Binswanger disease) (chaps. 10 and 11). Thus, chronic abnormalities of blood pressure function as distal causation in many cases of VaD, both with and without actual cerebral infarction.

Other Possible Risk Factors Implicated in Noninfarct Vascular Dementia

Whereas the proximate cause of vascular dementia in persons with multiinfarct or stroke is cerebral infarction, we have seen that when one starts to track causes farther back in the chain of pathogenic vascular events, or causes of the proximate cause of infarction, arteriosclerosis and abnormal blood pressure come into focus as important factors. Arteriosclerosis and long-standing abnormalities of blood pressure have been found to be critical risk factors not only for VaD in patients with cerebral infarction, but also in patients with VaD, who have never had cerebral infarction (i.e., patients with what we have termed noninfarct VaD) (chap. 10; Emery, Gillie, and Ramdev 1995; Emery, Gillie, and Smith 1996, 2000).

Other possible risk factors implicated in the pathogenic vascular chain preceding noninfarct VaD include diabetes mellitus, ischemic heart disease, abnormal electrocardiogram, myocardial infarction, peripheral vascular disease, chronic obstructive pulmonary disease, heart block, cardiomegaly, calcified iliac vessels, hypercholesterolemia, bradycardia, pacemaker complications, atrial fibrillation, ventricular hypertrophy, and right carotid stenosis (chaps. 10–12; Emery, Gillie, and Ramdev 1994, 1995; Emery, Gillie, and Smith 1996, 2000; Hachinski and Munoz 2000).

The long-term vascular patients represented by vascular conditions described above met criteria for dementia, but could not be diagnosed with vascular dementia because of lack of actual cerebral infarction (chap. 10). Why not classify them as having DAT? First, these particular patients did not meet criteria for probable AD because they had either higher ischemia scores than criteria permit or gait disorder early in illness (Hachinski 1983; McKhann, Drachman, and Folstein 1984; Reisberg et al. 1997; American Psychiatric Association 2000). But even more important, in terms of construct validity, it does not make sense to all of a sudden do an about face and ignore or deem unimportant or irrelevant the long-standing histories of vascular problems in order to come up with a diagnosis. Rather, classification criteria must be changed in order to accord with reality as evidenced by a broad spectrum of vascular patients. The nosologic criterial equation between VaD and cerebral infarction during the past three decades has resulted in standard practice by both researchers and clinicians whereby patients with long-standing histories of serious vascular disease, who lack actual cerebral infarction, are placed, or in our view, forced into the diagnostic category of DATs where they might not belong. Possible ramifications of this standard practice include years of contaminated Alzheimer research samples, inflated incidence and prevalence figures for DAT, and lack of appropriate medical treatment for vascular patients carrying the misdiagnosis of DAT.

Other Infarct and Noninfarct Mechanisms

The authors of chapters 11 and 12 discuss multiple paths and vascular mechanisms that can lead to vascular dementia: atherothrombotic stroke, cardiogenic embolic stroke, lacunar stroke, ischemic white matter lesions, and hemodynamic mechanisms. These authors also emphasize that multiple brain mechanisms exist which involve volume of total brain tissue lost because of infarcts, location of infarcts, and functional disconnection of cortex because of lacunar infarcts and white matter destruction (see chap. 12). More specific vascular mechanisms underlying VaD include inflammatory and noninflammatory arteriopathies of brain vessels and also mechanisms inhering in hereditary diseases (chaps. 11 and 12). Kirshner (chap. 7) discusses the critical mechanisms of edema and diaschisis in the conversion of focal brain insults into dementia.

The focus on noninfarct factors in the pathogenesis of vascular dementia is a particular contribution of this volume's authors. The authors of chapter 12 concluded that the following noninfarct factors may play a role in the pathogenesis of VaD: hypoperfusion, vessel wall changes leading to blood-brain barrier or carrier dysfunction, dysfunction of oligodendrocytes leading to defective myelination, and functional inactivity of nerve cells. Lack of adequate oxygenation is at the core of many noninfarct factors. The definition and methodology of studying these noninfarct factors is far from adequate. Other noninfarct factors in the pathogenesis of noninfarct VaD can be found in the data of chapter 10. It is clear that pathophysiologic mechanisms underlying noninfarct VaD exist that are as yet unidentified. The study of noninfarct factors in the vascular sequence leading to dementia is just beginning.

Conceptualization of a Preinfarct State

The term *preinfarct state* was introduced by Emery and colleagues (chap. 10) to assist in the definition of the spectrum of vascular dementia. Whereas not all white matter changes, for example, are infarcts per se, it is possible that some that are not actually infarcts constitute and define a preinfarct state. Generally, infarcts don't come out of nowhere. Thus, it is useful to envision both white matter changes and gray matter changes as part of a spectrum, from the preinfarct state at one end to a single infarct to multiple infarctions at the other. Not all brain matter changes are necessarily either lesions or infarcts, nor are lesions precisely the same as infarcts. The pathogenic processes leading to infarction constitute continua. However, we conclude that although the idea of a preinfarct state adds to the explanatory power of the infarct concept, VaD is broader than can be accounted for with the infarct concept, even when that concept is expanded to include a preinfarct state.

Focal versus Diffuse Lesions

The distinction between focal and generalized or diffuse disease is in reality not absolute and signifies a false dichotomy; again, the continuum perspective serves us better. Although VaD has by convention been associated with focality, focal lesions are in reality not purely localized. Focal lesions, such as stroke, can precipitate a diffuse encephalopathy or dementia in the aging brain (chap. 7). Focal lesions can disrupt functions of other brain areas through a number of mechanisms, including disruption of cortical connections, edema, and diaschisis (reduced metabolic activity of distant but synaptically connected areas of brain) (chaps. 7, 10, 12). Multiinfarct dementia, the definitional and nosologic prototype of focal vascular disorders, in reality, is a multifocal disorder (i.e., multiple infarction equals multiple focality). And where does one draw the line between multifocality and diffuse or generalized disease?

Interface between Vascular Dementia and Alzheimer Dementia

Of essence in the spectrum of vascular dementias and dementias of the Alzheimer type is the ambiguous transition between these two syndromes, which parallels the ambiguous transition between multifocality and diffuse disease.

Our previous discussion of arteriosclerosis in the distal causality of vascular disorders is relevant here. Atherosclerosis, a subtype of the broader category of arteriosclerosis (Stedman 1990), is basically an inflammatory disease, which can lead to ischemia of the brain, heart, or extremities (Ross 1993, 1999). The underlying mechanisms of atherosclerosis are fundamentally no different from those in other inflammatory syndromes (chap. 10; Ross 1993, 1999; Tormey et al. 1997). Accordingly, inflammation has pathogenic function in substantial numbers of cases of VaD; the exact percentage is not yet clear.

What is of interest is the common function of inflammation at the interface of vascular dementias and dementias of the Alzheimer type. The underlying process of inflammation in essence is the same irrespective of syndrome. Consequently, there is great similarity between VaD and DAT in how the inflammatory process contributes to brain disintegrity. Immunohistological data show many inflammatory markers newly appear or are upregulated in brain with DAT. Activated complement cascade, activated microglia, and other inflammatory factors play a major role in converting DAT into a malignant inflammatory process (chap. 5). In sum, although initial causes of pathology in vascular and Alzheimer dementias may be said to be different (e.g., plaque deposits in vessel walls for VaD and amyloid deposits in cerebral vascular walls, tangles, and plaques in DAT), a secondary process involving inflammation is common to both.

Evidence for other common factors in the vascular dementia-dementia of the Alzheimer type spectrum comes from recent research on the role of blood vessels in producing pathological changes in Alzheimer brain tissue. It is only recently understood that microvessels in Alzheimer brain are highly involved in deposition of amyloid-beta protein found in brains of persons with DAT (Miyakawa et al. 2000), underscoring common vascular pathogenesis in vascular and DATs.

At this point it is relevant to mention cystatin C amyloid (chap. 11). Cystatin C amyloid is associated with impairment of cerebral vascular autoregulation, which can be found in vascular-Alzheimer dementias (chaps. 10 and 11).

Other data indicate cerebral capillary ultrastructure is significantly more damaged in persons with dementia of the Alzheimer type than in normal elderly persons (Farkas et al. 2000). Decreased blood supply and cerebrovascular alterations appear to contribute to both vascular and Alzheimer dementias (chap. 10; Farkas et al. 2000).

Relatedly, emerging findings indicate that a significant percentage of persons with dementia of the Alzheimer type evidence chronic ischemic white matter leukoaraiosis (Brown et al. 2000). Periventricular veins in substantial numbers of persons with DAT were occluded by multiple layers of collagen in vessel walls; this collagen deposition was especially excessive in leukoaraiosis lesions.

Also, severe loss of oligodendrocytes in leukoaraiosis lesions due to extensive apoptosis was found in patients with DAT (Brown et al. 2000).

Finally, another investigation found aberrant nitric oxide synthase-3 expression in cerebrovascular degeneration and vascular-mediated injury in dementia of the Alzheimer type (De La Monte et al. 2000). This contributes to diminished capacity to remove respiratory waste products and toxins from extracellular space due to reduced capillary permeability and cerebral hypoperfusion due to impaired vasodilation (chap. 10; De La Monte et al. 2000).

To conclude, there is evidence that quite a few common factors of pathogenesis crosscut vascular and Alzheimer dementias. Vascular dementias and dementias of the Alzheimer type appear to represent two end-point phenotypic presentations of the overarching class of dementia, which share a number of underlying pathomechanisms. What we have termed *Alzheimer-type (alzheimerized) vascular dementia* could be identified as a noninfarct VaD subtype at the interface of VaD and DAT.

Cortical and Frontosubcortical Dementias

Differential Diagnosis

Assal and Cummings (chap. 9) present evidence for the construct validity and clinical utility of the cortical-frontosubcortical distinction. Some methodologic weaknesses of investigations comparing the two, such as lack of controls over disease severity, have posed a challenge to the validity of this construct (e.g., Mayeux and Stern 1987). However, recent controlled studies provide evidence for significant differences between cortical and frontosubcortical dementias and support the validity, reliability, and utility of this distinction for differential diagnosis and treatment (chap. 9).

Data presented by Assal and Cummings point to two distinguishable patterns of dementia. Cortical dementias, such as the DATs, are characterized by cognitive impairments in selective attention, language, visuospatial skills, and executive functions of category fluency, delayed alternation, delayed response, and set planning. Overall severity of memory impairment in cortical dementias is greater than in frontosubcortical dementias. However, procedural memory as well as flow of speech and speed of cognitive processing are better preserved in cortical than in frontosubcortical dementias. Cortical dementias are not typically characterized by motor impairments and anomalies as are frontosubcortical dementias. In contrast, frontosubcortical dementias are characterized by slowed attention, slow cognitive processing, dysarthric speech, perseveration and poor planning on visuospatial tasks, severely impaired executive functions of verbal fluency, set planning, and set shifting. Frontosubcortical dementias have at their core disorders of movement, posture, gait, and other motor processing (chap. 9).

As with other dichotomous distinctions discussed, we conclude that the cortical-frontosubcortical distinction has utility so long as it is understood that the distinction is not absolute but rather subserves a cortical-frontosubcortical continuum. The construct indicates predominance of brain regions of involvement and syndrome patterns rather than absolute exclusions implied by dichotomy.

Phylogenesis provides an added context for understanding the cortical-frontosubcortical distinction. Phylogenetic theory and data place evolution of subcortical functions earlier in phylogenesis than evolution of cortical/higher cortical functions (chap. 8). Consistent with the findings of chapter 9, we have stated that DAT (a cortical dementia) seems to involve *retrophylogenesis*, whereby functions last to evolve in phylogenesis are first to deteriorate (chap. 8). Thus, DAT, a prototype of cortical dementia, undergoes first a deterioration of higher cortical function; motor functions, having evolved earlier in species development, remain better preserved and deteriorate later than cortical functions (chap. 8).

Diseases Associated with Frontosubcortical Dementias

There are a number of categories of diseases associated with frontosubcortical dementia, and concomitantly, even more diseases (chaps. 7, 9, and 13). Categories of diseases include degenerative diseases, nondegenerative diseases, demyelinating diseases, infectious diseases, and miscellaneous (chap. 9). *Degenerative diseases* associated with frontosubcortical dementia include Parkinson disease, Huntington disease, progressive supranuclear palsy, Wilson disease, Fahr disease, multiple system atrophy, neuroacanthocytosis, Hallervorden-Spatz disease, spinocerebellar ataxias, frontotemporal dementia, amyotrophic lateral sclerosis, and progressive subcortical gliosis. *Vascular dementias* also involve features of the frontosubcortical dementias (chap. 9). Demyelinating diseases, such as multiple sclerosis and inherited leukoencephalopathies, can result in frontosubcortical dementia. Also, a miscellaneous collection of other diseases, such as normal pressure hydrocephalus, sarcoidosis, and Behcet disease are associated with frontosubcortical dementing. Finally, a number of *infectious dementias* evidence a frontosubcortical symptom pattern, including Whipple disease, neurosyphillis, Creutzfeldt-Jakob disease, and AIDS dementia complex (chaps. 3, 9, and 13).

The pioneering author of chapter 13 examines the acquired immunodeficiency syndrome dementia complex in detail. Nervous system involvement early in HIV-1 infection, neurologic complications during acute and "asymptomatic" phases, and late nervous system involvement, along with medical management, are discussed. Finally, major clinical manifestations of AIDS dementia complex with a frontosubcortical pattern affecting cognition, motor performance, and behavior are delineated.

We previously introduced the idea that there are more diseases and assaults to the organism than there are ways for the organism to respond: a "finite response model." This model is instructive here because it helps us understand the necessity of viewing the major types of dementia as syndromes or end-point phenotypic presentations with multiple pathways toward that phenotypic configuration.

Starting Locus, Brain Predominance, and Direction of Disease Course

We can conclude that the cortical-frontosubcortical distinction is most useful when viewed from a diachronic perspective. The distinction has most utility when it serves as an indicator of starting locus, brain predominance, and direction of disease course across time.

Increasing Brain Involvement, Overlap, and Elements of Similarity

With both frontosubcortical and cortical dementing, progression in disease course over time results in movement of one toward the other. Put another way, nature of progression (when it occurs) is toward more generalized and increasingly diffuse neurodegeneration. As differing dementias progress in their disease course across time, they move toward one another as more brain areas become involved. Movement is toward a more global terminus. There exists a finite number of brain areas, and as the different dementias increase their areas of involvement and overlap, they also increase in some elements of similarity.

Depressive Dementias

Prepermanent Intermediate-stage Dementia

The term *depressive dementia* was used first by McHugh and Folstein (1978) and refers to the syndrome that historically was called *depressive pseudodementia* (chap. 14). Because many patients with depressive dementia have cognitive deficits severe enough to meet diagnostic criteria for dementia (chaps. 1 and 3), the term *depressive dementia* is more reflective of the reality of the syndrome than is depressive pseudodementia. In this volume, the empirically based conceptualization is developed that depressive dementia is a "*prepermanent intermediate-stage dementia*" in the multiphasic long-term disease course between major depression without dementia to irreversible or permanent dementia. Accordingly, depressive dementia represents a *transitional stage* in the conversion of an initially-reversible or prepermanent dementia into a nonreversible or permanent end-stage dementia (e.g., DAT) (chap. 14).

The Concept of Pseudodementia

In viewing the history of the concept of pseudodementia, one finds an effort dating back at least several hundred years to differentiate nonreversible dementias from what on the surface appeared to be *reversible dementias* (chaps. 14–16). Data presented in chapter 14 suggest that depressive dementia is only *initially reversible* in many instances with progression to nonreversibility.

Investigators of pseudodementia have revealed that a presentation of dementia can be approximated by patients with a variety of disorders, including Ganser syndrome, conversion reaction, dissociative disorders, depersonalization, mania, malingering, schizophrenia, delirium, deafness, and normal pressure hydrocephalus (chaps. 3 and 14–16). Although the frequency distribution of disorders presenting with dementialike presentations remains unclear, what is clear is that, historically depressive-spectrum disorders constituted a substantial core in any series of patients with so-called reversible dementia.

The Continuity Framework

Both historical and present-day clinical case series have mainly used a dichotomous approach to dementia and pseudodementia. Parameters of irreversibility-reversibility and organic-nonorganic (or, put another way, structure-function) comprise the dichotomies around which dementia and pseudodementia historically have been defined. In contrast, the perspective taken by the authors of this volume is a continuity perspective. Organic deterioration is viewed as a continuous variable. We conclude that essential questions related to dementialike presentations cannot be resolved using a dichotomy model of dementia-pseudodementia. Difficult questions begin to yield once it is recognized that a continuum of organic degeneration exists.

As a concomitant to the degenerative continuum, there also appears to be a continuum of irreversibility-reversibility. Degrees of reversibility exist. Also, reversibility must be placed in a diachronic context. Hence, symptoms of a pseudodementia might be "reversed," but for how long? Reversibility is subject to time-limited variability. In this context, depressive dementia is found to be an initially-reversible dementia that in many instances later converts into permanent dementia (chap. 14).

Subgroups of the Dementia Spectrum of Depression

When organizing and interpreting data on the dementia spectrum of depression, a major methodologic problem is the ambiguous and changing use of terminology across both time and investigations. Definitions and diagnostic criteria for both affective and dementing disorders have undergone changes with time (see chaps. 6, 10, and 14), making it difficult to compare studies from different decades. There are also problems in comparing studies from the same time frame because of sampling ambiguities, such as the problem of phenomenal identity (i.e., different populations are identified by the identical term and identical populations are identified by differing terms). In many investigations of depression, no distinction is made between depression with and without dementia, thereby resulting in confounded data (see chap. 2).

With clarification of such heterogeneity in mind, Emery and Oxman (chap. 14) delineate prototypic groups of the dementia spectrum of depression. Five points along the continua of depression, cognitive impairment, and degenerative pathology are used to define five groups: (1) major depression without dementia; (2) depressive dementia; (3) degenerative dementia without depression; (4) degenerative dementia with depression; and (5) independent co-occurrence of depression and degenerative dementia.

Fundamental Connection between Depression and Dementia

Although there has been clinical interest in the differential diagnosis between depressive dementia and "organic" dementias for many years (chaps. 14–17), the idea that some fundamental relationship might exist between these nosologically distinct categories is relatively new and represents a major paradigm shift. The association between major depression without dementia, depressive dementia, and neurodegenerative "irreversible" dementia represents a new clinical and research focus. Whether depression without dementia, and its possible devolution into depressive dementia, represents a risk factor for irreversible dementia; or whether the cognitive deficits of depression represent an early preclinical phase of irreversible dementia are questions that bring into focus two sides of a fundamental continuity or spectrum relationship. Two sides of the same coin, one being the obverse of the other; these issues point to a fundamental connection between depression and dementia, which historically was not known and which represents a breakthrough perspective.

Depression as a Risk Factor for Dementia

Recent investigations converge on the idea that lifetime history of depression increases risk for irreversible dementia, regardless of genetic predisposition or family history (chaps. 14 and 15; van Duijn et al. 1994; Devanand et al. 1996; Wetherell et al. 1999).

A model pattern culled from longitudinal data is as follows: (1) several episodes of major depression/unipolar without significant cognitive impairment; (2) one or more episodes of major depression/unipolar during which cognitive function is significantly impacted with subsequent return to "normal"; (3) an episode of apparent depression during which the patient presents with an Alzheimer-type profile, with cognitive symptoms subsequently appearing to "reverse" (i.e., depressive dementia); and (4) a presentation with an Alzheimer-type profile without remission of cognitive symptoms, and with subsequent progressive neurodegeneration consistent with DAT. This pattern was found in 79% of forty-four patients with depressive dementia after follow-up of eight-year average duration. Where postmortems permitted (nine patients), neuropathological examination revealed typical markers of DAT: neuronal loss, neurofibrillary tangles, and neuritic plaques (chap. 14; Emery 1988, 1999; Kral and Emery 1989).

Recent longitudinal epidemiological data indicate that after 2.54 years of follow-up, depressed mood at baseline is associated with an increased risk of irreversible dementia (relative risk, 2.94; p 5 0.001). The increased risk relates primarily to development of DAT (relative risk, 2.05). This effect remained after study controls for age, gender, education, language of assessment, and "all major clinical risk factors" (Devanand et al. 1996, p. 180). There are numerous other recent investigations suggesting depression is a risk factor for dementia (chaps. 14 and 15).

Curvilinearlike Relationship between Depression and Degenerative Dementia

Important data suggest that the statistical effect of decreased depression in late life disappears when organic cases are excluded from analysis (e.g., Saunders et al. 1993). For lack of a better term, we will introduce the term *curvilinearlike* to try to explain this phenomenon. The relationship between depression and dementia, in some instances, appears to be curvilinearlike because there appears to be a threshold for central cholinergic function below which expression of clinical depression is not possible (chap. 17). Because degenerative dementia is defined in part by progressive loss of cholinergic function in the central nervous system (chaps. 3, 4, 15, and 17), it follows that major depression decreases as degenerative dementia increases. For heuristic purposes, we are proposing there is a positive correlation between depression and cognitive impairment, possibly until around the spectrum point of depressive dementia, after which the relationship starts to become negative, with depression ceasing clinical expression at the threshold point below which clinical depression can no longer be expressed (chap. 14). This curvilinearlike relationship between depression and degenerative dementia, which is based on threshold values for central cholinergic function, can explain the data, which hitherto have been so puzzling, that depression decreases as dementia increases (chap. 14).

Anticholinergics in the Conversion of Depression into Dementia of the Alzheimer Type

What factors constitute a diathesis for dementia of the Alzheimer type in patients with depression? We have indicated that depressive dementia appears to be a prepermanent intermediate-stage dementia in the long-term, multiphasic disease course of DAT in many, but not all cases (chap. 14). Why in some but not in all cases is the critical question that requires more systematic investigation.

What are some risk factors? One risk factor appears to be medications with anticholinergic effects (chaps. 3 and 14; Emery 1988, 1999; Kral and Emery 1989; Emery and Oxman 1997). A defining characteristic of DAT is the progressive loss of cholinergic function in the central nervous system (chaps. 3, 4, 15, and 17). The use of anticholinergics by patients with already fragile cholinergic function constitutes a risk for cognitive impairment. Of importance here is the use of antidepressants with anticholinergic side effects in the potential conversion of depression into depressive dementia, which in turn can progress to DAT.

In chapter 3, Patterson and Clarfield examine a variety of other medications that also can impact cognition negatively. The informed and judicious prescribing of medications is especially important in disorders in which progressive deterioration of cognition can occur (e.g., the depression-dementia spectrum).

Inflammation at the Interface of Depression and Dementia of the Alzheimer Type

We have already discussed the role of neural inflammatory mechanisms in dementia of the Alzheimer type (chap. 5). Further, the common function of inflammation at the interface between DAT and VaD has been examined (chap. 10). We look now at the role of cytokines and other inflammatory mediators of the immune system at the interface of depression and DAT. It is well known that psychiatric illness, such as depression, can compromise immune function (e.g., Kandel 2000; Leonard 2001; Snowdon 2001). Emerging evidence implicates pro-inflammatory cytokines in the pathological changes that occur in both depression and DAT. Data suggest that both activation (e.g., macrophage activity, acute phase proteins) and inhibition (e.g., natural killer cell activity) of the immune system occur in association with major depression (e.g., Leonard 2001). Many symptoms of depression are simulated by three proinflammatory cytokines (IL-1, IL-6, and TNF-α), which may impact brain function by activating cyclooxygenase, nitric acid synthase, and corticotrophin releasing factor (De La Monte et al. 2000; Leonard 2001). Effective antidepressant treatments largely attenuate immune changes, thus raising the possibility that normalization of central biogenic amine function implicated in the cause of depression may concomitantly involve the function of proinflammatory cytokines (chaps. 17 and 18; Leonard 2001). In relation to DAT, evidence for the function of neural inflammatory mechanisms has already been detailed (chap. 5).

To conclude, the role of inflammatory mechanisms thus appears to be important in the conversion of dementia of the Alzheimer type from a benign to a malignant disorder (chap. 5), at the interface of dementia of the Alzheimer type and vascular dementia (chap. 10), and at the interface of depression and dementia of the Alzheimer type.

Nondepressive "Pseudodementias"

Our decision to reconceptualize and reclassify depressive dementia outside the historically defining parameters of the pseudodementias resulted in a need to examine other disorders in the pseudodementia category through a new lens. In reworking defining parameters of the syndrome, chapter 16 emphasizes the heterogeneity of the pseudodementias. Analogous to the way this volume's authors have reconceptualized depressive dementia, Sachdev and Reutens reconceptualize the cognitive impairments of schizophrenia, introducing the concept of *schizophrenic dementia.* Just as the cognitive impairments of depressive dementia are real and not "pseudo," the cognitive impairments of schizophrenia are real. Sachdev and Reutens present evidence for biological abnormalities in association with the cognitive impairment profile of schizophrenic dementia.

Examining the material of chapter 16, what stands out is how few empiric data exist for any of the "pseudodementias," excepting depression and schizophrenia. Our study of depressive dementia alerts us to the possibility of long-term multiphasic disease courses with end-stage conversion to irreversible dementia. It is possible that other "pseudodementias" also represent initially-reversible, prepermanent intermediate-stage dementias in the transition to irreversible dementia. We conclude that all of the other disorders comprising the historical category of pseudodementia require long-term follow-up to see if, indeed, any "pseudodementias" exist at all.

Conclusion

The authors of this volume have discussed the presentations, differential diagnosis, nosology, and treatment of the spectra of the dementias from empirical, clinical, and theoretical perspectives. There has been an effort to contribute to the definition of the various dementias and the relationships between them. It is our conclusion that each dementing illness involves a spectrum: an array of varied but related presentations that form a continuous series. We have tried to do some groundwork and point toward future research that is needed to better understand the nature of these interrelationships between the dementias and, more important, to improve present approaches to rational treatment of the spectra of the dementias and of the excess disability existing in the context of those spectra.

REFERENCES

Alzheimer, A. 1907. Uber eine eigenartige Erkrankung de Hirnrinde. *Allgemeine Zeitschrift für Psychiatrie und Psychisch-Gerichliche Medizin* 64:146–48.

American Psychiatric Association. 1952. *Diagnostic and Statistical Manual of Mental Disorders.* Washington, D.C.: American Psychiatric Association.

American Psychiatric Association. 1968. *Diagnostic and Statistical Manual of Mental Disorders.* 2nd ed. Washington, D.C.: American Psychiatric Association.

American Psychiatric Association. 2000. *Diagnostic and Statistical Manual of Mental Disorders.* 4th ed., text revision. Washington, D.C.: American Psychiatric Association.

Baltes, P. 1993. The aging mind: Potential and limits. *Gerontologist* 33:580–94.

Birren, J.E., A. Woods, and M. Williams. 1980. Behavioral slowing with age: Causes, organization, and consequences. In *Aging in the 1980s*, edited by L. Poon. Washington, D.C.: American Psychological Association, pp. 293–308.

Brown, W., D. Moody, C. Thore, et al. 2000. Cerebrovascular pathology in Alzheimer's disease and leukoaraiosis. *Annals of the New York Academy of Sciences* 903:39–45.

Corder, E.H., A. Saunders, W. Strittmatter, et al. 1993. Gene dose of apolipoprotein E type 4 allele and the risk of Alzheimer's disease in late-onset families. *Science* 261: 921–23.

Cunningham, W., and J. W. Brookbank. 1988. *Gerontology.* New York: Harper and Row.

Cutler, R. G. 1976. Evolution of longevity in primates. *Journal of Human Evolution* 5: 169.

Darwin, C. 1955 [1859]. *The Origin of Species.* New York: Modern Library.

De La Monte, S., Y. Sohn, D. Etienne, et al. 2000. Role of aberrant nitric oxide synthase-3 expression in cerebrovascular degeneration and vascular-mediated injury in Alzheimer's disease. *Annals of the New York Academy of Sciences* 903:61–71.

Devanand, D., M. Sano, M. Tang, et al. 1996. Depressed mood and the incidence of Alzheimer's disease in the elderly living in the community. *Archives of General Psychiatry* 53:175–82.

Dobzhansky, T. 1964. *Heredity and the Nature of Man.* New York: Harcourt, Brace, and World.

Emery, V.O.B. 1985. Language and aging. *Experimental Aging Research Monograph Series* 11 (1):3–63.

Emery, V.O.B. 1988. *Pseudodementia: A Theoretical and Empirical Discussion.* Cleveland: Case Western Reserve University School of Medicine.

Emery, V.O.B. 1999. On the relationship between memory and language in the dementia spectrum of depression, Alzheimer syndrome, and normal aging. In *Language and Communication in Old Age: Multidisciplinary Perspectives*, edited by H. Hamilton. New York: Garland Publishing, pp. 25–62.

Emery, V.O.B. 2000. Language impairment in dementia of the Alzheimer type: A hierarchical decline? *International Journal of Psychiatry in Medicine* 30:145–64.

Emery, V.O.B., and L.B. Breslau. 1987. The acceleration process in Alzheimer's disease: Thought dissolution in Alzheimer's disease early-onset and senile dementia Alzheimer's type. *American Journal of Alzheimer's Care* 2:24–32.

Emery, V.O.B., E.X. Gillie, and P.T. Ramdev. 1994. Vascular dementia redefined. In *Dementia: Presentations, Differential Diagnosis, and Nosology*, edited by V.O.B. Emery and T.E. Oxman. Baltimore: Johns Hopkins University Press, pp. 162–94.

Emery, V.O.B., E.X. Gillie, and P.T. Ramdev. 1995. Noninfarct vascular dementia. In *Treating Alzheimer's and Other Dementias*, edited by M. Bergener and S. Finkel. New York: Springer, pp. 184–203.

Emery, V.O.B., E.X. Gillie, and J.A. Smith. 1996. Reclassification of the vascular dementias: Comparisons of infarct and noninfarct vascular dementias. *International Psychogeriatrics* 8:33–61.

Emery, V.O.B., E.X. Gillie, and J.A. Smith. 2000. Interface between vascular dementia and Alzheimer syndrome: Nosologic redefinition. *Annals of the New York Academy of Sciences* 903:229–38.
Emery, V.O.B., and T.E. Oxman. 1997. Depressive dementia: A "transitional dementia"? *Clinical Neuroscience* 4:23–30.
Farkas, E., G. DeJong, E. Apro, et al. 2000. Similar ultrastructural breakdown of cerebrocortical capillaries in Alzheimer's disease, Parkinson's disease, and experimental hypertension. *Annals of the New York Academy of Sciences* 903:72–82.
Guyton, A.C. 1981. *Basic Human Physiology.* Philadelphia: W. B. Saunders.
Guyton, A. C. 2000. *Medical Physiology.* New York: Mosby.
Hachinski, V. 1983. Multi-infarct dementia. *Neurologic Clinics* 1:27–36.
Hachinski, V., and D. Munoz. 2000. Vascular factors in cognitive impairment: Where are we now? *Annals of the New York Academy of Sciences* 903:1–6.
Kandel, E.R. 2000. Disorders of mood: Depression, mania, and anxiety disorders. In *Principles of Neural Science,* edited by E.R. Kandel, J. Schwartz, and T.M. Jessell. New York: McGraw-Hill, pp. 1209–26.
Kandel, E.R., J. Schwartz, and T.M. Jessell (Eds.). 2000. *Principles of Neural Science.* New York: McGraw-Hill.
Kral, V., and V.O.B. Emery. 1989. Long-term follow-up of depressive pseudodementia of the aged. *Canadian Journal of Psychiatry* 34:445–47.
Kuchna, I., J. Wegiel, M. Tarnawski, et al. 2001. Alzheimer type pathology in the memory system of people with Down syndrome. *Journal of Neuropathology and Experimental Neurology* 60:545–50.
Lee, V.M.Y. 2001. Tauists and Baptists united. *Science* 293:1446–47.
Leonard, B.E. 2001. Changes in the immune system in depression and dementia: Causal or co-incidental effects? *International Journal of Developmental Neuroscience* 19:305–12.
Lucca, U., M. Comelli, M. Tettamanti, et al. 1993. Rate of progression and prognostic factors in Alzheimer's disease: A prospective study. *Journal of the American Geriatrics Society* 41:45–49.
Mayeux, R., and Y. Stern. 1987. Subcortical dementia. *Archives of Neurology* 34:642–46.
McHugh, P., and M.F. Folstein. 1978. *Research Publication for the Association for Research in Nervous and Mental Disease* 57:17–30.
McKhann, G., D. Drachman, M. Folstein, et al. 1984. Clinical diagnosis of Alzheimer's disease. *Neurology* 34:939–44.
Miyakawa, T., T. Kimura, S. Hirata, et al. 2000. Role of blood vessels in producing pathological changes in the brain with Alzheimer's disease. *Annals of the New York Academy of Sciences* 903:46–54.
Mortimer, J.A., B. Ebbitt, S.P. Jun, et al. 1992. Predictors of cognitive and functional progression in patients with probable Alzheimer's disease. *Neurology* 42:1689–96.
National Academy on an Aging Society. 2000. *Challenges for the 21st Century: Chronic and Disabling Conditions.* Washington, D.C.: Gerontological Society of America.
Nicolas, A.S., S. Andrieu, F. Nourhashemi, et al. 2001. Successful aging and nutrition. *Nutrition Reviews* 59:88–92.
Peterson, R.C. 2000. Aging, mild cognitive impairment, and Alzheimer's disease. *Neurologic Clinics* 18:789–806.
Reisberg, B., A. Burns, H. Brodaty, et al. 1997. Diagnosis of Alzheimer's disease. *International Psychogeriatrics* 9:11–38.

Ross, R. 1993. The pathogenesis of atherosclerosis. *Nature* 362:801–9.
Ross, R. 1999. Mechanisms of disease: Atherosclerosis—an inflammatory disease. *New England Journal of Medicine* 340:115–26.
Rowe, J.W., and R.L. Kahn. 1998. *Successful Aging.* New York: Pantheon.
Rydel, R., A. Kurdowska, K. Johnson-Wood, et al. 1992. Secreted forms of the beta-amyloid precursor protein stimulate IL-6 release in cultures of human fibroblasts. *Neurobiology of Aging* 13 (Suppl. 1):S85.
Sacher, G.A. 1975. Maturation and longevity in relation to cranial capacity in hominid evolution. In *Antecedents of Man and After,* edited by T. Tuttle. The Hague: Moulton, pp. 115–23.
Salthouse, T. 1985. Speed of behavior and its implications for cognition. In *Handbook of the Psychology of Aging,* edited by J.E. Birren and K.W. Schaie. New York: Van Nostrand, pp. 400–422.
Saunders, P., J. Copeland, M. Dewey, et al. 1993. The prevalence of dementia, depression, and neurosis in late life: The Liverpool MRC-ALPHA study. *International Journal of Epidemiology* 22:838–47.
Schaie, K., and S. Willis. 1991. *Adult Development and Aging.* New York: HarperCollins.
Selkoe, D.J. 1992. Beta-amyloidosis: A seminal pathogenetic event in Alzheimer's disease. *Neurobiology of Aging* 13 (Suppl. 1):S74.
Selkoe, D.J. 2001. Alzheimer's disease: Genes, proteins, and therapy. *Physiological Reviews* 81:741–66.
Shihabuddin, L., P. Horner, J. Ray, et al. 2000. Adult spinal cord stem cells generate neurons after transplantation in the adult dentate gyrus. *Journal of Neuroscience* 20: 8727–35.
Sjögren, M., L. Rosengren, L. Minthon, et al. 2000. Cytoskeleton proteins in CSF distinguish frontotemporal dementia from AD. *Neurology* 54:1960–64.
Snowdon, D. 2001. *Aging with Grace.* New York: Bantam Books.
Stedman, T. 1990. *Stedman's Medical Dictionary.* Baltimore: Williams & Wilkins.
Tormey, V., J. Paul, C. Leonard, et al. 1997. T-cell cytokines may control the balance of functionally distinct macrophage populations. *Immunology* 90:463–69.
Udalova, G., and A. Karas. 1996. Learning, memory, and motivation in ants. *Russian Contributions to Invertebrate Behavior,* edited by C. Abramson, Z. Shuranova, and Y. Burmistrov. Westport, Conn.: Praeger, pp. 145–75.
vanDuijn, C., D. Clayton, V. Chandra, et al. 1994. Interaction between genetic and environmental risk factors for Alzheimer's disease: A reanalysis of case-control studies. *Genetic Epidemiology* 11:539–51.
Wetherell, J., M. Gatz, B. Johansson, et al. 1999. History of depression and other psychiatric illness as risk factors for Alzheimer disease in a twin sample. *Alzheimer Disease and Associated Disorders* 13:47–52.
Wisniewski, H.M., J. Wegiel, and E.R. Popovitch. 1994. Age-associated development of diffuse and thioflavine-S-positive plaques in Down syndrome. *Developmental Brain Dysfunction* 7:330–39.
World Health Organization. 1993. *The ICD-10 Classification of Mental and Behavioral Disorders: Diagnostic Criteria for Research.* Geneva: World Health Organization.

Index

Abrupt onset, 40, 64, 76, 307, 317, 318, 324, 325, 386, 399, 414. *See also* Onset
Abstraction, 11, 180, 194, 221, 222, 244–46, 270, 318, 319, 338, 381, 385. *See also* Cognitive evaluation; Mental status
Acetylcholinesterase inhibitors, 66, 69, 139, 141, 255, 409, 465, 466, 473, 480
Acetylcholine transferase, xxxi, 66, 69, 139, 141, 377–79, 387, 409, 444–46, 465, 466, 467, 474, 517. *See also* Cholinergic system; Cholinomimetic agents
Acquired immunodeficiency syndrome (AIDS), xxviii, 68, 69, 247, 249, 252–53, 336–58, 495
Activities of daily living (ADLs), 8, 12, 35, 36, 37, 43, 44, 45, 51, 62, 70, 210, 313, 322, 323, 338, 384, 408, 424, 425, 476, 47. *See also* Functional impairment
Affective disorders, xxix–xxxii, 7, 67, 68, 247, 361, 362, 363–88, 398–412, 417, 418, 419, 430–32, 437, 438, 444–57, 469, 470, 472, 474, 475, 480, 490, 502–3, 513–18. *See also* Depressive dementia; Major depressive disorder; Manic pseudodementias
Age-associated cognitive decline, xxi, 5, 6, 8, 12, 13, 20, 40–41, 45–46, 50, 491–93
Age-associated memory impairment, xxi, 4–5, 6, 8, 12, 13, 20, 40–41, 45–46, 50, 491–93. *See also* Memory
Age correlation, xix, xx, 4, 5, 39, 62–63, 294, 295, 368–70, 491–92, 493, 499–500
Aggression, 64, 180, 206, 207, 210, 247, 248, 427, 432, 468, 469, 470–74, 476
Aging, normal, xix, xxi, xxii, 3–5, 6–20, 32–35, 41, 43, 45–46, 50–53, 61–64, 140, 491–95
Agnosia, 7, 62, 64, 142, 143, 145, 207–8, 209–10, 239–40, 424–29. *See also* Cognitive evaluation; Mental status
AIDS dementia, myelopathic, 342–43
AIDS dementia complex, xxviii, 7, 68–69, 249, 252–53, 336–58, 495
AIDS staging system, 337–38. *See also* Memorial Sloan-Kettering (MSK) AIDS staging system
Alzheimer dementia. *See* Dementia of Alzheimer type (DAT)
Alzheimer disease. *See* Dementia of Alzheimer type (DAT)
Alzheimer disease type I, xxiii–xxiv, 142–43, 150, 499–501
Alzheimer disease type II, xxiii–xxiv, 142–43, 150, 499–501
Alzheimer syndrome. *See* Dementia of Alzheimer type (DAT)
Alzheimer(ized) vascular dementia, 284, 505, 506, 511
Amygdala, 205–10, 224–26
Amyloid-β protein, xxii–xxiii, 13–16, 89–108, 445–55, 496–98. *See also* Neuropathology
Amyloid fibrils, xxii–xxiii, 89, 90–91, 93–98, 99, 101–4, 448–50. *See also* Amyloid-β protein; Neuropathology
Amyloid interface, 281–83, 298, 509–10
Amyotrophic lateral sclerosis (ALS), 169–70, 248–50
Anticholinergic side effects, xxx, 69, 387, 474–75, 517–18. *See also* Acetylcholine transferase; Cholinergic system; Cholinomimetic agents
Anticonvulsants, 474

Antidepressant medications, xxxi, 69, 387, 399–400, 408–9, 410–11, 474–75, 517–18. *See also* Treatment
Antipsychotic drugs, 471, 472, 473, 474. *See also* Neuroleptics
Antiretroviral therapy, 336, 348–51
Anxiety pseudodementias, 362–63, 398–400, 436–37
Aphasia, 62, 156–70, 271–76, 277, 317, 323, 384–86, 399–401, 418. *See also* Language
Apoptosis, 283, 450–52
Approximate answers, 68, 399, 424, 426, 429
Apraxia, 12, 62, 64, 71, 163, 165, 204, 239, 272–73, 274–77, 317, 323, 387
Arithmetic, 194, 223, 272–73, 274–77, 401
Arteriosclerosis, 265, 268–70, 278–81, 282–84, 294–98, 302, 506–9
Arteriosclerotic psychosis, 265–66, 294
Aspirin, xxiii, 131–34
Ataxia, 71, 76, 99, 145, 201, 202, 204, 205, 214, 244–46, 252, 325. *See also* Gait; Movement disorders
Atherosclerosis, 265, 268–70, 278–81, 282–84, 510. *See also* Arteriosclerosis
Attention, 11, 241–42, 244–46, 270, 272–77, 384–86. *See also* Cognitive evaluation; Cognitive impairment; Concentration; Mental status
Autobiographical memory, 181, 189–93, 196, 205–10, 223–26. *See also* Memory
Autoimmunity, pathomechanisms of, xxiii, 121–33, 503–4
Autotoxicity, pathomechanisms of, xxiii, 121–33, 503–4

B_{12} deficiency, 7, 68, 71, 72, 73
Balance, 211, 212, 214
Basal ganglia disorders, 7, 66, 163–64, 167–68, 248–51, 253–55, 471–72. *See also* Subcortical dementias
Basal nucleus of Meynert, 445, 447–50, 451–53, 502
Behavioral assessment, 8–9, 12–13, 32, 35–37, 40, 41, 43–45, 51, 62, 70, 71, 72, 78, 245, 246–48, 325, 338, 339–42, 420, 424–30, 467–69. *See also* Functional impairment
Behavioral consistency, 384, 417, 424, 425, 426. *See also* Behavioral assessment
Behavioral disturbances, treatment of, 467–70, 471, 475–79, 480. *See also* Behavioral assessment
Behçet syndrome, 70, 249
β-protein amyloidosis, xxii–xxiii, 13–16, 89–108, 445–55, 496–98. *See also* Neuropathology
Binswanger disease, xxvii–xxviii, 251–52, 268–70, 278–81, 291–302, 307–9, 311–15, 318–20, 327–28, 506. *See also* White matter changes
Blood-brain barrier, xxiv, 142–43, 150, 282–83, 499–501, 508, 510. *See also* Alzheimer disease type I; Alzheimer disease type II
Blood pressure, 268–69, 278–79, 291–302, 310, 319, 322, 506–7. *See also* Hypertension; Hypotension
Boundaries, normal aging and dementia, xix, xxi, xxii, 3–20, 32–44, 45–47, 50–52, 78, 267, 270–75, 276–78, 491–95
Bradyphrenia, 239, 240, 246
Brain imaging, xxi, 13–15, 16–19, 20, 46, 47, 50, 75–77, 143–46, 159, 161, 167–68, 187–88, 196–97, 320–22, 344–45, 403–5, 407–8, 425, 434, 435–36. *See also* Neuroimaging
Brain infarct concept, xxv–xxvii, 263–67, 278–80, 281, 283–84, 505–11. *See also* Infarct
Brain weight, 13, 14–16

CAMDEX Mental Status Exam, 36–37
CERAD, 36–37, 90–91, 144
Cerebral capillary ultrastructure, xxvii, xxviii, 281–83, 509–11
Cerebral hemorrhage, xxvii, xxviii, 297–99. *See also* Cerebrovascular disease; Cystatin C amyloid; Infarct
Cerebrovascular disease, xxvi–xxviii, 65–66, 251–52, 263–84, 291–302, 306–28, 501–2, 505–11. *See also* Arteriosclerosis; Blood pressure; Gray matter lesions;

Hemodynamic mechanisms; Infarct; Preinfarct state; Vascular dementia; White matter changes
Choline acetyl transferase, xxxi, 46, 47, 66, 69, 139, 141, 255, 377–79, 387, 409, 444–56, 465–66, 473, 474, 480, 517. *See also* Acetylcholine transferase; Cholinergic system; Cholinomimetic agents
Cholinergic system, xxxi, 46, 47, 66, 69, 139, 141, 255, 377–79, 387, 409, 444–56, 465–66, 473, 480, 517
Cholinomimetic agents, 465–67
Chronic obstructive pulmonary disease (COPD), 267–70
Circulatory disturbances, xxvi–xxviii, 65–66, 251–52, 263–84, 291–302, 306–28, 501–2, 505–11. *See also* Arteriosclerosis; Hemodynamic mechanisms; Hypertension; Hypotension; Infarct; Noninfarct vascular dementia; Vascular dementia
Clinical history, 8, 12, 35–37, 43–45, 51, 62, 70, 76, 78, 210, 312, 313, 322–23, 325, 338, 384, 408, 409–12, 424–25, 476, 477
Cognitive enhancers, 463–67
Cognitive evaluation, 5–14, 32–35, 36–37, 40–53, 61–67, 71, 72, 78, 144, 204–5, 244–46, 255, 267–72, 273–78, 307, 312–19, 323–25, 337–41, 370, 373–79, 383–86, 400–2, 408–12, 423, 424–25. *See also* Attention; Concentration; Language; Memory; Mental status; Visuospatial function
Cognitive impairment, treatment of, 69, 131–34, 348–50, 387, 463–67, 474–75, 476–80, 517–18
Complement system, xxiii, 123–27, 129–32, 503–4
Concentration, 11, 241–42, 245–46, 270, 272–77, 384–86. *See also* Attention; Mental status
Confusional symptoms, 68, 142–43, 338, 424–25, 433–34
Construct validity, xxii, 31–32, 40–52, 178, 180, 183, 184, 188–96, 198, 199–200, 202–3, 263–67, 278–81, 361–66, 495–96, 505–6, 511–12, 513–17. *See also* Operational definition
Continuity model, xix–xxii, xxv–xxvii, xxix–xxx, xxxii, xxxiii, 31–53, 191–93, 210–27, 278–84, 361–83, 490–519. *See also* Spectrum model
Conversion disorder, xxxi, 398, 421, 424–26, 427, 428–30
Cortical dementias, xxv–xxvi, 89–108, 121–33, 139–50, 157–59, 165–66, 199–227, 239–41, 243, 255, 410, 425, 444–57, 465–69, 495–505
Creutzfeldt-Jakob disease, 67, 73–74, 164, 253
Curvilinear-like depression-dementia relation, xxix–xxx, 377–79, 516–17
Cystatin C amyloid, xxvii, 298–300, 510

Degenerative dementia: with depression, 376–79, 444–57, 515–16; without depression, 376, 515–16
Delirium, 40, 44–45, 62–63, 68, 71, 76, 78, 241, 420, 430–32, 433, 463–64, 514
Delusions, 70, 248, 398, 399, 400, 424–25, 427, 430–37, 452–54, 469–70, 471–73. *See also* Psychosis
Dementia of Alzheimer type (DAT), xxii–xxv, 6, 9–19, 31–33, 35, 38–40, 47–48, 64–65, 89–108, 121–33, 139–50, 157–59, 165–67, 183–84, 186–88, 190–91, 193–96, 198–99, 203–5, 209–10, 213–15, 217, 219–20, 221–23, 225–27, 244–45, 281–84, 306–8, 310, 313, 323, 364–67, 375–79, 385–87, 401, 404, 444–57, 465–69, 495–505; age of onset, xxiii–xxiv, 101, 74, 91, 140–46, 447, 448, 499–502 (*see also* Onset); atypical presentations, 165–67, 168–70, 204–5, 250–51, 502–3; clinical subgroups, xxiii–xxiv, 139–50, 498–503; definition, 32, 33, 35, 37–39, 40–43, 61–62, 90–91, 203–4, 495–96; epidemiology, 6–7, 49, 61–63, 72–74, 306–8, 364–67; familial incidence, 74, 91, 103–07, 146–48; heterogeneity, xxiii–xxiv, 74, 91, 98, 101, 139–50, 204–5, 250–51, 499–503, 509–11; immune system response, xxiii, 123–33, 503–4;

Dementia of Alzheimer type (DAT) (*continued*): language, 10, 11, 14–15, 157–59, 221–23, 225–26, 242, 385–86, 400–2, 424–25; life expectancy, 101–2, 141, 150, 447, 452, 456; memory, xxiv–xxv, 10–11, 98–99, 183–84, 186–88, 190–91, 193–96, 198–99, 203–5, 209–10, 213–15, 217–20, 221–23, 225–27, 243–46, 504–5; neuropathology, xxii–xxiii, 13–16, 89–108, 445–55, 496–98; prevalence, 6–7, 49, 61–63, 72–74, 306–8, 364–67, 445–47; stages, xxi, 5–8, 97, 98, 200- 27, 513–14, 516–17; subtypes, xxiii–xxiv, 74, 91, 98, 101, 103–107, 281–83, 284, 376–77, 447–50, 498–99, 509–11

Dementia rating scale, 7, 9, 32–37, 44, 78, 213, 270, 271, 272, 274–77

Dementia syndrome of depression. *See* Depressive dementia

Depression, xxix–xxxii, 7, 67, 68, 247, 323, 361, 362, 363–88, 398–412, 417, 418, 419, 430–32, 437, 438, 444–57, 469, 470, 472, 474, 475, 480, 490, 502–3, 513–18; stages of, xxix–xxx, 367–68, 372–80, 513–16. *See also* Affective disorders; Depressive dementia; Depressive-spectrum disorders

Depression-executive dysfunction syndrome, xxix–xxx, xxi, 373–75, 405–10

Depressive dementia, xxix–xxxii, 361–87, 398–411, 513–19; cognitive impairment, 370, 373–76, 380–81, 384–86, 398, 399, 400–403, 513–19; definition, xxix, 361–67, 373–76, 380–83, 398, 400–403, 513–19 ; language, 380–81, 385–86, 399–400, 401–3; long-term disease course, xxix–xxx, 361–67, 373–83, 402–5, 406, 513–19; memory, 380–81, 384–85, 370, 373–76, 398, 400, 401–3; neurobiology, 364–67, 377–79, 380–83, 386–87, 406–8, 517–19; neuropathology, xxxi, 364–67, 370–72, 373, 405–7, 517–19; onset, 361–67, 368–72, 373–76, 399–405, 513–19; prevalence, 362–67, 368–76, 378–380, 383, 399–405, 513–19; risk factors, xxix–xxxii, 361–67, 372–77, 378–80, 381–83, 399–405, 513–19; stages, xxix–xxx, 367–79, 513–19; treatment, 387–88, 399–400, 405–11, 515–19

Depressive pseudodementias. *See* Depressive dementia

Depressive-spectrum disorders. *See* Affective disorders; Depressive dementia; Manic pseudodementias; Spectrum model

Diabetes mellitus, 68, 70–71, 73, 267–70, 296, 310, 321, 322

Diachronic, xix, xxiv–xxv, 179, 180, 192, 193, 199–201, 226–27, 277, 490–91, 504–5, 514–17

Diagnostic and Statistical Manual of Mental Disorders, first edition (DSM I), 265, 266

Diagnostic and Statistical Manual of Mental Disorders, second edition (DSM II), 265, 266

Diagnostic and Statistical Manual of Mental Disorders, third edition (DSM III), 38, 65, 265, 266, 402–3

Diagnostic and Statistical Manual of Mental Disorders, fourth edition (DSM IV), 7, 20, 61, 65, 214, 240, 265, 266, 314, 402–3

Diagnostic and Statistical Manual of Mental Disorders, fourth edition revised (DSM IV-TR), 32, 33, 61, 65, 66, 240, 265, 266, 314, 402–3

Diaschisis, xxvii, 156–57, 278–79, 508, 509–10

Diffuse disease, xix–xx, xxiv–xxv, 156–57, 161–65, 170, 278–84, 509–10

Dissociative pseudodementias, 399–400, 427–29, 514

Distal causality, xxvii–xxviii, 156–57, 278–81, 509–10

Dopamine, 254–55, 448–50, 451–57. *See also* Neurotransmitters

Down syndrome, xxi, xxii–xxiii, 101–4, 498–99

Drug abuse pseudodementias. *See* Nondepressive pseudodementias

Drug toxicity, xxii, 68, 69, 70, 73, 387, 467, 471–73, 474, 475, 517–18. *See also* Iatrogenic factors

Dysarthria, 157, 204, 245, 248, 249, 273–76, 319–20, 323. *See also* Aphasia; Language
Dysthymic disorders. *See* Affective disorders; Depression; Depressive-spectrum disorders; Neurosis

Echoic memory, 212
Echolalia, 158, 159
Electroencephalogram (EEG), 46, 47, 67, 143–44, 160, 161, 313, 327, 386, 387, 425, 426. *See also* brain imaging
Emotional incontinence, 167, 168, 318, 319, 427, 428, 431, 432, 468, 469
Emotional memory, xxiv–xxv, 200, 205–10, 223, 224, 225, 226, 227, 504–5. *See also* Three-tiered evolutionary memory model
Environmental interventions, 463, 464, 465, 471, 475–80
Epidemiology, 350, 351, 364, 365, 366, 367, 368, 369, 370, 372, 376, 402–5
Epilepsy, 164, 165
Episodic memory, 188–91, 192, 193, 219, 220, 224, 226. *See also* Stage 4 memory
Evolutionary memory model, xxiv, xxv, 199–226, 504–5. *See also* Three-tiered evolutionary memory model
Excess disability, xxxii, 68, 387, 463, 464, 471, 473, 474, 475, 478–80, 519. *See also* Drug toxicity; Iatrogenic factors
Executive function, xxix, xxx, xxi, 11, 12, 64, 70, 240, 244–46, 319, 323, 373–75, 405–9
Extracranial carotid artery disease, 508, 509
Extrapyramidal symptoms, xxiv, 166, 167, 198, 199, 245, 249, 250, 251, 252, 502, 503

Factitious disorder, 426, 427, 428
Fahr disease, 248, 249, 251
Familial incidence, 74, 91, 103, 104, 105, 106, 107, 108, 146, 147, 148, 162, 163, 366, 367, 375, 404, 405, 447, 448. *See also* Epidemiology; Genetics; Prevalence
Fibrillar amyloid-β protein. *See* Dementia of Alzheimer type, neuropathology; Neuropathology
First-degree relatives, 74, 101, 103, 104, 105, 162, 163, 366, 367, 404, 405. *See also* Genetics
First-order criteria for dementia, xxii, 32, 33–40, 42, 43, 44, 45
fMRI. *See* Brain imaging, Neuroimaging
Focality vs. diffuse disease, xix, xx, xxiv, xxv, 156, 157, 161–65, 170, 278–84, 509, 510
Forgetfulness. *See* Age-associated memory impairment; Memory; Mild cognitive impairment
Frontostriatal dysfunction, 196, 197, 198, 199, 201, 202, 203, 204, 205, 406
Frontosubcortical dementia (FSCD), xix, xxiv, 64, 66, 67, 74, 156, 157, 167, 168, 169, 198, 239–55, 313, 406, 432, 511, 512, 513
Frontotemporal dementia, xix, xxiv, 64, 66, 67, 74, 156, 157, 167, 168, 169, 170, 198, 239–55, 313, 406, 432, 511, 512, 513
Fugue states, 427, 428, 429
Functional impairment, 8, 12, 32, 33, 35, 36, 37, 43, 44, 45, 51, 62, 64, 70, 210, 313, 322, 323, 337, 338, 384, 408, 424, 428, 476, 477

Gait, 71, 76, 99, 100, 145, 201, 202, 204, 205, 214, 244–46, 252, 325, 338, 340, 341. *See also* Ataxia; Basal ganglia disorders
Ganser syndrome, xxxi, 398, 417, 419, 426, 427, 429–30
General paresis, 69, 70, 73, 249, 345, 432, 514
Genetic memory, 178, 179, 180, 203. *See also* Memory
Genetic mutations. *See* Genetics
Genetics, xxi, 51, 52, 74–75, 91, 101–8, 146–49, 150, 162, 163, 249–50, 251, 252, 322, 366, 367, 375, 404, 405, 446, 447, 448, 454, 455, 497, 498, 499, 517–18
Granulovascular degeneration. *See* Neuropathology
Gray matter lesions, 14, 15, 37, 38, 76, 90, 91, 92–101, 121, 122, 145, 268, 269, 280–84, 445–51, 496, 497, 503, 504. *See also* Neuropathology

Hallucinations. *See* Psychosis
Hemodynamic mechanisms, 268, 269, 270, 278–81, 292–95, 308, 309, 318, 319, 506–10
Hepatic dementia, 68, 75, 472
Hereditary dysphasic dementia, 162, 163, 164, 165
Higher cortical memory, 199, 200, 201, 210–27. *See* Evolutionary memory model; Three-tiered evolutionary memory model
Highly active antiretroviral therapy (HAART), 336, 342, 348–51
Hippocampus, 13, 14, 15, 16–20, 130, 141–44, 165, 187–88, 197, 208, 215, 220, 221, 223, 224, 319, 373, 374, 435, 451. *See also* Neuropathology
HIV encephalopathy. *See* AIDS dementia complex
HIV-related cognitive motor complex. *See* AIDS dementia complex
Human immunodeficiency virus (HIV), xxviii, 7, 68–69, 249, 252, 253, 336–58, 495
Huntington disease, 196–205, 240, 241, 242–51. *See also* Subcortical dementias
Hyperactivity, 431–33, 468–72
Hypercalcemia, 68
Hypertension, xxvii, 268–70, 278–79, 291–302, 310, 322, 506–7
Hypotension, xxvii, 268–70, 278–79, 319, 322, 506–7
Hysterical infantilism, 428–29
Hysterical pseudodementias, 398, 421, 426–29, 514
Hysterical puerilism, 428–29

Iatrogenic factors, xxii, xxx, 68, 69, 70, 73, 387, 467, 471–73, 474, 475, 479, 517–18
Iconic memory, 212, 213
Idiopathic Parkinson disease. *See* Parkinson disease
Immune system response, xxiii, 121–33, 178, 203, 281–84, 340–50, 503, 504, 509–11, 518
Impulse control , 431–33, 463, 465, 468–72, 477
Infarct, xxvi–xxvii, 65–66, 251–52, 263–84, 291–302, 306–28, 501, 502, 505–11. *See* Multi-infarct dementia (MID); Preinfarct state
Inflammation, xxiii, 121–33, 178, 203, 281–84, 503, 504, 509–11
Information-processing theory, 184–188
Initially-reversible dementia. *See* Depressive dementia; Nondepressive pseudodementias
Insidious onset, 40, 64, 76, 307, 316, 317, 318, 323, 324, 325, 327, 328, 386, 399, 414, 424, 425. *See also* Onset
Institutionalization, 478, 479
Intermediate-stage dementia. *See* Depressive dementia; Nondepressive pseudodementias; Prepermanent dementia
Irreversible dementia. *See* Degenerative dementia; Dementia of Alzheimer type

Kluver-Bucy syndrome, 169

Lacunar state. *See* Vascular dementia; White matter changes
Language, xxiv, 10, 11, 62, 66–67, 156–70, 191–96, 271–76, 277, 317, 323, 384–86, 399–401, 418; in Alzheimer syndrome, xxiii–xxiv, 10, 11, 14, 15, 142–43, 150, 157–59, 193–96, 221–23, 225–27, 242, 385–86, 400–2, 424–25, 499–501; in depressive dementia, 380–81, 384–86, 399–403; in frontosubcortical dementia, 240, 242, 244–46; in major depressive disorder, 380–81, 384–86, 399, 403; in vascular dementia, 242, 245, 270–72, 273–77
Leukoaraiosis. *See* White matter changes
Leukopenia, 472
Lewy body disease, 39, 66, 241, 242–51, 313, 314, 371, 452, 453, 472
Life expectancy, xix, xx, 101–2, 141, 150, 447, 452, 456, 491–93. *See also* Epidemiology

Macroinfarct. *See* Infarct
Major depression with dementia. *See* Degenerative dementia, with depression; Depressive dementia

Major depression without dementia, 364–66, 367–70, 372–73, 377–79, 380–87, 402–5, 514–19. *See also* Affective disorders
Major depressive disorder. *See* Affective disorders; Degenerative dementia, with depression; Depressive dementia
Malingering, 398, 417–19, 423–26, 427–28, 514, 518–19
Mania. *See* Affective disorders; Manic pseudodementias
Manic pseudodementias, 398, 417–19, 430–32, 514, 518–19
Medications. *See* Acetylcholinesterase inhibitors; Anticonvulsants; Antidepressant medications; Antipsychotic drugs; Antiretroviral therapy; Cognitive enhancers; Highly active antiretroviral therapy; Neuroleptics; Noncogntive disturbance/psychopharmacology; Treatment
Membrane attack complex, xxiii, 125–33, 503, 504
Memorial Sloan Kettering (MSK) AIDS staging system, 337, 338
Memory, xxiv, xxv, 4–7, 8, 10, 11, 34, 62, 98, 99, 142–43, 150, 177–227, 243–46, 270–71, 272–76, 277, 370, 373–76, 380, 381, 384, 385, 398, 400, 401–3, 425, 499–501, 504–5; in Alzheimer syndrome, xxiv, xxv, 4–7, 10, 11, 98, 99, 142–43, 150, 183–88, 190, 191, 193–96, 198–99, 203–5, 209, 210, 213–15, 217–23, 225–27, 243–46, 499–501, 504–5; in depressive dementia, 365, 370, 373–76, 380, 381, 384, 385, 398, 400, 401–3; in major depressive disorder, 365, 370, 372, 373–76, 380, 381, 384, 385, 398, 400, 401–3; in vascular dementia, 8, 10, 243–46, 270, 271, 272–6, 277, 318, 319, 322, 323
Meningitis, 60, 70, 73, 345, 432
Mental status, 5–14, 32–35, 36, 37, 40–53, 61–67, 69, 71, 73, 78, 144, 204, 205, 241–46, 255, 270–76, 307, 312–19, 323–25, 337–41, 370, 373–79, 383–86, 400–5, 408–12, 423–25, 517–18. *See also* Abstraction; Attention, Cognitive evaluation; Concentration; Language; Memory; Visuospatial function
Metabolic disorders, xxvii, 46, 50, 51, 68, 70, 71–74, 75, 76, 78, 156–57, 268–70, 278, 281–83, 313, 319, 320, 463–65, 508–10
Metanaming tasks, 194, 195, 273
Microglia. *See* Neuropathology
Microinfarct. *See* Infarct
Mild cognitive impairment (MCI), xxi, 3–7, 8, 9–20, 67, 494–95
Mini-Mental State Exam (MMSE), 14, 15, 33, 34, 35, 64, 71–72, 78, 140, 159, 270, 271, 272, 274–77, 339–41, 402–3
Monckeberg arteriosclerosis, 268
Monoamine oxidase inhibitors (MAO inhibitors). *See* Antidepressant medications; Treatment
Mood changes, 62, 67, 68, 205–10, 245, 246, 247, 248, 252, 319, 323, 324, 468, 469, 470. *See also* Affective disorders; Emotional incontinence; Major depressive disorder
Mood disorders. *See* Affective disorders; Major depressive disorder
Mortality, xix, xx, 101–2, 141, 150, 447, 452, 456, 491–93
Motor dementias. *See* Basal ganglia disorders; Movement disorders; Subcortical dementias
Motor disorders. *See* Movement disorders
Motor function, 7, 12, 62, 64, 66, 71, 76, 99, 100, 145, 163–65, 167, 168, 201, 202, 204, 205, 214, 244, 245, 246, 248–51, 252, 253, 255, 272–77, 325, 338, 340, 341, 471, 472. *See also* Apraxia; Ataxia; Basal ganglia disorders; Gait; Movement disorders
Motor memory, xxiv, xxv, 200, 201–5, 504–5. *See* Evolutionary memory model; Three-tiered evolutionary memory model
Motor neuron disease, 169, 170, 248, 249, 250
Movement disorders, xxv–xxviii, 35, 36, 37, 38, 39, 46, 47, 201–5, 239–55. *See also* Apraxia; Ataxia; Basal ganglia disorders; Gait; Motor function

Movement memory, xxiv, xxv, 200, 201–5, 504–5. *See* Evolutionary memory model, Three-tiered evolutionary memory model
Multi-infarct dementia (MID), xxv–xxviii, 38, 39, 265–83, 291–302, 308–16, 317–18, 320, 322, 326, 327, 328, 505–10
Multiphasic disease course, xxi, xxix–xxxii, 361, 362, 363, 364–84, 387, 400–9, 513–18
Multiple sclerosis, 198–99, 242, 243, 248–51, 252, 254–55
Myelopathic AIDS dementia complex, 342–43
Myoclonus, xxiii–xxiv, 164, 165, 166, 167, 204, 205, 245, 246, 250, 251

National Institute of Neurological and Communicative Disorders and Stroke criteria, 20, 32, 33, 39, 65, 66, 90, 204, 205, 251, 268, 269, 314, 316, 317, 323–24
Near-miss answers, 68, 399, 421, 424, 426, 429, 430
Neocortical memory, xxiv, xxv, 199, 200, 201, 210–27, 504–5. *See also* Higher cortical memory
Neoplasm, 73, 76, 463
Neural inflammation, xxiii, 121–33, 178, 203, 281–84, 503, 504, 509–11
Neural inflammatory mechanisms, xxiii, 121–33, 178, 203, 281–84, 503, 4, 509–11
Neural plasticity, 179, 200, 182, 216
Neuritic plaques. *See* Dementia of Alzheimer type, neuropathology; Neuropathology
Neurofibrillary tangles. *See* Dementia of Alzheimer type, neuropathology, Neuropathology
Neurogenesis, 3, 493, 494
Neuroimaging, xxi, 13, 14, 15, 16–19, 20, 46, 47, 50, 75–77, 143–46, 159–61, 167–68, 187–88, 196–97, 320–22, 372, 406–8, 425, 434–36
Neuroleptics , 69, 132–33, 387, 399–400, 401, 408–9, 410, 411, 465–67, 469–75, 517–18. *See also* Treatment
Neuronal loss. *See* Neuropathology
Neuropathology, xxxi, xxii, xxiii, 13–15, 37–40, 42–45, 89–108, 121–33, 140, 145, 146, 161–66, 168–70, 240, 241, 248–51, 252–55, 281–84, 292–95, 299–301, 309–12, 314, 315, 316, 320–21, 364–67, 370, 371, 373, 403, 406, 407, 445–54, 496–97, 498, 503, 504, 509–13, 517–19; and cognitive impairment, 42, 43, 44, 370, 371; as criteria for Alzheimer diagnosis, 37, 38, 42, 43, 44, 370, 371, 496, 497; and functional impairment, 37, 38, 43, 44, 371; and HIV, 346–48; and infarction, 38, 39, 251–52, 292–95, 299–301, 309–13, 314–16, 320–28; and neurochemical correlates of major depression, 445, 446, 448–54; of progressive aphasia, 161–166; and studies of schizophrenia, 432–36; and white matter changes, 15, 251–52, 292–95, 299–301, 309–16, 320–21, 327, 328
Neurosarcoidosis, 248, 249, 250, 251
Neurosis, 361, 363, 364, 398, 417, 427–28, 436
Neurosyphilis, 69, 70, 249, 250
Neurotransmitters, xxxi, 139, 141, 142, 149, 281–84, 369–70, 374, 377–79, 386, 387, 388, 408, 409–11, 444–57, 465–67, 468, 470–75, 500, 516–18
Noncognitive disturbances, 467, 468, 470–75, 477–80
Noncognitive disturbances/nonpharmacologic intervention, 475–78
Noncognitive disturbances/psychopharmacology, 470–75
Nondepressive pseudodementias, xxx–xxxi, 417–37, 518–19
Noninfarct vascular dementia, xxvi–xxvii, 263–84, 506–11
Nonsteroidal anti-inflammatory drugs, 121–23, 132, 133
Normal aging, xix, xxi, xxii, 3–5, 6–20, 32–35, 41, 43, 45–46, 50–53, 61–64, 140, 453, 454, 491–95
Normal pressure hydrocephalus, 71, 75, 313, 364, 514
Nosology, xix–xxxiii, 4–7, 31–52, 61–64, 156, 157, 177–80, 188–90, 191–93, 198,

199–201, 226–27, 263–67, 278–84, 361–64, 367, 377–79, 380–84, 490–519

Obsessive compulsive pseudodementias, 364, 398, 419, 436, 437, 514
Oculomotor function, 211–14
Olfaction, 211, 212, 214, 215, 387
Oligodendrocytes, xxvii–xxviii, 311, 346, 347
Onset, 10, 40, 64, 76, 104, 105, 148, 166, 177, 307, 316, 317, 318, 323, 324, 325, 327, 328, 343, 386, 399, 414, 424, 425, 427, 448, 452
Operational definition, 4–7, 8, 31, 33, 35–52, 180, 183, 184, 188–96, 198, 199–200, 202–3, 263–67, 268–71
Orientation, 8, 9, 14, 15, 33, 34, 35, 62, 64, 71–72, 78, 140, 159, 199–201, 223–27, 270, 271, 272, 274–77, 339, 402, 403. *See also* Mental status
Overlearned material, 185, 187, 188, 199–201, 223–27. *See also* Memory; Stage 6 memory; Tertiary memory

Pallilalia, 242
Paradigm shift, xxi, 263–67, 278–84, 361–64, 367, 377–79, 380–84, 405–8, 490–519
Paraphasia, 242. *See also* Aphasia; Language
Paraphrenia, 364, 432–36. *See also* Schizophrenia
Parkinson disease, 7, 38, 39, 100, 163, 196–205, 240, 241, 242–46, 247–51, 255, 313, 409, 455, 456, 472, 505
Peripheral vascular disease (PVD), 269, 278–81, 506, 507
Personality changes, 167, 168, 239, 240, 247, 248, 251, 255, 318, 319, 323, 420, 426, 427, 428, 431, 436, 465, 467, 468, 469, 471–75
Phenotype, 362, 364, 381, 382
Phylogenetics, xxiv, xxv, 177–80, 199–227, 504–5
Pick bodies. *See* Pick disease
Pick complex, 164. *See also* Frontotemporal dementia; Pick disease
Pick disease, 7, 66, 67, 160, 161, 162, 164, 167, 168–70. *See also* Frontotemporal dementia
Preinfarct state, 278–81, 283–84, 509
Prepermanent dementia. *See* Depressive dementia; Intermediate-stage dementia; Nondepressive pseudodementias; Transitional dementias
Presenilin mutations, 91–92, 104–8
Prevalence, 49, 65, 67, 68, 69, 71, 74, 75, 131, 132, 350, 351, 364, 368, 369, 370, 371, 376, 377, 379, 380
Primary degenerative dementia. *See* Degenerative dementia; Dementia of Alzheimer type
Primary gain, 420, 427, 429
Primary memory, 181, 184–86, 210, 211, 215–18. *See also* Information-processing theory; Stage 2 memory
Primary progressive aphasia, 156–57, 159–65, 170
Problem behaviors, 468–69, 470
Procedural vs. declarative memory, 181, 196–99
Progressive aphasia, 156–57, 159–65, 170
Progressive supranuclear palsy, 167–68, 198–99, 239–41, 242–51, 313
Proximal causality, xxvii, xxviii, 156–57, 278–81, 509–10
Pseudodementias. *See* Depressive dementia; Nondepressive pseudodementias
Psychosis, 70, 71, 245, 246–48, 364, 398, 424–25, 430–37, 452, 463, 464, 465, 469–70, 471–74

Quality of life, 51, 465, 469, 470, 471, 475–79

Rapid eye motion (REM) activity, 384, 386, 387
Reactive depression, 398. *See also* Affective disorders
Reading, 158, 163, 242, 271–72, 273–77, 400–403, 436. *See also* Language
Renal failure, 68
Retro-ontogenesis, xxv, 177–78, 210, 221, 222–23, 226, 227, 504–5

Retrophylogenesis, xxv, 177–78, 199–227, 504–5
"Reversible" dementias. *See* Depressive dementias; Nondepressive pseudodementias
Reversibility, concept of, xxix, xxx, 361–67, 373–76, 380–84, 398–405, 417–19, 513–19

Sarcoidosis, 248, 249, 250, 251
Schizophrenia, 62, 432–36, 437, 455–56, 518, 519. *See also* Psychosis; Schizophrenic dementia
Schizophrenic dementia, xxxi, 432–36, 437, 455–56, 518, 519
Schizophrenic pseudodementias, xxxi, 432–36, 437, 455–56, 518, 519
Secondary gain, 420, 427
Secondary memory, 181, 184–88. *See also* Information-processing theory
Second-order criteria for dementia, 31, 32, 40, 41, 42. *See also* First order-criteria for dementia
Semantic memory, 10, 11, 181, 188, 191–96, 220–23
Semantics, 191–92, 193, 271–72, 273–76, 385–86, 400–401
Semiotic hierarchy (linguistic classification), 191–92
Senile neuritic plaques. *See* Dementia of Alzheimer type; Neuropathology
Sensory memory, 183, 199–201, 210–15. *See also* Higher cortical memory; Stage 1 memory
Sensory-motor deficits. *See* Apraxia; Basal ganglia disorders; Higher cortical memory; Motor dementias; Motor function; Movement disorders; Stage 1 memory; Subcortical dementias
Serotonin. *See* Antidepressant medications; Neurotransmitters
Sexuality, 169, 350–51, 430, 431, 432, 468, 469
Short-term memory, 181, 182–84, 185
Simulated dementia. *See* Nondepressive pseudodementias, Pseudodementias
Sleep disturbance, 71, 253, 384, 386, 387, 400, 408, 409, 465, 468, 469
Small vessels, 278–81, 282, 283, 291–302, 308, 309–16, 318, 319, 505–9, 510, 511. *See also* Cerebrovascular disease; Infarct; Noninfarct vascular dementia; Vascular dementia
Social and occupational function. *See* Behavioral assessment; Behavioral disturbances; Functional impairment
Social environment assessment, 463, 464, 465, 467–70, 475–80
Somatosenses, 211, 212
Spectrum model, xix–xxxiii, 31–53, 191–93, 210–27, 278–84, 327, 328, 361–83, 387, 490–519
Stage 1 memory (sensory), xxi, xxiv–xxv, 183, 199–201, 210–15, 226, 227, 504–5. *See also* Sensory memory
Stage 2 memory, xxi, xxiv–xxv, 199–201, 210, 211, 215–18, 226, 227, 504–5. *See also* Higher cortical memory; Primary memory; Short-term memory
Stage 3 memory (new learning), xxi, xxiv–xxv, 199–201, 218–20, 226, 227, 504–5. *See also* Episodic memory; Higher cortical memory
Stage 4 memory (delayed new learning), xxi, xxiv–xxv, 199–201, 218–20, 226, 227, 504–5. *See also* Higher cortical memory
Stage 5 memory (knowledge), xxi, xxiv–xxv, 199–201, 220–23, 226, 227, 504–5. *See also* Higher cortical memory; Semantic memory
Stage 6 memory (overlearned material), xxi, xxiv–xxv, 185, 187, 188, 199–201, 210–11, 223–227, 504–5. *See also* Higher cortical memory; Tertiary memory
Stepwise deterioration, 315, 316, 317, 323, 324, 325, 328
Stroke. *See* Infarct; Multi-infarct dementia; Preinfarct state; Vascular dementia
Subcortical dementias, xxv–xxvi, 7, 66, 163–64, 167–68, 198, 199, 239–55, 291–302, 307, 308–10, 313, 318–21, 326, 328, 340, 336–51, 374–75, 410, 471, 472, 505–10, 511–13

Subcortical memory, 199–201, 201–5, 243–46, 251–52, 374–75. *See also* Motor memory
Subcortical vascular dementia syndrome, 251–52, 291–302, 308–10, 318, 320, 321, 326, 328, 505–10. *See also* Vascular dementia
Subdural hematoma, 75
Sunset syndrome, 384, 386, 465, 468, 469
Survival value, 179, 180, 199, 200, 201
Synaptic potentiation, 178, 179, 182, 215–17, 218, 220, 221, 223, 224, 225
Syntax, 191–92, 195, 196, 222, 385–86, 400–401

Tauopathies, 162, 168
Tertiary memory, 181, 184–85, 187, 188, 210, 211, 223–27. *See also* Information-processing theory; Stage 6 memory
Thalamic degeneration, 253, 254, 255
Three-tiered evolutionary memory model, xxiv, xxv, 199–226, 504–5
Threshold concept, xxix–xxx, xxxi, 41, 369, 377–79, 449, 450, 456, 457, 515–18
Thyroid disease, 68, 73, 75
Transitional dementias. *See* Depressive dementias; Nondepressive pseudodementias
Transient ischemic attack (TIA), 268–70. *See also* Cerebrovascular disease; Vascular dementia
Treatment, xix, xxi, xxii, xxvii, xxviii, xxxii, 19, 20, 50–52, 61–78, 107–8, 121–23, 131–33, 149–50, 170, 225–27, 255, 300–302, 326–28, 337–39, 348–50, 374, 387–88, 399–400, 405–11, 437, 456–57, 463–80, 517, 518
Tricyclic antidepressants. *See* Antidepressant medications; Treatment
Trisomy of chromosome 21, xxi, xxii, xxiii, 101–4, 498–99. *See also* Down syndrome

Unconscious, 427, 428, 429, 430

Validity, xxii, 31–32, 40–52, 178, 180, 183, 184, 188–96, 198–200, 202–3, 263–67
Vascular Dementia, xxv–xxviii, 65–66, 263–84, 291–302, 306–28, 501–2, 505–11, 251–52; definition of, xxvi–xxviii, 39, 263–67, 278–86, 307, 327, 328; language, 271, 272, 273, 274–76, 277; memory, 8, 10, 270, 272, 273, 274–76, 277, 322, 323; mental status, 270, 272, 273, 274–76, 277, 322, 323; neuropathology, xxviii, 38, 39, 65, 66, 251, 252, 267, 268, 269, 270, 278–84, 293–302, 310–12, 320–21; onset and course of illness, 39, 251, 252, 307, 312–20, 322–28; prevalence, 65, 66, 251, 252, 264, 292, 306, 307; subtypes, xxvi–xxviii, 249, 251, 252, 263–84, 308–12, 315, 317–20, 322, 326
Vacuolar myelopathy, 342, 343
Vesanic dementia, 363
Vessel wall changes, 291–302, 308, 309–13, 319, 320–28. *See also* Noninfarct vascular dementia; Vascular dementia
Vestibular senses, 211, 212, 214
Visuospatial function, 12, 64, 144, 166, 240, 242–43, 245–46, 270, 274–77, 317, 323, 385, 425. *See also* Cognitive evaluation
Vitamins, 4, 7, 68, 71, 72, 73
Vorbeireden, 429. *See also* Approximate answers; Near-miss answers

Wandering, 384, 386, 465, 468, 469. *See also* Sunset syndrome
Western Aphasia Battery (WAB), 271, 272, 273, 274–77
Whipple disease, 70, 248–50
White matter changes, 38, 39, 75, 76, 142, 143, 268, 269, 270, 278–84, 291–301, 309–13, 315, 328, 319, 320, 321, 324, 326, 345
Wilson disease, 248, 249, 250, 251
Writing, 158, 163, 242, 245, 270, 323, 400–403. *See also* Language